Nursing
A Concept-Based Approach to Learning

PREPUBLICATION EDITION

North Carolina Concept-Based Learning Editorial Board

Pearson
New York Boston San Francisco
London Toronto Sydney Tokyo Singapore Madrid
Mexico City Munich Paris Cape Town Hong Kong Montreal

Publisher: Julie Levin Alexander
Assistant to Publisher: Regina Bruno
Editor-in-Chief: Maura Connor
Assistant to the Editor-in-Chief: Marion Gottlieb
Executive Acquisitions Editor: Kim Mortimer
Assistant Editor: Sarah Wrocklage
Director of Development: Stephanie Klein
Director of Marketing: Karen Allman
Marketing Specialist: Michael Sirinides
Managing Editor, Production: Patrick Walsh
Production Editor: GEX Publishing Services
Production Liaison: Anne Garcia
Media Project Manager: Rachel Collett
Manufacturing Manager: Ilene Sanford
Senior Design Coordinator: Maria Guglielmo-Walsh
Interior Design: GEX Publishing Services
Cover Design: Mary Siener
Composition: GEX Publishing Services
Printer/Binder: Courier Kendallville
Cover Printer: Lehigh-Phoenix Color/Hagerstown
Manager, Rights and Permissions: Zina Arabia
Manager, Visual Research: Beth Brenzel
Manager, Cover Visual Research & Permissions: Karen Sanatar
Image Permission Coordinator: Vickie Menanteaux

10 9 8 7 6 5 4 3 2 1

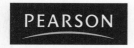

www.pearsonhighered.com

ISBN-13: 978-0-13-507795-5
ISBN-10: 0-13-507795-8

INTRODUCTORY LETTER

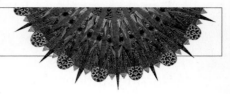

By Charlotte E. Blackwell

During the years 2006–2008, the associate degree nursing faculty in 55 community colleges was involved in a curriculum improvement project, a collaborative restructuring and revision of the associate degree nursing education curricula. The outcomes of the curriculum improvement project included a multi-institutional effort that led to the adaptation and implementation of one associate degree nursing curriculum that meets the standards of all the accrediting agencies and reflects the advances in nursing and health care practices.

Nurse educators across North Carolina investigated issues concerning the large volume of content included in their curricula. The educators agreed that the curriculum was experiencing content overload. After much research and consultation, the statewide team decided that a paradigm shift from a content-laden curriculum to a more conceptual approach to curriculum development and teaching was appropriate.

Much time and research was devoted to identifying and defining the specific concepts to be included in the statewide concept-based curriculum. Best examples of each concept—exemplars—were identified using research data derived from the Healthy People 2010 Report, the Institute of Medicine, the Centers for Disease Control and Prevention, the Joint Commission, the National Institute of Mental Health, the National Institutes of Health, and the NCLEX-RN® Test Plan, among others. Using data from these organizations, the statewide team identified exemplars that had high incidence and prevalence throughout the life span, across the health–illness continuum, and in various environmental settings.

Once the exemplars were identified, the team assigned them to the most appropriate concept and then arranged the concepts into the classifications of Individual, Nursing, and Health Care. Then the statewide project representatives assigned the identified concepts and exemplars to specific courses. In each of the concept-based nursing courses, concepts are presented across the life span, the health–illness continuum, and environmental settings.

Providing a concept-based curriculum is only a single component of the complete curriculum restructuring process needed to implement conceptual learning. By shifting from teacher-centered instructional methods to facilitating centered activities, the students emerge from an active, learner-centered environment able to identify the relationships among exemplars and concepts. Using exemplars to facilitate a deeper understanding of a concept facilitates abstract thinking, promotes schema construction, and allows the learner to transfer knowledge to various situations. Once a student is able to understand the connection between and among concepts, then, and only then, conceptual learning and deep understanding occurs.

Many nurse educators from North Carolina made important contributions to the concept-based curriculum. Sincere appreciation is extended to all my professional colleagues throughout the community college system who have supported the efforts of this work. As project director, I gratefully acknowledge the tireless, unselfish efforts of the Curriculum Improvement Project Steering Committee members: Carol Boles, Colleen Burgess, Linda Smith, Kathy Williford, and Linda Wright. Sincere appreciation is extended to Barbara Knopp, educational consultant for the North Carolina Board of Nursing, for her support with the project. Dr. Jean Giddens provided invaluable advice and consultation with the curriculum improvement project team, and I will always be grateful for her significant contributions.

The standardization of the associate degree nursing education curricula at 55 community colleges in North Carolina was a collaborative effort of many educators. The search for conceptually written texts and resources was important to the educators as they envisioned the implementation of the new conceptual curriculum and the student-centered learning activities. It is with great optimism that this conceptually written text will meet the needs of nurse educators and nursing students, not only in North Carolina, but across the United States as other states develop concept-based, standardized curricula.

Features That Help You Use This Book Successfully

Nursing students face challenges in their education—managing demands on their time, applying research findings, evaluating components of evidence-based practice, and developing their critical-thinking skills. Thus instructors and students alike value the in-text learning aids that we include in our textbooks to meet the challenges of nursing in today's world. We developed a textbook that is easy to learn from and easy to use as a professional reference. The following guide will help you use the text's features and resources to succeed in the classroom, in the clinical setting, on the NCLEX-RN® examination, and in nursing practice.

Each Concept begins with an **overview** of normal presentation and **exemplars** to help students navigate through the concept content.

The **Key Terms** and **Learning Outcomes** at the beginning of each concept highlight important terminology and provide an introductory overview of what will be covered in the concept.

Each Concept Chapter begins with an **"About"** section to give students a foundational introduction to the concept.

Oxygenation

10

Concept at-a-Glance
About Oxygenation, 287

Concept Learning Outcomes

After reading about this concept, you will be able to do the following:

1. Summarize the structure and physiologic processes of the respiratory system related to oxygenation.
2. List factors affecting oxygenation.
3. Identify commonly occurring alterations in oxygenation and their related treatments.
4. Explain common physical assessment procedures used to evaluate respiratory health of clients across the life span.
5. Outline diagnostic and laboratory tests and expected findings to determine the individual's oxygenation status.
6. Explain management of respiratory health and prevention of respiratory illness.
7. Demonstrate the nursing process in providing culturally competent care across the life span for individuals with common alterations in oxygenation.
8. Identify pharmacologic interventions in caring for the individual with alterations in respiratory function.

Concept Key Terms

Arterial blood gas (ABG), 298
Apnea, 293
Atelectasis, 294
Auscultation, 288
Bradypnea, 293
Bronchoscopy, 302
Bronchovesicular, 288
Chemistry panels, 305
Chest x-ray (CXR), 302
Chronic obstructive pulmonary disease (COPD), 290
Crackles, 294
Cyanosis, 290
Dyspnea, 293
Eupnea, 288
Expiration, 287
Hypercarbia, 290
Hypoxemia, 290
Incentive spirometry, 299
Inspiration, 287
Orthopnea, 293
Oxygenation, 287

Palpation, 294
Patent airway, 290
Peak expiratory flow rate (PEFR), 299
Pulmonary function tests (PFTs), 299
Pulse oximetry, 299
Percussion, 294
Pneumothorax, 293
Respiration, 287
Rhonchi, 294
Stridor, 294
Surfactant, 289
Symmetry, 294
Tachypnea, 293
Thoracentesis, 302
Tubular, 288
Ventilation, 288
Ventilation-perfusion (V-Q), 290
Vesicular, 289
Wheezing, 294

About Oxygenation

Oxygenation can be defined as the mechanisms that facilitate or impair the body's ability to supply oxygen to all cells of the body. The function of the respiratory system is to obtain oxygen from atmospheric air, to transport this air through the respiratory tract into the alveoli, and ultimately to diffuse oxygen into the blood that carries oxygen to all the cells of the body. The respiratory system achieves all this through **respiration**, the act of inhaling (**inspiration**) and exhaling (**expiration**) air to transport oxygen to the alveoli so

The concept overview provides the **normal presentation** of the concept, review of anatomy & physiology, assessment & diagnostic tests, alterations from normal, generic nursing care interventions, developmental considerations, and general collaborative care. Each concept overview provides a comprehensive introduction to the concept for the beginning student.

NORMAL PRESENTATION

Adequate oxygenation of the body depends on a healthy, intact respiratory system. The respiratory system obtains oxygen from atmospheric air and transports it into the alveoli, where oxygen diffuses into a capillary and is carried by the blood to all the cells of the body. The respiratory system also passes carbon dioxide from the body.

The upper respiratory system is the inlet for air into the body. The nose is the typical inlet. The nose is midline on the face, with the same color as facial skin. The nose is divided into two nares that are moist, pink, mucosa-lined passageways. The purpose of the nares is to warm, humidify, and filter air as it is breathed into the nose. The upper respiratory tract has two protective mechanisms to prevent foreign matter from entering the lower respiratory tract: sneezing and cilia. Foreign matter that enters the nose irritates the nasal passages and induces sneezing. Sneezing is a reflexive action that clears the upper airway. This reflexive action is active even in the neonatal period. Cilia are microscopic fine hairs within the posterior portion of the nares that

in the alveoli sacs. These passageways for air dilate and contract. The trachea and larger bronchi are supported by C-shaped cartilage rings, as well as by smooth muscle. The smaller bronchioles are supported by smooth muscles only. Bronchioles deliver air to the alveoli. These air passageways dilate and contract as the autonomic nervous system regulates the smooth muscles supporting them. The movement of air within the bronchial tree creates a mixture of sounds of air flowing through a tube and the breeziness of the open alveolar lung fields. This is termed **bronchovesicular** sound.

The lungs are also described in terms of their lobes. The lobes lie obliquely in the thoracic cavity. The right lung has three lobes; the left lung has two lobes. The inferior lobes are the largest. Most of the inferior lobes lie in the posterior thoracic cavity. Each lung has a pleural lining to aid respiration and separate it from the other lung. The pleural lining has two layers, and a minute amount of fluid between the layers allows the structures to glide across one another during respiration.

The final portion of the lower respiratory system is the air sacs. The outcroppings of the air sacs are called alveoli. The alveoli are the portion of the lungs that fulfill the function of

---

DEVELOPMENTAL CONSIDERATIONS Respiratory Development

INFANTS
- Respiratory rates are highest and most variable in newborns. The respiratory rate of a neonate is 40 to 80 breaths per minute.
- Infant respiratory rates average about 30 breaths per minute.
- Because of the structure of the ribcage infants rely almost exclusively on diaphragmatic movement for breathing. This is seen as abdominal breathing, as the abdomen rises and falls with each breath.

CHILDREN
- The respiratory rate gradually decreases, averaging around 25 breaths per minute in the preschooler and reaching the adult rate of 12 to 18 breaths per minute by late adolescence.
- During infancy and childhood, upper respiratory infections are common but usually not serious. Infants and preschoolers also are at risk for airway obstruction by foreign objects, such as coins and small toys. Cystic fibrosis, a chronic disease usually identified in early childhood, is a congenital disorder that affects the lungs, causing them to become congested with thick, tenacious (sticky) mucus. Asthma is another chronic disease often identified in childhood. The airways of the asthmatic child react to stimuli such as allergens, exercise, or cold air by constricting, becoming edematous, and producing excessive mucus. Airflow is impaired, and the child may wheeze as air moves through narrowed air passages.

OLDER ADULTS
- Older adults are at increased risk for acute respiratory diseases such as pneumonia and chronic diseases such as emphysema

and chronic bronchitis. COPD may affect older adults, particularly after years of exposure to cigarette smoke or industrial pollutants.
- Pneumonia may not present with the usual symptom of a fever, but may present with atypical symptoms, such as confusion, weakness, loss of appetite, and increased heart rate and respiration.

Nursing interventions should be directed toward achieving optimal respiratory effort and gas exchange:
- Always encourage wellness and prevention of disease by reinforcing the need for good nutrition, exercise, and immunizations, such as for influenza and pneumonia.
- Increase fluid intake, if not contraindicated by other problems such as cardiac or renal impairment.
- Encourage proper positioning and frequent changing of position to allow for better lung expansion and air and fluid movement.
- Teach the client to use breathing techniques for better air exchange.
- Pace activities to conserve energy.
- Encourage the client to eat more frequent, smaller meals to decrease gastric distention, which can cause pressure on the diaphragm.
- Teach the client to avoid extreme hot or cold temperatures that will further tax the respiratory system.
- Teach actions and side effects of drugs, inhalers, and treatments.

Source: Berman, A., Snyder, S. J., Kozier, B., *fundamentals of nursing: Concepts, process,* Upper Saddle River, NJ: Pearson Education.

Developmental Considerations boxes provide caring interventions for different lifespan groups such as infants, children, adolescents, the elderly, and pregnant women.

For the concepts in the Individual Domain, there is a presentation of **physical assessment** techniques that includes both normal and abnormal findings to help students differentiate between the two.

Oxygenation Assessment

Technique/Normal Findings	Abnormal Findings
Nasal assessment Inspect the nose symmetry. Inspect the nasal cavity using a flashlight. The septum should fall midline and intact. The mucosa of the nares is pink and moist without drainage. Both nares should be patent. (see Figure 10–5 ■)	■ Asymmetry indicates trauma or surgery. ■ Redness and/or swelling is observed. ■ Deviated septum narrows or occludes one naris. ■ Foreign bodies may be found in the nares, especially of infants, toddlers, and preschoolers. ■ Purulent drainage occurs. ■ Watery nasal drainage occurs. ■ Pale turbinates are seen.
Thoracic assessment Measure respiratory rate:	■ Bradypnea ■ Tachypnea ■ Apnea
Assess quality of breathing: Determine regularity in timing I:E ratio is 1:2. Assess depth of inspiration. Observe effort to breath.	■ Shortness of breath ■ Dyspnea ■ Orthopnea
Inspection of thoracic cavity Anteroposterior diameter is half the transverse diameter. *Normal ratio is 1:2.* (see Figures 10–6 ■ and 10–7 ■)	■ Anteroposterior equals transverse thoracic diameter measurements, called a barrel chest.
Inspection of the muscles of breathing The chest walls gently rise and fall with each breath. The muscles in the neck are relaxed. The trachea is midline. The intercostal muscles raise the chest upward and outward with inhalation, then calmly relax with exhalation.	■ Retraction of the intercostals occurs. ■ Sternocleidomastoid muscles of the neck contract. ■ Posturing occurs.
...f the thoracic wall for symmetry ...nds is observed with ...the chest wall. The tra-	■ Asymmetry of movement occurs. ■ Decreased expansion occurs. ■ The trachea shifts from midline.
...n to the respiratory system ...nation of the cell	Cyanosis is a blue tinge to the skin in fair individuals and gray coloration of the skin in darker pigmented individuals.
...finger and are normally ...il bed to the finger.	Clubbed nail beds have an angle of 180° or greater, depending on the duration of time an individual has had hypoxemia.

Assessment Interview Oxygenation

CURRENT RESPIRATORY PROBLEMS
- Have you noticed any changes in your breathing pattern (e.g., shortness of breath, difficulty in breathing, need to be in upright position to breathe, or rapid and shallow breathing)?
- If so, which of your activities might cause these symptoms to occur?
- How many pillows do you use to sleep at night?

HISTORY OF RESPIRATORY DISEASE
- Have you had colds, allergies, asthma, tuberculosis, bronchitis, pneumonia, or emphysema?
- How frequently have these occurred? How long did they last? And how were they treated?
- Have you been exposed to any pollutants?

LIFESTYLE
- Do you smoke? If so, how much? If not, did you smoke previously, and when did you stop?
- Does any member of your family smoke?
- Is there cigarette smoke or other pollutants (e.g. fumes, dust, coal, asbestos) in your workplace?
- Do you drink alcohol? If so, how many drinks (mixed drinks, glasses of wine, or beers) do you usually have per day or per week?
- Describe your exercise patterns. How often do you exercise and for how long?

PRESENCE OF COUGH
- How often and how much do you cough?
- Is it productive, that is, accompanied by sputum, or nonproductive, that is, dry?
- Does the cough occur during certain activity or at certain times of the day?

DESCRIPTION OF SPUTUM
- When is the sputum produced?
- What is the amount, color, thickness, and odor of the sputum?
- Is it ever tinged with blood?

PRESENCE OF CHEST PAIN
- How does going outside in the heat or the cold affect you?
- Do you experience any pain with breathing or activity?
- Where is the pain located?
- Describe the pain. How does it feel?
- Does it occur when you breathe in or out?
- How long does it last, and how does it affect your breathing?
- Do you experience any other symptoms when the pain occurs (e.g., nausea, shortness of breath or difficulty breathing, lightheadedness, palpitations)?
- What activities precede your pain?
- What do you do to relieve the pain?

Assessment Interviews provide students with sample questions to ask during an assessment, thus helping students to prepare for the patient encounter.

DIAGNOSTIC TESTS Respiratory System

NAME OF TEST Sputum studies
- Culture and sensitivity
- Acid-fast smear and culture
- Cytology

PURPOSE AND DESCRIPTION Culture and sensitivity of a single sputum specimen is done to diagnose bacterial infections, identify the most effective antibiotic, and evaluate treatment.

Sputum is examined for presence of acid-fast bacillus, specifically tuberculosis. A series of three early morning sputum specimens is used.

Sputum is examined for presence of abnormal (malignant) cells. A single sputum specimen is collected in a special container of fixative solution.

NURSING CONSIDERATIONS Sputum specimens may also be obtained during bronchoscopy (described later) if the client is unable to provide a specimen. If collecting a specimen from client with infectious disease, such as tuberculosis, the nurse should wear personal protective equipment, and the specimen may be collected outdoors to dilute droplet nuclei if negative airflow is not available in the client's room.

Developmental Considerations Sputum may be collected from infants and young children, who cannot cooperate enough to expectorate into a cup, by performing deep suctioning of the pharynx to induce a cough reflex and produce sputum.

NAME OF TEST Arterial blood gases (ABGs)

PURPOSE AND DESCRIPTION This test of arterial blood is done to assess alterations in acid–base balance caused by a respiratory disorder, a metabolic disorder, or both. A pH of less than 7.35 indicates acidosis, and a pH of more than 7.45 indicates alkalosis. To determine a respiratory cause, assess the $PaCO_2$: If pH is decreased and $PaCO_2$ is increased, respiratory acidosis is indicated.

Normal values:
pH: 7.35–7.45
$PaCO_2$: 35–45 mmHg
PaO_2: 75–100 mmHg
HCO_3: 24–28 mEq/L
BE: ± 2 mEq/L

NURSING CONSIDERATIONS Arterial blood is collected in a heparinized needle and syringe. Sample is placed on an icebag and taken immediately to the laboratory. If client is receiving oxygen, indicate on laboratory slip. Apply pressure to puncture site for 2–5 min, or longer if needed. Do not collect blood from the same arm used for an intravenous (IV) infusion.

Developmental Considerations When performing arterial puncture on infants and young children, only the radial artery should be used after verifying ulnar perfusion via an Allen's test. The Allen's test is performed by having the client elevate the hand and make a fist for 30 s. Pressure is applied to the ulnar and radial artery, the client opens the hand, which should appear blanched from lack of perfusion, and then pressure is removed from the ulnar artery while pressure on the radial artery is maintained. If the hand does not become pink and perfused, it indicates damage to the ulnar artery and the radial artery in that arm should not be used for arterial puncture.

NAME OF TEST Pulse oximetry

PURPOSE AND DESCRIPTION This noninvasive test is used to evaluate or monitor oxygen saturation of the blood. A device that uses infrared light is attached to an extremity (most commonly the finger, but can also be used on the toe, earlobe, or nose) and light is passed through the tissues or reflected off bony structures.

Normal values: 90%–100%

NURSING CONSIDERATIONS Assess for factors that may alter findings, including faulty placement, movement, diminished perfusion (such as cool skin), dark skin color, and acrylic nails.

Developmental Considerations Fingers and toes are not appropriate sites for young infants because they are so small. Probes are available that wrap around the palm of the hand or sole of the foot with a piece of tape to hold them in place, and they work well.

NAME OF TEST Chest x-ray

PURPOSE AND DESCRIPTION Chest x-ray is used to identify abnormalities in chest structure and lung tissue, for diagnosis of diseases and injuries of the lungs, and to monitor treatment.

NURSING CONSIDERATIONS No special preparation is needed.

NAME OF TEST Computed tomography (CT)

PURPOSE AND DESCRIPTION CT of the thorax may be performed when x-rays do not show some areas well, such as the pleura and mediastinum. It is also done to differentiate pathologic conditions (such as tumors, abscesses, and aortic aneurysms), to identify pleural effusion and enlarged lymph nodes, and to monitor treatment. Images are shown in cross-section.

NURSING CONSIDERATIONS No special preparation is needed. Caution should be provided to cover the genitals of young children and avoid radiation of any cells with rapid turnover, especially the gonads. If x-rays must be obtained, shield the neck region and the lower abdomen.

The concept overview introduces the student to all the **Diagnostic Tests** that could be used for that concept. For each test, the table summarizes the purpose, description, client preparation required, related nursing care, and family/client health education as applicable.

Alterations and Treatments

Once the students understand the normal presentation of the concept, the chapter describes the commonly seen alterations from normal and possible treatments. This provides students with a general overview for the concept as a whole.

ALTERATIONS AND TREATMENTS Respiratory System

Alteration	Description	Treatment
Chronic obstructive pulmonary disease (COPD)	COPD is a preventable, treatable disease of compromised airflow within the respiratory system. COPD is a progressive disorder that alters the structures of the respiratory system over time. Inflammation of the mucous membranes of the bronchial tubes occurs as well as loss of elasticity in lung parenchyma.	- Smoking cessation - Avoidance of secondhand smoke - Administration of bronchodilators - Administration of corticosteroids - Use of breathing exercises - Respiratory therapy consult - Administration of pulmonary function tests - Spirometry - Complete blood count (CBC), chemistries, and arterial blood gases - Taking sputum specimen - Administration of oxygen - Physical therapy consult - Nutritional consult
Asthma	Asthma is a chronic inflammatory disease of the airways. Asthma presents with coughing, wheezing, shortness of breath, chest tightness, and sputum production. Asthma is defined in relation to severity and control as well as to impairments and risk.	- Smoking cessation - Avoidance of secondhand smoke - Avoidance of aggravating factors - Respiratory therapy consult - Measuring daily peak expiratory flow rate - Administration of maintenance bronchodilators - Administration of maintenance corticosteroids - Exercise planning by physical therapy - Administration of short-acting bronchodilators for exercise - Measuring CBC, chemistry panels, and arterial blood gases - Taking a sputum specimen
Respiratory syncytial virus (RSV)	RSV is a highly contagious lower respiratory infection that affects nearly 100% of children younger than 2 years of age. Repeated infections of RSV occur throughout the life span, though subsequent infections tend to be milder.	- Smoking cessation by caregivers - Avoidance of secondhand smoke - Separating sick individuals from well individuals - Observation of breathing pattern including, rate, rhythm, and quality - Teaching the parents or caregiver how to observe breathing patterns - Maintaining adequate fluid volume and calories - Oral and nasal suctioning - Possible use of bronchodilators and corticosteroids
Sudden infant death syndrome (SIDS)	SIDS is the leading cause of death of infants beyond the neonatal period. SIDS occurs most often between the first and the fourth months of life, but may occur up to 1 year of age. The cause of SIDS is not known. Infants who appear healthy are found dead by parents or caregivers. Preventive measures have reduced the incidence of SIDS in developed countries, including the United States.	- Placing infant on his or her back to sleep - Smoking cessation by caregivers - Avoidance of secondhand smoke - Ensuring a totally smoke-free environment - Co-sleeper or same-room sleeping of infant and parents - Avoiding bed sharing - Maintaining adult-comfort room temperature - Breastfeeding - Using a pacifier
Acute respiratory distress syndrome (ARDS)	ARDS is a disorder with rapid onset of progressive malfunction of the lungs' ability to take in oxygen. Extensive lung tissue inflammation and small blood vessel injury occurs, followed by malfunction of other organs.	- Measuring CBC, chemistry panels, and arterial blood gases - Taking sputum specimen - Administration of oxygen - Providing ventilator support - Administration of hemodynamic intravenous drugs

Medications After students understand the possible alterations from normal in the Individual Domain concepts, the chapter summarizes pharmacologic management commonly used for those alterations along with related nursing responsibilities, followed by other collaborative care.

MEDICATIONS	Pharmacologic Interventions: Glaucoma			
Drug Classifications	**Mechanism of Action**	**Commonly Prescribed Drugs**	**Nursing Considerations**	
Antiglaucoma Drugs				
■ Prostaglandins	Drugs for glaucoma work by one of two mechanisms: increasing the outflow of aqueous humor at the canal of Schlemm or decreasing the formation of aqueous humor at the ciliary body. Many agents for glaucoma act by affecting the autonomic nervous system	■ bimatoprost (Lumigan) ■ latanoprost (Xalatan) ■ travoprost (Travatan) ■ unoprostone isopropyl (Rescula)	■ Assess and note eye color, presence of inflammation, exudates, or pain. ■ Note vital signs and most recent liver function test results because these may be altered by the drug.	
■ Beta-adrenergic blockers		■ betaxolol (Betoptic) ■ carteolol (Ocupress) ■ levobunolol (Betagan) ■ metipranolol (OptiPranolol) ■ timolol (Betimol, Timoptic, and others)	■ Assess the client for allergies or contraindications to beta-blocker therapy, including asthma, chronic obstructive pulmonary disease (COPD), heart block, and heart failure. ■ Maintain pressure over the lacrimal sac after administration to prevent systemic absorption. ■ Assess for side effects such as bradycardia, hypotension, and depression. ■ Teach about the drug, its dose, administration, and desired and side effects.	
■ Alpha₂-adrenergic agonists		■ apraclonidine (Iopidine) ■ brimonidine tartrate (Alphagan)	■ Assess the client for contraindications and adverse reactions to adrenergic agonists, including acute angle-closure glaucoma, hypertension, cardiac dysrhythmias, and coronary heart disease. ■ Assess for central nervous system side effects of anxiety, nervousness, and muscle tremors. If these side effects are severe, notify the physician. ■ Assess for a hypersensitivity reaction, including itching, lid edema, and discharge from the eyes. Notify the physician if you notice these signs.	
■ Carbonic anhydrase inhibitors		■ acetazolamide (Diamox) ■ brinzolamide (Azopt) ■ methazolamide (Neptazane)	■ Assess for allergies or other contraindications to the use of carbonic anhydrase inhibitors, including known allergy to sulfa, or severe renal or hepatic disease. ■ Monitor for increased drug interactions of amphetamines, procainamide, quinidine, tricyclic antidepressants, and ephedrine	

1.1 CONFUSION

KEY TERMS
Confusion, *15*
Delirium, *15*

BASIS FOR SELECTION OF EXEMPLAR
Standards of Nursing Practice
NCLEX

LEARNING OUTCOMES
1. Describe the pathophysiology, etiology, and clinical manifestations of confusion.
2. Identify risk factors associated with confusion.
3. Illustrate the nursing process in providing culturally competent and caring interventions across the life span for individuals with confusion.
4. Formulate priority nursing diagnoses appropriate for an individual with confusion.
5. Create a plan of caring interventions for an individual with confusion.
6. Employ evidence-based caring interventions (or prevention) for an individual with confusion.
7. Assess expected outcomes for an individual with confusion.
8. Discuss therapies used in the collaborative care of an individual with confusion.

OVERVIEW
Confusion is an alteration in cognition that makes it difficult to think clearly, focus attention, or make decisions. It may come on suddenly or gradually, depending on the cause. It can be a one-time event, recurrent, or a constant state of mind. The most important thing to understand about confusion is that it is frequently a symptom and not a diagnosis. Any number of things can cause confusion, including hypoxia, poor perfusion, medications, and disease. The onset of confusion requires thorough assessment to determine the causative agent and improve client outcomes.

Delirium is an acute disorder of cognition that affects functional independence. Confusion, a loss of orientation and memory, can occur in clients of all ages, but it is most commonly seen in older people. The terms *acute confusion* and delirium are used interchangeably by most health professionals, with nurses favoring the use of acute confusion and physicians the term delirium (McCurren & Cronin, 2003, p. 319). Confusion often presents with subtle symptoms, but an attempt should be made to differentiate between acute confusion (delirium) and chronic confusion (dementia) (Table 1–7).

PATHOPHYSIOLOGY AND ETIOLOGY
Delirium often has an abrupt onset; it can be reversed by treating its cause. This contrasts with dementia, often called chronic confusion, which has symptoms that are gradual and irreversible (e.g., Alzheimer's disease). Clients who are confused often know something is wrong and want help. It is important to pay special attention to sudden changes in mood or personality, as these may be signs of delirium related to recent changes in medication, onset of undetected illness, or exacerbation of chronic illness.

Age-related cognitive decline, resulting from slower information processing, mild memory impairment, and decreases in brain volume secondary to loss of some neurons place older clients at increased risk for confusion when they face additional stressors of illness, loss, or change in environment. Depression or other emotional problems can also act as stressors, increasing the likelihood of delirium. It is important to remember that delirium is usually caused by a treatable physical or mental health illness and, when treated typically results in full recovery. Delirium is associated with increased mortality, increased hospital costs, and long-term cognitive and functional impairment (Tullmann, Mion, Fletcher, & Foreman, 2008).

Etiology
Delirium occurs in 6% to 30% of the general hospital population and 7% to 52% of postsurgical clients (Edwards, 2003, p. 347). Delirium in the intensive care unit (ICU) setting is a common problem and has been described as sundown syndrome, ICU psychosis, and ICU syndrome. Delirium or acute confusional state, superimposed on Alzheimer's disease, was found in 8 of 20 older adults with documented dementia (Fick & Foreman, 2000). It is estimated that anywhere from 14% to 80% of all older persons hospitalized for the treatment of an acute physical illness experience an episode of delirium (Foreman, Wakefield, Culp, & Milisen, 2001). Unfortunately, delirium is unrecognized or misdiagnosed by both the physician and the nurse in up to two-thirds of cases (Hanley, 2004, p. 218).

It is not uncommon to think of older adults as the only people who become confused, but this is incorrect. Confusion can occur at any stage of the developmental process and may be caused by alcohol intoxication, low blood sugar, head trauma, fluid and/or

After providing the student with an introduction to the concept, each chapter provides modules for all the **exemplars**.

The exemplars are set up as discreet modules within the chapter so that students can refer to them easily and work through the related learning activities. Each exemplar begins with its own set of Key Terms, Learning Outcomes, and Evidence-Based Selection Criteria for its use as an exemplar within that concept.

At the end of each exemplar module, the student can work through **Review** activities that help the student relate to other concepts, apply critical thinking, analyze case studies, and more. There is also a cross-referenced link to the **Companion Skills Manual**, which contains all the step-by-step skills for students to practice in the lab.

 REVIEW Confusion

RELATE: LINK THE CONCEPTS

Linking the concepts of Accountability, Advocacy, Ethics, and Safety with the concept of Cognition:

1. What special responsibilities is the nurse accountable for when caring for a client who is confused?
2. How does the nurse advocate for the confused client?
3. The nurse is caring for a client who is confused and displaying trouble with decision making. If the client declines a treatment essential to obtaining a positive outcome for the client, considering the client's bill of rights, what is the nurse's ethical obligation?
4. What interventions are important for the nurse to initiate in order to maintain safety for the confused client?

READY: GO TO COMPANION SKILLS MANUAL

1. Applying body mechanics
2. Assisting the client with ambulation
3. Assessing appearance and mental status
4. Assessing the neurologic system
5. Bathing an adult client
6. Administering medication
7. Evaluating client safety

REFLECT: CASE STUDY

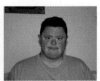

Clifford is a 64-year-old male who has been married to his wife, Pam, for 40 years. Their only child, 24-year-old Gary, has Down syndrome and lives with them. Clifford is a middle manager for a small manufacturing company where he has worked over the last 20 years.

Overall, Clifford is in good health, although he has recently been undergoing conservative treatment for benign prostate hypertrophy. He has a history of depression. He had a brief episode during college, for which he did not seek treatment. He had another episode shortly after Gary was born, and at the encouragement of his wife, he sought treatment, which consisted of counseling and antidepressant agents. He quit taking the medications after about 6 months and decided he would just learn to deal with depression on his own. Although he has had mild episodes of depression over the years since that time, Clifford has been unwilling to seek

---

 CLIENT TEACHING **Fetal Alcohol Syndrome**

Fetal alcohol syndrome (FAS) is a preventable cause of mental retardation. About 10% of women consume alcohol while pregnant, and 2% engage in frequent or binge drinking (Suellentrop, Morrow, Williams, D'Angels, 2006). This indicates that all women must receive clear messages about the dangers of drinking while pregnant. Teach all pregnant women that total abstention from alcohol for the entire length of pregnancy is the only completely effective method of preventing FAS. Include this in teaching to all adolescent girls, so they are aware of how alcohol can harm their infant if they become pregnant. Emphasize that the most dangerous time may be early in pregnancy before women commonly know they are pregnant.

Additional boxed features help students make linkages to other concepts, such as **Client Teaching, Diversity, Culture, Alternative Therapies,** and others.

The textbook highlights **Evidence-Based Practice** throughout to provide students with the research-based rationales for their nursing care interventions.

EVIDENCE-BASED PRACTICE **Parental Presence During Procedures**

Increasingly, parents are permitted to be present during medical procedures performed on their children. Previous resistance to parental presence has been based on the fear that parents would delay or interfere with the procedure, distract or increase the anxiety of the health professionals performing the procedure, or experience heightened anxiety of their own. Studies have investigated parental presence in various situations involving medical procedures such as anesthesia induction, intravenous (IV) starts, and resuscitation (Meyers, Eichhorn, & Guzzetta, 1998; Munro & D'Errico, 2000; Powers & Rubenstein, 1999). In most cases, parents are less anxious if they are able to be present when their child has a procedure, and the ability of health professionals to perform procedures is not affected (Lewandowski & Tesler, 2003; Sacchetti, Paston, & Carraccio, 2005).

PRACTICE ALERT

To determine the impact of the child with mental retardation on the family, the nurse asks parents to describe (1) family activities that include the child, (2) strategies that parents and siblings use to deal with community attitudes about the child, and, (3) in the case of a child with other disabilities, methods of managing the child's care and planning for future care needs.

Other boxes integrated into the exemplars teach students about clinical implications that will help them be successful in their clinical experiences.

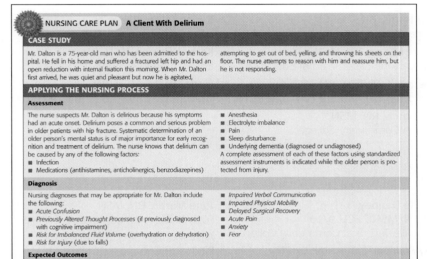

NURSING CARE PLAN   A Client With Delirium

CASE STUDY

Mr. Dalton is a 75-year-old man who has been admitted to the hospital. He fell in his home and suffered a fractured left hip and had an open reduction with internal fixation this morning. When Mr. Dalton first arrived, he was quiet and pleasant but now he is agitated, attempting to get out of bed, yelling, and throwing his sheets on the floor. The nurse attempts to reason with him and reassure him, but he is not responding.

APPLYING THE NURSING PROCESS

Assessment

The nurse suspects Mr. Dalton is delirious because his symptoms had an acute onset. Delirium poses a common and serious problem in older patients with hip fracture. Systematic determination of an older person's mental status is of major importance for early recognition and treatment of delirium. The nurse knows that delirium can be caused by any of the following factors:
- Infection
- Medications (antihistamines, anticholinergics, benzodiazepines)

- Anesthesia
- Electrolyte imbalance
- Pain
- Sleep disturbance
- Underlying dementia (diagnosed or undiagnosed)

A complete assessment of each of these factors using standardized assessment instruments is indicated while the older person is protected from injury.

Diagnosis

Nursing diagnoses that may be appropriate for Mr. Dalton include the following:
- *Acute Confusion*
- *Previously Altered Thought Processes* (if previously diagnosed with cognitive impairment)
- *Risk for Imbalanced Fluid Volume* (overhydration or dehydration)
- *Risk for Injury* (due to falls)

- *Impaired Verbal Communication*
- *Impaired Physical Mobility*
- *Delayed Surgical Recovery*
- *Acute Pain*
- *Anxiety*
- *Fear*

Expected Outcomes

The expected outcomes for the plan of care specify that Mr. Dalton will
- be free from injury.
- begin to exhibit resolution of his symptoms of delirium.
- experience correction of the underlying mechanisms causing his delirium.

- receive consultation, assessment, and treatment from appropriate members of the interdisciplinary team, including physicians, nurses, physical therapists, dietitians, social workers, and others as appropriate to resolve and improve his delirium.

Planning and Implementation

The following nursing interventions may be appropriate for Mr. Dalton:
- Establish a therapeutic relationship by being present and using gentle touch and a soft voice for communication.
- Review all current medications.
- Evaluate basic laboratory studies (complete blood count, serum electrolytes, and urinalysis).
- Provide supportive and restorative care.
- Treat behavioral symptoms.
- Correct sensory deficits (place glasses and hearing aids if used by the older person).

- In consultation with the physician, consider further testing as appropriate that may include chest radiology, blood culture, drug levels, serum B12, thyroid function tests, pulse oximetry, electrocardiogram, brain imaging, lumbar puncture, or electroencephalogram.
- Administer medications as ordered by the physician (haloperidol 0.5 to 2.0 mg or lorazepam 0.5 to 2.0 mg every 4 to 6 hours).
- Reassure, educate, and involve family.
- Maintain a quiet and peaceful environment, reducing stimuli to the extent possible.

Evaluation

The nurse will consider the plan a success based on the following criteria:
- Mr. Dalton will return to normal cognitive and physical function.

- He will be free from injury.
- He will cooperate with a rehabilitation plan and be discharged to home or a rehabilitation facility.

For applicable exemplars, students learn to apply the **Nursing Process** and use **Nursing Care Plans**.

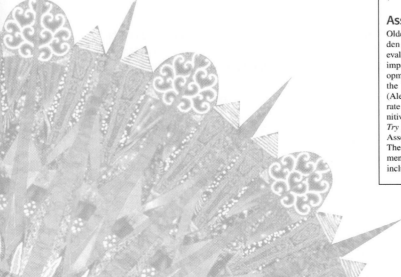

NURSING PROCESS

The goal of nursing care is to reduce the incidence of delirium in the client at risk and prevent complications in the delirious client. Routine screening for delirium should be part of the comprehensive plan of care for the older adult or the client at risk. Delirium can be prevented by recognizing high-risk clients and implementing a standardized protocol (Tullmann et al., 2008).

Assessment

Older persons do not develop dementia overnight, so any sudden change in mental status needs to be aggressively evaluated. Delirium must be ruled out because cognitive impairment caused by delirium may be reversible. The development of delirium may indicate decreased reserve capacity of the brain and signal an increased risk for dementia (Alexopoulos, Silver, Kahn, Frances, & Carpenter, 2004). To rate delirium and distinguish delirium from other types of cognitive impairment, the Hartford Institute for Geriatric Nursing *Try This* Assessment Series recommends use of the Confusion Assessment Method (CAM) (Inouye et al., 1990) (Box 1–3). The CAM includes two parts: Part 1 is an assessment instrument that screens for overall cognitive impairment; Part 2 includes only those four features that distinguish delirium. The

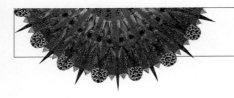

CONTRIBUTORS

ADVISORY BOARD

Charlotte Blackwell, RN, BSN, MSEd
Wake Technical College

Carol Hardin Boles, RN, MSN
Surry Community College

Colleen Burgess,
RN, MSN, APRN, BC, EdD (candidate)
Catawba Valley Community College

Delia Frederick, RN, MSNEd
Southwestern Community College

Robin Harris, BNS, MSEd
College of the Albemarle

Barbara Knopp, RN, MSN
North Carolina State Board of Education

Katherine K. Phillips, RN, MSN
Guilford Technical Community College

Linda Smith, RN, MSN
Johnston Community College

Renee Taylor, RN, BSN
Robeson Community College

Kathy Williford, MSN, RN
Edgecombe Community College

Linda Wright, MSN, RN
Western Piedmont Community College

CONTRIBUTOR TEAM

Catherine Borysewicz, MSN, RN, BC, CNE
Carolinas College of Health Sciences

Colleen Burgess,
RN, MSN, APRN, BC, EdD (candidate)
Catawba Valley Community College

Barbara Callahan RN, NCC, BSN, MEd,
Lenoir Community College

Sheryl Cornelius, MSN, RN
Mitchell Community College

Amy G. Crittenden, RN, MSN, CEN
Guilford Technical Community College

Rachelle Denney,
RN, BSN, MSNC ECU 9/10
Fayetteville Technical Community College

Cathy Franklin-Griffin, RN, CHPN
Surry Community College

Delia Frederick, RN, MSNEd
Southwestern Community College

Martha Freeze, MSN, ACNSBC
Rowan Cabarrus Community College

Barbara Knopp, RN, MSN
North Carolina State Board of Education

June Martin, RN, MSN
Forsyth Technical Community College

Alisa Montgomery, RN, MSN, CNE
Piedmont Community College

Camille Reese, EdD, MSN, RNC
Mitchell Community College

Marilyn Springle, RN, MSN, FNPBC
Carteret Community College

EDITORIAL CONSULTANTS

Adelaide R. McCulloch, BA
Editor

Debra S. McKinney, MSN, MBA/HCM, RN
Writer

Kim Wyatt, BSN, MFA
Writer

REVIEWER PANEL

Barbara Callahan, RN, NCC, BSN, MEd
Lenoir Community College

Colleen Burgess,
RN, MSN, APRN, BC, EdD (candidate)
Catawba Valley Community College

Joyce Estes, RN, MSN
Catawba Valley Community College

Susan M. Fowler, RN, BSN, MHS
Tri-County Community College

Delia Frederick, RN, MSNEd
Southwestern Community College

Gail A. Garren, MSN, RN
University of Phoenix

Robin Harris, BNS, MSEd
College of the Albemarle

Barbara Knopp, RN, MSN
North Carolina State Board of Education

Camille Reese, EdD, MSN, RNC
Mitchell Community College

Linda Smith, RN, MSN
Johnston Community College

Marie Thomas, PhD, RN
Forsyth Technical Community College

Kathy Williford, MSN, RN
Edgecombe Community College

Nursing: A Concept-Based Approach to Learning
PREPUBLICATION EDITION CONTENTS

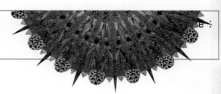

Cognition

1

Concept at-a-Glance

Concept Learning Outcomes

After reading about this concept, you will be able to do the following:

1. Summarize the structure and physiologic processes of the neurological system related to cognition.

2. List factors affecting cognition.

3. Identify common alterations in cognition and their related treatments.

4. Explain common physical assessment procedures used to evaluate the cognitive health of clients across the life span.

5. Outline diagnostic and laboratory tests to determine the individual's cognitive status.

6. Explain management of cognitive health and prevention of cognitive dysfunction.

7. Demonstrate the nursing process in providing culturally competent care across the life span for individuals with common alterations in cognition.

8. Identify pharmacologic interventions in caring for the individual with alterations in cognitive function.

Concept Key Terms

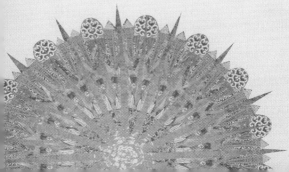

About Cognition

Cognition is a complicated process by which an individual learns, stores, retrieves, and uses information. Cognitive processing supports reasoning, problem solving, remembering, interpreting, and communicating. The nervous system is responsible for control of cognitive function and both voluntary and involuntary activities.

Joan is a 58-year-old registered nurse working in a busy urban emergency department. Sometimes Joan has to think to remember a term she has used frequently throughout her nursing career, and she jokes that she's having a "senior moment." She tells stories and laughs about not being able to find her keys, searching for her eyeglasses only to find they are propped up on her head, or calling her children by the wrong name. Though she may joke about her memory and growing older, Joan is an excellent nurse who has a great deal of experience and acts as a resource for new staff members in the emergency department. Joan's situation raises two very important questions: Is cognitive loss an inevitable result of the aging process or is it an indication of a disease process that requires further diagnostic testing? Do all older people lose cognitive function? ●

NORMAL PRESENTATION

The ability to think and learn makes us human. It enables us to be rational, to make good judgments, to interpret the world around us, and to learn new skills. **Cognitive development** refers to the manner in which people learn to think, reason, and use language. It involves a person's intelligence, perceptual ability, and ability to process information. Cognitive development represents a progression of mental abilities from illogical to logical thinking, from simple to complex problem solving, and from concrete thinking to understanding abstract concepts. It is important to note that sensory alterations can cause changes in cognitive functioning (Wahl & Heyl, 2003).

Cognitive Theories

All developmental theories are simply that—theories. A theory is developed to explain a collection of observations or facts and to predict future occurrences. As such, no one theory can explain all of reality, and all theories have some strengths and some weaknesses.

The most widely known cognitive theorist is Jean Piaget. His theory of cognitive development has contributed to other theories, such as Kohlberg's theory of moral development and Fowler's theory of the development of faith. According to Piaget (1966), based on his observations and work with children, cognitive development is an orderly, sequential process in which a variety of new experiences (stimuli) are needed before intellectual abilities can develop. He believed that age and maturational ability largely influence the child's view of the world. Given nurturing experiences, the child's ability to think matures naturally (Ginsberg & Opper, 1988; Piaget, 1972). Piaget's cognitive developmental process is divided into four major phases: the sensorimotor phase, the preoperational phase, the concrete operational phase, and the formal operational phase. These phases are explained in detail in the Development concept.

Although Piaget's theory of cognitive development provides a useful framework for examining and understanding the thought process of young children, like all theories it is not perfect. He developed the theory mainly by observation of his own three children. It may lack some applicability in cross-cultural contexts, and it does not explain the importance of social contexts in learning. Two other important cognitive theories expand the work of Piaget and may provide assistance for nurses:

1. Lev Vygotsky (1896–1934) agreed with Piaget's theory of a child's cognition. However, he believed that children are embedded in social contexts that influence learning. With guidance and assistance from parents and others, children learn tasks that are impossible for them to master alone. Vygotsky also viewed the social structure of language as essential to development of thought (Santrock, 2005; Vygotsky, 1962).

2. Information processing is another theory of cognitive development that views attention and memory as the most important parts of learning, rather than the structures Piaget described. Infants tend to habituate or become bored with the same stimuli and therefore are more attentive to, and learn from, new stimuli that are introduced to them. Long-term and short-term memory both are important to learning. The older child actively engages in strategies to assist with memorization, thereby playing an active part in learning (Meltzoff & Gopnick, 1997; Santrock, 2005).

Nursing Practices

Cognitive theory is essential to pediatric nursing. The nurse must understand a client's thought processes in order to design stimulating activities and meaningful, appropriate teaching plans. Health teaching is tailored to the understanding of cognitive stages. For example, a nurse can expect a toddler to be egocentric and literal; therefore, explanations to the toddler should focus on the needs of the toddler rather than on the needs of others. A child's concept of time suggests how far in advance the nurse should prepare that child for procedures. Similarly, the nurse's decision to offer manipulative toys, read stories, draw pictures, or give the child reading material to explain health care measures depends on the child's cognitive stage of development. A teenager can be expected to use rational thinking and to reason; therefore, when explaining the need for a medication to a teen, a nurse can outline the consequences of taking and not taking the medication, enabling the adolescent client to make a rational decision. Nurses must remember, however, that the range of normal cognitive development is broad, despite the age ranges attributed to each level. When teaching adults, nurses may become aware that some adults are more comfortable than others with concrete thought and some are slower to acquire and apply new information.

PRACTICE ALERT

Any change or deviation from normal in an individual's cognitive function should be evaluated. Because a number of factors can influence cognition, it can take time to determine the reason behind a change or impairment in cognitive function. Stress, grief, impairment of oxygenation, head injury, obstructive sleep apnea, stroke, embolism, and alcohol and drug abuse are just some of the conditions that can result in impaired cognitive ability.

Cognitive Abilities and Aging

Piaget's phases of cognitive development end with the formal operations phase. However, considerable research on cognitive abilities and aging is already beginning to provide insight into changes in cognition experienced by older adults, both as part of the normal aging process and through alterations that sometimes develop as people age. The brain loses mass with aging. In addition, blood flow to the brain decreases, the meninges thicken, and brain metabolism slows. Little is known about the effect of these physical changes on the cognitive functioning of the older adult. Lifelong mental activity, particularly verbal activity, helps the older adult retain a high level of cognitive function and maintain long-term memory.

Intellectual capacity includes perception, cognitive agility, memory, and learning. Declines in any of these abilities can affect cognition.

PERCEPTION   **Perception**, or the ability to interpret the environment, depends on the acuteness of the senses. If the aging person's senses are impaired, the ability to perceive the environment and react appropriately is diminished. Changes in the nervous system may also affect perceptual capacity.

COGNITIVE ABILITY   In older adults, changes in cognitive abilities are more often a difference in speed than in ability. Overall, the older adult maintains intelligence, problem solving, judgment, creativity, and other well-practiced cognitive skills. Intellectual loss generally reflects a disease process (e.g., atherosclerosis) that causes the blood vessels to narrow and diminishes perfusion of nutrients to the brain. Most older adults do not experience cognitive impairments; only 15% of older men and 11% of older women manifest moderate or severe memory impairment (FIFAS, 2004). Cognitive impairment that interferes with normal life is not considered part of normal aging. A decline in intellectual abilities that interferes with social or occupational functions should always be regarded as abnormal. Family members should be advised to seek prompt medical evaluation.

MEMORY   Memory is also a component of intellectual capacity and involves the following steps:

1. Momentary perception of stimuli from the environment, referred to as **sensory memory**.
2. Storage in **short-term memory** (information held in the brain for immediate use or what one has in mind at a given moment). An example of this type of memory is when an individual calls directory assistance for a telephone number and remembers the number only for the brief time needed to dial the number. Short-term memory also deals with the recent past few minutes to a few hours, which is often referred to as **recent memory**.
3. Encoding, in which the information leaves short-term memory and enters **long-term memory**, the repository for information stored for periods longer than 72 hours and usually weeks and years. Memories of childhood friends, teachers, and events are stored in long-term memory. Older people who remember the flowers in their wedding bouquet or the names of the boys on their dance card are drawing from long-term memory.

In older adults, retrieval of information from long-term memory can be slower, especially if the information is not frequently used. Most age-related differences, however, occur in short-term memory. Older adults tend to forget the recent past. This forgetfulness can be improved by using memory aids, making notes or lists, and placing objects in consistent locations.

LEARNING   Older people need additional time for learning, largely because of problems in retrieving information. Motivation is also important. Older adults have more difficulty in learning information they do not consider meaningful; therefore, the nurse should be particularly careful to discover what is meaningful to the older adult before attempting client education.

Cognitive Function in Older Adults

Normal, healthy aging is not characterized by cognitive and mental disorders (U.S. Department of Health and Human Services, 2001). Some cognitive abilities may decline with age, some may improve, and some stay relatively stable. These changes are highly variable from one person to another as a person ages and may even vary within a person over time. Most older people will not have significant memory impairment, but many may experience slight problems with word finding and remembering names. Usually, these problems are mild and the older person can compensate for them. Levels of educational attainment within the older population have increased significantly and are projected to continue to increase over the next decade. Higher education levels are linked to better health outcomes and a higher standard of living in retirement. However, even though older people share similar generational experiences, there may be considerable diversity among them. Life experiences, health status, race, culture, sexual orientation, and a variety of other factors can make an older person who did not finish high school think and act more like a college professor and vice versa.

Normally, an older person's mental health and cognition remain relatively stable. For those functions that do change, the change is usually not severe enough to cause significant impairment in daily life or social ability. Severe changes and sudden loss of cognitive function are usually symptoms of a physical or mental illness, such as Alzheimer's disease, stroke, or serious depression. The following are some general cognitive changes that are considered normal age-related changes (American Psychological Association, 2008):

■ Information-processing speed declines with age, resulting in a slower learning rate and greater need for repetition of information.
■ The ability to divide attention between two tasks shows age-related decline.
■ The ability to switch attention rapidly from one auditory input to another shows age-related decline (visual input switching ability does not change significantly with age).
■ The ability to maintain sustained attention or perform vigilance tasks appears to decline with age.
■ The ability to filter out irrelevant information appears to decline with age.

- Short-term or primary memory remains relatively stable.
- Long-term or secondary memory exhibits more substantial age-related changes, with a greater decline for recall than for recognition. (Cueing improves performance of long-term memory.)
- Most aspects of language are well preserved, such as use of language sounds and meaningful combinations of words. Vocabulary improves with age. However, word finding, naming ability, and rapid word list generation decline with age.
- Visuospatial task ability such as drawing and construction ability declines with age.
- Abstraction and mental flexibility show some age-related decline.
- Accumulation of practical experience, or wisdom, continues until the very end of life.

PRACTICE ALERT

Normal healthy older persons who forget where they put the keys can be assured there is no significant memory problem, but if they forget what a key is for or how to use it, they should be referred for further evaluation and treatment.

Decline of intellectual function is generally greater in older people who develop disease and disability than in those who remain healthy. Many impairments in cognitive capacity, mood, and performance that formerly were attributed to "normal aging" are now known to be associated with psychiatric illness or physical disease. Significant changes in mood, cognitive ability, and personality should never be dismissed as normal aging, but always aggressively assessed and referred for treatment.

Late adulthood is no longer seen as a period of growth cessation and arrested cognitive development, but rather a period of continued growth with the opportunity for development of unique capacities (Ebersole, Hess, & Lugfen, 2004). Education, pulmonary health, general health, and activity levels all influence cognitive activity in later life. Older adults often have a positive outlook and seek challenges and activities that maintain their well-being. Since most changes of aging are gradual, the older person adjusts to the changes over time. Methods for coping with age-associated cognitive changes follow:

- Making lists, posting appointments on calendars, and writing "notes to self"
- Using memory training and memory enhancement techniques (for instance, when meeting a new person for the first time, trying to link his or her name to a common object or easily remembered item)
- Playing computer games that emphasize eye–hand coordination and memory of shapes, colors, and objects
- Keeping the mind challenged and mentally active (reading daily, completing a crossword puzzle, playing bridge, etc.)
- Using assistive devices such as pill boxes and preprogrammed telephones, and reliance on habits such as parking in the same place in the mall parking lot to reduce chances of forgetting vital information
- Seeking support and encouragement from others

- Staying positive and hopeful for the future, including laughing at oneself when appropriate. ("You won't believe what I did today. I showed up for my doctor's appointment with one brown and one black shoe! Oh well, at least I'm not a slave to fashion!")

A nurse who is beginning to notice changes in an older client's cognitive activity can suggest and encourage use of these methods and other coping techniques to assist the client in adjusting to the changes and maintaining a positive outlook.

Older adults must be able to monitor their cognitive abilities and adapt to changes in their memory skills to function safely in their everyday lives. Some people with severe cognitive deficits may continue to engage in behaviors that are unsafe for them, such as driving, cooking, and trying to live independently. Others with good memories may live in continual fear that they are developing Alzheimer's disease whenever they forget a name or an appointment.

It is difficult to predict whether an older person who has mild problems with memory will develop more severe memory loss. Some older people try to hide or cover up memory problems because they fear restrictions on their freedoms and living situation. Memory changes may result from a variety of causes, including Alzheimer's disease, depression, underlying psychiatric illness, physical illness, medications, vitamin deficiencies, and sensory impairments. Any alteration or concern over cognitive abilities should be assessed to identify reversible causes of memory loss and institute appropriate safety measures in a supportive environment.

ALTERATIONS
Pediatric Cognitive Disorders

A wide array of cognitive conditions occur in childhood. Some are mild and not diagnosed until a child has difficulty in school, while others may be associated with physical signs that are visible at birth.

LEARNING DISABILITIES **Learning disabilities** involve neurological conditions in which the brain cannot receive or process information in the normal manner. They are common in young children, affecting approximately 8–10% of school children. Often the impairment is in only one or two types of learning, making diagnosis difficult. Common types of learning disorders are listed and described in Box 1–1. Children may have difficulty in processing visual information that is manifested in reading, writing, and mathematics performance. Others may have more difficulty with oral information, leading to problems in language development and reading (Kelly & Aylward, 2005; National Center for Learning Disabilities, 2004).

The causes of learning disorders are complex. Sometimes they are related to low birth weight or problems during the perinatal period. Children suspected of having a disability should be evaluated and diagnosed by a learning specialist such as a psychologist with specialty training. A series of cognitive and developmental tests are most commonly used. Brain scanning with magnetic resonance imaging (MRI) is showing promise for providing diagnostic clues, but is not yet commonly used or

Box 1–1 Learning Disorders

DISORDER	CLINICAL MANIFESTATIONS
Dyslexia	Difficulty with writing, reading, spelling
Dyscalculia	Difficulty with mathematics and computation
Dysgraphia	Difficulty with writing, spelling, and composition
Dyspraxia	Difficulty with manual dexterity and coordination

Source: Ball, J. W., & Bindler, R. C. (2008). *Pediatric nursing* (4th ed., p. 1137). Upper Saddle River, NJ: Pearson Education.

available in most communities. Some disabilities may have a genetic component, since their occurrence is more common when other family members are affected. Treatments generally involve teaching children how to compensate for the difficulties by using capabilities that are intact. Some children will require accommodations, such as having all material presented in class provided to them in writing, or being given extra time to complete tests. Children with learning disabilities should have individualized education plans (IEPs) established with realistic goals for school performance. These plans are normally developed collaboratively by the classroom teacher, a learning specialist, and the child's parents.

Nursing Management

Nurses play a major role in identifying children with learning disabilities. In fact, the pediatrician's office is frequently the first place a parent will take a child if the parent suspects something is wrong with the child's development. Nurses may also encounter families during health promotion visits or in other settings when parents relay concerns about the child's behavior at home or in day care or about the child's performance or difficulty in some aspect of school. The nurse should ask whether there is a family history of learning problems, and evaluate the child's history for prematurity, low birth weight, head injury, seizure activity, and other chronic health conditions. The nurse assesses the child for the following developmental milestones, which can indicate a learning disability:

- Inability to phrase sentences together by 2.5 years of age
- Inability to use speech that is understandable at least 50% of the time by age 3 years
- Inability to tie shoes, button clothes, hop, or cut with scissors by kindergarten
- Inability to sit for a short story by 3–5 years (Kelly & Aylward, 2005)

A number of screening tools exist to help nurses and other professionals screen children for suspected learning disabilities in order to determine whether a referral is necessary.

A nurse who suspects a child may have a learning disability should refer the family to the school or other testing resource. The nurse should partner with the family to plan for the child's learning needs. This includes helping the family to work closely with the child, providing a setting at home to maximize potential for learning, building healthy self-esteem in the child, and assisting the family in working with the school to establish annual goals for the child. A multidisciplinary team, including teachers, therapists, and the family, commonly works within the school to plan for the child's learning needs (Lambros & Leslie, 2005). In some states, a special agency or network exists for diagnosing children younger than kindergarten age, and a nurse or primary care provider can refer a family for diagnostic procedures before a child enters school. Because most children with learning disabilities can learn to perform well in their areas of strength and compensate for areas of difficulty, early intervention is key to their success and to building a positive self-image regarding their abilities.

MENTAL RETARDATION **Mental retardation** is defined as significant limitation in intellectual functioning and adaptive behavior. It is manifested in differences in conceptual, social, and practical life skills and begins before the age of 18 years (American Association of Mental Retardation, 2004). Later events that lead to limitations in function are referred to as brain injury. Intellectual functioning is generally characterized by an IQ below 70–75 and significant impairment in **adaptive functioning** (the ability of an individual to meet the standards expected for his or her cultural group). The individual with mental retardation has adaptive deficits in at least two areas, such as communication, self-care, home living, social/interpersonal skills, use of community resources, self-direction, functional academic skills, work, leisure, health, or safety. A low IQ score by itself does not necessarily correlate with impairment in adaptive skills. The child should be evaluated within the contexts of the individual's cultural and community environments. The IQ score and the level of adaptive skills together determine the severity of mental retardation.

Mental retardation is one type of developmental disability. A **developmental disability** is any of a variety of chronic conditions that are characterized by mental and/or physical impairment. Other examples are pervasive developmental disorder, cerebral palsy, and sensory loss. A developmental disability begins by the age of 21 years and lasts throughout life (Bhasin, Brocksen, Avchen, & Braun, 2006). Early detection, diagnosis, and treatment can greatly increase the chances of a successful and productive life for an individual with a developmental disability.

Mental retardation occurs in 12 per 1,000 children, a decrease from 15.5 per 1,000 one decade ago (Bhasin et al., 2006). The causes of mental retardation can be grouped into three general categories: prenatal errors in the development of the central nervous system (CNS), prenatal or postnatal changes in the biologic environment of the person, and external forces leading to CNS damage. In each instance, the precipitating factor causes a change in the form, function, and adaptation of the CNS. Table 1–1 provides examples of common causes of mental retardation for each category.

Three common conditions associated with mental retardation from the prenatal category are Down syndrome, fragile X syndrome, and fetal alcohol syndrome. In the United States, about 1 in 1,000 infants, or 5,500 infants each year, are born with **Down syndrome** (Centers for Disease Control and Prevention,

TABLE 1–1 Common Conditions Associated With Mental Retardation

PRENATAL CONDITIONS	BIOLOGIC ENVIRONMENT	EXTERNAL FORCES
Down syndrome	Inborn errors of metabolism (e.g., phenylketonuria, hypothyroidism)	Traumatic brain injury (e.g., accident)
Fragile X syndrome		Poison ingestion (acute or chronic)
Fetal alcohol syndrome		Hypoxia/anoxic insult
Maternal infection (e.g., rubella, cytomegalovirus)		Infection (e.g., meningitis)
		Environmental deprivation

Source: Ball, J. W., & Bindler, R. C. (2008). *Pediatric nursing* (4th ed., p. 1138). Upper Saddle River, NJ: Pearson Education.

2006). The condition is caused by an extra chromosome; the child has 47 rather than 46 chromosomes. The most common chromosome affected is 21, so that the child often has trisomy 21, or three copies instead of two of chromosome 21. In addition to mental retardation and physical signs, the child with Down syndrome is at higher risk of developing other conditions such as cardiac defects, hearing loss, strabismus, gastrointestinal problems, orthodontic conditions, thyroid disease, dermatologic conditions, and leukemia (Van Cleve, Cannon, & Cohen, 2006).

Fragile X syndrome is caused by a single recessive gene abnormality on the X chromosome. The faulty gene creates a deficiency in the FMR1 protein that leads to brain changes. The condition is often associated with other conditions such as attention deficit/hyperactivity disorder (ADHD), anxiety, and autism (Hagerman, 2006).

Fetal alcohol syndrome (FAS) is caused by the effect of ethyl alcohol on the developing fetus. The term *fetal alcohol spectrum disorder* (FASD) describes the wide range of effects from the condition, which can range from FAS to a milder condition called fetal alcohol effects (FAE) (Caley, Shipkey, Winkelman et al., 2006). Alcohol ingestion by the pregnant woman can influence the development of many body organs, and its effects can range from mild to severe. In spite of the warnings regarding use of alcohol during pregnancy, alcohol use remains a leading cause of mental retardation, affecting 2 in 1,000 births in the United States, or 8,000 to 12,000 infants annually (Troshinksy, 2004).

Fetal alcohol syndrome is more common in groups with a higher intake of alcohol. The rate in Native American and Alaskan Native communities is 10 times the rate in the general population (Troshinksy, 2004). Because some Native American tribes have a high rate of alcoholism, the federal government has joined with them to lower that risk among this ethnic group. On some reservations, such as the Yakama Nation in Washington State, alcoholic beverages are not sold and educational programs are in place to discourage use of alcohol among pregnant women.

Phenylketonuria and hypothyroidism are two common biochemical causes of mental retardation. Other causes are traumatic brain injury and infections of the CNS.

Clinical Manifestations Mild mental retardation was originally described as an IQ between 50 and 70, with moderate retardation between 35 and 50, severe retardation between 20 and 35, and profound retardation below 20. Although an IQ below 70 is considered indicative of retardation, the functional assessment of the child is now considered a more accurate identification of children's performance and needs. **Functional assessments** can include diagnostic testing, but they primarily involve detailed observations of the behavior, responses, and abilities a child uses in both the home and school settings. In other words, these assessments look at how a child functions on a daily basis in his or her environment. Children who are mentally retarded manifest delays in all areas of development, including motor movement, language, and adaptive behavior. They usually achieve developmental milestones more slowly than the average child. These developmental delays may be the first indication to parents and care providers of the child's condition.

Mental retardation is sometimes accompanied by sensory impairment, speech problems, motor and orthopedic disabilities, and seizure disorders. Of children with mental retardation, 10–30% manifest at least one such disorder. Table 1–2 lists several physical characteristics associated with Down syndrome, fragile X syndrome, and fetal alcohol syndrome.

Diagnostic Tests Mental retardation is diagnosed and initial treatment is planned in a multistep process that involves a multidisciplinary team that includes the parents. This team usually includes a developmental specialist, physician, geneticist, nurse, teacher, language therapist, and rehabilitation specialists. See Table 1–3 for a description of the *DSM-IV-TR* for mental retardation.

The team will begin by conducting a comprehensive history and evaluation of the child's physical characteristics, developmental level, and intellectual and adaptive functioning. Laboratory tests such as chromosome analysis, blood enzyme levels, and lead levels or cranial imaging may be ordered to provide additional information. A three-generation family history is generally performed (Moeschler, Shevell, & American Academy of Pediatrics, 2006).

Developmental screening using a test such as the Denver II can help to identify children who may be at risk of developmental delay. A neurologic examination may indicate asymmetry of movement or strength, irritability or lethargy, or abnormal pitch to an infant's cry. Because mental retardation may be accompanied by physical abnormalities, it is important to observe the child for facial symmetry, distance between the

TABLE 1–2 **Characteristics of Three Common Conditions Associated With Mental Retardation**

DOWN SYNDROME (See Figure 1–1 ■)	FRAGILE X SYNDROME	FETAL ALCOHOL SYNDROME (See Figure 1–2 ■)
Small head (microcephaly)	Long face	Flat midface
Flattened forehead	Prominent jaw	Low nasal bridge
Wide, short neck	Large ears	Long philtrum with narrow upper lip
Epicanthal eye folds	Frequent otitis media	Short upturned nose
White spots on eye iris (Brushfield spots)	Large testicles	Poor coordination
Congenital cataracts	Epicanthal eye folds	Failure to thrive
Flat nose	Strabismus	Skeletal and joint abnormalities
Small, low-set ears	High-arched palate	Hearing loss
Protruding tongue	Scoliosis	
Short broad hands	Pliable joints	
Simian line on palm		
Wide space between first and second toes		
Hearing loss		
Increased incidence of diabetes, congenital heart defect, and leukemia		
Hypotonia		

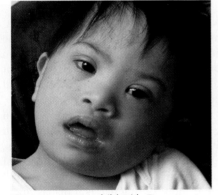

Figure 1–1 ■ A child with Down syndrome.

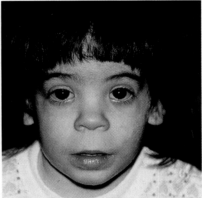

Figure 1–2 ■ A child with fetal alcohol syndrome.

Courtesy of Dr. Sterling Clarren, Seattle, WA, and Vancouver, BC. From Clarren, S. F. H. Smith, D.W. (1978). The fetal alcohol syndrome. *New England Journal of Medicine, 298,* 1063–1067.

Source: Ball, J. W., & Bindler, R. C. (2008). *Pediatric nursing* (4th ed., p. 1140). Upper Saddle River, NJ: Pearson Education.

eyes, level of the ears, hair growth, and palmar creases. These abnormalities may be cues to other health problems.

Clinical Therapy Based on the results of the evaluation, the multidisciplinary team will plan the support needed to maximize the child's potential for development. Management focuses on early intervention to improve the degree of adaptive functioning. Simultaneous treatment of associated physical, emotional, and behavioral problems is provided. Depending on the child's condition, special education programs and physical or occupational therapy may be necessary. At all stages, the multidisciplinary team obtains the permission of, discusses test results with, and makes recommendations to the parent. Parents' understanding of and participation in this process are critical to the success of any treatment plan, and the parents' permission is required for any treatment to be provided.

TABLE 1–3 *DSM-IV-TR* Diagnostic Criteria for Mental Retardation

A. Significantly subaverage intellectual functioning: an IQ of approximately 70 or below on an individually administered IQ test (for infants, a clinical judgment of significantly subaverage intellectual functioning).

B. Concurrent deficits or impairments in present adaptive functioning (i.e., the person's effectiveness in meeting the standards expected for his or her age by his or her cultural group) in at least two of the following areas: communication, self-care, home living, social/interpersonal skills, use of community resources, self-direction, functional academic skills, work, leisure, health, and safety.

C. The onset is before age 18 years.

Source: Reprinted with permission from the *Diagnostic and Statistical Manual of Mental Disorders,* Text Revision, Fourth Edition, (Copyright © 2000). American Psychiatric Association.

PRACTICE ALERT

Prematurity and low birth weight place the child at risk of displaying below-normal cognitive development. Premature and low-birth-weight infants need frequent, thorough neurologic and developmental examinations, particularly in the first 2 years of life. Premature infants are expected to reach developmental milestones at approximately the same age as infants born at normal gestational age. For example, an infant born 2 months prematurely should be evaluated on milestones of an infant 2 months younger than the infant's current chronological age. The infant gradually catches up and reaches the chronological age milestones by about 2 years of age. Nurses should encourage parents to keep health promotion appointments and be sure the child receives developmental screening at each visit.

The child may require supportive care and assistance with activities of daily living (ADLs). The plans for intervention change as the child grows and family situations evolve. Some classes and community agencies offer transitional classes when children who are mentally retarded reach adolescence and young adulthood. These services help teach self-care skills that may enable some youth to live in group homes or other community settings. Families can receive help in planning for the child's future as parents look toward retirement. Information is provided on living options, health insurance, work opportunities, and other needs. Agencies that provide these services can also offer respite services for parents and other family members who have spent much time with the child for many years.

Nursing Management   Nurses can help to identify children with mental retardation through history taking, observation, and developmental screening during early childhood. The history should provide information about the mental and adaptive functioning of birth parents and other family members, as mental retardation can have a genetic component. The pregnancy and birth history can provide important information relating to the mother's alcohol and drug use during pregnancy. Nurses should be alert for a history of difficult pregnancy and problems during delivery.

When genetic conditions in the family predispose family members to mental retardation, careful assessment of the child is needed. Children from deprived environments or those at risk from environmental hazards, such as lead poisoning, are more likely to manifest mental retardation.

Many children with mental retardation are not diagnosed with the condition until they reach school age, particularly if the condition is mild or moderate. Early intervention, however, can help to enhance the child's functioning later. During home visits or clinic appointments, in child care centers, and during hospitalization, nurses should be alert for signs of developmental delays, multiple (more than three) physical anomalies associated with a specific condition, or neurologic alterations. Developmental assessment should be part of each health care visit.

Once the diagnosis of mental retardation has been made, the nurse assesses the adaptive functioning of the child and family. A functional assessment of the child should be performed, including toileting, dressing, and feeding skills. The child's language, sensory, and psychomotor functioning are assessed, as well as the home and community for safety hazards. The nurse observes how the family is managing with the child. The availability of services, such as support groups for parents and special education opportunities for children, is assessed. The coping skills of family members are evaluated.

Several nursing diagnoses may be appropriate for the child with mental retardation, depending on the degree, cause, and outcome of the condition. Diagnoses that relate to impairments in adaptive functioning and family impact include the following:

- Delayed growth and development related to neonatal disease or condition
- Imbalanced nutrition (less than body requirements) related to inability to ingest sufficient food
- Self-care deficit (dressing, toileting, bathing) related to developmental disability
- Impaired verbal communication related to developmental disability
- Risk for injury related to lack of understanding of environmental hazards
- Compromised family coping related to the child's developmental variations

Prevention is important for some types of mental retardation. All pregnant women or those who are trying to become pregnant should stop ingestion of alcohol and nonprescription drugs. Encourage regular prenatal visits; these help to prevent premature births, which have a higher association with mental retardation than birth at term.

Nearly all children with mental retardation are cared for in the community; however, they may have conditions that require periodic hospitalization or frequent health care visits. When needed, nursing care focuses on providing emotional support and information to family members, assisting the child with adaptive functioning, and fostering parental management of the child's activities. When possible, the nurse uses preventive teaching to lower the risk of mental retardation.

Family members need empathy and support both at the time of diagnosis and in the ensuing years. Following initial diagnoses, parents may enter an acute or chronic state of grief over the loss of the perfect child. The nurse should encourage them to verbalize their feelings. Introducing them to parents of other mentally retarded children may provide assistance and support as they learn how to manage the child's needs. The availability of respite care to provide parents with a break from caretaking is discussed. Other family members may also be experiencing grief or guilt and should be given an opportunity to talk about their feelings.

Parents need honest information and answers to their questions about the child's condition. The nurse should reinforce information provided by genetic counselors and other health care professionals. Parents need help accessing information about community resources designed to assist children with mental retardation. Such resources include the Zero to Three Project, special education preschools and schools, county health services, and respite care. The nurse refers parents to Internet sources and helps them to interpret information received and analyze its strengths and limitations. The nurse should ask parents if they

CLIENT TEACHING Fetal Alcohol Syndrome

Fetal alcohol syndrome (FAS) is a preventable cause of mental retardation. About 10% of women consume alcohol while pregnant, and 2% engage in frequent or binge drinking (Suellentrop, Morrow, Williams, D'Angels, 2006). This indicates that all women must receive clear messages about the dangers of drinking while pregnant. Teach all pregnant women that total abstention from alcohol for the entire length of pregnancy is the only completely effective method of preventing FAS. Include this in teaching to all adolescent girls, so they are aware of how alcohol can harm their infant if they become pregnant. Emphasize that the most dangerous time may be early in pregnancy before women commonly know they are pregnant.

have questions about individualized education plans (IEPs), and review federal and state laws and services that might be helpful to the family, including the following:

- Administration on Developmental Disabilities (ADD) is the U.S. organization that ensures that the Developmental Disabilities Act goals are met. The agency implements the Developmental Disabilities and Bill of Rights Act of 2000 and seeks to enhance life through training activities, educating the community, eliminating barriers, and influencing policy (Administration for Children and Families, 2004).
- State councils on developmental disabilities (SCDDs) are present in each state to increase integration of children with developmental disabilities.
- Public Law (PL) 94–142 of 1975 mandates that all children, even those with handicaps, be provided with public education and related services (Box 1–2).
- PL 99–457 of 1986 expanded the services of PL 94–142 to include children from birth to 5 years who need special education. Its focus is the importance of fostering development and enhancing the capacity of families to meet the needs of children.
- PL 101–336 of 1990 is known as the American Disabilities Act (ADA). It prohibits discrimination and ensures equal opportunity for persons with disabilities in employment, state and local government services, public accommodations, commercial facilities, and transportation.
- Individuals with Disabilities Education Act Amendments (IDEA) of 1997 strengthened the academic expectations and accountability for children with disabilities.

Box 1–2 Education for All Handicapped Children Act

The Education for All Handicapped Children Act, P.L. 94–142, provides free appropriate public education to all handicapped children between 2 and 21 years of age. Amendments to this act in 1986 (P.L. 99–457) encouraged states to provide early intervention services for infants and toddlers with developmental delay by providing federal funding. This act and its amendments also include language specifically designed to protect the rights of parent and child and to ensure parent participation in the educational process.

PRACTICE ALERT

To determine the impact of the child with mental retardation on the family, the nurse asks parents to describe (1) family activities that include the child, (2) strategies that parents and siblings use to deal with community attitudes about the child, and, (3) in the case of a child with other disabilities, methods of managing the child's care and planning for future care needs.

Children with mental retardation require close supervision because they may lack an understanding of common hazards. The nurse ensures safety in the hospital environment. The nurse assists parents in providing safety at home and school and teaching their child such necessary skills as pedestrian safety. Both physical and emotional safety should be considered. This type of child may be overly trusting of others and can be at risk for physical or sexual abuse.

Parents should be encouraged in efforts to maximize the child's areas of strength and identify needs related to adaptive behaviors. The nurse refers parents to resources to assist in the areas of adaptive functioning in which the child has impairment, such as communication, self-care activities, or social skills. During hospitalization, the nurse can support parents' efforts to maintain the child's skills in toileting, dressing, and self-care by planning interventions to use the skills being taught at home.

The child with mental retardation needs ongoing care throughout childhood, and adaptation of interventions as development occurs and the family's needs evolve. Parents often act as case managers for the child's care. The nurse can assist parents as necessary to acquire the skills required to coordinate the child's plan of care. The child's needs should be evaluated regularly and the parents asked to assist with the treatment plan as necessary. The nurse assists with plans for education and services such as physical or speech therapy. Most children with mental retardation have an IEP designed to meet their specific learning needs. Parents, nurses, and other professionals such as teachers and language therapists are part of the team that establishes this plan. All team members work together to promote optimal development and socialization. As the child reaches adolescence, education is directed toward a vocation, issues of sexuality, and the goal of independent living, when appropriate.

Specific guidelines for care are available for the child with Down syndrome. These guidelines suggest times for evaluation of hearing, growth, cardiac function, and other areas designed for early identification and treatment of associated disorders (Van Cleve & Cohen, 2006). There are specific growth grids for children with Down syndrome, and specific topics to suggest for anticipatory guidance during health care visits.

The expected outcomes of nursing care depend on the child's needs and developmental level. Early in the diagnostic phase, desired outcomes may involve the family's understanding of the diagnosis and the child's special needs. Later outcomes may focus on the child's communication and self-help skills. Outcomes related to cognitive performance and adaptive skills may be developed during childhood.

PRACTICE ALERT

Children with learning disabilities or mental retardation are at greater risk of abuse than their typically developing peers. They may also have more difficulty verbalizing or explaining the abuse. The reasons for this risk are many, including the increased emotional and economic stress these children place, unintentionally of course, on their parents. Nurses working with children with these special needs should be alert for any evidence of abuse, but should also be aware that some disabilities can cause injuries that mimic abuse. After careful assessment, a nurse who suspects a child has been abused should immediately report her suspicions to the local child protective services agency.

Dementia

Dementia is a progressive loss of cognitive function. It is critical that dementia be differentiated from delirium, an acute and reversible syndrome. Both may be characterized by changes in memory, judgment, language, mathematic calculation, abstract reasoning, and problem-solving ability.

Dementia affects multiple cortical functions. Impairments of cognitive function are usually accompanied by deterioration in emotional control, social behavior, and motivation. People with dementia lose their ability to solve problems and may experience personality changes including agitation and hallucinations. All forms of dementia result from death of neurons and/or the loss of communication among the cells. Although the exact cause is not always known, many forms of dementia are characterized by abnormal structures in the brain called inclusions. While a genetic component clearly exists in the development of some kinds of dementia, there may be no known family history of the condition in an individual who develops dementia.

It is estimated that as many as 6.8 million people in the United States have dementia, and at least 1.8 million of those are severely affected. Studies of some communities have found that almost half of all people age 85 and older have some form of dementia. However, despite increased incidence in older people, dementia is not a normal part of aging (National Institute of Neurological Disorders and Stroke, 2005b).

Many diseases and conditions may cause dementia, including Alzheimer's disease, vascular dementia, Huntington's disease, Creutzfeldt-Jakob disease, metabolic disorders, poisoning and anoxia, and medications. Table 1–4 provides an overview of its most common causes. Doctors do not diagnose dementia unless two or more brain functions (such as memory, language skills, perception, reasoning, or judgment) are significantly impaired without loss of consciousness. The most common type of dementia is Alzheimer's disease (AD).

Even though the actual cause of all dementias may not be known, risk factors for developing one or more kinds of dementia have been identified. These include advancing age, a family history of a disease that causes dementia, smoking and alcohol use, atherosclerosis, high cholesterol and plasma homocysteine levels, diabetes, mild cognitive impairment, and Down syndrome.

People often experience other conditions that may mimic dementia. These include the following:

- Age-related cognitive decline, resulting from slower information processing and mild memory impairment. With aging, the brain often decreases in volume and some neurons are lost. These changes are normal and are not considered a part of dementia.
- Mild cognitive impairment, which may progress to dementia, but is not severe enough to be initially diagnosed as such.
- Depression or other emotional problems that cause people to be passive, slow, confused, or forgetful.
- Delirium, characterized by confusion, rapidly altering mental states, disorientation, and possible personality changes. Delirium is usually caused by a treatable physical or mental health illness and, when treated, results in a full recovery.

Dementia can be difficult to diagnose in its early stages, primarily because an individual experiencing dementia may not notice these slight gradual changes until they become more pronounced or he or she may deny experiencing any changes. This can present challenges for family members: An older person with early dementia may blame others for hiding or stealing his or her belongings when, in reality, he or she has simply misplaced them. These delusions can be hurtful to family and friends who are attempting to assist the older person and may result in increased social isolation and conflict within the family.

TABLE 1–4 Common Causes of Dementia

NAME	CAUSE AND PRIMARY PATHOPHYSIOLOGY
Alzheimer's disease (the most common cause of dementia in people age 65 and older)	Cause is unknown; characterized by two abnormalities in the brain: amyloid plaques and neurofibrillary tangles.
Vascular dementia (the second most common cause of dementia)	Caused by brain damage from cerebrovascular and cardiovascular problems (usually strokes). May also be caused by cerebral blood vessel damage from genetic disorders, endocarditis, myeloid angiopathy, vasculitis, and profound hypotension.
Lewy body dementia	Cause is usually unknown, although familial cases have been reported. Cells die, and remaining cells in the substantia nigra contain abnormal structures called Lewy bodies.
Frontotemporal dementia	Nerve cells, especially in the frontal and temporal lobes, degenerate. In many people, abnormal tau protein accumulates in neurofibrillary tangles.

Source: Burke, K., & LeMone, P. (2008). *Medical surgical nursing care* (4th ed., p. 1618), Upper Saddle River, NJ: Pearson Education.

TABLE 1–5 **Common Deficits Associated With Dementia**

DEFICIT	CLINICAL MANIFESTATIONS
Akathisia	Inability to keep still; feeling of restlessness
Anomia	Difficulty naming persons or objects; no impairment of comprehension
Aphasia/paraphasia	Impairment of comprehension and expression of language (both verbal and written)
Ataxia	Poor muscle control during voluntary movement, poor balance
Carphologia/floccillation	Involuntary, repeated picking at bedding and clothing
Constructional difficulty	Difficulty assembling blocks, drawing or copying three-dimensional figures
Dysphagia	Difficult or painful swallowing
Echolalia	Involuntary repetition of words or sentences just spoken by another person

An individual with dementia may experience one or more of several cognitive deficits. These can be mild, as in the case of anomia, or more pronounced, as with paraphasia. Some of these deficits are listed in Table 1–5.

Other alterations related to cognition that are not addressed as part of this concept include, but are not limited to, mental illness.

PHYSICAL ASSESSMENT

A physical assessment should be conducted at each office visit or health care interaction to determine any potential changes in the cognitive state of an older person. Nurses should conduct a cognitive assessment using tools such as those listed in Table 1–6. One of the most frequently used is the Mini-Mental State Exam (MMSE), a short, 30-question test used to assess the extent of cognitive impairment. The MMSE can be used to assess for changes in cognitive function over time. Frequently used as a screening tool for Alzheimer's disease, the MMSE assesses cognitive function in a number of areas, including language, mathematics, memory, and motor skills.

Nurses should also be alert for any need to assess for depression in the older individual, particularly one who has recently

(text continues on p. 14)

Cognitive Assessment

Techniques and Normal Findings	Abnormal Findings Special Considerations
Mental Status	
The nurse assesses the mental status of the client when meeting the client for the first time. This process begins with taking the health history and continues with each client contact.	A variety of tools are available to conduct mental status assessment. These tools are described in Table 1–6.

TABLE 1–6 **Tools for Assessment of Mental Status**

TOOL	ASSESSMENT
Mini-Mental State Examination (MMSE)	Cognitive status—conducted via interview
Addenbrooke's Cognitive Examination	Detects early dementia
Confusion Assessment Method (CAM)	Tests for delirium
Telephone Interview for Cognitive Status (TICS)	Similar to MMSE, cognitive function assessed via telephone interview
Cornell Scale for Depression in Dementia	Assessment of behavioral problems
Dementia Symptoms Scale	Assessment of behavioral problems
Psychogeriatric Dependency Rating Scale	Assessment of behavioral problems
Hopkins Competency Assessment Test	Assessment of ability to make decisions about health care
General Health Questionnaire	Assessment of emotional disturbance in those with normal cognitive ability
Hamilton Depression Rating Scale	Assessment of depression in clients with impaired cognition
Short Portable Mental Status Questionnaire (SPMSQ)	Assessment of organic brain deficit

(continued)

Cognitive Assessment (continued)

Techniques and Normal Findings   **Abnormal Findings Special Considerations**

1. Instruct the client.

- Explain to the client that you will be conducting a variety of tests. Tell the client that you will provide instructions before beginning each examination. Explain that moving about and changing position during the examination will be required. Provide reassurance that the tests will not cause discomfort; however, the client must inform you of problems if they arise during any part of the assessment. Identify the types of equipment you will use and describe the purpose in relation to neurologic function. Tell the client that you will begin the assessment with some general questions about the present and past. Then you will ask the client to respond to number and word questions.

2. Position the client.

- The client should be sitting on the examination table wearing an examination gown (see Figure 1–3 ■).

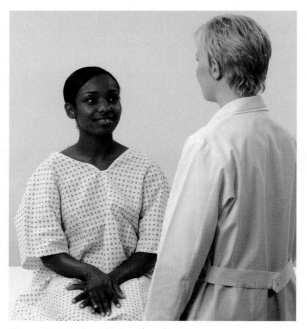

Figure 1–3 ■ Positioning the client.

3. Observe the client.

- Look at the client and note hygiene, grooming, posture, body language, facial expressions, speech, and ability to follow directions.

Changes could be indicative of depression, schizophrenia, organic brain syndrome, or obsessive-compulsive disorder.

4. Note the client's speech and language abilities.

- Throughout the assessment, note the client's rate of speech, ability to pronounce words, tone of voice, loudness or softness (volume) of voice, and ability to speak smoothly and clearly.
- Assess the client's choice of words, ability to respond to questions, and ease with which a response is made.

Changes in speech could reflect anxiety, Parkinson's disease, depression, or various forms of aphasia.

5. Assess the client's sensorium.

- Determine the client's orientation to date, time, place, and reason for being here. Grade the level of alertness on a scale from full alertness to coma.

Neurologic disease can produce a sliding or changing degree of alertness. Change in the level of consciousness may be related to cortical or brain stem disease. A stroke, seizure, or hypoglycemia could also contribute to a change in the level of consciousness.

Cognitive Assessment (continued)

Techniques and Normal Findings	Abnormal Findings Special Considerations

6. Assess the client's memory.

- Ask for the client's date of birth, Social Security number, names and ages of any children or grandchildren, educational history with dates and events, work history with dates, and job descriptions. Ask questions for which the response can be verified.

Loss of long-term memory may indicate cerebral cortex damage, which occurs in Alzheimer's disease.

7. Assess the client's ability to calculate problems.

- Start with a simple problem, such as $4 + 3$, $8 \div 2$, and $15 - 4$.
- Progress to more difficult problems, such as $(10 \times 4) - 8$, or ask the client to start with 100 and subtract 7 ($100 - 7 = 93$, $93 - 7 = 86$, $86 - 7 = 79$, and so on).
- Remember to use problems that are appropriate for the developmental, educational, and intellectual level of the client.
- Asking the client to calculate change from one dollar for the purchase of items costing 25, 39, and 89 cents is a quick test of calculation.

Inability to calculate simple problems may indicate the presence of organic brain disease, or it may simply indicate lack of exposure to mathematical concepts, nervousness, or an incomplete understanding of the examiner's language. In an otherwise unremarkable assessment, a poor response to calculations should not be considered an abnormal finding.

8. Assess the client's ability to think abstractly.

- Ask the client to identify similarities and differences between two objects or topics, such as wood and coal, king and president, orange and apple, and pear and celery. Quote a proverb and ask the client to explain its meaning. For example:
  - "A stitch in time saves nine."
  - "The empty barrel makes the most noise."
  - "Don't put all your eggs in one basket."
- Be aware that age and culture influence the ability to explain American proverbs and slang terms.

Responses made by the client may reflect lack of education, mental retardation, or dementia. Clients with personality disorders such as schizophrenia or depression may make bizarre responses.

9. Assess the client's mood and emotional state.

- Observe the client's body language, facial expressions, and communication technique. The facial expression and tone of voice should be congruent with the content and context of the communication.
- Ask if the client generally feels this way or if he or she has experienced a change and if so over what period of time.
- Ask the client if it is possible to identify an event or incident that fostered the change in mood or emotional state.
- The client's mood and emotions should reflect the current situation or response to events that trigger mood change or call for an emotional response (e.g., a change in health status, a loss, or a stressful event).

Lack of congruence of facial expression and tone of voice with the content and context of communication may occur with neurologic problems, emotional disturbance, or a psychogenic disorder such as schizophrenia or depression.

Lack of emotional response, lack of change in facial expression, and flat voice tones can indicate problems with mood or emotional responses. Other abnormal findings in relation to mood and emotional state include anxiety, depression, fear, anger, overconfidence, ambivalence, euphoria, impatience, and irritability. Mood disorders are associated with bipolar disorder, anxiety disorders, and major depression.

10. Assess perceptions and thought processes.

- Listen to the client's statements. Statements should be logical and relevant. The client should complete his or her thoughts.
- Determining the client's awareness of reality assesses perception.

Disturbed thought processes can indicate neurologic dysfunction or mental disorder.
Disturbances in sense of reality can include hallucination and illusion. These are associated with mental disturbances as seen in schizophrenia.

11. Assess the client's ability to make judgments.

- Determine if the client is able to evaluate situations and to decide upon a realistic course of action. For example, ask the client about future plans related to employment.
- The plans should reflect the reality of the client's health, psychological stability, and family situation and obligations. The client's responses should reflect an ability to think abstractly.

Impaired judgment can occur in emotional disturbances, schizophrenia, and neurologic dysfunction.

Source: Adapted from D'Amico, D., & Barbarito, C. (2007). *Health and physical assessment in nursing* (pp. 744–746). Upper Saddle River, NJ: Pearson Education.

Assessment Interview   Cognition

The following questions are helpful in gathering additional information. The nurse should preface these questions by explaining to the client that some of them may seem silly or unimportant, but they are helpful in assessing memory.

- What is your name?
- How old are you?
- Where were you born?
- Where are you right now?
- What day of the week is it? What is the date?
  Questions 1 through 5 determine whether the client is oriented to person, place, and time.
- What would you take with you if a fire broke out?
  This tests the client's ability to make a judgment.
- Count backward from 10 to 1.
  This question tests cognitive function.
- What did you have for breakfast?
  This question tests recent memory.
- Who were the last two presidents?
  This tests remote memory.
- Describe what the following statement means: People who live in glass houses shouldn't throw stones.
  This question tests the client's ability to do abstract or symbolic thinking.
- Are you having any problems thinking? If so, describe what happens.
  The client may not be able to answer this question if a thought disorder is present. Clients with bipolar disorders and who are manic describe their thoughts as "racing."
- Do you have trouble making decisions? Describe what happens when you have to make a decision.
  The inability to make decisions may indicate depression or low self-esteem.

- Do you ever hear voices, see objects, or experience other sensations that don't make sense? If so, describe your experiences.
  The client who is out of touch with reality may experience auditory, visual, gustatory, somatic, and olfactory hallucinations (hearing, seeing, tasting, feeling, and smelling stimuli that are not real). Discussing hallucinatory experiences in detail may reinforce them for the client; therefore, it is important not to dwell on these symptoms with the client.
- If you hear voices, do they tell you what you must do?
  The nurse asks this question to determine if the client is experiencing command hallucinations. These are dangerous hallucinations that may lead the client to self-destructive behavior or to harm others.
- Do you ever misinterpret objects, sounds, or smells? If so, please describe.
  Clients who are very anxious or out of contact with reality may experience illusions (misinterpretation of environmental stimuli).

It is important to assess the content of a client's hallucinations and delusions in order to provide for the client's safety and the safety of others. Command hallucinations tell clients to carry out acts against themselves or others that are usually harmful. These command hallucinations may be part of an elaborate delusional system in which clients feel persecuted or in danger. In some cases, clients are disturbed by these thoughts and share them with others. In other situations, clients keep their thoughts to themselves, and these thoughts do not become apparent until they commit some violent act. A client who demonstrates these symptoms should be referred to a psychiatric/mental health nurse or clinical specialist who has the skill and expertise needed to uncover hallucinatory and delusional thinking without exacerbating the symptoms.

---

experienced a dramatic life change. Typical changes that can result in depression include moving out of a lifelong home to a new environment and the loss of a spouse or family member. The Geriatric Depression Scale (GDS) is a screening instrument used in many clinical settings to assess depression in older people. The GDS is a 30-item (long version) or 15-item (short version) instrument with questions that can be answered "yes" or "no." An older person can complete the GDS alone by circling the correct answer, or have it read to him or her. When tested in various groups of older people, the GDS was found to distinguish successfully between depressed and nondepressed older people (Yesavage et al., 1983). The GDS can be used for screening physically healthy or ill individuals and those with cognitive impairment (Hartford Institute for Geriatric Nursing, 2008). Older people scoring above 10 should be referred for further assessment. The Cornell Depression Scale (CDS) can be used to screen for depression in older adults with severe cognitive impairments (MMSE below 15).

The Senses and Cognition

Clients who are out of contact with reality may display illusional, delusional, and hallucinatory speech and behaviors, such as talking to themselves (auditory hallucinations); reacting to objects, noises, or other people in strange ways

(illusions); or discussing false beliefs (delusions). Direct questioning may increase the client's anxiety and escalate the abnormal behavior or cause confusion. The nurse should use direct questioning only when the client appears to be in control and in touch with reality.

PHARMACOLOGIC THERAPIES

Pharmacologic treatment and research of chemicals to treat cognitive disorders are primarily aimed at reducing the effect of Alzheimer's disease, which is discussed in the Confusion exemplar. Though acetylcholinesterase inhibitors have been the mainstay in the treatment of Alzheimer's dementia, several other agents are being investigated for their possible benefit in delaying the progression of Alzheimer's, including anti-inflammatory agents, cyclooxygenase 2 (COX-2) inhibitors, estrogen, ginkgo biloba, and antioxidants. Agitation accompanying delusions, dementia, and delirium may be treated with antipsychotic agents, such as risperidone (Risperdal) and olanzapine (Zyprexa). Conventional antipsychotics such as haloperidol (Haldol) are occasionally prescribed, although extrapyramidal side effects often limit their use. Anxiety and depression, which may occur less frequently than agitation with delusions, dementia, and delirium, may be treated with anxiolytics, including buspirone (BuSpar) or some of the benzodiazepines, to control unease and apprehension. Mood stabilizers such as sertraline (Zoloft), citalopram (Celexa), or fluoxetine (Prozac) are given when major depression interferes with daily activities. Although Alzheimer's is the most common cause of dementia, there are other causes as well. A physician working with a client who exhibits dementia will likely conduct a number of tests to rule out other causes, and prescribe other or additional medications as necessary to address other or additional conditions that may cause dementia. One example is excess calcium, which has been found to cause lesions and narrow blood vessels in the brain. A physician may prescribe a calcium channel blocker in addition to acetylcholinesterase inhibitors for a client with dementia.

1.1 CONFUSION

KEY TERMS
Confusion, 15
Delirium, 15

BASIS FOR SELECTION OF EXEMPLAR
Standards of Nursing Practice
NCLEX®-RN

LEARNING OUTCOMES

1. Describe the pathophysiology, etiology, and clinical manifestations of confusion.
2. Identify risk factors associated with confusion.
3. Illustrate the nursing process in providing culturally competent and caring interventions across the life span for individuals with confusion.
4. Formulate priority nursing diagnoses appropriate for an individual with confusion.
5. Create a plan of caring interventions for an individual with confusion.
6. Employ evidence-based caring interventions (or prevention) for an individual with confusion.
7. Assess expected outcomes for an individual with confusion.
8. Discuss therapies used in the collaborative care of an individual with confusion.

OVERVIEW

Confusion is an alteration in cognition that makes it difficult to think clearly, focus attention, or make decisions. It may come on suddenly or gradually, depending on the cause. It can be a one-time event, recurrent, or a constant state of mind. The most important thing to understand about confusion is that it is frequently a symptom and not a diagnosis. Any number of things can cause confusion, including hypoxia, poor perfusion, medications, and disease. The onset of confusion requires thorough assessment to determine the causative agent and improve client outcomes.

Delirium is an acute disorder of cognition that affects functional independence. Confusion, a loss of orientation and memory, can occur in clients of all ages, but it is most commonly seen in older people. The terms *acute confusion* and delirium are used interchangeably by most health professionals, with nurses favoring the use of acute confusion and physicians the term delirium (McCurren & Cronin, 2003, p. 319). Confusion often presents with subtle symptoms, but an attempt should be made to differentiate between acute confusion (delirium) and chronic confusion (dementia) (Table 1–7).

PATHOPHYSIOLOGY AND ETIOLOGY

Delirium often has an abrupt onset; it can be reversed by treating its cause. This contrasts with dementia, often called chronic confusion, which has symptoms that are gradual and irreversible (e.g., Alzheimer's disease). Clients who are confused often know something is wrong and want help. It is important to pay special attention to sudden changes in mood or personality, as these may be signs of delirium related to recent changes in medication, onset of undetected illness, or exacerbation of chronic illness.

Age-related cognitive decline, resulting from slower information processing, mild memory impairment, and decreases in brain volume secondary to loss of some neurons place older clients at increased risk for confusion when they face additional stressors of illness, loss, or change in environment. Depression or other emotional problems can also act as stressors, increasing the likelihood of delirium. It is important to remember that delirium is usually caused by a treatable physical or mental health illness and, when treated typically results in full recovery. Delirium is associated with increased mortality, increased hospital costs, and long-term cognitive and functional impairment (Tullmann, Mion, Fletcher, & Foreman, 2008).

Etiology

Delirium occurs in 6–30% of the general hospital population and 7–52% of postsurgical clients (Edwards, 2003, p. 347). Delirium in the intensive care unit (ICU) setting is a common problem and has been described as sundown syndrome, ICU psychosis, and ICU syndrome. Delirium or acute confusional state, superimposed on Alzheimer's disease, was found in 8 of 20 older adults with documented dementia (Fick & Foreman, 2000). It is estimated that anywhere from 14–80% of all older persons hospitalized for the treatment of an acute physical illness experience an episode of delirium (Foreman, Wakefield, Culp, & Milisen, 2001). Unfortunately, delirium is unrecognized or misdiagnosed by both the physician and the nurse in up to two-thirds of cases (Hanley, 2004, p. 218).

It is not uncommon to think of older adults as the only people who become confused, but this is incorrect. Confusion can occur at any stage of the developmental process and may be caused by alcohol intoxication, low blood sugar, head trauma, fluid and/or

TABLE 1–7 Differentiating Between Delirium and Dementia

CHARACTERISTIC	DELIRIUM	DEMENTIA
Distinguishing feature	Acute, fluctuating change in mental status	Memory impairment
Onset	Sudden, acute	Slow, insidious
Duration	Temporary; may last hours to days	Chronic, gradual, irreversible
Time of day	Worsens at night	No change with time of day
Sleep-wake cycles	Disturbed; cycles often reversing	Disturbed; fragmented; frequent awakening during the night
Alertness	Fluctuating; may be alert and oriented during the day but becoming confused and disoriented at night	Generally normal
Thinking	Disorganized, distorted; impaired attention; alterations in memory	Judgment impaired; difficulty with abstraction and word finding
Delusions/hallucinations	May have visual, auditory, and tactile hallucinations; misinterpretation of real sensory experiences	Delusions; usually no hallucinations
Causative and risk factors	Cerebral and cardiovascular disease, infections, reduced hearing and vision, environmental change, stress, sleep deprivation, polypharmacy, dehydration	Alzheimer's disease; multiple infarct dementia

electrolyte imbalances, nutritional deficiencies, hypothermia, hypoxia, medications, sepsis, or sleep deprivation. In older adults, onset of illness may also cause mental confusion.

Risk Factors

Older adults are at risk for delirium, especially when hospitalized, because they often have other chronic medical problems (e.g., chronic obstructive pulmonary disease, hypertension, stroke). Many elders also take numerous medications with anticholinergic, narcotic, or sedative effects that increase the risk for delirium. Undertreating pain can contribute to the risk as well. Many older adults have vision or hearing loss, which makes it easy to misunderstand what they see or hear, further contributing to confusion. All of these risks plus the unfamiliar surroundings and routine of a hospital, possible sleep deprivation, stress, and sensory overload compound the older adult's risk for developing delirium.

Clinical Manifestations

Manifestations of confusion can range from very subtle symptoms, such as forgetting where one is or what one is doing, to acute loss of cognitive function. Clients may be unable to correctly answer questions related to time, place, person, or thing. They may become agitated, aggressive, fearful, anxious, or withdrawn. Symptoms may come on suddenly, or at specific times of the day. Sundown syndrome is manifested by confusion that occurs after sunset and usually resolves when the sun rises in the morning.

Features of delirium include fluctuations in alertness ranging from stuporous to hypervigilance. Clients are often inattentive, are easily distractible, have difficulty shifting attention from one focus to another, and often have difficulty keeping track of what is being said. They are disoriented to time and place but should not be disoriented to person. Memory testing reveals inability to recall recent events, instructions, names, events, activities, and current news. Thinking is disorganized and speech is often rambling, irrelevant, incoherent, unclear or showing an illogical flow of ideas. Confused clients will switch unpredictably from topic to topic and have difficulty expressing needs or concerns. Speech may be garbled. Severe delirium may include perceptual disturbances such as illusions and visual or auditory hallucinations and misperceptions that lead clients to call a stranger by a relative's name. Psychomotor activity may be hypoactive, hyperactive, or mixed subtypes (Tullmann et al., 2008).

NURSING PROCESS

The goal of nursing care is to reduce the incidence of delirium in the client at risk and prevent complications in the delirious client. Routine screening for delirium should be part of the comprehensive plan of care for the older adult or the client at risk. Delirium can be prevented by recognizing high-risk clients and implementing a standardized protocol (Tullmann et al., 2008).

Assessment

Older persons do not develop dementia overnight, so any sudden change in mental status needs to be aggressively evaluated. Delirium must be ruled out because cognitive impairment caused by delirium may be reversible. The development of delirium may indicate decreased reserve capacity of the brain and signal an increased risk for dementia (Alexopoulos, Silver, Kahn, Frances, & Carpenter, 2004). To rate delirium and distinguish delirium from other types of cognitive impairment, the Hartford Institute for Geriatric Nursing *Try This* Assessment Series recommends use of the Confusion Assessment Method (CAM) (Inouye et al., 1990) (Box 1–3). The CAM includes two parts: Part 1 is an assessment instrument that screens for overall cognitive impairment; Part 2 includes only those four features that distinguish delirium. The

Box 1–3 The Confusion Assessment Method for the Intensive Care Unit (CAM-ICU)

FEATURES AND DESCRIPTIONS	ABSENT	PRESENT

I. ACUTE ONSET OR FLUCTUATING COURSE*

A. Is there evidence of an acute change in mental status from the baseline?
B. Or, did the (abnormal) behavior fluctuate during the past 24 hours, that is, tend to come and go or increase and decrease in severity as evidenced by fluctuations on the Richmond Agitation Sedation Scale (RASS) or the Glasgow Coma Scale?

II. INATTENTION†

Did the patient have difficulty focusing attention as evidenced by a score of less than 8 correct answers on either the visual or auditory components of the Attention Screening Examination (ASE)?

III. DISORGANIZED THINKING

Is there evidence of disorganized or incoherent thinking as evidenced by incorrect answers to three or more of the 4 questions and inability to follow the commands?
Questions
  1. Will a stone float on water?
  2. Are there fish in the sea?
  3. Does 1 pound weigh more than 2 pounds?
  4. Can you use a hammer to pound a nail?
Questions and Commands
  1. Are you having unclear thinking?
  2. Hold up this many fingers. (Examiner holds 2 fingers in front of the patient.)
  3. Now do the same thing with the other hand (without holding the 2 fingers in front of the patient). (If the patient is already extubated from the ventilator, determine whether the patient's thinking is disorganized or incoherent, such as rambling or irrelevant conversation, unclear or illogical flow of ideas, or unpredictable switching from subject to subject.)

IV. ALTERED LEVEL OF CONSCIOUSNESS

Is the patient's level of consciousness anything other than alert, such as being vigilant or lethargic or in a stupor or coma?
Alert: spontaneously fully aware of environment and interacts appropriately
Vigilant: hyperalert
Lethargic: drowsy but easily aroused, unaware of some elements in the environment or not spontaneously interacting with the interviewer; becomes fully aware and appropriately interactive when prodded minimally
Stupor: difficult to arouse, unaware of some or all elements in the environment or not spontaneously interacting with the interviewer; becomes incompletely aware when prodded strongly; can be aroused only by vigorous and repeated stimuli and as soon as the stimulus ceases, stuporous subject lapses back into unresponsive state
Coma: unarousable, unaware of all elements in the environment with no spontaneous interaction or awareness of the interviewer so that the interview is impossible even with maximal prodding

Overall CAM-ICU Assessment (Features 1 and 2 and either Feature 3 or 4):	Yes____	No____

*The scores included in the 10-point RASS range from a high of 4 (combative) to a low of _5 (deeply comatose and unresponsive). Under the RASS system, patients who were spontaneously alert, calm, and not agitated were scored at 0 (neutral zone). Anxious or agitated patients received a range of scores depending on their level of anxiety: 1 for anxious, 2 for agitated (fighting ventilator), 3 for very agitated (pulling on or removing catheters), or 4 for combative (violent and a danger to staff). The scores _1 to _5 were assigned for patients with varying degrees of sedation based on their ability to maintain eye contact: _1 for more than 10 seconds, _2 for less than 10 seconds, and _3 for eye opening but no eye contact. If physical stimulation was required, then the patients were scored as either_4 for eye opening or movement with physical or painful stimulation or _5 for no response to physical or painful stimulation. The RASS has excellent interrater reliability and intraclass correlation coefficients of 0.95 and 0.97, respectively, and has been validated against visual analog scale and geropsychiatric diagnoses in 2 ICU studies.
†In completing the visual ASE, the patients were shown 5 simple pictures (previously published) at 3-second intervals and asked to remember them. They were then immediately shown 10 subsequent pictures and asked to nod "yes" or "no" to indicate whether they had or had not just seen each of the pictures. Since 5 pictures had been shown to them already, for which the correct response was to nod "yes," and 5 others were new, for which the correct response was to nod "no," patients scored perfectly if they achieved 10 correct responses. Scoring accounted for either errors of omission (indicating "no" for a previously shown picture) or for errors of commission (indicating "yes" for a picture not previously shown). In completing the auditory ASE, patients were asked to squeeze the rater's hand whenever they heard the letter A during the recitation of a series of 10 letters. The rater then read 10 letters from the following list in a normal tone at a rate of 1 letter per second: S, A, H, E, V, A, A, R, A, T. A scoring method similar to that of the visual ASE was used for the auditory ASE testing.

Source: The Confusion Assessment Method for the Intensive Care Unit (CAM-ICU). Ely, E. W., Inouye, S. K., Bernard, G. R., Gordon, S., Francis, J., May, L., Truman, B., Speroff, T., Gautam, S., Margolin, R., Hart, R. P., & Dittus, R. (2001). Delirium in mechanically ventilated patients: Validity and reliability of the confusion assessment method for the intensive care unit (CAM-ICU). JAMA, 286(21), 2703–2710. Table 1, p. 2705.

NURSING CARE PLAN A Client With Delirium

CASE STUDY

Mr. Dalton is a 75-year-old man who has been admitted to the hospital. He fell in his home and suffered a fractured left hip and had an open reduction with internal fixation this morning. When Mr. Dalton first arrived, he was quiet and pleasant but now he is agitated, attempting to get out of bed, yelling, and throwing his sheets on the floor. The nurse attempts to reason with him and reassure him, but he is not responding.

APPLYING THE NURSING PROCESS

Assessment

The nurse suspects Mr. Dalton is delirious because his symptoms had an acute onset. Delirium poses a common and serious problem in older patients with hip fracture. Systematic determination of an older person's mental status is of major importance for early recognition and treatment of delirium. The nurse knows that delirium can be caused by any of the following factors:

- Infection
- Medications (antihistamines, anticholinergics, benzodiazepines)

- Anesthesia
- Electrolyte imbalance
- Pain
- Sleep disturbance
- Underlying dementia (diagnosed or undiagnosed)

A complete assessment of each of these factors using standardized assessment instruments is indicated while the older person is protected from injury.

Diagnosis

Nursing diagnoses that may be appropriate for Mr. Dalton include the following:

- *Acute Confusion*
- *Previously Altered Thought Processes* (if previously diagnosed with cognitive impairment)
- *Risk for Imbalanced Fluid Volume* (overhydration or dehydration)
- *Risk for Injury* (due to falls)

- *Impaired Verbal Communication*
- *Impaired Physical Mobility*
- *Delayed Surgical Recovery*
- *Acute Pain*
- *Anxiety*
- *Fear*

Expected Outcomes

The expected outcomes for the plan of care specify that Mr. Dalton will

- be free from injury.
- begin to exhibit resolution of his symptoms of delirium.
- experience correction of the underlying mechanisms causing his delirium.

- receive consultation, assessment, and treatment from appropriate members of the interdisciplinary team, including physicians, nurses, physical therapists, dietitians, social workers, and others as appropriate to resolve and improve his delirium.

Planning and Implementation

The following nursing interventions may be appropriate for Mr. Dalton:

- Establish a therapeutic relationship by being present and using gentle touch and a soft voice for communication.
- Review all current medications.
- Evaluate basic laboratory studies (complete blood count, serum electrolytes, and urinalysis).
- Provide supportive and restorative care.
- Treat behavioral symptoms.
- Correct sensory deficits (place glasses and hearing aids if used by the older person).

- In consultation with the physician, consider further testing as appropriate that may include chest radiology, blood culture, drug levels, serum B12, thyroid function tests, pulse oximetry, electrocardiogram, brain imaging, lumbar puncture, or electroencephalogram.
- Administer medications as ordered by the physician (haloperidol 0.5–2.0 mg or lorazepam 0.5 to 2.0 mg by mouth every 4–6 hours).
- Reassure, educate, and involve family.
- Maintain a quiet and peaceful environment to decrease noise stimuli to the extent possible.

Evaluation

The nurse will consider the plan a success based on the following criteria:

- Mr. Dalton will return to normal cognitive and physical function.

- He will be free from injury.
- He will cooperate with a rehabilitation program and be discharged to home or a rehabilitation facility (as appropriate).

NURSING CARE PLAN   A Client With Delirium (continued)

ETHICAL DILEMMA

Mr. Dalton's daughter requests that he be restrained to prevent falls. She has seen older persons with waist restraints and feels the use of this device will keep her father safe from injury. The nurse wishes to be responsive to the daughter's request, but professional standards indicate that restraints can worsen delirium and injure the older person. The ethical dilemma involves threats to the older person's and surrogate's autonomy versus nonmaleficence or the desire to do no harm. The nurse should educate and inform the daughter regarding the risks of entrapment and strangulation that accompany the use of restraints. Agitation and anxiety can be exacerbated as the older person fights to free himself from the restraints, and larger doses of medication may be needed to reduce symptoms. Physical restraints should be used cautiously (if at all) and only as a last resort. Additionally, a delirious physically restrained older person will need constant observation to prevent injury, entrapment, and strangulation.

Critical Thinking and the Nursing Process

1. How would you explain the diagnosis of Alzheimer's disease to a family?
2. What resources are available in your community or professional setting to assist older persons and their families caring for a loved one with dementia?
3. Identify three major changes you would like to see implemented in your clinical agency that would facilitate the care of older persons with dementia.
4. Caring for older persons with cognitive impairments (dementia and delirium) can be stressful for nurses and other health care providers. What types of support services and resources in the clinical setting would assist you to provide the highest quality care to older persons with cognitive impairments?

tool can be administered in less than 5 minutes. It closely correlates with DSM-IV criteria for delirium. See the Best Practices feature: The Confusion Assessment Method for the Intensive Care Unit (CAM-ICU). When the older client's cognitive status appears to be impaired, the nurse should request the client's permission to include a family member or caregiver in the assessment to supplement and verify the information the patient reports.

Because of the role depression can play in increasing the risk for delirium, it is important to screen the older adult. The GDS and the CDS can be used to screen for depression in older clients as previously described.

The client should be assessed for risk factors including baseline cognitive function, medication history, and environment. The nurse looks for manifestations of pain, metabolic disturbances, dehydration, infection, or impaired mobility that can contribute to the development of confusion. The nurse should assess for evidence of delirium at least every 8 hours (Tullmann et al., 2008).

Diagnosis

Nursing diagnoses are individualized based on client needs and cause of confusion, but may include the following:

- Insomnia
- Disturbed Sleep Patterns
- Self-care Deficit
- Acute or Chronic Confusion
- Wandering
- Impaired Memory
- Impaired Verbal Communication
- Caregiver Role Strain

Planning

Nursing care is planned based on client needs and must consider factors such as safety, support systems, and ability to provide self-care. Potential outcomes may include the following:

- Absence of confusion
- Cognitive status returned to baseline
- Discharged to same destination as prehospitalization
- Able to perform activities of daily living

Implementation

The nurse must provide a therapeutic environment for the confused client. Interventions include fostering orientation by frequently reassuring and reorienting the client through the use of calendars, clocks, caregiver identification, explanation of all activities, and clear communication. Appropriate sensory stimulation is provided by reducing noise, maintaining adequate lighting, and performing one task at a time. The nurse helps the client to obtain adequate sleep, maximize mobility, and create an environment that contains familiar objects from home. Family and friends should be encouraged to stay at the bedside, and consistency of caregivers is optimum. The nurse should communicate clearly, provide simple explanations,

Box 1–4 Promoting a Therapeutic Environment for a Client With Acute Confusion/Delirium

- Wear a readable name tag.
- Address the person by name and introduce yourself frequently: "Good morning, Mr. Richards. I am Betty Brown. I will be your nurse today."
- Identify time and place as indicated: "Today is December 5, and it is 8:00 in the morning."
- Ask the client, "Where are you?" and orient the client to place (e.g., nursing home) if indicated.
- Place a calendar and clock in the client's room. Mark holidays with ribbons, pins, or other means.
- Speak clearly and calmly to the client, allowing time for your words to be processed and for the client to respond.
- Encourage family to visit frequently unless this activity causes the client to become hyperactive.
- Provide clear, concise explanations of each treatment procedure or task.
- Eliminate unnecessary noise.
- Reinforce reality by interpreting unfamiliar sounds, sights, and smells; correct any misconceptions of events or situations.
- Schedule activities (e.g., meals, bath, activity and rest periods, treatments) at the same time each day to provide a sense of security. If possible, assign the same caregivers.
- Provide adequate sleep.
- Keep glasses and hearing aid within reach.
- Ensure adequate pain management.
- Keep familiar items in the client's environment (e.g., photographs), and keep the environment uncluttered. A disorganized, cluttered environment increases confusion.
- Keep room well lit during waking hours.

reassure and educate the family, and minimize invasive procedures. Pharmacological interventions for confusion should be the last resort and used only when all other measures have proven ineffective (Tullmann et al., 2008). Box 1–4 lists nursing interventions to help promote a therapeutic environment for the client with acute confusion/delirium.

Evaluation

Clients are evaluated based on ability to meet outcomes; the nursing plan of care is adapted as indicated. In addition to evaluating client outcomes, a decrease in the occurrence of delirium should become a measure of the quality of care delivered by all facilities that care for older adults.

REVIEW   Confusion

RELATE: LINK THE CONCEPTS

Linking the concepts of Accountability, Advocacy, Ethics, and Safety with the concept of Cognition:

1. What special responsibilities is the nurse accountable for when caring for a client who is confused?
2. How does the nurse advocate for the confused client?
3. The nurse is caring for a client who is confused and displaying trouble with decision making. If the client declines a treatment essential to obtaining a positive outcome for the client, considering the client's bill of rights, what is the nurse's ethical obligation?
4. What interventions are important for the nurse to initiate in order to maintain safety for the confused client?

READY: GO TO COMPANION SKILLS MANUAL

1. Applying body mechanics
2. Assisting the client with ambulation
3. Assessing appearance and mental status
4. Assessing the neurologic system
5. Bathing an adult client
6. Administering medication
7. Evaluating client safety

REFLECT: CASE STUDY

Clifford is a 64-year-old male who has been married to his wife, Pam, for 40 years. Their only child, 24-year-old Gary, has Down syndrome and lives with them. Clifford is a middle manager for a small manufacturing company where he has worked over the last 20 years.

Overall, Clifford is in good health, although he has recently been undergoing conservative treatment for benign prostate hypertrophy. He has a history of depression. He had a brief episode during college, for which he did not seek treatment. He had another episode shortly after Gary was born, and at the encouragement of his wife, he sought treatment, which consisted of counseling and antidepressant agents. He quit taking the medications after about 6 months and decided he would just learn to deal with depression on his own. Although he has had mild episodes of depression over the years since that time, Clifford has been unwilling to seek

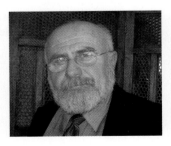

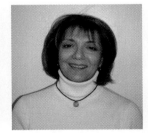

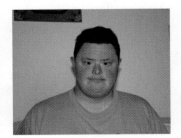

CLIENT TEACHING   Using the Assimilation Process

Whatever the client's cultural background, use the assimilation process to help the client learn a new skill that will be needed at home:

- Introduce a new skill by having the client observe as it is demonstrated.
- Explain each step of using the new skill.
- Have the client perform the new skill while the nurse observes and helps.

- Have the client practice the new skill to improve his or her performance.
- Have the client perform the skill at home without assistance from a nurse.
- When the skill has been assimilated, the client can perform it at home without having to think about how to do it.

help clients learn new skills, see the Client Teaching feature.) **Acculturation** is the process of not only adapting to another culture but also accepting the majority group's culture as one's own. Language, customs, religious practices, or traditions can be adapted from one culture to another. Because culture is complex, members of a cultural group may engage in many behaviors and habits unconsciously, making them difficult to explain to others.

Sometimes, smaller cultural groups within a larger society maintain their customs and other cultural traits. **Subculture groups** are minority groups characterized by specific norms, beliefs, and values that coexist with a dominant culture. The members of a subculture group may share distinct dress, rituals, or language. Examples of subculture groups are street gangs, mountain folk, and pop-group followers (e.g., "Dead Heads").

MULTICULTURALISM **Multiculturalism** is defined as many subcultures coexisting within a given society in which no one culture dominates. In a multicultural society, human differences are accepted by most people, leading to a desire to overcome racism, sexism, and other forms of discrimination (Multiculturalism Definitions, 2008). Classrooms in these communities are culturally diverse, and students have different levels of socialization and learning styles.

In the United States, one driver of multiculturalism has been immigration. People from nearly every country in the world have come to the United States in search of a new way of life. Many, such as the Hmong people immigrating from Asia, sought freedom from an oppressive government. Others sought religious freedom, and still others freedom from poverty. Each family or group of immigrants brings its own culture with it, adding to what has been called the "melting pot" that is the United States. The ideal of the melting pot is the assimilation of multiple ethnic groups with their cultural practices into an American national identity with national allegiance and values.

Typically, families and groups from the same country will relocate to a specific area or neighborhood, which helps them to maintain their native language, traditions, and ways of worship. These **ethnic groups** have common racial characteristics—for example, nationality, language, values, and customs—and they share a cultural heritage. Examples of ethnic groups are the large Cuban-American population living in and around Miami, Florida; the Lakota Sioux, one of three major ethnic groups that

make up the Great Sioux Nation; and the Hmong populations living in western North Carolina.

Immigrant groups often maintain use of their native language in their homes and places of worship for several generations. Children may speak their native language in the home and English at school, and families retain ties to their country of origin and continue native cultural practices. As these families have children and grandchildren, however, customs such as food preparation and eating habits, dress, and celebration of holidays survive, but other cultural traditions become lost as the descendants of the original immigrants assimilate further into American culture. Today, the multiple cultures in the United States may be better described as "a tossed salad"— each group intermingles with other cultures but maintains its own separate identity and cultural heritage. These differences can impact how individuals and families interact with health care providers and other professionals. Nurses working in areas with people of many cultures must be careful to respect each client's culture.

RACE **Race** refers to socially defined populations that have in common genetically transmitted physical characteristics, such as skin color, bone structure, and other genetic traits. Today, the U.S. Bureau of the Census recognizes six categories of race: Native American, African American, Asian American, Native Hawaiians or Other Pacific Islanders, White (European American), and Some Other Race (available to people who do not think they belong in the other race categories). The Census Bureau asks questions to determine Hispanic/Latino status separate from race.

STEREOTYPING **Stereotyping** refers to generalizing that all individuals in a group are the same. Stereotyping does help to provide a frame of reference regarding people from other cultures, but it also can lead to misunderstandings and miscommunication. One example is the still pervasive tendency that Americans have to group all Asian Americans together despite the many countries that they represent and the fact that many Asian-American families have been U.S. citizens for several generations (for more information on this tendency, see the Asian-Nation Web site at http://www.asian-nation.org).

Use of stereotypes also can have grave, long-standing effects on the people of a culture or an ethnic group. Nowhere is this more clear than in the effects of segregation in the American South. Segregation and racial prejudices

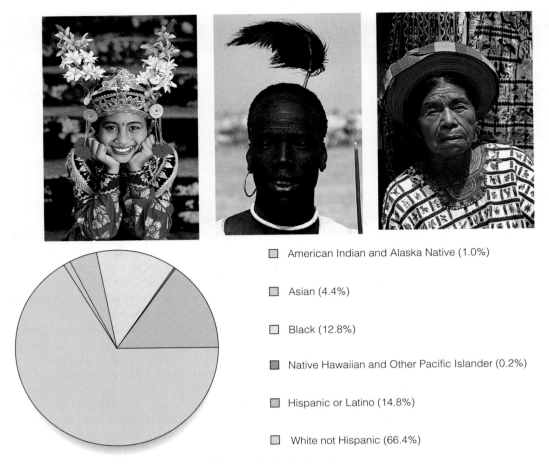

American Indian and Alaska Native (1.0%)

Asian (4.4%)

Black (12.8%)

Native Hawaiian and Other Pacific Islander (0.2%)

Hispanic or Latino (14.8%)

White not Hispanic (66.4%)

Figure 2–1 ■ Different cultural heritages are parts of the population in America.

Source: Graph from U.S. Bureau of the Census. (2007). State & County QuickFacts. Retrieved from http://quickfacts.census.gov/qfd/states/00000.html; Steve Vidler/SuperStock; Robert Caputo/Stock Boston; Arvind Garg/Getty Images, Inc.—Liaison.

have contributed to a general lack of trust and apprehension among some African Americans in the South related to accepting and following medical recommendations (Betancourt & Ananeh-Firemping, 2004). While less prevalent today, it remains a factor in how some African Americans view working with health care professionals. Regardless of the reason why a client may be reluctant to follow treatment recommendations, the best way the nurse can address this reluctance is by building a relationship of respect and trust. Often, respectful communication and a sincere desire for the client's health and well-being can overcome any cultural misunderstandings.

Culture in the United States

According to the U.S. Census (2007) Bureau, the estimated population of United States in 2006 was 299,398,484. In addition to the six races defined by the Census Bureau and the ethnicity known as Hispanic/Latino, there are an uncountable number of cultures, subcultures, and ethnic groups. Some of these are easily defined, but many are not. Children whose parents come from different cultures may not identify with either parent's culture (Figure 2–1 ■).

The culture of the United States is Western, and Western culture often is associated with economic liberalization (free trade), democratization (or representative government), and scientific advancement (technology and gadgets). As a result of large numbers of immigrants arriving from many countries throughout this country's history, the culture of the United States also is multicultural. These various cultures are represented by numerous professional, ethnic, religious, recreational, demographic, or social groups with which individuals may identify or to which they may belong. Some examples are the National Association for the Advancement of Colored People (NAACP), a civil rights organization; the American Irish Historical Society, a cultural organization; and the National Association of Hispanic Nurses, a professional organization.

Within the United States, the federal government as well as state and local governments have instituted any number of policies supporting this multicultural population. Some of these government multicultural policies (modified from Multiculturalism, 2004) are as follows:

- Acceptance of multiple citizenship
- Support for minority holidays and celebrations
- Support for music and arts from minority cultures
- Acceptance of traditional and religious dress in schools and public places (Figure 2–2 ■)
- Encouragement of minority representation in education, politics, and the workforce

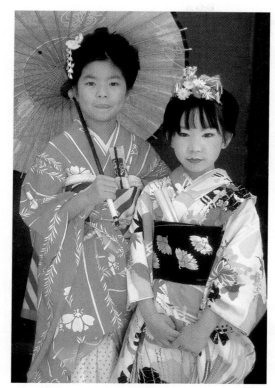

Figure 2–2 ■ Subcultures can maintain heritage and identity through dress, foods eaten, and daily activities.

Government at the federal, state, and local levels supports education. The primary unofficial language is American English, although government agencies frequently offer programs and print publications in other languages. Many religions are practiced, including Protestant Christianity, Catholicism, Judaism,

Hinduism, Islam, and Buddhism. **Religion** refers to a set of doctrines accepted by a group of people who gather together regularly to worship that offer a means to relate to God or a higher power, nature, and their spiritual being. Religion plays a greater role in some communities than in others: One town may sponsor a living nativity at Christmas, while the next may ban religious spectacles on government property altogether. Family arrangements in the United States are exceedingly diverse, including the nuclear family, single-parent families, childless couples, and blended families (Figures 2–3 ■ and 2–4 ■).

Influenced by many of the cultures within its borders, American culture includes a few general values and attitudes toward social behaviors (Essortment, 2008):

- Importance placed on punctuality and time sensitivity
- Distaste for pushiness, condescension, and bullying
- Intolerance of line jumping or not waiting one's turn
- Acceptance of casual and formal attire at the same events
- Liberation of women (feminism)
- Acceptance of political discussions (if not specific)
- Appreciation of efficiency at work and in social situations

CULTURAL DIFFERENCES
Variations in Social Behavior

People learn the social behaviors practiced in their cultures. These behaviors differ from culture to culture, which can present challenges when cultures interact. Some common social behavioral variations among people of different cultures involve communication, environmental control, hygiene, space, time, and social organization.

COMMUNICATION Each culture may speak a different language or a variation of another language. The meaning of words can differ among various groups of people, and misunderstandings may result from lack of common communication.

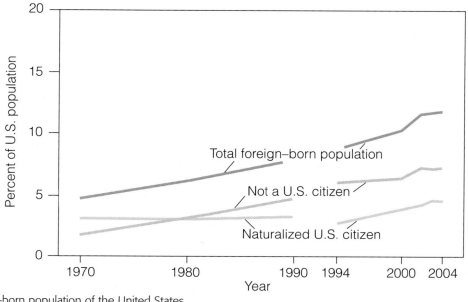

Figure 2–3 ■ Foreign-born population of the United States.

Source: Centers for Disease Control and Prevention. U. S. Census Bureau.

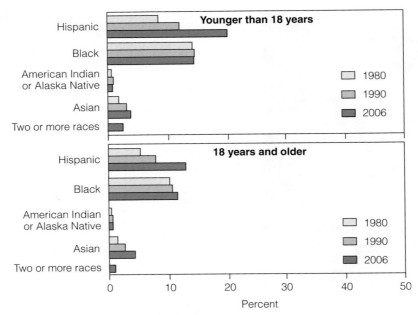

Figure 2–4 ■ Population of the United States by race and ethnicity.

Source: Centers for Disease Control and Prevention, National Center for Health Statistics. (2006). Health, United States, 2006, Figure 3. Data from U.S. Bureau of the Census.

Misinterpretation of nonverbal communication also may lead to problems. For example, direct eye contact may show disrespect in some cultures and be a sign of interest and active listening in others.

ENVIRONMENTAL CONTROL An individual's relationship to nature varies among cultures. Different health practices, values, and experiences with illness also are found.

HYGIENE Cleanliness practices vary among cultures. For example, body odors and the way people respond to them are different among various societies. Cultural practices determine whether body odors are disguised, ignored, or enhanced.

SPACE Culture defines a person's perception of personal space. Comfort can result from honoring the boundaries of personal space, whereas anxiety can result when these boundaries are not followed. Practices regarding proximity to others, body movements, and touch differ among cultures.

TIME The concepts of time, duration of time, and points in time vary among cultures. Past-oriented cultures, for example, value tradition. Individuals from cultures that closely follow tradition may not be receptive to new procedures or treatments. Present-oriented cultures focus on the here and now, and individuals from these cultures may not be receptive to preventive health care measures. Some cultures have no focus on time, and individuals from these cultures may miss appointments or be late.

SOCIAL ORGANIZATION Societies are influenced by many factors, such as religion, sexual orientation, socioeconomic status, gender, age, and geography, and life-cycle factors relative to families and individuals differ among cultures. The role of older adults, the head of the household, and men and women in the society may determine the behaviors of these individuals.

Disparities in Health Care

In 2002, the Institute of Medicine (IOM) released a report on disparities in the United States regarding the types and quality of health services that racial and ethnic minorities receive. The IOM report explored factors that might contribute to inequities in care and contained recommended policies and practices to eliminate these inequities.

The IOM found significant variation in the rates of medical procedures by race even when income, age, and severity of conditions were comparable. This research indicates that U.S. racial and ethnic minorities are less likely to receive medical care, and when they do, receive lower quality of services (Figures 2–5 ■ and 2–6 ■). Nurses should be alert to practices (formal and informal) in their work environment that impact the quality of care offered to individuals of any ethnic group and should work to ensure quality care and provision of best practice methods to all clients.

The recommendations for reducing these disparities in health care include increasing awareness of them among the public, health care providers, insurance companies, and policy makers. More minority health care providers are needed in underserved communities, and more interpreters are needed in clinics and hospitals to improve the quality of care. The IOM report suggests educating health care professionals to increase their cultural competence with different populations and inform them of how discrimination and racism affect the

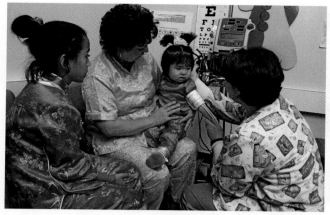

Figure 2–5 ■ Although much has been done to improve the quality of health services received by American cultural and ethnic minorities, these services are still in need of continued reform.

provision of health care. Including information about health care disparities in the curriculum is one way to educate nurses early in their careers (IOM, 2002).

PHYSICAL ASSESSMENT

Cultural differences can affect the physical assessment in several ways. Biological variations in cultural groups are the simplest and most obvious differences that nurses will deal with in their professional careers. Differences in values, beliefs, and religions can be more challenging, however, and often require nurses to go the extra mile to ask the right questions to obtain very important information regarding a client's health and perceptions of Western medicine.

Differences in Values and Beliefs

The assessment process includes asking questions about mental status and psychological disorders. The beliefs and values of a culture define normal and abnormal behaviors and thinking processes, so the client's culture may view mental status and psychological disorders as having psychological, physical, social, spiritual, or emotional origins. Learning about cultural expectations of behaviors and ways of thinking helps nurses to understand the client's mental status.

Cultures may explain mental problems in different ways. People from some cultures may believe that those with mental problems need to be avoided because of mystical, magical, or evil powers. Some cultures believe mental problems are punishments for sins or wrong deeds done in this life or, as sometimes is the case among Indian and Asian populations that practice Hinduism, a previous life. Culturally sensitive nurses ask questions to determine how family members and others from the client's culture may view someone with a mental illness.

Biological Variations

People differ genetically and physiologically. These biological variations among individuals, families, and races produce differences in susceptibility and response to various diseases among people of different cultures and all walks of life (Figure 2–7 ■).

SUSCEPTIBILITY TO DISEASE Certain ethnic groups or races may tend toward developing specific diseases. African Americans, for example, have a higher incidence of hypertension and sickle cell anemia. Cardiovascular disease is the number-one killer of American women, and African-American women are at greater risk from this disease compared to women from any other ethnic group (Centers for Disease Control and Prevention, 2009). Native Americans have a higher incidence of tuberculosis. Sometimes, however,

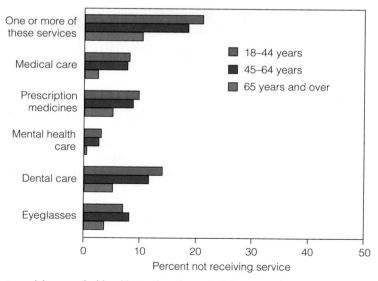

Figure 2–6 ■ Percentage not receiving needed health services because of cost, 2005.

Source: Centers for Disease Control and Prevention, National Center for Health Statistics, Health, United States, 2007, Figure 21. Data from National Health Interview Survey.

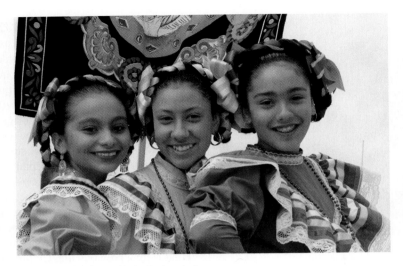

Figure 2–7 ■ Those of different cultures also have biological variations.

Source: Skjold Photographs.

an individual's susceptibility to disease is not so obvious but may be discerned as a nurse takes a health history, including the health of any parents, grandparents, and siblings.

GROWTH AND DEVELOPMENT   Average adult size, growth rate, and shape vary among individuals because of genetic and environmental factors. Nutritional status influences growth as well: Children with inadequate diets may have slowed development.

LABORATORY VALUES   Japanese Americans, Hispanic Americans, and Native Americans usually have higher blood glucose levels than the general population.

NUTRITION   All cultural groups have food preferences, and these preferences often can be an indicator or even the cause of a health issue. Cultures in which sugar cane is a major crop (e.g., Latin America and the Philippines) have an increased incidence of diabetes mellitus. Regional food preferences also can endanger the health of populations already susceptible to

a disease. African-American women in the southern United States, for example, should avoid some of the traditional foods of that region, including fried chicken and fish and greens cooked in lard or pork fat, which increase their risk of heart disease.

SKELETAL FRAME   Even skeletons show differences in racial and ethnic backgrounds. Native Americans have an increased incidence of back problems. African-American and white men usually are taller than Asian-American and Mexican-American men. Small-framed white women of European descent are predisposed to osteoporosis.

SKIN COLOR   This most obvious difference among individuals has important implications for health care providers. Darker skin tones require closer inspection to observe changes (as when assessing for changes in oxygenation). African Americans and Native Americans have lower incidences of skin cancer because of higher levels of melanin.

2.1 VALUES AND BELIEFS

KEY TERMS

Belief system, *31*
Cultural competence, *33*
Cultural values, *31*
World view, *31*

LEARNING OUTCOMES

After learning about this exemplar, you will be able to do the following:
1. Describe the role of belief systems in the development of culture.
2. Discuss common rules reflecting basic values found in many cultures.
3. Identify ways in which religion influences cultural beliefs and behaviors.
4. Relate characteristics of culture by observing behaviors within a culture.

OVERVIEW

Culture includes a society's values, beliefs, assumptions, principles, myths, legends, and norms. People use these to help them define meaning, identify acceptable behaviors, choose emotional reactions, and determine appropriate actions in given

situations. Values and belief systems are part of a culture, as are family relationships and roles (Figure 2–8 ■). To understand client behaviors better, the nurse must identify which cultures are present demographically in a given area, learn more about those cultures by reading or attending a class about them, and apply that knowledge and experiences in providing client care.

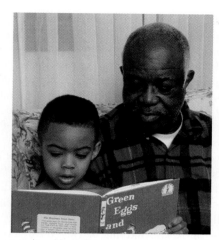

Figure 2–8 ■ Cultural beliefs and practices include family relationships and roles.

Values reflect an underlying system of beliefs. **Cultural values** describe preferred ways of behaving or thinking that are sustained over time and used to govern a cultural group's actions and decisions. When people live together in a society, cultural values determine the rules they live by each and every day. These rules may be variously stated, but they basically address the same values. Examples of these rules include the following:

■ Don't steal from others.
■ Respect other people's property.
■ Don't hurt people in your own culture.
■ Don't take another's mate.
■ Share your food and clothing with those who are in need.
■ Speak truthfully based on what you see.
■ Respect your elders for their wisdom and experience.
■ Respect God or a higher power.
■ Respect nature and your environment.

Characteristics of culture include observable behaviors as well as the unseen values that influence those behaviors. Cultural practices have meaning that gives the group its world view and that reflects the social organization of the culture as a whole. The organization of a culture or society includes the following elements:

■ A physical element: the geographic area in which the society is located
■ An infrastructure element: the framework of the systems and processes that keep the society functioning
■ A behavioral element: the way people in the society act and react to each other
■ A cultural element: all the values, beliefs, assumptions, and norms that comprise a code of conduct for acceptable behaviors within the society

Each culture has its own world view or understanding of the world. A **world view** refers to how the people in a culture perceive ideas and attitudes about the world, other people, and life in general.

A culture's world view supports its overall **belief system**, which is developed to explain the mysteries of the universe and of life that each society tries to understand (Figure 2–9 ■). What is the meaning of life? How do individuals know their purpose in life? What is reality? How much can be known about values and beliefs? Some world-view questions concern God or a higher power. Is there a God? How was the universe created? What happens after death? A culture's belief systems influence an individual's decisions and actions in society regarding everything from the preparation of food to rituals of death and burial (for an example, see the Focus on Diversity and Culture feature that follows). Scientific and medical advancements may or may not impact a culture's belief systems.

Beliefs systems differ in every culture. The beliefs of a society are passed from generation to generation by word of mouth. As cultures interact with other cultures and assimilate, some cultural beliefs become lost, some are kept, and others adapt to incorporate parts of other cultures.

Children learn the belief system of their culture from parents and other family members who teach them any number of values and beliefs, including those about what is "right or wrong." Multicultural societies like the that of the United States have a mix of traditional moral basics. The differences may originate from religious beliefs or social conditions. People make decisions about "right or wrong," and as things change, people adapt and the culture evolves.

Belief systems are based on people's experiences of the world. As people's knowledge and understanding grow, their belief systems expand. Knowing why we believe what we believe builds self-awareness and understanding of differences in our own beliefs compared with the beliefs of others.

One way people develop beliefs is by analyzing and critically thinking about causation. How does one thing cause

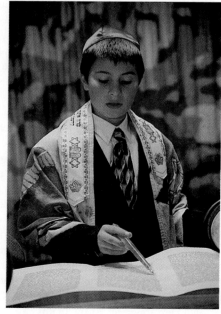

Figure 2–9 ■ Cultures try to understand and give meaning to life through spiritual beliefs, social values, and acceptable behaviors.

FOCUS ON DIVERSITY AND CULTURE
The Peoplehood Model

An example of cultures having distinct beliefs and practices can be found with Native American tribes. Each tribe has a distinct language, territory, specific ceremonial cycles, and sacred history that tells how it came into existence and incorporates expected interactions with the environment, ceremony guidelines, and expected behaviors with others within the community. Figure 2–10 ■ shows Tom Holm's Peoplehood Model, in which the four factors overlap and interact with each other (Cornsilk and Blythe, 2008).

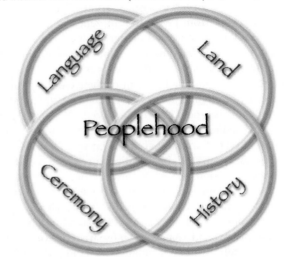

Figure 2–11 ■ The Peoplehood model of Native Americans.

Source: Cornsilk, C., & Blythe, F. (Executive Producers). (2006, November). *Indian country diaries.* Peoplehood. New York and Washington, DC: Public Broadcasting Service. Retrieved from http://www.pbs.org/indiancountry.

another? This is logical thinking and rational problem solving. The skills of evidence-based believing develop as individuals mature and learn. Events are measurable, and facts are supported by scientific studies.

Another method of developing beliefs is by adopting traditional beliefs. Family and cultural traditions influence our belief systems through family bias, societal prejudices, and social culture. These beliefs are passed on through generations and often are accepted without questions. What was necessary in an earlier generation may no longer be useful for later generations but still be retained because of tradition (Figure 2–11 ■).

How might generations continue a practice based on tradition rather than necessity? Consider a certain family that always cut roasts in half before cooking the meat. The third-generation daughter said she did it because she thought it made the meat more tender. The second generation woman (the daughter's mother) said she had learned it from her own mom, and she thought it was done to reduce cooking time and save energy. And the first-generation woman (the daughter's grandmother) said the oven she had when she was raising her family was very small, so she always had to cut the roast in half to fit inside (Inspired Personal Development, 2007). In this case, the practice of cutting the roast in half was based on a tradition passed down through the years rather than on the size of the family oven.

Beliefs can be adopted from people who have authority in our lives. In addition to giving us traditional beliefs, parents play an early role of authority. Other people in authority roles include teachers, religious leaders, doctors, or charismatic people.

Clubs, gangs, and groups have common beliefs that are integrated into the members' belief systems. Members adopt the identity of the group through mutual influence of values and beliefs. Personal attitudes become reflections of the group, giving beliefs by association.

Another influence on beliefs is enlightenment or revelation. Enlightenment may come from the experience of "a gut feeling" or from intuition. This inspiration is not predictable and may give us insight (Inspired Personal Development, 2007).

Culturally based beliefs and traditions can affect the course and outcome of disease and illness. Health care providers and clients bring their respective cultural backgrounds and expectations to a medical interview. Their cultural differences can present barriers to necessary care. Some areas in which barriers can arise include the following:

- The importance of family in managing illness and disease
- The belief that illnesses are not always strictly a biological problem
- Cultural assumptions about disease and illness that may influence the presentation of symptoms or the response to treatments
- Failure of clients to see a pattern of repeated illness as a chronic condition rather than their symptoms as unrelated occurrences
- Cultural beliefs that discussing prognosis and risks with clients can influence outcomes or be dangerous

While cultural beliefs and behaviors change over the years as a cultural group adapts to new ideas and conditions, some individuals may retain traditional behaviors and thinking and continue to follow the beliefs and practices as always. Tension may increase when different health belief systems conflict with each other. The result may be anxiety, anger, or fear. The health care provider's cultural sensitivity may reduce this discomfort by showing a nonjudgmental attitude of respect.

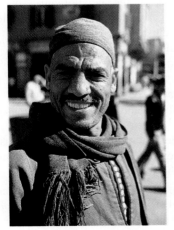

Figure 2–11 ■ Cultural beliefs are passed on through generations as traditions.

Source: Frank Siteman/Photolibrary.com.

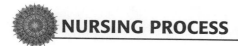

NURSING PROCESS

Assessment

During the initial assessment interview with clients and their families, include focused questions to identify cultural behaviors, health beliefs, illness practices, and cultural needs. This information can be used in planning culturally sensitive care. A helping relationship with clients and families involves spending time with them, building trust, and showing a desire to better understand their values and beliefs.

Assessment questions may include the following areas:

- Does the client follow culturally specific traditions? If so, how closely? Where does the client see himself or herself on a heritage continuum ranging from strict devotion to a mix of cultural influences? To what extent has the client been socialized to an American lifestyle?
- Are there specific practices regarding types of foods eaten or not eaten? How are foods prepared? At what times are meals scheduled?
- Are unique customs followed in the home that the client needs to maintain while he or she is away? Are there specific times for these practices?
- What does the family consist of for the client? What members of the family stay in the home with the client? How will family members participate in the client's care?
- Does the client speak and understand the English language? Is another language spoken in the home?

Physical cues can guide a nurse in choosing assessment questions. For example, consider the following:

- *Clothing.* If a client is wearing clothes that are traditional in his or her native land, the nurse may want to ask additional questions to identify cultural practices impacting health care.
- *Adult family members present for the assessment.* This signals an increased possibility for family involvement in decision making related to health care practices
- *Young children present for an assessment of their mother.* This may indicate the family lacks sufficient supports for the mother to come alone, and it may prompt the nurse to ask questions related to self-care and caregiver role strain. This can be true among families regardless of cultural background.

When clients speak languages other than English or are not proficient in English, minimal assessment information from clients can be obtained with the following questions:

- What language do you speak? Do you speak any English?
- How long have you lived here?
- What do you think caused your problem?
- When did it start?
- Why do you think it started when it did?
- What does your sickness do to you?
- How severe is your sickness?
- What do you fear about your sickness?
- What kind of treatment do you think you need?
- Are there any religious practices we need to know about?
- Who is your family?
- Who makes decisions most of the time?
- Who can you go to for help when you need it?

Diagnosis

No NANDA nursing diagnoses exclusively address culture. However, differences in cultural behaviors, beliefs, and values could potentially cause clients many problems. Cultural misunderstandings or miscommunications also may occur result from different perceptions of health and of the illness diagnosed. The following are examples of NANDA nursing diagnoses that may be appropriate for clients of different cultures (depending on individual situations):

- Powerlessness
- Spiritual Distress
- Risk for Impaired Religiosity
- Disturbed Thought Processes
- Fear
- Decisional Conflict
- Noncompliance
- Anxiety
- Ineffective Health Maintenance
- Ineffective Coping
- Acute Pain
- Impaired Social Interaction

Planning

DEVELOPING CULTURAL COMPETENCE Nurses provide care to individuals from many different cultures. To be culturally sensitive, nurses must have cultural information and be able to apply this knowledge to improve the quality of their nursing care. Nurses need to avoid stereotyping and personal bias, which may raise barriers to culturally sensitive behaviors. Nurses need to understand their own world views to appreciate differences in their client's cultural world view.

Cultural competence is the ability to apply the knowledge and skills needed to provide quality care for clients from different cultures. Culture competence has some basic characteristics, including the following:

1. Valuing diversity
2. Capacity for cultural self-assessment
3. Awareness of the different dynamics present when cultures interact
4. Knowledge about different cultures
5. Adaptability in providing nursing care that reflects an understanding of cultural diversity

The Focus on Diversity and Culture feature that follows will help you examine your own cultural competence and sensitivity.

In the United States, there are plenty of opportunities to encounter differences resulting from cultural diversity, and these encounters require cultural competence. Some demographic areas have experienced culturally varied client populations for decades, and other areas of the country have only recently seen increases in immigrant populations. Health practices, beliefs about illness and disease, decisions to enter health care systems, and responses to health care providers are some of the topics influenced by cultural differences. Understanding these differences and being able to communicate will enhance the nurse's effectiveness in eliminating barriers to providing health care.

FOCUS ON DIVERSITY AND CULTURE   How Culturally Sensitive Are You?

To help you identify areas where you can improve when providing nursing care to culturally different people, answer the following questions by checking Yes or No:

____ Yes ____ No   I accept values of others even when different from my own.
____ Yes ____ No   I accept beliefs of others even when different from my own.
____ Yes ____ No   I accept that the male and female roles may vary among different cultures.
____ Yes ____ No   I accept that religious practices may influence how a client responds to illness, health problems, and death.
____ Yes ____ No   I accept that alternative medicine practices may influence a client's response to illness and health problems.
____ Yes ____ No   I accept cultural diversity in my clients.
____ Yes ____ No   I attend educational programs to enhance my knowledge and skills in providing care to diverse cultural groups.
____ Yes ____ No   I understand that clients who are unable to speak English may be very proficient in their own languages.
____ Yes ____ No   I try to have written materials in the client's language available when possible.
____ Yes ____ No   I use interpreters when available to improve communication.

If you have more No responses than Yes responses, you may not be as culturally sensitive as you could be. The purpose of this self-assessment is to increase your awareness of areas where you can improve to develop your cultural sensitivity.

Diversity also has increased within the health care professions. In the United States, these professions were once open only to whites, but over time, all the health care professions, including nursing, have opened to students and practitioners from all races and cultures. This increasing diversity among health care professionals is slowly impacting how Western health care is perceived among individuals from other cultures, but there are still gains to be made and barriers to be overcome.

Developing cultural competence is a continuous process. The LEARN model (American Medical Student Association, 2007) is a tool for developing cultural competency. Below is a modification of this model to help the nurse include cultural behaviors in a client's health care:

Listen to the client's perception of the problem.

Explain your perception of the problem and of the treatments ordered by the physician.

Acknowledge and discuss the differences and similarities between these two perceptions.

Review the ordered treatments while remembering the client's cultural parameters.

Negotiate agreement. Assist the client in understanding the medical treatments ordered by the physician, and have the client help to make decisions about those treatments as appropriate (e.g., choosing cultural foods that are permitted on an ordered diet).

Box 2–1 provides a chance to put the LEARN model into practice.

No one becomes culturally aware or culturally sensitive overnight. There is a process by which nursing students (and other individuals) learn cultural confidence, with learning taking place in a fairly predictable sequence:

1. Students begin by developing cultural awareness of how culture shapes beliefs, values, individual power, and social power.
2. Students develop cultural knowledge about the differences, similarities, and inequalities in experience and practice among various societies.
3. Students develop cultural understanding of problems and issues facing societies and cultures when values, beliefs, and behaviors are compromised by another culture.
4. Students develop cultural sensitivity to the cultural beliefs, values, and behaviors of their clients. This reflects an awareness of their own cultural beliefs, values, and behaviors that may influence their nursing practice.
5. Students develop cultural competence and provide care that respects the cultural values, beliefs, and behaviors of their clients.

Hopefully, at the end of this sequence, nursing students will have developed a model of ethical multiculturalism, as described in the Evidence-Based Practice feature that follows.

Box 2–1 Critical Thinking Exercise: The LEARN Model

An Arab couple has come to Nurse Smith's clinic because the wife, who is 6 months pregnant, is not feeling well. The husband speaks English well, but the wife's proficiency in English is more limited. Both are dressed in American-style clothes. During the assessment, Nurse Smith determines that the couple has a 9-month-old and a 2-year-old at home. Nurse Smith also learns that the husband is the head of the household, making most of the major decisions for the family, and that the wife has sole responsibility for the family's care and daily living needs. The wife presents with exhaustion and elevated blood pressure. After obtaining a urine specimen, the physician diagnoses toxemia and orders the wife to be on strict bed rest and to return in two weeks. While the husband conveys concern for his wife's health, he is reluctant to have her treatment disrupt the household routine.

1. What NANDA diagnoses might Nurse Smith identify for this family?
2. Using the LEARN model, describe how Nurse Smith could discuss the situation and the doctor's recommendations with both the husband and wife.

EVIDENCE-BASED PRACTICE   A Model of Ethical Multiculturalism

The Harper Model is an evidenced-based model of ethical multiculturalism (Figure 2–12 ■) developed and presented at the 34th Annual Transcultural Nursing Society Conference (Harper, 2008). This model includes key attributes of cultural competence and the relationship to a continuum of ethical philosophies. Dr. Harper has said, "Cultural competence occurs on a continuum. Even when you believe you are competent, you can always learn more!" (Harper, 2008).

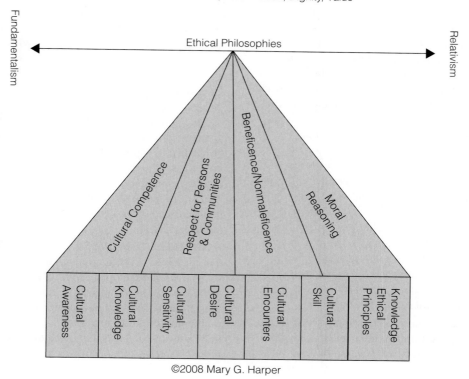

Revised Model of Ethical Multiculturalism
Balance = Protection, Preservation, Dignity, Value

©2008 Mary G. Harper

Figure 2–12 ■ This model shows how components of cultural competence are obtained through ethical influences, knowledge, and experience with the culture.

Source: Mary Harper, University of Central Florida. Reprinted with permission.

MAINTAINING CULTURAL COMPETENCE   Maintaining cultural competence is an ongoing process. Nurses continually assess, modify, and evaluate the care provided to culturally diverse clients. Reframing questions can show sensitivity and respect for different cultural beliefs. Active listening can assist nurses in understanding cultural differences. Four significant factors need to be considered:

- Clinical differences among people of different cultures and ethnic groups. For example, African Americans have a higher incidence of hypertension, and some Native-American tribes have a higher incidence of diabetes.
- A need both to have interpreters when languages differ and to understand differences in the meaning of words when communicating with clients who speak various languages.
- Respect for the belief systems of others and the effects of those beliefs on well-being, including when clients use alternative health care practices instead of traditional Western medicine.

- Trust between clients and nurses as part of the helping relationship. Authority figures are not accepted readily in some cultures. Trust both in the nurse and in the care provided need to be established.

Implementation

Implementation of cultural competence involves many aspects of the nursing process. These aspects include communication, using an interpreter, and collaboration. Institutions such as hospitals also need to develop and implement cultural competence to address the cultural and language needs of an increasingly multicultural client population.

COMMUNICATION   The United States is a country of many cultures, and health care professionals need to have a basic understanding of how language impacts health care delivery systems. Clients with limited proficiency in English often run into barriers when they try to enter the health care system.

They may delay making an appointment because of difficulties communicating over the telephone, for example, and during this delay, the health problem may become more severe, requiring more expensive treatment. If the client does make an appointment, there may be misunderstandings about the scheduled date, time, or location. If the client makes it to the appointment, he or she may have difficulty speaking with the registration person, causing additional delay and frustration. At the appointment, there may be confusion and misunderstanding during the medical interview and examination. A complete medical history may not be possible with language barriers. Alternatively, if inaccurate information is received as a result of the client misunderstanding the questions, inappropriate diagnostic tests may be done unnecessarily. If the client does not understand take-home instructions, he or she may take inappropriate actions. Clients must understand clearly what is required of them.

The brain interprets and gives meaning to what we see, hear, taste, smell, and feel. People from different cultures have different experiences and points of reference, however, so two people from different cultures who are experiencing the same reality will interpret it in entirely different ways. For example, someone makes the "OK" gesture. How would this be interpreted? What if the person is from a culture in which this gesture is obscene? Or what if the person is from a culture in which this gesture has romantic connotations? Behavior has no meaning unless the observer interprets the behavior and gives it meaning. The mind has been culturally trained, so different cultures will produce different interpretations.

USING AN INTERPRETER Many clients do not speak English, and even if clients do speak English, their speech may be limited or lack proficiency. Any facility receiving federal funding from the U.S. Department of Health and Human Services is required to communicate effectively with clients or risk the loss of that funding (American Medical Student Association, 2007). Having bilingual nurses available is one strategy to address the language barrier. Another strategy is providing access to language banks through electronic or telephone systems nurses can dial up for interpreter services. Unless a client brings an interpreter with her, however, an interpreter may not have any previous knowledge of the client. Nurses can ask a client or family with limited English proficiency if the family works with any area service organizations that provide interpreters. These organizations attempt to provide competent interpreters who build relationships with families over time.

Guidelines for using an interpreter include the following:
- When possible, use an interpreter to translate and provide meaning behind the words.
- To protect client confidentiality, avoid using a family member as an interpreter.
- If possible, use an interpreter of the same sex as the client.
- Address your questions to the client, not the interpreter, but maintain eye contact with both the client and the interpreter.
- Avoid using metaphors, medical jargon, similes, and idiomatic phrases.
- Observe the client's nonverbal communication.

- Plan what to say, and avoid rephrasing or hesitating.
- Use short questions and comments. Ask one question at a time.
- Speak slowly and distinctly, but not loudly.
- Provide written materials in the client's language as available.

COLLABORATION A number of professionals can assist a nurse in providing culturally appropriate care for a family. The most obvious of these, as already discussed, is the interpreter. Nurses also may collaborate with a client's religious leader, particularly when the client wants clarification on how a treatment may be viewed under the laws of his or her religion or when a client needs some assistance with activities of daily living (as in the case of the Arab couple with whom Nurse Smith was working). Churches, synagogues, and mosques can provide support and often services to their members.

Nurses should take a holistic approach to their nursing care and recognize the wholeness of all clients, regardless of their diverse cultural, racial, ethnic, religious, or other background or heritage (Figure 2–13 ■). Accepting clients as they are can give comfort to the families as well as to the clients, which can increase compliance with the treatment regimen. The Client Teaching feature that follows discusses how communication between parents and nurses can help to bring about a collaborative relationship.

HOSPITALS, LANGUAGE, AND CULTURE The Joint Commission (2008) conducted a study called *Hospitals, Language, and Culture: A Snapshot of the Nation* that investigated how 60 hospitals across the United States were addressing cultural and language needs among an increasingly multicultural client population. The Joint Commission found there was no one-size-fits-all solution; the process of becoming more culturally competent was unique to each organization.

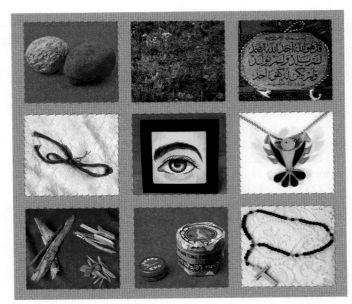

Figure 2–13 ■ Cultures use various symbols and traditions for health beliefs and practices.

CLIENT TEACHING **Communication Between Parents and Nurses**

When children enter the health care system, it is usually the parents that provide information about what is wrong with the child, how long a problem has been occurring, what they have tried to do to help the problem, and so on. Taking care of children is a collaborative effort between parents, nurses, and other health care providers. Mutual respect and support are healthy attitudes that will facilitate the child's health care experience.

Parents may need to learn how best to communicate with nurses and other health care professionals. Some suggestions that can be given to parents to support this communication include the following:

■ Keep records of all medical treatments, immunizations, major illnesses, routine medications, hospitalizations, diagnostic tests results, and screening results.

■ Write down any questions about the care or treatment of childhood conditions, illnesses, developmental progress, behavioral or mental concerns, or preventive measures.

■ Become familiar with a child's daily habits of eating, sleeping, playing, learning activities, social interactions, usual schedule each day, emotional expressions, and interactions with pets and other family members.

Some suggestions for nurses to support this communication include the following:

■ Provide information to parents, and be available to answer any questions they might have.

■ Be honest and real with the parents.

■ Respect family dynamics and values, and find opportunities for using them in the care of the child.

■ Maintain open communication with parents and other family members.

Based on the data gathered, the Joint Commission identified some issues and offered recommendations for how organizations could develop cultural competence:

■ Identify the needs of client populations served in the community, and assess how well current practices are meeting these needs.

■ Bring various health care providers in the organization together to gain their perspectives on and experiences with providing care, barriers to working with different cultures, and gaps in the services delivered.

■ Initiate a continuous monitoring process for assessment and evaluation of cultural and language needs.

■ Improve the services provided to meet the needs of clients using the resources available to the organization.

The case of a middle-aged Chinese client refusing pain medication following nasal surgery illustrates cultural competence. When asked why he refused, he replied his discomfort was bearable and he could survive without any medication. Later, the nurse found him restless and uncomfortable and again offered pain medication. Again, he refused, explaining that her responsibilities at the hospital were far more important than his comfort, and that he did not want to impose. Only after the nurse firmly insisted that the client's comfort was one of her most important responsibilities did he finally agree to take the medication.

Among Asian people, health is considered a state of spiritual and physical harmony with nature. There is a need for balance between yin and yang. When an imbalance occurs, illness results. Asian clients do not usually complain about pain or physical problems because they are taught self-restraint and the priority of group over individual needs. Another factor that may be involved in this case is that initial refusal of something offered is seen as a gesture of courtesy; this client may have considered it impolite to agree to the pain medication the first time it was offered. The best approach for the nurse is to consider the client's need for pain medication even if the client has not requested or even refuses relief from pain. Then, if the client still refuses, the nurse should respect his or her wishes.

Evaluation

Nursing care is evaluated by comparing client outcomes with goals established for nursing diagnoses that are identified following appropriate assessment. The nursing process includes cultural sensitivity specific to the client. Nurses should consider the impact of the client's beliefs and behaviors on achievement of the goals established. If cultural differences are a factor, the nursing care plan needs to be modified to include cultural influences that support the client in reaching expected outcomes.

The nursing process organizes the nursing care of clients, beginning with assessment and ending with evaluation. Cultural sensitivity can be included in every phase of the nursing process to support both clients and their families. The following cultural issues need to be addressed throughout the nursing process (modified from Russell Consulting, 2005):

■ Routines of daily life both in and out of the home
■ Customs and practices
■ Level of education and training
■ Ceremonies, celebrations, and events that clients follow
■ How health care decisions are made
■ The head of the household's role
■ Verbal and nonverbal communication
■ Physical environment and boundaries of personal space
■ Organizational structure of the home

ALTERNATIVE HEALTH CARE

Health practices involving exercise, diet, and environment are beneficial to clients. However, some clients may believe in health care practices that fall outside the scope of Western medicine. Acupuncture and yoga are two excellent and increasingly familiar examples.

Cultural health practices must be respected and not ignored, because they are important to clients. If nontraditional health practices have no negative impact on the client, it may be important for the client to continue using them.

Alternative medical health and mental health treatments are becoming increasingly popular among the general population as well. Many people are adopting alternative healing practices from different cultures, such as Buddhist meditation, Asian acupuncture, Native-American sweat lodges, and Chinese herbal medicines. The importance in the healing process of body, mind, and spirit and of being in harmony with nature are common themes in many cultural healing practices and rituals (Corkindale, 2008).

REVIEW **Values and Beliefs**

RELATE: **LINK THE CONCEPTS**

You are a nurse working in a children's rehabilitation center. A 6-year-old girl who is recovering from a car accident comes to your center for an extended stay. She speaks a little English. Her family has recently moved here from China, and her parents speak very little English. Although, they are grateful for the help they are receiving, they are very stressed about their daughter's situation.

Linking the concepts of Family, Stress and Coping, and Communication with the concept of Culture:

1. How will you communicate with her parents?
2. Does the communication barrier increase the chances of error in caring for this child?
3. What will you do to reassure the child and help her be more at ease?

REFLECT: **CASE STUDY**

Jesus Hernandez is a 5-year-old boy and a client at the pediatric clinic at which you are employed. His family are immigrants from Mexico; he speaks a little English. His mother, Senora Hernandez, speaks very little English. Her older daughter, Maria, is 15 and speaks English fairly well. Maria usually acts as interpreter for the family.

Jesus is diagnosed with allergic asthma. His pediatrician prescribes Singulair once a day, to be taken at night; a steroid inhaler to be taken morning and night; and an albuterol inhaler to be used before recess and whenever he is short of breath, but not more than two puffs every 6 hours. The pediatrician also refers Jesus to an allergist for further evaluation.

1. How can you, as the nurse, be sure that his mother understands the medication instructions?
2. How can you be sure she understands his condition and at what point she may need to take him to the emergency room if his breathing deteriorates?
3. How can you be sure he will take his inhaler before recess at school each day?
4. How can you assist the family with following up on the referral to the allergist?

REFERENCES

American Academy of Family Physicians. (2007). Cultural competence self-test. Retrieved May 14, 2009, from http://www.aafp.org/fpm/20001000/58cult.html#boxb

American Association of Colleges of Nursing. (2006). Cultural competency in baccalaureate nursing education. Retrieved May 14, 2009, from http://www.aacn.nche.edu

American Medical Student Association. (2007). Cultural competency in medicine. Retrieved May 14, 2009, from http://www.amsa.org/programs/gpit/cultural.cfm

Berman, A., Snyder, S. J., Kozier, B., & Erb, G. (2008). Kozier & Erb's fundamentals of nursing: Concepts, process, and practice (8th ed.). Upper Saddle River, NJ: Pearson Education.

Betancourt, J. R., & Ananeh-Firemping, O. (2004). Not me! Doctors, decisions and disparities in health care. Retrieved May 14, 2009, from http://www.medscape.com/viewarticle/480602

Centers for Disease Control and Prevention, U.S. Department of Health and Human Services. (2007). Health, United States, 2007. Chartbook on trends in the health of Americans. Retrieved May 14, 2009, from http://www.cdc.gov/nchs/data/hus/hus07.ped#contents

Centers for Disease Control and Prevention, U.S. Department of Health and Human Services. (2009). Women and heart disease fact sheet. Retrieved May 14, 2009, from http://www.cdc.gov/DHDSP/library/fs_women_heart.htm

Collins, S. D. (2006). Is cultural competency required in today's nursing care? NSNA IMPRINT, Feb/Mar, 52–54. Retrieved May 14, 2009, from http://www.nsna.org/pubs/imprint/febmar06/impfeb_feat_collins.pdf

Corkindale, D. F. (2008). Healing traditions in multi-cultural America. Retrieved May 14, 2009, from http://www.debbiecorkindale.com/multicultural.html

Comsilk, C., & Blythe, F. (Executive Producers). (2006, November). Indian country diaries. Peoplehood. New York and Washington, DC: Public Broadcasting Service. Retrieved from http://www.pbs.org/indiancountry

Craven, R. F., & Himle, C. J. (2007). Fundamentals of nursing human health and function (5th ed.). Philadelphia: Lippincott Williams & Wilkins.

Cultural Diversity in Nursing. Transcultural Nursing. (2008). Cultural competence. Retrieved May 14, 2009, from http://www.culturediversity.org/cultcomp.htm

Culturally sensitive nursing care. (2008). Retrieved May 14, 2009, from http://www.megaessays.com/viewpaper/88079.html

Department of Education, Science, and Training. (2008). Current models of multicultural education. Retrieved May 14, 2009, from http://www.dest.gov.au/archive/HIGHERED/nursing?pubs?multi_cultural/5.htm

DiversityRx. (2008). Why language and culture are important. Retrieved May 14, 2009, from http://www.diversityrx.org/htmL/ESLANG.htm

essortment. (2008). American culture for foreigners. Retrieved May 14, 2009, from http://www.essortment.com/all/americanculture_rtjl.htm

Harper, M. G. (2008). Evaluation of the antecedents of cultural competence. University of Central Florida. Retrieved from http://www.tcns.org

Hooker, R. (2008). World civilizations. Retrieved May 14, 2009, from http://wsu.edu/~dee/WORLD.HTM

Inspired Personal Development. (2007). The big 5 that develop your belief system. Retrieved May 14, 2009, from http://www.inspired-personal-development.com/belief-system.html

Institute of Medicine of the National Academies. (2002). Unequal treatment: Confronting racial and ethnic disparities in health care. Washington, DC: National Academy of Sciences.

Jay, G. (2008). What is multiculturalism? Milwaukee, WI: University of Wisconsin.

The Joint Commission. (2008). Hospitals, language, and culture: A snapshot of the nation. Retrieved May 14, 2009, from http://www.jointcommission.org/PatientSafety/HLC

Management Sciences for Health. (2008). The provider's guide to quality and culture. Retrieved from http://erc.msh.org/

Multicultural Nursing Education. (2008). National review of nursing education. Retrieved from http://www.dest.gov.au/archive/HIGHERED/nursing/pubs/multi_cultural/5.htm

Multiculturalism. (2004). Retrieved June 3, 2009, from http://www.wikinfo.org/index.php/Multiculturalism

Multiculturalism definition. (2008). Retrieved from http://www.answers.com/topic/multiculturalism

Peace Corps. (2003). Culture matters: The Peace Corps cross cultural workbook. Retrieved from http://peacecorps.gov/multimedia/pdf/library/T0087_culturematters.pdf

Persistent Stereotypes About Asian Americans. (2009). Retrieved from http://www.asian-nation.org/

Potter, P. A., & Perry, A. G. (2009). Fundamentals of nursing (7th ed.). St. Louis, MO: Mosby.

Rusbult, C. (2007). What is a worldview?—Definition & introduction. Retrieved from http://www.asa3.org/ASA/education/views/index.html

Russell Consulting Cooperation. (2005). Understanding organizational cure. Retrieved from http://www.russellconsultinginc.com/docs/white/culture.html

Society of the United States. (2008).. Retrieved from http://en.wikipedia.org/wiki/Society_of_the_United_States

Transcultural Nursing Society. (2008). Retrieved from http://www.tcns.org

U.S. Bureau of the Census. (2007). State & County QuickFacts. Retrieved from http://quickfacts.census.gov/qfd/states/00000.html

Values and Beliefs as Components of Culture: An Introduction (2008). Retrieved from http://www.wsu.edu/gened/learn-modules/top_culture/values-beliefs/values-beliefs-intro.html

What is culture? (2008). Retrieved from http://dictionary.reference.com/browse/culture

Wilkinson, J. M., & Van Leuven, K. (2007). Fundamentals of nursing theory, concepts & applications. Philadelphia: F.A. Davis.

Wilson-Stronks, A., Galvez, E., & The Joint Commission (2007). Exploring cultural and linguistic services in the nation's hospitals: A report of findings. Retrieved from http://www.jointcommission.org/PatientSafety

Development

3

Concept at-a-Glance

Concept Learning Outcomes

After reading about this concept, you will be able to do the following:

1. Differentiate between the terms *growth* and *development*.
2. Describe essential principles related to growth and development.
3. List factors that influence growth and development.
4. Describe the stages of growth and development according to various theorists.
5. Compare Peck's and Gould's stages of adult development.
6. Compare Kohlberg's and Gilligan's theories of moral development.
7. Compare Fowler's and Westerhoff's stages of spiritual development.
8. Explain contemporary developmental approaches such as temperament theory, ecologic theory, and the resilience framework.
9. Recognize major developmental milestones for clients at each stage of development.
10. Identify normal age-related changes.
11. Discuss the importance of developmentally appropriate care in meeting client's needs.

About Development

The terms *growth* and *development* both refer to dynamic processes. Often used interchangeably, these terms have different meanings. **Growth** refers to physical change and increase in size. It can be measured quantitatively. Indicators of growth include height,

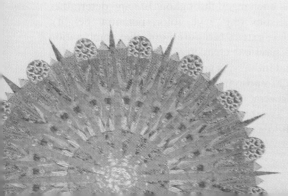

weight, bone size, and dentition. The pattern of physiologic growth is similar for all people. However, growth rates vary during different stages of growth and development. The growth rate is rapid during the prenatal, neonatal, infancy, and adolescent stages and slows during childhood. Physical growth is minimal during adulthood.

Development is an increase in the complexity of function and skill progression, the capacity and skill of a person to adapt to the environment. Development is the behavioral aspect of growth (e.g., a person develops the ability to walk, to talk, and to run). ●

Growth and development are independent, interrelated processes. For example, an infant's muscles, bones, and nervous system must grow to a certain point before the infant is able to sit up or walk. Growth generally takes place during the first 20 years of life; development takes place throughout the life span. The following are principles of growth and development:

- Growth and development are continuous, orderly, sequential processes influenced by maturational, environmental, and genetic factors.
- All humans follow the same pattern of growth and development.
- The sequence of each stage is predictable, although the time of onset, the length of the stage, and the effects of each stage vary with each person.
- Learning can either help or hinder the maturational process, depending on what is learned.
- Each **developmental stage** (level of achievement) has its own characteristics. For example, Piaget suggested that in the sensorimotor stage (birth to 2 years) children learn to coordinate simple motor tasks.
- Growth and development occur in a **cephalocaudal** direction, that is, starting at the head and moving toward the trunk, legs, and feet (Figure 3–1 ■). This pattern is particularly obvious at birth, when the head of the infant is disproportionately large.
- Growth and development occur in a **proximodistal** direction, that is, from the center of the body outward (see Figure 3–1). For example, infants can roll over before they can grasp an object with the thumb and second finger.
- Development proceeds from simple to complex, or from single acts to integrated acts. To accomplish the integrated act of drinking and swallowing from a cup, for example, the child must first learn a series of single acts: eye–hand coordination; grasping; hand–mouth coordination; controlled tipping of the cup; and then mouth, lip, and tongue movements to drink and swallow.
- Development becomes increasingly differentiated. Differentiated development begins with a generalized response and progresses to a specific skilled response. For example, an infant's initial response to a stimulus involves the total body, but a 5-year-old child can respond more specifically with laughter or fear.
- Certain stages of growth and development are more critical than others. It is known, for example, that the first 10–12 weeks after conception are critical. The incidence of congenital anomalies as a result of exposure to certain viruses, chemicals, or drugs is greater during this stage than during others.

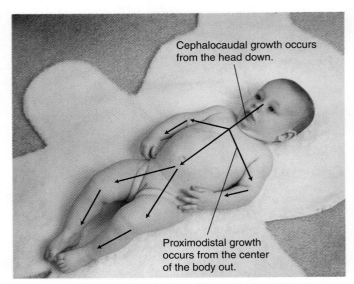

Cephalocaudal growth occurs from the head down.

Proximodistal growth occurs from the center of the body out.

Figure 3–1 ■ In normal cephalocaudal growth, the child gains control of the head and neck before the trunk and limbs. In normal proximodistal growth, the child controls arm movements before hand movements. For example, the child reaches for objects before being able to grasp them. Children gain control of their hands before their fingers; that is, they can hold things with the entire hand before they can pick something up with just their fingers.

- The pace of growth and development is uneven. It is known that growth is greater during infancy than during childhood. Asynchronous development is demonstrated by rapid growth of the head during infancy and the extremities at puberty.

STAGES OF GROWTH AND DEVELOPMENT

The rate of a person's growth and development is highly individual; however, the sequence of growth and development is predictable. Stages of growth usually correspond to certain developmental changes (Table 3–1).

INFLUENCES ON DEVELOPMENT

Many factors can influence growth and development. Knowledge of these factors helps the nurse to intervene to promote positive growth and development of the individual. Both genetic and environmental factors contribute to individual differences.

Genetics

The genetic inheritance of an individual is established at conception. It remains unchanged throughout life and determines physical characteristics (e.g., eye color, potential height); gender; and, to some extent, **temperament**, that combination of biological and physical characteristics that is specific to each individual and influences personality and behavior. Each child inherits 23 chromosomes from the mother's egg and 23 from the father's sperm, resulting in a unique individual with 46 chromosomes. Two of these are **sex chromosomes**, which determine the child's gender; the rest, called **autosomal chromosomes**, govern all remaining characteristics. Every

TABLE 3-1 Stages of Growth and Development

STAGE	AGE	SIGNIFICANT CHARACTERISTICS	NURSING IMPLICATIONS
Neonatal	Birth to 28 days	Behavior is largely reflexive and develops to more purposeful behavior.	Assist parents to identify and meet unmet needs.
Infancy	1 month to 1 year	Physical growth is rapid.	Control the infant's environment so that physical and psychological needs are met.
Toddlerhood	1 to 3 years	Motor development permits increased physical autonomy. Psychosocial skills increase.	Safety and risk-taking strategies must be balanced to permit growth.
Preschool	3 to 6 years	The preschooler's world is expanding. New experiences and the preschooler's social role are tried during play. Physical growth is slower.	Provide opportunities for play and social activity.
School age	6 to 12 years	Stage includes the preadolescent period (10–12 years). Peer group increasingly influences behavior. Physical growth is slower.	Allow time and energy for the school-age child to pursue hobbies and school activities. Recognize and support child's achievement.
Adolescence	12 to 18 years	Self-concept changes with biological development. Values are tested. Physical growth accelerates. Stress increases.	Assist adolescents to develop coping behaviors. Help adolescents develop strategies for resolving conflicts.
Young adulthood	18 to 40 years	A personal lifestyle develops. Person establishes a relationship with a significant other and a commitment to something.	Accept adult's chosen lifestyle and assist with necessary adjustments relating to health. Recognize the person's commitments. Support change as necessary for health.
Middle adulthood	40 to 65 years	Lifestyle changes due to other changes; for example, children leave home, occupational goals change.	Assist clients to plan for anticipated changes in life, to recognize the risk factors related to health, and to focus on strengths rather than weaknesses.
Older adulthood			
Young-old	65 to 74 years	Adaptation to retirement and changing physical abilities is often necessary. Chronic illness may develop.	Assist clients to keep mentally, physically, and socially active and to maintain peer group interactions.
Middle-old	75 to 84 years	Adaptation to decline in speed of movement, reaction time, and increasing dependence on others may be necessary.	Assist clients to cope with loss (e.g., hearing, sensory abilities and eyesight, death of loved one). Provide necessary safety measures.
Old-old	85 and older	Increasing physical problems may develop.	Assist clients with self-care as required, and with maintaining as much independence as possible.

Source: Berman, A., Snyder, S. J., Kozier, B., & Erb, G. (2008). *Kozier & Erb's fundamentals of nursing: Concepts, process, and practice* (8th ed., p. 351). Upper Saddle River, NJ: Pearson Education.

chromosome carries many genes that determine physical characteristics, intellectual potential, personality type, and other traits. Children are born with the potential for certain features; however, their interaction with the environment influences how and to what extent particular traits are manifested. For example, a child may have the potential for a high level of intellectual performance, but if he or she lives in an environment without access to supports such as education and proper nutrition, that potential may never be reached.

Since chromosomes and genes carry messages that encode for certain characteristics, they also can carry diseases. Children can be affected by chromosomal disorders, such as fragile X or Down syndrome, which involve either altered numbers or altered structure of chromosomes. Although some of these mutations are incompatible with life and result in fetal death, live births can occur with others. Chromosomal disorders may be caused by an array of factors, such as radiation exposure, parental age, or parental disease states; however, sometimes their causes cannot be determined.

Some children inherit genes that lead to diseases such as cystic fibrosis; others may have a mutation that manifests in the disease. A family history of these diseases is usually present, but because genes sometimes mutate, an initial incidence of a genetic disorder may appear with no identifiable history.

Prenatal Influences

Some Asian cultures calculate age from the time of conception. This practice acknowledges the profound influence of the prenatal period.

The mother's nutrition and general state of health play a part in pregnancy outcome. Poor nutrition can lead to low-birth-weight infants and infants with compromised neurologic performance, slow development, or impaired immune status with resultant high disease rates. Low maternal stores of iron can result in anemia in the infant (American Academy of Pediatrics, 2004). Maternal smoking is associated with low-birth-weight infants. Ingestion of alcoholic beverages, including beer and wine, during pregnancy may lead to fetal alcohol syndrome or fetal alcohol effects. Substance abuse by the mother may result in neonatal addiction, convulsions, hyperirritability, poor social responsiveness, and other neurologic disturbances of the infant, as well as changes in neurobehavioral and cognitive function of children (Huizink & Mulder, 2006).

Even prescription or nonprescription drugs may adversely affect the fetus. This was brought to general attention when the drug thalidomide, commonly prescribed in Europe to treat nausea during the 1950s, resulted in the birth of infants with limb abnormalities to women who had taken the drug during pregnancy. Differences in physiology related to gastric emptying, renal clearance, drug distribution, and other factors contribute to variations in pharmacokinetics during pregnancy. Drugs can cause teratogenesis (abnormal development of the fetus) or mutagenesis (permanent changes in the fetus' genetic material) (McCarter-Spaulding, 2005). Certain drugs can cause bleeding, stained teeth, impaired hearing, or other defects in the infant. The U.S. Food and Drug Administration (FDA) has established risk categories for drugs in pregnancy.

Some maternal illnesses are harmful to the developing fetus. One example is rubella (German measles), which is rarely a serious disease for adults but can cause deafness, vision defects, heart defects, and mental retardation in the fetus if it is acquired by a pregnant woman. A fetus can also acquire diseases such as AIDS and HIV infection or hepatitis B from the mother.

Chronic maternal distress or depression can affect the fetus. Excess stress hormones such a cortisone pass through the placenta, and can result in lower birth weight and size. Recent studies indicate that maternal distress during pregnancy can also affect a baby's temperament and neurobehavioral development (Diego, 2006).

Radiation, chemicals, and other environmental hazards may adversely affect a fetus when the mother is exposed to these influences during her pregnancy. The best outcomes for infants occur when mothers eat well; exercise regularly; seek early prenatal care; refrain from use of drugs, alcohol, tobacco, and excessive caffeine; and follow general principles of good health.

Family and Parenting

An environmental factor that is extremely important in the development of children is the profile of family characteristics. The family is an important component in every child's life and plays an essential role in fostering the development of youth. Parenting is a significant concept in families. The effects of parenting interact with a child's individual characteristics to influence risk and protective factors, personality characteristics, and developmental outcomes.

The families into which individuals are born influence them profoundly. Children are supported in different ways and acquire different world views depending on such factors as whether they have one or two parents or stepparents, whether one or both parents work, how many siblings are present, and whether an extended family is close. When working with a child or family, the nurse should take note of variations in family structure such as single parent, homosexual parents, extended family, and stepparents.

Cultural Influences

Another factor that influences development is culture, both through traditional practices and due to genetic variations among some ethnic groups. The traditional customs of the many cultural groups represented in North America influence the development of children in these groups. Nutritional practices of various ethnic groups may influence the rate of growth for infants. In addition, development may be influenced by childrearing practices. For example, the Native American practice of carrying infants on boards often delays walking compared to the norm measured in some developmental tests. Children who are carried by straddling the mother's hips or back for extended periods have a low incidence of developmental hip dysplasia since this keeps their hips in an abducted position. It is important for nurses to take cultural practices into account when performing developmental screening; some tests may not be culturally sensitive and can inaccurately label a child as delayed when the pattern of development is simply different in the group, perhaps due to family's childrearing practices. In these cases there is no lasting delay in any milestone, but variation in acquiring skills may occur.

All cultural groups have rules regarding patterns of social interaction. Schedules of language acquisition are determined by the number of languages spoken and the amount of speech in the home. The particular social roles men and women assume in the culture affect school activities and ultimately career choices. Attitudes toward touching and other methods of encouraging developmental skills vary among cultures.

Genetic traits common in certain ethnic or cultural groups may predispose children to being at the upper or lower ranges of growth and may influence other physical characteristics. Genetic variations also make certain groups more prone to develop certain diseases.

Nutrition

Adequate nutrition is an essential component of growth and development. For example, poorly nourished children are more likely to get infections than are well-nourished children. In addition, poorly nourished children may not attain their full height potential. Inadequate nutrition during pregnancy and the first few years of life may also impact brain development. If the brain is not properly nourished children will fall behind on development. Children who are severely malnourished may have permanent brain damage and may even die.

Environment

A few environmental factors that can influence growth and development are the living conditions of the child (e.g., homelessness), socioeconomic status (e.g., poverty versus financial stability), climate, and community (e.g., providing developmental support versus exposing the child to hazards).

Health

Illness or injury can affect growth and development. Being hospitalized is stressful for a child and can affect the child's coping mechanisms. Prolonged or chronic illness may affect normal developmental processes, including psychosocial development.

GROWTH AND DEVELOPMENT THEORIES

Growth and development are commonly thought of as having five major components: psychosocial, cognitive, moral, spiritual, and biophysical. Researchers have advanced several theories about the various stages and aspects of growth and development, particularly with regard to infant and child development. A discussion of some of the major theories follows.

Psychosocial Theories

Psychosocial development refers to the development of personality. **Personality**, a complex concept that is difficult to define, can be considered as the outward (interpersonal) expression of the inner (intrapersonal) self. It encompasses a person's temperament, feelings, character traits, independence, self-esteem, self-concept, behavior, ability to interact with others, and ability to adapt to life changes.

Many theorists have attempted to account for psychosocial development in humans. These theories often explain the development of a person's personality and the causes of behavior.

FREUD (1856–1939) Sigmund Freud introduced a number of concepts about development that are still used today. The **unconscious mind** is the part of a person's mental life of which he or she is unaware. This concept of the unconscious is one of Freud's major contributions to the field of psychiatry. The **id** resides in the unconscious and, operating on the pleasure principle, seeks immediate pleasure and gratification. The

ego, the realistic part of the person, balances the gratification demands of the id with the limitations of social and physical circumstances. The methods the ego uses to fulfill the needs of the id in a socially acceptable manner are called defense mechanisms or adaptive mechanisms. **Defense mechanisms**, or **adaptive mechanisms** as they are more commonly called today, are the result of conflicts between the id's impulses and the anxiety created by the conflicts due to social and environmental restrictions. The third aspect of the personality, according to Freud, is the superego. The **superego** contains the conscience and the ego ideal. The conscience consists of society's "do not's," usually resulting from parental and cultural expectations. The ego ideal comprises the standards of perfection toward which the individual strives. Freud also proposed that the underlying motivation to human development is a dynamic, psychic energy, which he called **libido**. According to Freud's theory of psychosexual development, the personality develops in five overlapping stages from birth to adulthood. The libido changes its location of emphasis within the body from one stage to another. Therefore, a particular body area has special significance to a client at a particular stage. The first three stages (oral, anal, and phallic) are called *pregenital stages*. The culminating stage is the *genital stage*. Table 3–2 indicates characteristics for each stage.

Freudian theory asserts that the individual must meet the needs of each developmental stage to move successfully to the next. For example, during the oral stage, nurses can assist an infant's development by making feeding a pleasurable experience. This provides comfort and security for the infant. Freud

TABLE 3–2 Freud's Five Stages of Development

STAGE	AGE	CHARACTERISTICS	IMPLICATIONS
Oral	Birth to 1 1/2 years	Mouth is the center of pleasure (major source of gratification and exploration). Security is primary need. Major conflict: weaning.	Feeding produces pleasure and a sense of comfort and safety. Feeding should be pleasurable and provided when required.
Anal	1 1/2 to 3 years	Anus and bladder are the sources of pleasure (sensual satisfaction, self-control). Major conflict: toilet training.	Controlling and expelling feces provide pleasure and sense of control. Toilet training should be a pleasurable experience.
Phallic	4 to 6 years	The child's genitals are the center of pleasure. Masturbation offers pleasure. Other activities can include fantasy, experimentation with peers, and questioning of adults about sexual topics. Major conflict: the Oedipus or Electra complex, which resolves when the child identifies with parent of same sex. (The Oedipus complex refers to the male child's attraction to his mother and hostile attitudes toward his father. The Electra complex refers to the female child's attraction to her father and hostile attitudes toward her mother.)	The child identifies with the parent of the opposite sex and later takes on a love relationship outside the family. Encourage identity.
Latency	6 years to puberty	Energy is directed toward physical and intellectual activities. Sexual impulses tend to be repressed. Relationships between peers of the same sex develop.	Encourage child with physical and intellectual pursuits. Encourage sports and other activities with same-sex peers.
Genital	Puberty and after	Energy is directed toward full sexual maturity and function and development of skills needed to cope with the environment.	Encourage separation from parents, achievement of independence, and decision making.

Source: Murray, R. B., & Zentner, J. P. (2001). *Health promotion strategies through the life span* (7th ed., p. 238). Upper Saddle River, NJ: Merrill/Prentice Hall. Adapted with permission.

also emphasized the importance of infant–parent interaction. Therefore, the nurse, as a caregiver, should provide a warm, caring atmosphere for an infant and assist parents to do so when the infant returns to their care.

If the person does not achieve a satisfactory progression at one stage, the personality becomes fixated at that stage. **Fixation** is immobilization or the inability of the personality to proceed to the next stage because of anxiety. For example, making toilet training a positive experience during the anal stage enhances the child's feeling of self-control. If, however, the toilet training was a negative experience, the resulting conflict or stress can delay or prolong progression through that stage or cause a person to regress to a previous stage. Ideally, an individual progresses through each stage with balance between the id, ego, and superego.

ERIKSON (1902–1996) Erik H. Erikson (1963, 1968) adapted and expanded Freud's theory of development to include the entire life span, believing that people continue to develop throughout life. He described eight stages of development (Table 3–3).

Erikson's theory proposes that life is a sequence of developmental stages or levels of achievement. Each stage signals a task that must be accomplished. The resolution of the task can be complete, partial, or unsuccessful. Erikson believed that the more successful an individual is at each developmental stage, the healthier the personality of the

individual will be. Failure to complete any developmental stage interferes with the person's ability to progress to the next level. These developmental stages can be viewed as a series of crises. Successful resolution of these crises supports healthy ego development. Failure to resolve the crises damages the ego.

Erikson's eight stages reflect both positive and negative aspects of the critical life periods. The resolution of the conflicts at each stage enables the person to function effectively in society. Each phase has its own developmental task, and the individual must find a balance between, for example, trust and mistrust (Stage 1) or integrity and despair (Stage 8). See Figures 3–2 ■ and 3–3 ■.

When using Erikson's developmental framework, nurses should be aware of indicators of positive and negative resolution of each developmental stage. According to Erikson, the environment is highly influential to development. Nurses can enhance a client's development by being aware of the individual's developmental stage and assisting with the development of coping skills related to stressors experienced at that specific level. Nurses can strengthen a client's positive resolution of a developmental task by providing the individual with appropriate opportunities and encouragement. For example, a 10-year-old child (industry versus inferiority) can be encouraged to be creative, to finish schoolwork, and to learn how to accomplish these tasks within the limitations imposed by health status. An older adult can be encouraged to maintain generativity (care for and connection

TABLE 3–3 **Erikson's Eight Stages of Development**

STAGE	AGE	CENTRAL TASK	INDICATORS OF POSITIVE RESOLUTION	INDICATORS OF NEGATIVE RESOLUTION
Infancy	Birth to 18 months	Trust versus mistrust	Learning to trust others	Mistrust, withdrawal, estrangement
Early childhood	18 months to 3 years	Autonomy versus shame and doubt	Self-control without loss of self-esteem; ability to cooperate and to express oneself	Compulsive self-restraint or compliance; willfulness and defiance
Late childhood	3 to 5 years	Initiative versus guilt	Learning the degree to which assertiveness and purpose influence the environment; beginning ability to evaluate one's own behavior	Lack of self-confidence; pessimism, fear of wrongdoing; overcontrol and overrestriction of own activity
School age	6 to 12 years	Industry versus inferiority	Beginning to create, develop, and manipulate; developing sense of competence and perseverance	Loss of hope, sense of being mediocre; withdrawal from school and peers
Adolescence	12 to 20 years	Identity versus role confusion	Coherent sense of self; plans to actualize one's abilities	Feelings of confusion, indecisiveness, and possible antisocial behavior
Young adulthood	18 to 25 years	Intimacy versus isolation	Intimate relationship with another person; commitment to work and relationships	Impersonal relationships; avoidance of relationship, career, or lifestyle commitments
Adulthood	25 to 65 years	Generativity versus stagnation	Creativity, productivity, concern for others	Self-indulgence, self-concern, lack of interests and commitments
Maturity	65 years to death	Integrity versus despair	Acceptance of worth and uniqueness of one's own life; acceptance of death	Sense of loss, contempt for others

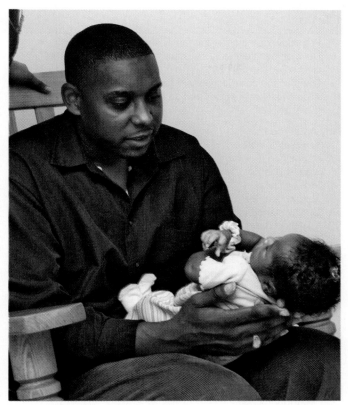

Figure 3–2 ■ Note that the parent and infant faces are in the same plane. This "en face" position enables both to examine the other's face and establish eye contact, fostering attachment between parent and child.

with others) in order to avoid a sense of stagnation, or a feeling of disconnectedness that increases self-absorption and loneliness.

Erikson emphasized that people must change and adapt their behavior to maintain control over their lives. In his view, no stage in personality development can be bypassed, but

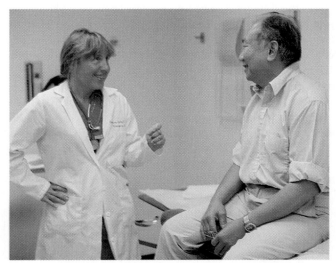

Figure 3–3 ■ Regular assessments can help older adults maintain their health and independence, contributing to achievement of integrity versus despair.

people can become fixated at one stage or regress to a previous stage under anxious or stressful conditions. For example, a middle-aged woman who has never satisfactorily resolved the identity versus role confusion task might regress to an earlier stage when stressed by an illness with which she cannot cope.

HAVIGHURST (1900–1991) Robert Havighurst believed that learning is basic to life and people continue to learn throughout life. He described growth and development as occurring in six stages, each associated with 6–10 tasks to be learned (Table 3–4).

Havighurst promoted the concept of developmental tasks in the 1950s. A **developmental task** is "a task which arises at or about a certain period in the life of an individual, successful achievement of which leads to his happiness and to success with later tasks, while failure leads to unhappiness in the individual, disapproval by society, and difficulty with later tasks" (Havighurst, 1972, p. 2).

Havighurst's developmental tasks provide a framework that the nurse can use to evaluate a person's general accomplishments. However, some nurses find that the broad categories limit its usefulness as a tool in assessing specific accomplishments, particularly those of infancy and childhood. In a multicultural society, the definition of successful completion of tasks may vary with values and belief systems as well (e.g., not all individuals may wish to marry or bear children), making these tasks less relevant for some.

VYGOTSKY (1896–1934) Lev Vygotsky, referred to as a "social constructivist," explored the concept of cognitive development within a social, historical, and cultural context, arguing that adults guide children to learn, and that development depends on the use of language, play, and extensive social interaction. These ideas have been used in treatment of children with learning disorders, autism, mental handicaps, and other disabilities (Edwards, 2002). These ideas also support the benefit of adult social learning opportunities through group interaction and observation. Vygotsky truly supported social learning and reinforcement through work, group discussion, and other means.

PECK (1968–) Theories and models about adult development are relatively recent compared with theories of infant and child development. Research into adult development has been stimulated by a number of factors, including increased longevity and healthier old age. In the past, development was viewed as complete by the time of physical maturity, and aging was considered a decline following maturity. The emphasis was on the negative aspects rather than the positive aspects of aging. However, Robert Peck believes that, although physical capabilities and functions decrease with old age, mental and social capacities tend to increase in the latter part of life.

Peck proposes three developmental tasks during old age, in contrast to Erikson's one (integrity versus despair):

1. **Ego differentiation versus work-role preoccupation.** An adult's identity and feelings of worth are highly dependent on that person's work role. On retirement, people may

TABLE 3–4 Havighurst's Age Periods and Developmental Tasks

Infancy and Early Childhood
1. Learning to walk
2. Learning to take solid foods
3. Learning to talk
4. Learning to control the elimination of body wastes
5. Learning sex differences and sexual modesty
6. Achieving psychologic stability
7. Forming simple concepts of social and physical reality
8. Learning to relate emotionally to parents, siblings, and other people
9. Learning to distinguish right from wrong and developing a conscience

Middle Childhood
1. Learning physical skills necessary for ordinary games
2. Building wholesome attitudes toward oneself as a growing organism
3. Learning to get along with age-mates
4. Learning an appropriate masculine or feminine social role
5. Developing fundamental skills in reading, writing, and calculating
6. Developing concepts necessary for everyday living
7. Developing conscience, morality, and a scale of values
8. Achieving personal independence
9. Developing attitudes toward social groups and institutions

Adolescence
1. Achieving new and more mature relations with age-mates of both sexes
2. Achieving a masculine or feminine social role
3. Accepting one's physique and using the body effectively
4. Achieving emotional independence from parents and other adults
5. Achieving assurance of economic independence
6. Selecting and preparing for an occupation

7. Preparing for marriage and family life
8. Developing intellectual skills and concepts necessary for civic competence
9. Desiring and achieving socially responsible behavior
10. Acquiring a set of values and an ethical system as a guide to behavior

Early Adulthood
1. Selecting a mate
2. Learning to live with a partner
3. Starting a family
4. Rearing children
5. Managing a home
6. Getting started in an occupation
7. Taking on civic responsibility
8. Finding a congenial social group

Middle Age
1. Achieving adult civic and social responsibility
2. Establishing and maintaining an economic standard of living
3. Assisting teenage children to become responsible and happy adults
4. Developing adult leisure-time activities
5. Relating oneself to one's spouse as a person
6. Accepting and adjusting to the physiologic changes of middle age
7. Adjusting to aging parents

Later Maturity
1. Adjusting to decreasing physical strength and health
2. Adjusting to retirement and reduced income
3. Adjusting to death of a spouse
4. Establishing an explicit affiliation with one's age group
5. Meeting social and civil obligations
6. Establishing satisfactory physical living arrangements

Source: Havighurst, R. J. (1972). *Developmental tasks and education.* (3rd ed.). Boston, MA: Allyn and Bacon. Copyright © 1972 Pearson Education. Reprinted by permission of the publisher.

experience feelings of worthlessness unless they derive their sense of identity from a sufficient number of roles that one such role can replace the work role or occupation as a source of self-esteem. For example, a man who likes to garden or golf can obtain ego rewards from those activities, replacing rewards formerly obtained from his occupation.

2. **Body transcendence versus body preoccupation.** This task calls for the individual to adjust to decreasing physical capacities and at the same time maintain feelings of well-being. Preoccupation with declining body functions reduces happiness and satisfaction with life.

3. **Ego transcendence versus ego preoccupation.** Ego transcendence is the acceptance without fear of one's death as inevitable. This acceptance includes being actively involved in one's own future beyond death. Ego preoccupation, by contrast, results in holding onto life and a preoccupation with self-gratification.

GOULD (1935–) Roger Gould is another theorist who has studied adult development. He believes that transformation is a central theme during adulthood: "Adults continue to change over the period of time considered to be adulthood

and developmental phases may be found during the adult span of life" (Gould, 1972, p. 33). According to Gould, the 20s is the time when a person assumes new roles, in the 30s role confusion often occurs, in the 40s the person becomes aware of time limitations in relation to accomplishing life's goals, and in the 50s the acceptance of each stage as a natural progression of life marks the path to adult maturity.

- **Stage 1 (ages 16–18).** Individuals consider themselves part of the family rather than individuals; they begin to want to separate from their parents.
- **Stage 2 (ages 18–22).** Although individuals have established autonomy, they feel it is in jeopardy; they feel they could be pulled back into their families.
- **Stage 3 (ages 22–28).** Individuals feel established as adults and autonomous from their families. They see themselves as well-defined but still feel the need to prove themselves to their parents. They see this as the time for growing and building for the future.
- **Stage 4 (ages 29–34).** Marriage and careers are well established. Individuals question what life is all about and wish to be accepted as they are, no longer finding it necessary to prove themselves.

- **Stage 5 (ages 35–43).** This is a period of self-reflection. Individuals question long-held values as well as life itself. They see time as finite, with little time left to shape the lives of adolescent children.
- **Stage 6 (ages 43–50).** Personalities are seen as set. Time is accepted as finite. Individuals are interested in social activities with friends and spouse and desire both sympathy and affection from spouse.
- **Stage 7 (ages 50–60).** This is a period of transformation, with a realization of mortality and a concern for health. There is an increase in warmth and a decrease in negativism. The spouse is seen as a valuable companion (Gould, 1972, pp. 525–527).

JUNG'S THEORY OF INDIVIDUALISM This theory hypothesizes that as a person ages, the shift of focus is away from the external world (extroversion) toward the inner experience (introversion). At this stage of life, the older person will search for answers to many of life's riddles and try to find the essence of the "true self." To age successfully, the older person will accept past accomplishments and failures (Jung, 1960). Older persons subscribing to Jung's theory may spend a lot of time in contemplation and introspection.

DISENGAGEMENT THEORY Introduced by Cummings and Henry in 1961, this controversial theory asserts that the appropriate pattern of behavior in later life is for the older person and society at large to engage in a mutual and reciprocal withdrawal. Thus, when death occurs, neither the older individual nor society is disadvantaged, and social equilibrium is maintained. Mandatory retirement forces some older people to withdraw from work-related roles, accelerating the process of disengagement. In some cultures, older people remain engaged, active, and busy throughout their lives.

CONTINUITY THEORY This theory advances the idea that successful aging involves maintaining or continuing previous values, habits, preferences, family ties, and all other linkages that have formed the basic underlying structure of adult life. Older age is not viewed as a time that should trigger major life readjustment, but rather as just a time to continue being the same person (Havighurst et al., 1963). According to this theory, the pace of activities may be slowed. The older person may drop activities pursued in earlier life that did not bring satisfaction and genuine happiness. For some, relief from constant time pressures and deadlines is one of the benefits of old age.

Piaget's Theory of Cognitive Development

Cognitive development refers to the manner in which people learn to think, reason, and use language. It involves a person's intelligence, perceptual ability, and ability to process information. Cognitive development represents a progression of mental abilities from illogical to logical thinking, from simple to complex problem solving, and from understanding concrete ideas to understanding abstract concepts.

The most widely known cognitive theorist is Jean Piaget. His theory of cognitive development has contributed to other theories, such as Kohlberg's moral development and Fowler's development of faith theories, both discussed in this chapter.

According to Piaget (1966), cognitive development is an orderly, sequential process in which a variety of new experiences (stimuli) must exist before intellectual abilities can develop. Piaget divides cognitive development into five major phases: the sensorimotor phase, the preconceptual phase, the intuitive thought phase, the concrete operations phase, and the formal operations phase. A detailed discussion of these phases, and how the nurse can incorporate his or her knowledge of them into nursing plans and interventions, can be found in the Cognition concept.

A person develops through each of these phases; each phase has its own unique characteristics (Table 3–5). In each phase, the person uses three primary abilities: assimilation, accommodation, and adaptation. **Assimilation** is the process through which humans encounter and react to new situations by using the mechanisms they already possess. In this way, people acquire knowledge and skills as well as insights into the world around them. **Accommodation** is a process of change whereby cognitive processes mature sufficiently to allow the person to solve problems that were unsolvable before. This adjustment is possible chiefly because new knowledge has been assimilated. **Adaptation**, or coping behavior, is the ability to handle the demands made by the environment.

Nurses can use Piaget's theory of cognitive development when developing teaching strategies. For example, a nurse can expect a toddler to be egocentric and literal; therefore, explanations to the toddler should focus on the needs of the toddler rather than on the needs of others. A 13-year-old can be expected to use rational thinking and to reason; therefore, when explaining the need for a medication, a nurse can outline the consequences of taking and not taking the medication, enabling the adolescent to make a rational decision. Nurses must remember, however, that the range of normal cognitive development is broad, despite the ages arbitrarily associated with each level. When teaching adults, nurses may become aware that some adults are more comfortable with concrete thought and are slower to acquire and apply new information than are other adults.

Behaviorism

Behaviorist theory states that learning takes place when an individual's reaction to a stimulus is either positively or negatively reinforced. The more rapid, consistent, and positive the reinforcement, the more likely a behavior is to be learned and retained.

B.F. Skinner believed that organisms learn as they respond to or "operate on" their environment. His research led to the concept of *operant conditioning*, in which he maintained that rewarded or reinforced behavior will be repeated; behavior that is punished will be suppressed. Most of his work was with laboratory animals.

Social Learning Theory

Albert Bandura (1925–), a contemporary psychologist, believes that children learn attitudes, beliefs, customs, and values through their social contacts with adults and other children. Children imitate (or model) the behavior they see; if the behavior is positively reinforced, they tend to repeat it. However, Bandura also believes that people can consciously choose how

TABLE 3–5 Piaget's Phases of Cognitive Development

PHASES AND STAGES	AGE	SIGNIFICANT BEHAVIOR
Sensorimotor phase	Birth to 2 years	
Stage 1: Use of reflexes	Birth to 1 month	Most action is reflexive.
Stage 2: Primary circular reaction	1 to 4 months	Perception of events is centered on the body. Objects are extension of self.
Stage 3: Secondary circular reaction	4 to 8 months	The external environment is acknowledged. Changes in the environment are actively made.
Stage 4: Coordination of secondary schemata	8 to 12 months	A goal can be distinguished from a means of attaining it.
Stage 5: Tertiary circular reaction	12 to 18 months	Individual tries and discovers new goals and ways to attain goals. Rituals are important.
Stage 6: Inventions of new means	18 to 24 months	Individual interprets the environment by mental image; uses make-believe and pretend play.
Preconceptual phase	2 to 4 years	Individual uses an egocentric approach to accommodate the demands of an environment. Everything is significant and relates to "me." Individual explores the environment. Language development is rapid. Words are associated with objects.
Intuitive thought phase	4 to 7 years	Egocentric thinking diminishes. Individual thinks of one idea at a time, includes others in the environment. Words express thoughts.
Concrete operations phase	7 to 11 years	Individual solves concrete problems; begins to understand relationships such as size; understands right and left; is cognizant of viewpoints.
Formal operations phase	11 to 15 years	Individual uses rational thinking. Reasoning is deductive and futuristic.

Source: Adapted from Piaget, J. (1966). *The origin of intelligence.* Copyright © 1966 International Universities Press, Inc. Reprinted with permission.

to act, such as deciding to handle problems by talking rather than using violence. The external environment (the behavior of others) and the child's internal processes are both key elements in the behaviors the child manifests (Bandura, 1986, 1997a).

Bandura believes that an important determinant of behavior is **self-efficacy**, or the expectation that someone can produce a desired outcome. For example, if adolescents believe they can avoid use of drugs or alcohol, they are more likely to do so. A child who has confidence in his or her ability to exercise regularly or lose weight has a greater chance of success with these behavior changes. Parents who have confidence in their ability to care adequately for their infants are more likely to do so (Bandura, 1997b).

 EVIDENCE-BASED PRACTICE **Self-Efficacy**

Clinical Question
Nurses often provide information for parents and children that will encourage them to adopt healthy lifestyles. Providing information may not be enough; many of us know about healthy behaviors but do not consistently apply them. The concept of self-efficacy helps to explain why some people take on healthy behaviors, whereas others do not. People who are convinced they can make a positive change are more likely to do so. A number of research projects test and apply self-efficacy in teaching about health. Two examples follow.

Evidence
A federally funded study sought to measure the effectiveness of a preventive parent training program among low-income families with small children. The weekly sessions involved viewing a videotape and discussing positive and negative parenting skills observed. The researchers compared characteristics of the parents who chose to attend the sessions, including a measure of parental self-efficacy, or belief that they could manage a range of tasks and situations in caring for their young children. Parents with lower self-efficacy scores were significantly more likely to enroll in and attend the parenting training sessions (Garvey, Julion, Fogg, et al., 2006).

Mothers who have a greater degree of self-efficacy about their ability to breastfeed are significantly more likely to begin and to continue breastfeeding. A Breastfeeding Self-Efficacy Scale has been developed to identify both risk and protective factors that influence the self-efficacy of new mothers. Educational level, support from other women, quality of postpartum care, maternal anxiety, and plans made for feeding method all influence the breastfeeding self-efficacy scores of women (Dennis, 2006).

Best Practice
In addition to providing information about health behaviors, nurses need to integrate methods to increase self-efficacy in teaching projects with families. Assessments should be designed to identify self-efficacy of parents and children around health topics of interest. Interventions can then be planned to enhance the self-efficacy of family members.

Critical Thinking
Nurses can apply the concept of self-efficacy in teaching children and families.
1. Plan a teaching project for school-age children to foster healthy eating. Include expected outcomes for the children and interventions.
2. Could your outcome be improved if you focus not just on getting the content across, but also on increasing the belief and confidence that the children will be able to integrate the new behaviors into their lives?
3. What activities could your teaching plan include that would be likely to improve the self-efficacy of these school-age children?

TABLE 3–6 Nine Parameters of Personality—Chess and Thomas

PARAMETER	DESCRIPTION	SCORING
Activity level	Degree of motion during eating, playing, sleeping, bathing	High, medium, or low
Rhythmicity	Regularity of schedule maintained for sleep, hunger, elimination	Regular, variable, or irregular
Approach or withdrawal	Response to a new stimulus such as a food, activity, or person	Approachable, variable, or withdrawn
Adaptability	Degree of adaptation to new situations	Adaptive, variable, or nonadaptive
Threshold of responsiveness	Intensity of stimulation needed to elicit a response to sensory input, objects in the environment, or people	High, medium, or low
Intensity of reaction	Degree of response to situations	Positive, variable, or negative
Quality of mood	Predominant mood during daily activity and in response to stimuli	Positive, variable, or negative
Distractibility	Ability of environmental stimuli to interfere with the child's activity	Distractible, variable, or nondistractible
Attention span and persistence	Amount of time devoted to activities (compared with other children of the same age) and the degree of ability to stick with an activity in spite of obstacles	Persistent, variable, or nonpersistent

Source: Data from Chess, S., & Thomas, A. (1996). *Temperament: Theory and practice.* Philadelphia: Brunner/Mazel Publishers.

Temperament Theory

Chess and Thomas (1995, 1996) recognize the innate qualities of personality that each individual brings to the events of daily life. They view the child as an individual who both influences and is influenced by the environment. However, Chess and Thomas focus on one specific aspect of development—the wide spectrum of behaviors possible in children, identifying nine parameters of response to daily events (Table 3–6). Infants generally display clusters of responses, which Chess and Thomas have classified into three major personality types (Box 3–1). Although most children do not demonstrate all behaviors described for a particular type, they usually show a grouping indicative of one personality type (Chess & Thomas, 1995, 1996).

Box 3–1 Patterns of Temperament—Chess and Thomas

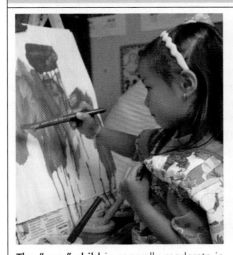 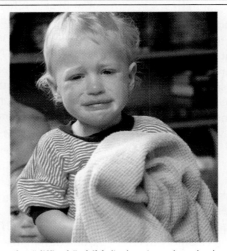 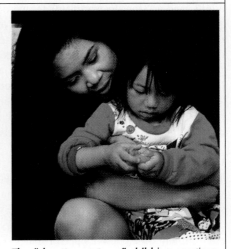

The **"easy" child** is generally moderate in activity; shows regularity in patterns of eating, sleeping, and elimination; and is usually positive in mood and when subjected to new stimuli. The easy child adapts to new situations and is able to accept rules and work well with others. About 40% of children in the New York Longitudinal Study displayed this personality type.

The **"difficult" child** displays irregular schedules for eating, sleeping, and elimination; adapts slowly to new situations and persons; and displays a predominantly negative mood. Intense reactions to the environment are common. The New York Longitudinal Study found that approximately 10% of children display this personality type.

The **"slow-to-warm-up" child** has reactions of mild intensity and is slow to adapt to new situations. The child displays initial withdrawal followed by gradual, quiet, and slow interactions with the environment. About 15% of children in the New York Longitudinal Study displayed this personality type.

The remaining 35% of children studied showed some characteristics of each personality type.

Source: Ball, J. W., Bindler, R. C., & Cowen, K. J. (2010). *Child health nursing: Partnering with children and families* (2nd ed.). Upper Saddle River, NJ: Pearson Education.

Longitudinal research has demonstrated that personality characteristics displayed during infancy are often consistent with those seen later in life. The ability to predict future characteristics is not possible, however, because of the complex and dynamic interaction of personality traits and environmental reactions.

Resiliency Theory

Why do some children have such different behavioral outcomes from others coming from similar backgrounds? A theory that examines the individual's characteristics as well as the interaction of these characteristics with the environment is the resiliency model. **Resilience** is the ability to function with healthy responses, even when experiencing significant stress and adversity (Stewart, Reid, & Mangham, 1997). In this model, the individual or family members experience a crisis that provides a source of stress, and the family interprets or deals with the crisis based on resources available. Families and individuals have **protective factors** that provide strength and assistance in dealing with crises and **risk factors** that promote or contribute to their challenges. Risk and protective factors can be identified in children, in their families, and in their communities. A typical crisis for a young child might be a transfer to a new child care provider. Protective factors for a child transferring to a new provider could involve past positive experiences with new people and an "easy" temperament. An additional protective factor might be the level of understanding the new child care provider has about the adaptation needs of young children to new experiences. Risk factors for a child experiencing this type of transition might include repeated moves to new care providers, limited close relationships with adults, and a "slow-to-warm-up" temperament.

Once confronted by a crisis, the child and family first experience the **adjustment phase**. This phase is characterized by disorganization and unsuccessful attempts at meeting the crisis. In the **adaptation phase**, the child and family meet the challenge and use resources to deal with the crisis (Malone, 1998). Adaptation may lead to increasing resilience, as the child and family learn about new resources and inner strengths and develop the ability to deal more effectively with future crises.

Ecologic Theory

The relative importance in human development of heredity versus environment—or nature versus nurture—is controversial among theorists. **Nature** refers to the genetic or hereditary capability of an individual. **Nurture** refers to the effects of the environment on a person's performance. Contemporary developmental theories increasingly recognize the interaction of nature and nurture in determining the child's development.

The ecologic theory of development was formulated by Urie Bronfenbrenner to explain the child's unique relationship in all of life's settings, from close to remote (Bronfenbrenner, 1986, 2005; Bronfenbrenner, McClelland, Ceci, Moen, & Wethington, 1996). **Ecologic theory** emphasizes the presence of mutual interactions between the child and these various settings. Neither nature nor nurture is considered more important. Bronfenbrenner believes each child brings a unique set of genes—and specific attributes such as age, gender, health, and other characteristics—to his or her interactions with the environment. The child then interacts in many settings at different levels or systems (Figure 3–4 ■). The five systems of ecologic theory are microsystem, mesosystem, exosystem, macrosystem, and chronosystem.

MICROSYSTEM This level is defined as the daily, consistent, close relationships such as home, child care, school, friends, and neighbors. For the child with a chronic illness requiring regular care, the health care providers may even be part of the microsystem. In the ecologic model, the child influences each of these settings in addition to being influenced by them, with reciprocal interactions.

MESOSYSTEM This level includes relationships of microsystems with one another. For example, two microsystems for most children are the home and the school. The relationships between these microsystems are shown by parents' involvement in their children's school. This involvement, in turn, influences the effects of both the home and school settings on the children.

EXOSYSTEM This level of ecologic theory is composed of those settings that influence the child even though the child is not in close daily contact with the system. Examples are the parents' jobs and the governing board of the local school district. Although the child may not go to the parents' workplaces, he or she can be influenced by policies related to health care, sick leave, inflexible work hours, overtime, travel, or even the mood of the boss (through its impact on the parent). The child's needs may influence a parent to give up a certain job or to work harder to obtain money for the child's education. Likewise, when a local school board votes to ban certain books or to finance a field trip, the child is influenced by these decisions; the child, in turn, can help establish an atmosphere that will guide future school board decisions.

MACROSYSTEM This level includes the beliefs, values, and behaviors expressed in the child's environment. Culture is a powerful influence on the macrosystem, as is the political system. For instance, a democratic system creates different beliefs, values, and even eating practices from those of an anarchic system.

CHRONOSYSTEM This final level brings the perspective of time to the previous settings. The time period during which the child grows up influences views of health and illness. For example, the experiences of children with influenza in the 19th versus 20th centuries were quite different.

Moral Theories

Moral development, a complex process not fully understood, involves learning what one should and should not do. It is more than merely the imprinting of parents' rules and virtues or values on children. The term **moral** means "relating to right and wrong." The terms *morality, moral behavior,* and *moral development* need to be distinguished from each other. **Morality** refers to the requirements necessary for people to live together in society, **moral behavior** is the way a person perceives and responds to those requirements, and **moral development** is the pattern of change in moral behavior with age.

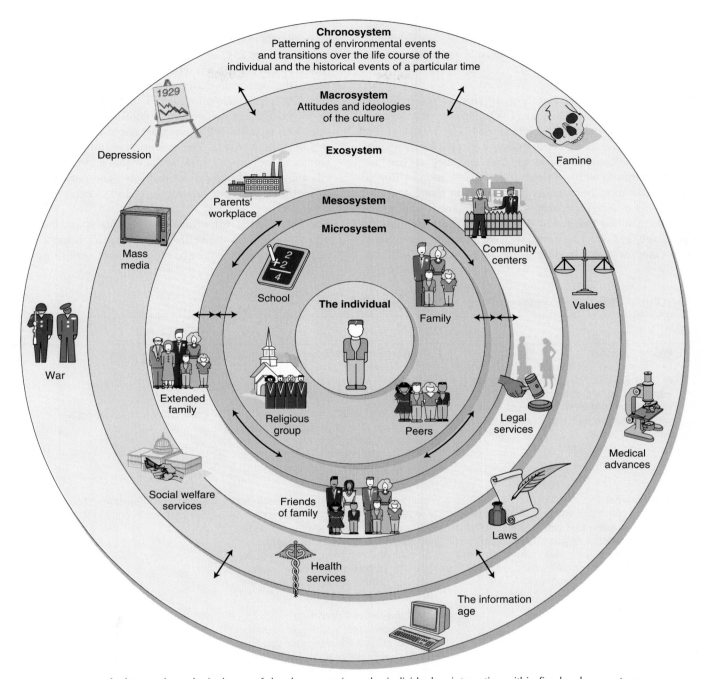

Figure 3–4 ■ Bronfenbrenner's ecologic theory of development views the individual as interacting within five levels or systems.

Source: Redrawn from Santrock, J. W. (2005). *Life span development.* Madison, WI: Brown & Benchmark. Based on Bronfenbrenner's (1979, 1986) works in Contexts of child rearing: Problems and prospects. *American Psychologist, 34,* 844–850; Ecology of the family as a context for human development: Research perspectives. *Developmental Psychology, 22,* 723–742.

KOHLBERG (1927–1987) Lawrence Kohlberg's theory specifically addresses moral development in children and adults (Kohlberg, 1981, 1984). The morality of an individual's decision was not Kohlberg's concern; rather, he focused on the reasons an individual makes a decision. According to Kohlberg, moral development progresses through three levels and six stages. Levels and stages are not always linked to a certain developmental stage, because some people progress to a higher level of moral development than others.

At Kohlberg's first level, called the *premoral* or *preconventional level,* children are responsive to cultural rules and labels of good and bad, right and wrong. However, children interpret these in terms of the consequences of their actions—punishment or reward. At the second level, the *conventional level,* the individual is concerned about maintaining the expectations of the family, group, or nation, and sees this as right. The emphasis at this level is on conformity and loyalty to one's own expectations as well as society's. Level III is called the *postconventional, autonomous*, or *principled level*. At this level, people make an effort to define valid values and principles without regard to outside authority or to the expectations of others (Table 3–7).

GILLIGAN (1936–) After more than 10 years of research with female subjects, Carol Gilligan (1982) reported that women often consider the dilemmas Kohlberg used in his research to be irrelevant. Women scored consistently lower on Kohlberg's scale of moral development despite the fact that they approached moral dilemmas with considerable sophistication. Gilligan believed that most frameworks for research in moral development do not include the concepts of caring and responsibility.

Gilligan found that moral development proceeds through three levels and two transitions, with each level representing a more complex understanding of the relationship of self and others and each transition resulting in a crucial reevaluation of the conflict between selfish and responsibility (Murray & Zentner, 2001, p. 251).

Stage 1: Caring for oneself In this first stage of development, the person is concerned only with caring for the self. The individual feels isolated, alone, and unconnected to others. There is no concern or conflict with the needs of others because the self is the most important. The focus of this stage is survival. The transition of this stage occurs when the individual begins to view this approach as selfish and moves toward responsibility. The person begins to realize a need for relationships and connections with other people.

Stage 2: Caring for others During this stage, the individual recognizes the selfishness of earlier behavior and begins to understand the need for caring relationships with

TABLE 3–7 Kohlberg's Stages of Moral Development

LEVEL	STAGE	AVERAGE AGE
I. Preconventional Person is responsive to cultural rules of labels of good and bad, right or wrong. Externally established rules determine right or wrong actions. Person reasons in terms of punishment, reward, or exchange of favors. **Egocentric focus**	**1. Punishment and Obedient Orientation** Fear of punishment, not respect for authority, is the reason for decisions, behavior, and conformity.	Toddler to 7 years
	2. Instrumental Relativist Orientation Conformity is based on egocentricity and narcissistic needs. There is no feeling of justice, loyalty, or gratitude. "I'll do something if I get something for it or because it pleases you."	Preschooler through school age
II. Conventional Person is concerned with maintaining expectations and rules of the family, group, nation, or society. A sense of guilt has developed and affects behavior. The person values conformity, loyalty, and active maintenance of social order and control. Conformity means good behavior or what pleases or helps another and is approved. **Societal focus**	**3. Interpersonal Concordance Orientation** Decisions and behavior are based on concerns about others' reactions; the person wants others' approval or a reward. An empathic response, based on understanding of how another person feels, is a determinant for decisions and behavior. ("I can put myself in your shoes.")	School age through adulthood (Most American women are in this stage.)
	4. Law-and-Order Orientation The person wants established rules from authorities, and the reason for decisions and behavior is that social and sexual rules and traditions demand the response. ("I'll do something because it's the law and my duty.")	Adolescence and adulthood (Most men are in this stage.)
III. Postconventional The person lives autonomously and defines moral values and principles that are distinct from personal identification with group values. He or she lives according to principles that are universally agreed on and that the person considers appropriate for life. **Universal focus**	**5. Social Contract Legalistic Orientation** The social rules are not the sole basis for decisions and behavior because the person believes a higher moral principle applies, such as equality, justice, or due process.	Middle-aged or older adult Only 20% or fewer of Americans achieve this stage.
	6. Universal Ethical Principle Orientation Decisions and behaviors are based on internalized rules, on conscience rather than social laws, and on self-chosen ethical and abstract principles that are universal, comprehensive, and consistent.	Middle-aged or older adult Few people attain or maintain this stage. Examples of this stage are seen in times of crisis or extreme situations.

Source: Murray, R. B., Zentner, J. P., & Yakimo, R. (2009). *Health promotion strategies through the life span* (pp. 32–33). Upper Saddle River, NJ: Pearson Prentice Hall. Adapted with permission.

others. Caring relationships bring with them responsibility. The definition of responsibility includes self-sacrifice, where "good" is considered to be "caring for others." The individual now approaches relationships with a focus on not hurting others. This approach causes the individual to be more responsive and submissive to others' needs, often to the exclusion of meeting one's own needs. A transition from goodness to truth occurs when the individual recognizes that the lack of balance between caring for oneself and caring for others in this approach can cause difficulties with relationships. The woman makes decisions on personal intentions and consequences of actions rather than on how she thinks others will react (Murray & Zentner, 2001, p. 253).

Stage 3: Caring for self and others During this last stage, a person sees the need for a balance between caring for others and caring for the self. The concept of responsibility now includes responsibility for the self and for other people. Care remains the focus on which decisions are based. However, the person recognizes the interconnections between the self and others and realizes that if one's own needs are not met, other people may also suffer.

Gilligan (1982) believes that because women often see morality in the integrity of relationships and caring, the moral problems they encounter are different from those of men. Men tend to consider what is right to be what is just, whereas for women what is right is taking responsibility for others as a self-chosen decision (p. 140). The ethic of justice, or fairness, is based on the idea of equality: Everyone should receive the same treatment. This is the development path usually followed by men and widely accepted by moral theorists. By contrast, the ethic of care is based on the premise of nonviolence: No one should be harmed. This is the path typically followed by women but given little attention in the literature of moral theory.

In discussing the development of maturity, Gilligan (1982) stated that both viewpoints blend "in the realization that just as inequality adversely affects both perspectives in an unequal relationship, so too violence is destructive for everyone involved" (p. 174). The blending of these two perspectives could give rise to a new view of human development and a better understanding of human relations.

Spiritual Theories

The spiritual component of growth and development refers to individuals' understanding of their relationship with the universe and their perceptions about the direction and meaning of life.

FOWLER James Fowler describes the development of faith as a force that gives meaning to a person's life. He uses the term *faith* as a form of knowing, a way of being in relation to "an ultimate environment." To Fowler, "faith is a relational phenomenon; it is an active 'mode-of-being-in-relation' to another or others in which we invest commitment, belief, love, risk and hope" (Fowler & Keen, 1985, p. 18). Fowler's stages in the development of faith are described in Table 3–8.

Fowler's theory and developmental stages were influenced by the work of Piaget, Kohlberg, and Erikson. Fowler believes that the development of faith is an interactive process between the individual and his or her environment (Fowler, Streib, & Keller, 2004). In each of Fowler's stages, new patterns of thought, values, and beliefs are added to those the individual already holds; therefore, the stages must follow in sequence. Faith stages, according to Fowler, are separate from Piaget's cognitive stages: They evolve from a combination of knowledge and values.

WESTERHOFF (1933–) John Westerhoff describes faith as a way of being and behaving that evolves from an experienced faith, guided by parents and others during a person's infancy and childhood, to an owned faith that is internalized in adulthood and serves as a directive for personal action (Table 3–9). For the client who is ill, faith—whether in a higher authority (e.g., God, Allah, Jehovah), in the client's own self, in the health care team, or in a combination of all—provides strength and trust.

TABLE 3–8 **Fowler's Stages of Spiritual Development**

STAGE	AGE	DESCRIPTION
0. Undifferentiated	0 to 3 years	Infant unable to formulate concepts about self or the environment
1. Intuitive-projective	4 to 6 years	A combination of images and beliefs given by trusted others, mixed with the child's own experience and imagination
2. Mythic-literal	7 to 12 years	Private world of fantasy and wonder; symbols referring to something specific; dramatic stories and myths used to communicate spiritual meanings
3. Synthetic-conventional	Adolescent or adult	World and ultimate environment structured by the expectations and judgments of others; interpersonal focus
4. Individuating-reflexive	After 18 years	Constructing one's own explicit system; high degree of self-consciousness
5. Paradoxical-consolidative	After 30 years	Awareness of truth from a variety of viewpoints
6. Universalizing	Maybe never	Becoming an incarnation of the principles of love and justice

Source: Fowler, J., & Keen, S. (1985). *Life maps: Conversations in the journey of faith.* Waco, TX: Word Books; and Hollander, A. (1980). *How to help your child have a spiritual life: A parents' guide to inner development.* New York: A and W Publishers. Adapted with permission.

TABLE 3–9 Westerhoff's Four Stages of Faith

STAGE	AGE	BEHAVIOR
Experienced faith	Infancy/early adolescence	Experiences faith through interaction with others who are living a particular faith tradition
Affiliative faith	Late adolescence	Actively participates in activities that characterize a particular faith tradition; experiences awe and wonderment; feels a sense of belonging
Searching faith	Young adulthood	Through a process of questioning and doubting own faith, acquires a cognitive as well as an affective faith
Owned faith	Middle adulthood/old age	Puts faith into personal and social action and is willing to stand up for what the individual believes, even against the nurturing community

Source: Westerhoff, J. *Will our children have faith?* (1976). New York: Seabury Press. Reprinted with permission from the author.

GROWTH AND DEVELOPMENT

Nurses use information about developmental milestones to assess children, to identify those with delays, and to plan interventions that will foster development. To do so requires a comprehensive understanding of expected physical growth and development, cognitive abilities, and psychosocial characteristics (Fine & Mayer, 2006; Johnson & Marlow, 2006). Potential risks—such as prematurity, international adoption, and presence of health problems—necessitate a more frequent and in-depth assessment of observed milestones. Nurses compare the expected findings with assessment results, making referrals for further evaluation when appropriate, and using the results to plan nursing interventions.

INFANT (BIRTH TO 1 YEAR)

Can you imagine tripling your present weight in a single year? Or becoming proficient in understanding fundamental words in a new language and even speaking a few? These and many more accomplishments take place in the first year of life. Starting as a mainly reflexive creature, the infant can walk and communicate by the year's end. Never again in life is development so swift.

Physical Growth and Development

The first year of life is one of rapid change for the infant. The infant's birth weight usually doubles by about 5 months and triples by the end of the first year (Figure 3–5 ■).

Height increases by approximately 1 foot during this year. Teeth begin to erupt at about 6 months, and by the end of the first year, the infant has six to eight deciduous teeth. Physical growth is closely associated with type and quality of feeding.

Body organs and systems, although not fully mature at 1 year of age, function differently than they did at birth. Kidney and liver maturation helps the 1-year-old excrete drugs or other toxic substances more readily than in the first weeks of life. The changing body proportions mirror changes in developing internal organs. Maturation of the nervous system is demonstrated by increased control over body movements, enabling the infant to sit, stand, and walk. Sensory function also increases as the infant begins to discriminate visual images, sounds, and tastes (Table 3–10).

Cognitive Development

The brain continues to increase in complexity during the first year of life. Most of the growth involves maturation of cells, with only a small increase in cell number. This growth of the brain is accompanied by development of its functions. One has only to compare the behavior of an infant shortly after birth with that of a 1-year-old to understand the incredible maturation of brain function. The newborn's eyes widen in response to sound; the 1-year-old turns to the sound and recognizes its significance. The 2-month-old cries and coos; the 1-year-old

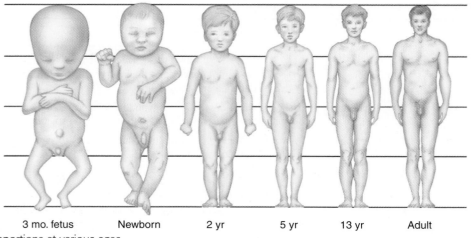

	3 mo. fetus	Newborn	2 yr	5 yr	13 yr	Adult

Figure 3–5 ■ Body proportions at various ages.

TABLE 3–10 Growth and Development Milestones During Infancy

AGE	PHYSICAL GROWTH	FINE MOTOR ABILITY	GROSS MOTOR ABILITY	SENSORY ABILITY
Birth to 1 month	Gains 5–7 oz (140–200 g)/ week. Grows 1.5 cm (1/2 in.) in first month. Head circumference increases 1.5 cm (1/2 in.)/month.	Holds hand in fist. Draws arms and legs to body when crying.	Inborn reflexes such as startle and rooting are predominant activity. May lift head briefly if prone. Alerts to high-pitched voices. Comforts with touch.	Prefers to look at faces and black-and-white geometric designs. Follows objects in line of vision.
2 to 4 months	Gains 5–7 oz (140–200 g)/ week. Grows 1.5 cm (1/2 in.)/ month. Head circumference increases 1.5 cm (1/2 in.)/month. Posterior fontanel closes. Eats 120 mL/kg/24 h (2 oz/lb/24 h).	Holds rattle when placed in hand. Looks at and plays with own fingers. Brings hands to midline.	Moro reflex fading in strength. Can turn from side to back and then return. Head lag when pulled to sitting position decreases; sits with head held in midline with some bobbing. When prone, holds head and supports weight on forearms.	Follows objects 180 degrees. Turns head to look for voices and sounds.
4 to 6 months	Gains 5–7 oz (140–200 g)/ week. Doubles birth weight 5–6 months. Grows 1.5 cm (1/2 in.)/month. Head circumference increases 1.5 cm (1/2 in.)/month. Teeth may begin erupting by 6 months. Eats 100 mL/kg/24 h (1 1/2 oz/lb/24 h).	Grasps rattles and other objects at will; drops them to pick up another offered object. Mouths objects. Holds feet and pulls to mouth. Holds bottle. Grasps with whole hand (palmar grasp). Manipulates objects.	Holds head steady when sitting. Has no head lag when pulled to sitting. Turns from abdomen to back by 4 months and then back to abdomen by 6 months. When held standing supports much of own weight.	Examines complex visual images. Watches the course of a falling object. Responds readily to sounds.
6 to 8 months	Gains 3–5 oz (85–140 g)/ week. Grows 1 cm (3/8 in.)/month. Growth rate slower than first 6 months.	Bangs objects held in hands. Transfers objects from one hand to the other. Pincer grasp begins at times.	Most inborn reflexes extinguished. Sits alone steadily without support by 8 months. Likes to bounce on legs when held in standing position.	Recognizes own name and responds by looking and smiling. Enjoys small and complex objects at play.
8 to 10 months	Gains 3–5 oz (85–140 g)/ week. Grows 1 cm (3/8 in.)/month.	Picks up small objects. Uses pincer grasp well.	Crawls or pulls whole body along floor by arms. Creeps by using hands and knees to keep trunk off floor. Pulls self to standing and sitting by 10 months. Recovers balance when sitting.	Understands words such as "no" and "cracker." May say one word in addition to "mama" and "dada." Recognizes sound without difficulty.
10 to 12 months	Gains 3–5 oz (85–140 g)/ week. Grows 1 cm (3/8 in.)/month. Head circumference equals chest circumference. Triples birth weight by 1 year.	May hold crayon or pencil and make mark on paper. Places objects into containers through holes.	Stands alone. Walks holding onto furniture. Sits down from standing.	Plays peek-a-boo and patty cake.

Source: Ball, J. W., & Bindler, R. C., (2008). *Pediatric nursing: Caring for children* (4th ed., p. 83). Upper Saddle River, NJ: Pearson Education.

says a few words and understands many more. The 6-week-old grasps a rattle for the first time; the 1-year-old reaches for toys and begins to feed himself or herself.

The infant's behaviors provide clues about thought processes. Piaget's work outlines the infant's actions in a set of rapidly progressing changes in the first year of life. The infant receives stimulation through sight, sound, and feeling, which the maturing brain interprets. This input from the environment interacts with internal cognitive abilities to enhance cognitive functioning.

Psychosocial Development

The infant relies on interactions with primary care providers to meet needs and then begins to establish a sense of trust in other adults and in children. As trust develops, the infant becomes comfortable in interactions with a widening array of people.

PLAY An 8-month-old infant is sitting on the floor, grasping blocks and banging them on the floor. When a parent walks by, the infant laughs and waves hands and feet wildly (Figure 3–6 ■). The infant plays primarily alone with toys (**solitary play**) but enjoys the presence of adults or other children. Physical capabilities enable the infant to move toward and reach for objects of interest.

Cognitive ability is reflected in manipulation of the blocks to create different sounds. Social interaction enhances play. The presence of a parent or other person increases interest in surroundings and teaches the infant different ways to play.

The play of infants begins in a reflexive manner. When infants move extremities or grasp objects, they experience the foundations of play. They gain pleasure from the feel and sound of these activities, and gradually perform them purposefully. For example, when a parent places a rattle in the hand of a 6-week-old infant, the infant grasps it reflexively. As the hands move randomly, the rattle makes an enjoyable sound. The infant learns to move the rattle to create the sound and then finally to grasp the toy at will to play with it.

The next phase of infant play focuses on manipulative behavior. The infant examines toys closely, looking at them, touching them, and placing them in his or her mouth. The infant learns a great deal about texture, qualities of objects, and all aspects of the surroundings. At the same time, interaction with others becomes an important part of play. The social nature of play is obvious as the infant plays with other children and adults.

Toward the end of the first year, the infant's ability to move in space enlarges the sphere of play. Once infants

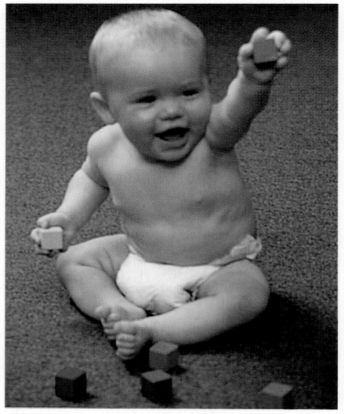

Figure 3–6 ■ Garrett shows us that an 8-month-old child can play with blocks, demonstrating physical, cognitive, and social capabilities.

crawl or walk, they can get to new places, find new toys, discover forgotten objects, or seek out other people for interaction. Play is a reflection of every aspect of development, as well as a method for enhancing learning and maturation (Table 3–11).

TABLE 3–11 Psychosocial Development During Infancy

AGE	PLAY AND TOYS	COMMUNICATION
Birth to 3 months	■ Prefers visual stimuli of mobiles, black-and-white patterns, mirrors ■ Responds to auditory stimuli such as music boxes, tape players, soft voices ■ Responds to rocking and cuddling ■ Moves legs and arms while adult sings and talks ■ Likes varying stimuli—different rooms, sounds, visual images	■ Coos ■ Babbles ■ Cries
3 to 6 months	■ Prefers noise-making objects that are easily grasped like rattles ■ Enjoys stuffed animals and soft toys with contrasting colors	■ Vocalizes during play and with familiar people ■ Laughs ■ Cries less ■ Squeals and makes pleasure sounds ■ Babbles multisyllabically (mamamamama)
6 to 9 months	■ Likes teething toys ■ Increasingly desires social interaction with adults and other children ■ Favors soft toys that can be manipulated and mouthed	■ Increases vowel and consonant sounds ■ Links syllables together ■ Uses speechlike rhythm when vocalizing with others
9 to 12 months	■ Enjoys large blocks, toys that pop apart and go back together, nesting cups and other objects ■ Laughs at surprise toys like jack-in-the-box ■ Plays interactive games like peek-a-boo ■ Uses push-and-pull toys	■ Understands "no" and other simple commands ■ Says "dada" and "mama" to identify parents ■ Learns one or two other words ■ Receptive speech surpasses expressive speech

Source: Ball, J. W., & Bindler, R. C., (2008). *Pediatric nursing: Caring for children* (4th ed., p. 87). Upper Saddle River, NJ: Pearson Education.

FOCUS ON DIVERSITY AND CULTURE
Reaching Developmental Milestones

In traditional Native American families, children are allowed to unfold and develop naturally at their own pace. Children wean and toilet train themselves with little interference or pressure from parents. The nurse should be sensitive to the childrearing practices of the family and support them in these culturally accepted practices, rather than imposing Western beliefs on reaching developmental milestones.

PERSONALITY AND TEMPERAMENT Why does one infant frequently awaken at night crying while another sleeps for 8 to 10 hours undisturbed? Why does one infant smile much of the time and react positively to interactions while another is withdrawn around unfamiliar people and frequently frowns and cries? Such differences in responses to the environment are believed to be inborn characteristics of temperament. Infants are born with a tendency to react in certain ways to noise and to interact differently with people. They may display varying degrees of regularity in activities of eating and sleeping, and manifest a capacity for concentrating on tasks for different amounts of time.

The nursing assessment identifies personality characteristics of the infant that the nurse can share with the parents. With this information, the parents can appreciate more fully the uniqueness of their infant and design experiences to meet the infant's needs. Parents can learn to modify the environment to promote adaptation. For example, an infant who does not adapt easily to new situations may cry, withdraw, or develop another way of coping when adjusting to new people or places. Parents might be advised to use one or two babysitters rather than engaging new sitters frequently. If the infant is easily distracted when eating, parents can feed the infant in a quiet setting to encourage a focus on eating. Although the infant's temperament is unchanged, the ability to fit with the environment is enhanced.

COMMUNICATION Even at a few weeks of age, infants communicate and engage in two-way interaction; they express comfort by soft sounds, cuddling, and eye contact. The infant displays discomfort by thrashing the extremities, arching the back, and crying vigorously. From these rudimentary skills, communication ability continues to develop until the infant speaks several words at the end of the first year of life (see

Table 3–9). Nonverbal methods continue to be a primary method of communication between parent and child.

Nurses assess communication to identify possible abnormalities or developmental delays. Language ability may be assessed with the Denver II Developmental Test or other specialized language screening tools. Normal infants and toddlers understand (**receptive speech**) more words than they can speak (**expressive speech**). Abnormalities may be caused by a hearing deficit, developmental delay, or lack of verbal stimulation from caretakers. Further assessment may be required to pinpoint the cause of the abnormality.

Nursing interventions focus on providing a stimulating and comforting environment. Parents are encouraged to speak to infants and teach words. Hospital nurses should include the infant's known words when providing care, and provide nonverbal support by hugging and holding. Nurses planning interventions should consider the family's cultural patterns for communications and development.

TODDLER (1 TO 3 YEARS)

Toddlerhood is sometimes called the first adolescence. The child, who months before was merely an infant, from 1–3 years is now displaying independence and negativism. Pride in newfound accomplishments emerges during this time.

Physical Growth and Development

The rate of growth slows during the second year of life. The child requires limited food intake during this time, a change that may cause concern to the parent. The nurse should reassure parents with these concerns that this is a normal occurrence in their child's development. By age 2 years, the birth weight has usually quadrupled and the child is about one-half of the adult height. Body proportions begin to change, with longer legs and a smaller head in proportion to body size than during infancy. The toddler has a pot-bellied appearance and stands with feet apart to provide a wide base of support. By approximately 33 months, eruption of deciduous teeth is complete, with 20 teeth present.

Gross motor activity develops rapidly (Table 3–12) as the toddler progresses from walking to running, kicking, and riding a tricycle. As physical maturation occurs, the toddler develops the ability to control elimination patterns.

TABLE 3–12 Growth and Development Milestones During Toddlerhood

AGE	PHYSICAL GROWTH	FINE MOTOR ABILITY	GROSS MOTOR ABILITY	SENSORY ABILITY
1–2 years	■ Gains 8 oz (227 g) or more per month. ■ Grows 3.5–5 in. (9–12 cm) during this year. ■ Anterior fontanel closes.	■ By end of second year, builds a tower of four blocks. ■ Scribbles on paper. ■ Can undress self. ■ Throws a ball.	■ Runs. ■ Walks up and down stairs. ■ Likes push- and pull-toys.	Visual acuity 20/50
2–3 years	■ Gains 1.4–2.3 kg (3–5 lb)/year. ■ Grows 5–6.5 cm (2–2.5 in.)/year.	■ Draws a circle and other rudimentary forms. ■ Learns to pour. ■ Is learning to dress self.	■ Jumps. ■ Kicks ball. ■ Throws ball overhand.	

Source: Ball, J. W., & Bindler, R. C., (2008). *Pediatric nursing: Caring for children* (4th ed., p. 88). Upper Saddle River, NJ: Pearson Education.

Cognitive Development

During the toddler years, the child moves from the sensorimotor to the preoperational stage of development. The early use of language awakens in the 1-year-old the ability to think about objects or people when they are absent. Object permanence is well developed.

At about 2 years of age, the increasing use of words as symbols enables the toddler to use preoperational thought. Rudimentary problem solving, creative thought, and an understanding of cause-and-effect relationships are now possible.

Psychosocial Development

The toddler is soundly rooted in a trusting relationship and feels more comfortable in asserting autonomy and separating from primary care providers. It is important for toddlers to begin asserting their autonomy within the context of safe places and relationships that promote their interaction with both adults and other children.

PLAY   Many changes in play patterns occur between infancy and toddlerhood. The toddler's motor skills enable him or her to bang pegs into a pounding board with a hammer. The social nature of toddler play is also readily seen. Toddlers find the company of other children pleasurable, even though socially interactive play may not occur. Toddlers tend to play with similar objects side-by-side, occasionally trading toys and words (Figure 3–7 ■). This is called **parallel play**. This playtime with other children assists toddlers to develop social skills. Toddlers engage in play activities they have seen at home, such as pounding with a hammer and talking on the phone. This imitative behavior helps them to learn new actions and skills.

Physical skills are manifested in play as toddlers push and pull objects, climb in and out and up and down, run, ride a Big Wheel, turn the pages of books, and scribble with a pen. Both gross motor and fine motor abilities are enhanced during this age period.

Cognitive understanding enables the toddler to manipulate objects and learn about their qualities. Stacking blocks and placing rings on a building tower teach spatial relationships and other lessons that provide a foundation for future learning. Various kinds of play objects should be provided for the toddler to meet play needs. These play needs can easily be met whether the child is hospitalized or at home (Table 3–13).

PERSONALITY AND TEMPERAMENT   The toddler retains most of the temperamental characteristics identified during infancy, but may demonstrate some changes. The normal developmental progression of toddlerhood also plays a part in responses. For example, the infant who previously responded positively to stimuli, such as a new babysitter, may appear more negative in toddlerhood. The increasing independence characteristic of this age is shown by the toddler's use of the word *no*. The parent and child constantly adapt their responses to each other and learn anew how to communicate with each other.

COMMUNICATION   Because the individual's capacity for development of language skills is greatest during the toddler period, adults should communicate frequently with children in

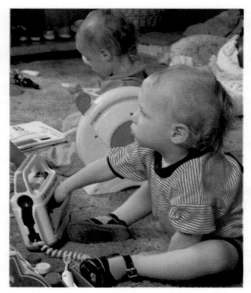

A

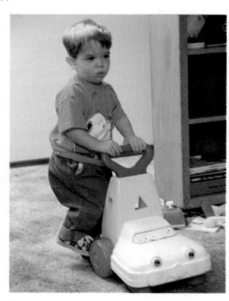

B

Figure 3–7 ■ *A*, Two children are displaying typical parallel play, since they enjoy playing near other children, but are not engaging in social interactions with each other. Which cognitive and motor skills are these children developing? *B*, Imitative play such as pushing and pulling a vacuum allows this toddler to develop gross and fine motor skills.

this age group. This communication is critical not only to the toddler's ability to communicate simple wants and needs, but also to cognitive and language development, as they affect the toddler's future literacy. Toddlers also begin to learn the subtleties of language, as they begin to imitate words and speech intonations, as well as the social interactions and nonverbal gestures that they observe.

At the beginning of toddlerhood, the child may use four to six words in addition to "mama" and "dada." Receptive speech (the ability to understand words) far outpaces expressive

TABLE 3–13 Psychosocial Development During Toddlerhood

AGE	PLAY AND TOYS	COMMUNICATION
1–3 years	■ Refines fine motor skills by use of cloth books, large pencil and paper, wooden puzzles. ■ Facilitates imitative behavior by playing kitchen, grocery shopping, toy telephone. ■ Learns gross motor activities by riding Big Wheel tricycle, playing with soft ball and bat, molding water and sand, tossing ball or bean bag. ■ Cognitive skills develop by educational television shows, music, stories, and books.	■ Increasingly enjoys talking. ■ Vocabulary grows expotentially, especially when spoken and read to. ■ Needs to release stress by pounding board, frequent gross motor activities, and occasional temper tantrums. ■ Likes contact with other children and learns interpersonal skills.

Source: Ball, J. W., & Bindler, R. C., (2008). *Pediatric nursing: Caring for children* (4th ed., p. 90). Upper Saddle River, NJ: Pearson Education.

speech. By the end of toddlerhood, however, the 3-year-old has a vocabulary of almost 1,000 words and uses short sentences.

Communication occurs in many ways, some of which are nonverbal. Toddler communication includes pointing, pulling an adult over to a room or object, and speaking in **expressive jargon** (using unintelligible words with normal speech intonations as if truly communicating in words). Other communication methods include crying, pounding or stamping feet, displaying a temper tantrum, or other means that illustrate dismay. These powerful communication methods can upset parents, who often need suggestions for handling them. Adults can best assist the toddler by verbalizing the feelings shown by the toddler, by saying things like, "You must be very upset that you cannot have that candy. When you stop crying you can come out of your room." Verbalizing the child's feeling and then ignoring further negative behavior ensures that the parent is not unintentionally reinforcing the inappropriate behavior. While the toddler's search for autonomy and independence creates a need for such behavior, an upset toddler may respond well to holding, rocking, and stroking.

Parents and nurses can promote a toddler's communication by speaking frequently, naming objects, giving single-step directions, explaining procedures in simple terms, expressing feelings that the toddler seems to be displaying, and encouraging speech. The toddler from a bilingual home is at an optimal age to learn two languages. If the parents do not speak English, the toddler will benefit from a child care experience that will expose him or her to English in addition to his or her native language.

The nurse who understands the communication skills of toddlers is able to assess expressive and receptive language and communicate effectively, thereby promoting positive health care experiences for these children. Parents often need ideas of strategies for communication with the young child.

PRESCHOOL CHILD (3 TO 6 YEARS)

The preschool years are a time of new initiative and independence. Most children are in a child care center or school for part of the day, and they learn a great deal from this social contact. Language skills are well developed, and the child is able to understand and speak clearly. Endless projects characterize the world of busy preschoolers. They may work with play dough to form animals, then cut out and paste paper, then draw and color.

Physical Growth and Development

Preschoolers grow slowly and steadily, with most growth taking place in long bones of the arms and legs. The short, chubby toddler gradually gives way to a slender, long-legged preschooler (Table 3–14).

Physical skills continue to develop. The preschooler runs with ease, holds a bat, and throws balls of various types. Writing ability increases, and the preschooler enjoys drawing and learning.

TABLE 3–14 Growth and Development Milestones During the Preschool Years

PHYSICAL GROWTH	FINE MOTOR ABILITY	GROSS MOTOR ABILITY	SENSORY ABILITY
Gains 1.5–2/5 kg (3–5 lb)/year. Grows 4–6 cm (1 1/2–2 1/2 in.)/year.	Uses scissors. Draws circle, square, cross. Draws at least a six-part person. Enjoys art projects such as pasting, stringing beads, using clay. Learns to tie shoes at end of preschool years. Buttons clothes. Brushes teeth. Eats three meals, with snacks. Uses spoon, fork, and knife.	Throws a ball overhand. Climbs well. Rides tricycle.	Visual acuity continues to improve. Can focus on and learn letters and numbers.

Source: Ball, J. W., & Bindler, R. C., (2008). *Pediatric nursing: Caring for children* (4th ed., p. 92). Upper Saddle River, NJ: Pearson Education.

The preschool period is a good time to encourage good dental habits. Children can begin to brush their own teeth with parental supervision and help in reaching all tooth surfaces. Parents should floss children's teeth, give fluoride as ordered if the water supply is not fluoridated, and schedule the first dental visit so the child can become accustomed to the routine of periodic dental care.

Cognitive Development

The preschooler exhibits characteristics of preoperational thought. Symbols or words are used to represent objects and people, enabling the young child to think about them. This is a milestone in intellectual development; however, the preschooler still has some limitations in thought (Table 3–15).

It is important to understand the preschooler's thought processes in order to plan appropriate teaching for health care and development of health habits.

Psychosocial Development

The preschooler is more independent in establishing relationships with others. The child interacts closely with children and adults as well as being able to plan and carry out activities.

PLAY The preschooler has begun to play in a new way (Figure 3–8 ■). Toddlers simply play side by side with friends, each engaging in his or her own activities; preschoolers interact with others during play. One child cuts out colored paper while his or her friend glues it on paper in a design. This new type of interaction is called **associative play**.

In addition to this social dimension, other aspects of play also differ. The preschooler enjoys large motor activities such as swinging, riding a tricycle, and throwing a ball. Increasing manual dexterity is demonstrated in greater complexity of drawings and manipulation of blocks and modeling. These changes necessitate planning of playtime to include appropriate activities. Preschool programs and child life departments in hospitals help meet this important need.

Materials provided for play can be simple but should guide activities in which the child engages. Because fine motor activities are popular, paper, pens, scissors, glue, and a variety of other such objects should be available. The child can use them to create important images such as pictures of people, hospital beds, or friends. A collection of dolls, furniture, and clothing can be manipulated to represent parents and children, nurses and physicians, teachers, or other significant people.

TABLE 3–15 **Characteristics of Thought Identified by Piaget**

CHARACTERISTIC	DEFINITION	DEVELOPMENT STAGE	NURSING IMPLICATIONS
Object permanence	Ability to understand that when something is out of sight it still exists	Sensorimotor period, especially in coordination of secondary schemes substage from 8–12 months	Before development of object permanence, babies will not look for toys or other objects out of sight; as the concept is developing they are concerned when a parent leaves, since they are not certain the parent will return.
Egocentrism	Ability to see things only from one's own point of view	Preoperational thought	Peers or others who have gone through an experience will not impress the preschooler; teaching should focus on what an experience will be like to the child.
Transductive reasoning	Connecting two events in a cause-effect relationship simply because they occur together in time	Preoperational thought	Ask the child what he or she thinks caused an occurrence; ask how the two events are connected; correct misconceptions to lessen child's guilt.
Centration	Focusing only on one particular aspect of a situation	Preoperational thought	Listen to the child's comments and deal with concerns in order to be able to present new concepts to the child.
Animism	Giving lifelike qualities to nonliving things	Preoperational thought	Ask preschool children to describe how a machine works, or how the trees move. Provide opportunities to learn about machines that may move and make noises (intravenous pumps, magnetic resonance imaging) to decrease fears.
Magical thinking	Believing that events occur because of one's thoughts or actions	Preoperational thought	Ask young children how they became ill, or what caused a parent's or sibling's illness. Correct misconceptions when the child blames self for causing problems by wishing someone ill or having bad behavior.
Conservation	Knowing that matter is not changed when its form is altered	Concrete operational thought	Before conservation of thought is reached, the child may think that gender can be changed when hair is cut, the leg under a cast is broken in separate pieces. Ask perceptions and clarify misconceptions.

Source: Ball, J. W., & Bindler, R. C., (2008). *Pediatric nursing: Caring for children* (4th ed., p. 93). Upper Saddle River, NJ: Pearson Education.

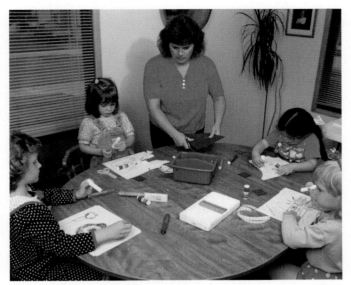

Figure 3–8 ■ Preschoolers have well-developed language, motor, and social skills, and they can work creatively together on an art project, as this group is doing at an in-home child care center.

Because fantasy life is so powerful at this age, the preschooler readily uses props to engage in **dramatic play**, that is, the living out of the drama of human life.

The nurse can use playtime to assess the preschooler's developmental level, knowledge about health care, and emotions related to health care experiences. Observations about objects chosen for play, content of dramatic play, and pictures drawn can provide important assessment data. The nurse can also use play periods to teach the child about health care procedures and offer an outlet for expressing emotions (Table 3–16).

PERSONALITY AND TEMPERAMENT Characteristics of personality observed in infancy tend to persist over time. The preschooler may need assistance as these characteristics are expressed in the new situations of preschool or nursery school. An excessively active child, for example, will need gentle, consistent handling to adjust to the structure of a classroom. Encourage parents to visit preschool programs to choose the one that would best foster growth in their child. Some preschoolers enjoy the structured learning of a program that focuses on cognitive skills, while others are happier and more open to learning in a small group that provides much time for free play. Nurses can help parents to identify their

child's personality or temperament characteristics and to find the best environment for growth.

COMMUNICATION Language skills blossom during the preschool years. The vocabulary grows to over 2,000 words, and children speak in complete sentences of several words and use all parts of speech. They practice these newfound language skills by endlessly talking and asking questions.

The sophisticated speech of preschoolers mirrors the development occurring in their minds and helps them to learn about the world around them. However, this speech can be quite deceptive. Although preschoolers use many words, their grasp of meaning is usually literal and may not match that of adults. These literal interpretations have important implications for health care providers. For example, the preschooler who is told she will be "put to sleep" for surgery may think of a pet recently euthanized; the child who is told that a dye will be injected for a diagnostic test may think he is going to die; mention of "a little stick" in the arm can cause images of tree branches rather than of a simple immunization.

Concrete visual aids such as pictures of a child undergoing the same procedure or a book to read together enhance teaching by meeting the child's developmental needs. Handling medical equipment such as intravenous bags and stethoscopes increases interest and helps the child to focus. Teaching may have to be done in several short sessions rather than one long session.

Some general approaches:
■ Allow time for the child to integrate explanations.
■ Verbalize frequently to the child.
■ Use drawings and stories to explain care.
■ Use accurate names for bodily functions.
■ Allow choices.

The preschooler's social growth and increased communication skills make these years the perfect time to introduce concepts related to problem solving and conflict resolution. Puzzles and manipulative toys help foster early problem-solving skills. Children in this age group can learn to calm themselves by learning how to take deep breaths and count to 3 or 5 when they are upset. Many preschool programs employ special curricula that help teachers and parents assist children in developing essential conflict resolution skills. Using language to resolve conflict is a protective factor that decreases the likelihood of children choosing inappropriate or violent behavior to try to get what they want or bring a distressing interaction to a close.

TABLE 3–16 Psychosocial Development During Preschool Years

AGE	PLAY AND TOYS	COMMUNICATION
3–6 years	Associative play is facilitated by simple games, puzzles, nursery rhymes, songs. Dramatic play is fostered by dolls and doll clothes, play houses and hospitals, dress-up clothes, puppets. Stress is relieved by pens, paper, glue, scissors. Cognitive growth is fostered by educational television shows, music, stories and books.	Developed and uses all parts of speech, occasionally incorrectly. Communicates with a widening array of people. Play with other children is a favorite activity. Health professionals can ■ verbalize and explain procedures to children. ■ use drawings and stories to explain care. ■ use accurate names for bodily functions. ■ allow the child to talk, ask questions, and make choices.

SCHOOL-AGE CHILD (6 TO 12 YEARS)

Errol, 10 years old, arrives home from school shortly after 3 p.m. each day. He immediately calls his friends and goes to visit one of them. They are building models of cars and collecting baseball cards. Endless hours are spent on these projects and on discussions of events at school that day.

Nine-year-old Karen practices soccer two afternoons a week and plays in games each weekend. She also is learning to play the flute and spends her free time at home practicing. Although practice time is not her favorite part of music, Karen enjoys the performances and wants to play well in front of her friends and teacher. Her parents now allow her to ride her bike unaccompanied to the store or to a friend's house.

These two school-age children demonstrate common characteristics of their age group. They are in a stage of industry in which it is important to the child to perform useful work. Meaningful activities take on great importance and are usually carried out in the company of peers. A sense of achievement in these activities is important to developing self-esteem and to preventing a sense of inferiority or poor self-worth.

Physical Growth and Development

School age is the last period in which girls and boys are close in size and body proportions. As the long bones continue to grow, leg length increases (see Figure 3–5). Fat gives way to muscle, and the child appears leaner. Jaw proportions change as the first deciduous tooth is lost at 6 years and permanent teeth begin to erupt. Body organs and the immune system mature, resulting in fewer illnesses among school-age children. Medications are less likely to cause serious side effects, because they can be metabolized more easily. The urinary system can adjust to changes in fluid status. Physical skills are also refined as children begin to play sports, and fine motor skills are well developed through school activities (Table 3–17).

Although it is commonly believed that the start of adolescence (age 12 years) heralds a growth spurt, the rapid increases in size commonly occur during school age. Girls may begin a growth spurt as early as 9 or 10 years of age and boys a year or so later (Figure 3–9 ■). Nutritional needs increase dramatically with this spurt.

The loss of the first deciduous teeth and the eruption of permanent teeth usually occur at about age 6 years, or at the beginning of the school-age period. Of the 32 permanent teeth, 22–26 erupt by age 12 years and the remaining molars follow during the teenage years. The school-age child should be closely monitored to ensure that brushing and flossing are ade-

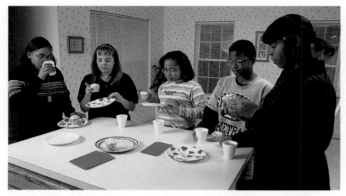

Figure 3–9 ■ Because girls have a growth spurt earlier than boys, girls often are taller than boys of the same age.

quate, that fluoride is taken if the water supply is not fluoridated, that dental care is obtained to provide for examination of teeth and alignment, and that loose teeth are identified before surgery or other events that may lead to loss of a tooth.

Cognitive Development

The child enters the stage of concrete operational thought at about age 7 years. This stage enables school-age children to consider alternative solutions and solve problems. However, school-age children continue to rely on concrete experiences and materials to form their thought content.

During the school-age years, the child learns the concept of conservation (that matter is not changed when its form is altered). At earlier ages, a child believes that when water is poured from a short, wide glass into a tall, thin glass, there is more water in the taller glass. The school-age child recognizes that, although it may look like the taller glass holds more water, the quantity is the same. The concept of conservation is helpful when the nurse explains medical treatments. The school-age child understands that an incision will heal, that a cast will be removed, and that an arm will look the same as before once the intravenous infusion is removed.

Psychosocial Development

The school-age child has many friends and cooperatively interacts with others to accomplish tasks. The child develops a sense of accomplishment from activities and relationships.

PLAY When the preschool teacher tries to organize a game of baseball, both the teacher and the children become frustrated. Not only are the children physically unable to hold a bat and hit a ball, but they seem to have no understanding of the rules

TABLE 3–17 Growth and Development Milestones During the School-Age Years

PHYSICAL GROWTH	FINE MOTOR ABILITY	GROSS MOTOR ABILITY	SENSORY ABILITY
Gains 1.4–2.2 kg (3–5 lb)/year.	Plays card and board games.	Roller skates or ice skates.	Is able to concentrate for longer periods.
Grows 4–6 cm (1 1/2–2 1/2 in.)/year.	Enjoys craft projects.	Jumps rope. Rides two-wheeler.	Can read.

Source: Ball, J. W., & Bindler, R. C., (2008). *Pediatric nursing: Caring for children* (4th ed., p. 96). Upper Saddle River, NJ: Pearson Education.

TABLE 3-18 Psychosocial Development During the School-Age Years

AGE	ACTIVITIES	COMMUNICATION
6–12 years	Gross motor development is fostered by ball sports, skating, dance lessons, water and snow skiing/boarding, biking. A sense of industry is fostered by playing a musical instrument, gathering collections, starting hobbies, playing board and video games. Cognitive growth is facilitated by reading, crafts, word puzzles, school work.	Use of language is mature. Is able to converse and discuss topics for increasing lengths of time. Spends many hours at school and with friends in sports or other activities. Health professionals can ■ assess child's knowledge before teaching. ■ allow the child to select rewards following procedures. ■ teach techniques such as counting or visualization to manage difficult situations. ■ include both parent and child in health care decisions.

Source: Ball, J. W., & Bindler, R. C., (2008). *Pediatric nursing: Caring for children* (4th ed., p. 97). Upper Saddle River, NJ: Pearson Education.

of the game and do not want to wait for their turn at bat. By 6 years of age, however, children have acquired the physical ability to hold the bat properly and may occasionally hit the ball. school-age children also understand that everyone has a role—the pitcher, the catcher, the batter, the outfielders. They cooperate with one another to form a team, are eager to learn the rules of the game, and want to ensure that these rules are followed exactly (Table 3–18).

The characteristics of play exhibited by the school-age child include cooperation with others and the ability to play a part in order to contribute to a unified whole. This type of play is called **cooperative play**. The concrete nature of cognitive thought leads to a reliance on rules to provide structure and security. Children have an increasing desire to spend much of their playtime with friends, which demonstrates the social component of play. Play is an extremely important method of learning and living for the school-age child. Active physical play has decreased in recent years as television viewing and playing of computer games have increased, leading to poor nutritional status and high rates of overweight among children.

When a child is hospitalized, the separation from playmates can lead to feelings of sadness and purposelessness. school-age children often feel better when placed in multibed units with other children. Games can be devised even for wheelchair-bound children. Normal, rewarding parts of play should be integrated into care. Friends should be encouraged to visit or call a hospitalized child. Discharge planning for the child who has had a cast or brace applied should address the activities in which the child can participate and those the child must avoid. Nurses should reinforce the importance of playing games with friends to both parents and children.

PERSONALITY AND TEMPERAMENT The enduring aspects of temperament continue to be manifest during the school years. The child classified as "difficult" at an earlier age may now have trouble in the classroom. Nurses may advise parents to provide a quiet setting for homework and to reward the child for concentration. For example, after completing homework, the child may watch a television show. Creative efforts and alternative methods of learning should be valued. Encourage parents to see their children as individuals who may not all learn in the same way. The "slow-to-warm-up" child may need encouragement to try new activities and to share experiences with others, whereas the "easy" child will readily adapt to new schools, people, and experiences.

COMMUNICATION During the school-age years, the child should learn how to correct any lingering pronunciation or grammatical errors. Vocabulary increases, and the child learns about parts of speech in school. school-age children enjoy writing and, while in the hospital, can be encouraged to keep a journal of their experiences as a method of dealing with anxiety. The literal translation of words characteristic of preschoolers is uncommon among school-age children.

Following are some communication strategies helpful with the school-age child:
- Provide concrete examples of pictures or materials to accompany verbal descriptions.
- Assess knowledge before planning the instruction.
- Allow child to select rewards following procedures.
- Teach techniques such as counting or visualization to manage difficult situations.
- Include child in discussions and history with parent.

Sexuality

Although children become aware of sexual differences between genders during preschool years, they deal much more consciously with sexuality during the school-age years. As children mature physically, they need information about their bodily changes so that they can develop a healthy self-image and an

---

 ALTERNATIVE THERAPIES   Music and Art Therapy

Most children are accustomed to listening to music via earphones or earbuds. They should be encouraged to bring their favorite music to the hospital as a means of stress reduction. It may also reduce the need for sedation during diagnostic tests or uncomfortable procedures (DeLoach Walworth, 2005). Musical instruments and artistic tools such as paints and brushes, markers, and clay are frequently used in hospital and other care settings to help children express fears and anxieties about their illnesses. Just as important, these tools can assist children in sharing their desires and dreams for health and wellness.

understanding of the relationships between their bodies and sexuality. Children become interested in sexual issues and are often exposed to erroneous information on television shows, in magazines, or from friends and siblings. Schools and families need to use opportunities to teach school-age children factual information about sex and to foster healthy concepts of self and others. It is advisable to ask occasional questions about sexual issues to learn how much the child knows and to provide correct information when answers demonstrate confusion.

Both friends and the media are common sources of erroneous ideas. Appropriate and inappropriate touch should be discussed, with lists of trusted people who can be approached (teachers, clergy, school counselors, family members, neighbors) to discuss any episodes with which the child feels uncomfortable. Because even these trusted people can be implicated in inappropriate episodes, the nurse should encourage the child to go to more than one person, an important approach if the child is uncomfortable about a relationship with any individual.

ADOLESCENT (12 TO 18 YEARS)

Adolescence is a time of passage signaling the end of childhood and the beginning of adulthood. Although adolescents differ in behaviors and accomplishments, they are all in a period of identity formation. If a healthy identity and sense of self-worth are not developed in this period, role confusion and purposeless struggling will ensue. The adolescents in your care will represent various degrees of identity formation, and each will offer unique challenges.

Physical Growth and Development

The physical changes ending in **puberty**, or sexual maturity, begin near the end of the school-age period. The prepubescent period is marked by a growth spurt at an average age of 10 years for girls and 13 years for boys, although there is considerable variation among children. The increase in height and weight is generally remarkable and is completed in 2–3 years (Table 3–19). The growth spurt in girls is accompanied by an increase in breast size and growth of pubic hair. Menstruation occurs last and signals achievement of puberty. In boys, the growth spurt is accompanied by growth in size of the penis and testes and by growth of pubic hair. Deepening of the voice and growth of facial hair occur later, at the time of puberty.

During adolescence children grow stronger and more muscular and establish characteristic male and female patterns of fat distribution. The apocrine and eccrine glands mature, leading to increased sweating and a distinct odor to perspiration.

All body organs are now fully mature, enabling the adolescent to take adult doses of medications.

The adolescent must adapt to a rapidly changing body for several years. These physical changes and hormonal variations offer challenges to identity formation.

Cognitive Development

Adolescence marks the beginning of Piaget's last stage of cognitive development, the stage of formal operational thought. The adolescent no longer depends on concrete experiences as the basis of thought but develops the ability to reason abstractly. Such concepts as justice, truth, beauty, and power can be understood. The adolescent revels in this newfound ability and spends a great deal of time thinking, reading, and talking about abstract concepts.

The ability to think and act independently leads many adolescents to rebel against parental authority. Through these actions, adolescents seek to establish their own identity and values. While this behavior is normal for adolescents, it can create a number of difficulties at home and school as adolescents try to balance their needs to express themselves and the expectations of parents, teachers, and other authority figures.

Psychosocial Development

The adolescent is mature in relationships with others. Establishing a meaningful identity is the key aspect that the teen is working on during relationships and activities.

ACTIVITIES Maturity leads to new activities. Adolescents may drive, ride buses, or bike independently. They are less dependent on parents for transportation and spend more time with friends. Activities include participation in sports and extracurricular school activities, as well as "hanging out" and attending movies or concerts with friends (Table 3–20). The peer group becomes the focus of activities, regardless of the teen's interests. Peers are important in establishing identity and providing meaning. Although same-sex interactions predominate, boy–girl relationships are more common than at earlier stages. Adolescents thus participate in and learn from social interactions fundamental to adult relationships.

PERSONALITY AND TEMPERAMENT Characteristics of temperament manifested during childhood usually remain stable in the teenage years. For instance, the adolescent who was a calm, scheduled infant and child often demonstrates initiative to regulate study times and other routines. Similarly, the adolescent who was an easily stimulated infant may now have a

TABLE 3–19 **Growth and Development Milestones During Adolescence**

PHYSICAL GROWTH	FINE MOTOR ABILITY	GROSS MOTOR ABILITY	SENSORY ABILITY
Variation in age of growth spurt During growth spurt, girls gain 7–25 kg (15–55 lb) and grow 2.5–20 cm (2–8 in.); boys gain approximately 7–29.5 kg (15–65 lb) and grow 11–30 cm (41/2–12 in.).	Skills are well developed.	New sports activities are attempted and muscle development continues. Some lack of coordination is common during growth spurt.	Sensory ability is fully developed.

Source: Ball, J. W., & Bindler, R. C., (2008). *Pediatric nursing: Caring for children* (4th ed., p. 99). Upper Saddle River, NJ: Pearson Education.

TABLE 3–20 Psychosocial Development During Adolescence

AGE	ACTIVITIES	COMMUNICATION
12–18 years	Sports—ball games, gymnastics, water and snow skiing/boarding, swimming, school sports School activities—drama, yearbook, class office, club participation Quiet activities—Reading, school work, television, computer, video games, music	Increasing communication and time with peer group—movies, dances, driving, eating out, attending sports events Applying abstract thought and analysis in conversations at home and school

Source: Ball, J. W., & Bindler, R. C., (2008). *Pediatric nursing: Caring for children* (4th ed., p. 100). Upper Saddle River, NJ: Pearson Education.

messy room, a harried schedule with assignments always completed late, and an interest in many activities. It is also common for an adolescent who was an easy child to become more difficult because of the psychological changes of adolescence and the need to assert independence.

As during the child's earlier ages, the nurse's role may be to inform parents of different personality types and to help them support the teen's uniqueness while providing necessary structure and feedback. Nurses can help parents understand their teen's personality type and work with the adolescent to meet expectations of teachers and others in authority.

COMMUNICATION All parts of speech are used and understood by the adolescent. Colloquialisms and slang are commonly used with the peer group. The adolescent often studies a foreign language in school, having the ability to understand and analyze grammar and sentence structure.

The adolescent increasingly leaves the home base and establishes close ties with peers. These relationships become the basis for identity formation. A period of stress or crisis generally occurs before a strong identity can emerge. The adolescent may try out new roles by learning a new sport or other skills, experimenting with drugs or alcohol, wearing different styles of clothing, or trying other activities. It is important to provide positive role models and a variety of experiences to help the adolescent make wise choices.

The adolescent also has a need to leave the past, to be different, and to change from former patterns to establish a self-identity. Rules that are repeated constantly and dogmatically will probably be broken in the adolescent's quest for self-awareness. This poses difficulties when the adolescent has a health problem that requires ongoing care, such as diabetes or a heart problem. Introducing the adolescent to other teens who manage the same problem appropriately is usually more successful in getting the adolescent to comply with a care plan than telling the adolescent what to do.

Privacy should be ensured during the taking of health histories or interventions with teens. Even if a parent is present for part of a history or examination, the adolescent should be given the opportunity to relay information to or ask questions of the health care provider alone. The adolescent should be given a choice of whether to have a parent present during an examination or while care is provided. Most information shared by an adolescent is confidential. Some states mandate disclosure of certain information to parents such as an adolescent's desire for an abortion. In these cases, the adolescent should be informed of what will be disclosed to the parent.

Setting up teen rooms (recreation rooms for use only by adolescents) or separate adolescent units in hospitals can provide necessary peer support during hospitalization. Most adolescents are not pleased when placed on a unit or in a room with young children. Nurses and care staff should allow adolescents the freedom of choice whenever possible, including preferences for evening or morning bathing, the type of clothes to wear while hospitalized, timing of treatments, and visitation guidelines. Use of contracts with adolescents may increase adherence with health care recommendations. Firmness, gentleness, choices, and respect must be balanced during care of adolescent clients.

Some specific communication strategies that help with the adolescent:

- Provide written and verbal explanations.
- Direct history and explanations to teen alone; then include parent.
- Allow for safe exploration of topics by suggesting that the teen is similar to other teens. ("Many teens with diabetes have questions about.... How about you?")
- Arrange meetings for discussions with other teens.

SEXUALITY With maturation of the body and increased secretion of hormones, the adolescent achieves sexual maturity. This complex process involves growing interactions with members of the opposite sex, an interplay of the forces of society and family, and identity formation. The early adolescent progresses from dances and other social events with members of the opposite sex to the late adolescent who is mature sexually and may have regular sexual encounters. About 47% of all high school students in the United States have had intercourse and 34% are currently sexually active. Only 63% used a condom at their last sexual encounter, putting this age group at high risk of acquiring sexually transmitted infections (Eaton, Kann, Kinchen, et al., 2006).

Teenagers need information about their bodies and emerging sexuality. They should understand the interests and forces they experience. Including sex education in school classes and health care encounters is important. Information on methods to prevent sexually transmitted diseases is given, with most school districts now providing some teaching on HIV. Far more common risks to teens, however, are diseases such as gonorrhea, herpes, and hepatitis. Health histories should include questions on sexual activity, sexually transmitted diseases, and birth control use and understanding. Most hospitals routinely perform pregnancy screening on adolescent girls before elective procedures.

Adolescents will benefit from clear information about sexuality, an opportunity to develop relationships with adolescents in various settings, an open atmosphere at home and school where problems and issues can be discussed, and previous experience in problem solving and decision making. Sexual issues should be among topics that adolescents can discuss openly in a variety of settings. Alternatives and support for their decisions should be available.

Some adolescents identify with a sexual minority group such as lesbian, gay, bisexual, or transgendered. These teens are at particular risk of being stigmatized and harassed by other youth or adults. They are more likely to suffer a variety of problems such as isolation, rejection by significant others, violence, suicide, and sexual risk-taking (Rew, Whittaker, Taylor-Seehafer, & Smith, 2005). Nurses are instrumental in helping these youths by providing information for them and their parents, integrating sexual minority content into sexual education curricula, and providing referrals for health and social care when needed. Nurses must examine their own beliefs and communication styles to provide culturally competent care. They can promote trust and acceptance among youth and in the general school community (Bakker & Cavender, 2003). Additionally, the nurse who encounters a sexually active teenager should remember that he or she may be the very first health care provider with whom the teenager discusses his or her sexuality. The nurse who refrains from asserting his or her own beliefs and who emphasizes open communication and active listening will strengthen the teen's confidence in the health care system and increase the likelihood that the teen will seek help from a health care professional in the future.

ADULT

The adult years commonly are divided into three stages: young adulthood (ages 18–40), middle adulthood (ages 40–65), and older adulthood (over age 65). Although developmental markers are not as clearly delineated in the adult as in the infant or child, specific changes in intellectual, psychosocial, and spiritual development, as well as in physical structures and functions do occur with aging (see Tables 3–3, 3–4, 3–7, 3–8 and Figure 3–10 ■). Applying a variety of developmental theories is important to the holistic care of the adult client as nurses perform assessments, implement care, and teach.

The Young Adult

From ages 18–25, the healthy young adult is at the peak of physical development. All body systems are functioning at maximum efficiency. During the 30s, some normal physiologic changes begin. A comparison of physical status for young adults during their 20s and 30s is shown in Table 3–21.

Many individualized psychosocial stressors may affect the young adult. Choices must be made about education, occupation, relationships, independence, and lifestyle. The young adult without adequate education or job skills may face unemployment, poverty, homelessness, and limited access to health care.

Physical assessment of the young adult includes height and weight, blood pressure, and vision. During the health history, the nurse should ask specific questions about substance use, sexual activity and concerns, exercise, eating habits, menstrual history and patterns, coping mechanisms, any familial chronic illnesses, and family changes.

The Middle Adult

The middle adult, ages 40–65, has physical status and function similar to that of the young adult. However, many changes take place between ages 40 and 65. Table 3–22 lists the physical changes that normally occur in the middle years.

Physical assessment of the middle adult includes all body systems, including blood pressure, vision, and hearing. Monitoring for risks and onset of cancer symptoms is essential. During the health history, the nurse should ask specific questions about food intake and exercise habits, substance abuse, sexual concerns, changes in the reproductive system, coping mechanisms, and family history of chronic illnesses.

TABLE 3–21 Physical Status and Changes in the Young Adult Years

ASSESSMENT	STATUS DURING THE 20S	STATUS DURING THE 30S
Skin	Smooth, even temperature	Beginning of wrinkles
Hair	Slightly oily, shiny	Beginning of graying
	Beginning of balding	Balding
Vision	Snellen 20/20	Some loss of visual acuity and accommodation
Musculoskeletal	Strong, coordinated	Some loss of strength and muscle mass
Cardiovascular	Maximum cardiac output	Slight decline in cardiac output
	60–90 beats/min	60–90 beats/min
	Mean BP: 120/80	Mean BP: 120/80
Respiratory	Rate: 12–20	Rate: 12–20
	Full vital capacity	Decline in vital capacity

Source: LeMone, P., & Burke, K. (2008). *Medical-surgical nursing: Critical thinking in client care* (4th ed., p. 26). Upper Saddle River, NJ: Pearson Education.

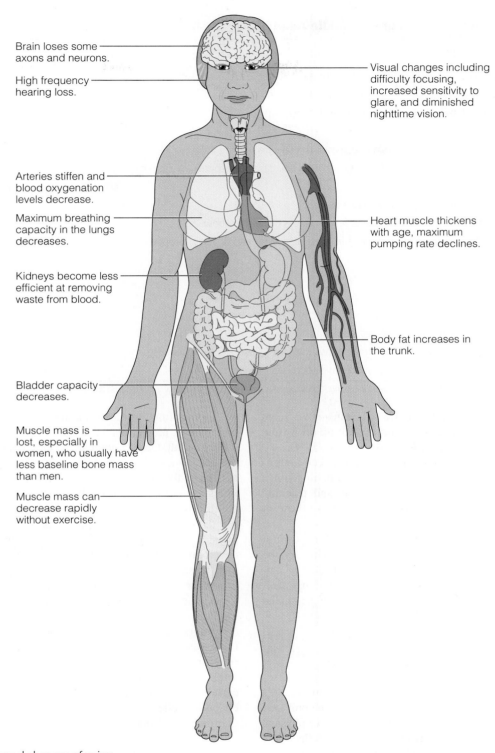

Brain loses some axons and neurons.

High frequency hearing loss.

Visual changes including difficulty focusing, increased sensitivity to glare, and diminished nighttime vision.

Arteries stiffen and blood oxygenation levels decrease.

Maximum breathing capacity in the lungs decreases.

Heart muscle thickens with age, maximum pumping rate declines.

Kidneys become less efficient at removing waste from blood.

Body fat increases in the trunk.

Bladder capacity decreases.

Muscle mass is lost, especially in women, who usually have less baseline bone mass than men.

Muscle mass can decrease rapidly without exercise.

Figure 3–10 ■ Normal changes of aging.

The Older Adult

The older adult period begins at age 65, but it can be further divided into three periods: the young-old (65–74 years), the middle-old (75–84 years), and the old-old (age 85 years and older). With increasing age, a number of normal physiologic changes occur, as listed in Table 3–23.

The older adult population is increasing more rapidly than any other age group. In the last century, the number of adults in the United States living to age 65 or older increased from 3.1 million in 1900 to an estimated 40.2 million in 2010. There will be 71 million older adults by the year 2030, more than twice the number in 2000 (35 million).

TABLE 3–22 Physical Changes in the Middle Adult Years

ASSESSMENT	CHANGES
Skin	Decreased turgor, moisture, and subcutaneous fat result in wrinkles.
	Fat is deposited in the abdominal and hip areas.
Hair	Loss of melanin in hair shaft causes graying.
	Hairline recedes in men.
Sensory	Visual acuity for near vision decreases (presbyopia) during the 40s.
	Auditory acuity for high-frequency sounds decreases (presbycusis); more common in men.
	Sense of taste diminishes.
Musculoskeletal	Skeletal muscle mass decreases by about age 60.
	Thinning of intervertebral discs results in loss of height (about 2.5 cm [1 in.]).
	Postmenopausal women may have loss of calcium and develop osteoporosis.
Cardiovascular	Blood vessels lose elasticity.
	Systolic blood pressure may increase.
Respiratory	Loss of vital capacity (about 1 L from age 20–60) occurs.
Gastrointestinal	Large intestine gradually loses muscle tone; constipation may result.
	Gastric secretions are decreased.
Genitourinary	Hormonal changes occur: menopause, women ($\downarrow$ estrogen); andropause, men ($\downarrow$ testosterone).
Endocrine	Gradual decrease in glucose tolerance occurs.

Source: LeMone, P., & Burke, K. (2008). *Medical-surgical nursing: Critical thinking in client care* (4th ed., p. 27). Upper Saddle River, NJ: Pearson Education.

The average life expectancy in the United States is 72 years for men and 79 years for women (Administration on Aging, 2003; American Association of Retired Persons, 2004).

The increasing number of older adults has important implications for nursing. Clients needing health care in all settings will be older, requiring nursing interventions and teaching specifically designed to meet needs that differ from those of young and middle adults.

Physical assessment of the older adult includes a careful examination of all body systems. During the health history, the nurse should ask specific questions about usual dietary patterns; elimination; exercise and rest; use of alcohol, nicotine, over-the-counter medications, and prescription drugs; sexual concerns; financial concerns; and support systems.

APPLYING GROWTH AND DEVELOPMENT CONCEPTS TO NURSING PRACTICE

Different theories explain one or more aspects of an individual's growth and development. Typically, theorists examine only one aspect of development, such as the cognitive, moral, or physical aspect. The area chosen for examination usually reflects the researcher's academic discipline and personal interest. The theorists may also limit the population that is studied to a particular part of the life span, such as infancy, childhood, or adulthood.

Although such theories can be useful, they have limitations. First, the theory chosen may explain only one aspect of the growth and development process. Yet a person does not develop in fragmented sections but rather as a whole human being. Thus, the nurse may find it necessary to apply several theories to gain an adequate understanding of the growth and development of a client.

Another limitation of some theories is the suggestion that certain tasks are performed at a specific age. In most cases, the child or adult does accomplish the task at the time specified by the guidelines. In other cases, however, the nurse may find that an individual does not accomplish the task or meet the milestone at the exact time the theory suggests. Such individual differences are not easily defined or categorized by a single theory. Human development is a complex synthesis of physiological, cognitive, psychological, moral, and spiritual development. Nurses should expect individual variations and take these into consideration when applying theories about growth and development. In so doing, they will be better able to understand a client's development and plan effective nursing interventions.

In nursing, developmental theories can be useful in guiding assessment, explaining behavior, and providing a direction for nursing interventions. An understanding of a child's intellectual ability helps a nurse to anticipate and explain certain reactions, responses, and needs. Nurses can then encourage client behavior that is appropriate for that particular developmental stage.

Theories are also useful in planning a nursing intervention. For instance, choosing the appropriate toy for a 3-year-old boy requires some knowledge of the physical and cognitive development of the child, as well as a sensitivity to individual preferences.

In adult care, knowledge about the physical, cognitive, and psychologic aspects of the aging process is a fundamental aspect of administering sensitive nursing care. For example, nurses can use their familiarity with the theories of development to help clients understand and anticipate the psychosocial changes that take place after retirement or the physical limitations that come with aging.

TABLE 3–23 **Physical Changes in the Older Adult Years**

ASSESSMENT	CHANGES
Skin	■ Decreased turgor and sebaceous gland activity result in dry, wrinkled skin. Melanocytes cluster, causing "age spots" or "liver spots."
Hair and nails	■ Scalp, axillary, and pubic hair thins; nose and ear hair thickens. Women may develop facial hair.
	■ Nails grow more slowly; may become thick and brittle.
Sensory	■ Visual field narrows, and depth perception is distorted.
	■ Pupils are smaller, reducing night vision.
	■ Lenses yellow and become opaque, resulting in distortion of green, blue, and violet tones and increased sensitivity to glare.
	■ Production of tears decreases.
	■ Sense of smell decreases.
	■ Age-related hearing loss progresses, involving middle- and low-frequency sounds.
	■ Threshold for pain and touch increases.
	■ Alterations in proprioception (sense of physical position) may occur.
Musculoskeletal	■ Loss of overall mass, strength, and movement of muscles occurs; tremors may occur.
	■ Loss of bone structure and deterioration of cartilage in joints results in increased risk of fractures and limitation of range of motion.
Cardiovascular	■ Systolic blood pressure rises.
	■ Cardiac output decreases.
	■ Peripheral resistance increases, and capillary walls thicken.
Respiratory	■ Loss of vital capacity continues as the lungs become less elastic and more rigid.
	■ Anteroposterior chest diameter increases; kyphosis occurs.
	■ Although blood carbon dioxide levels remain relatively constant, blood oxygen levels decrease by 10–15%.
Gastrointestinal	■ Production of saliva decreases, and declining number of taste buds reduces the number of accurate receptors for salt and sweet.
	■ Gag reflex is decreased, and stomach motility and emptying are reduced.
	■ Both large and small intestines undergo some atrophy, with decreased peristalsis.
	■ The liver decreases in weight and storage capacity; incidence of gallstones increases; pancreatic enzymes decrease.
Genitourinary	■ Kidneys lose mass, and the glomerular filtration rate is reduced (by nearly 50% from young adulthood to old age).
	■ Bladder capacity decreases, and the micturition reflex is delayed. Urinary retention is more common.
	■ Women may have stress incontinence; men may have an enlarged prostate gland.
	■ Reproductive changes in men occur:
	▪ Testosterone decreases.
	▪ Sperm count decreases.
	▪ Testes become smaller.
	▪ Length of time to achieve an erection increases; erection is less full.
	■ Reproductive changes in women occur:
	▪ Estrogen levels decrease.
	▪ Breast tissue decreases.
	▪ Vagina, uterus, ovaries, and urethra atrophy.
	▪ Vaginal lubrication decreases.
	▪ Vaginal secretions become alkaline.
Endocrine	■ Pituitary gland loses weight and vascularity.
	■ Thyroid gland becomes more fibrous, and plasma T_3 decreases.
	■ Pancreas releases insulin more slowly; increased blood glucose levels are common.
	■ Adrenal glands produce less cortisol.

Source: LeMone, P., & Burke, K. (2008). *Medical-surgical nursing: Critical thinking in client care* (4th ed., p. 29). Upper Saddle River, NJ: Pearson Education.

REFERENCES

Administration on Aging, U.S. Department of Health and Human Services. (2003). *Statistics: A profile of older Americans, 2003*. Retrieved May 4, 2009 from http://www.aoa.gov/AoAroot/Aging_Statistics/Profile/2003/4.aspx#figure1

American Academy of Pediatrics. (2004). *Pediatric nutrition handbook* (5th ed.). Elk Grove Village, IL: Author.

American Association of Retired Persons. (2004). *Profile of older Americans, 2004*. Washington, DC: Resource Services Group.

Bakker, L. J., & Cavender, A. (2003). Promoting culturally competent care for gay youth. *Journal of School Nursing, 19*, 65–72.

Bandura, A. (1986). *Social foundations of thought and actions: A social cognitive theory*. Englewood Cliffs, NJ: Prentice Hall.

Bandura, A. (1997a). *Self-efficacy: The exercise of control*. New York: W. H. Freeman.

Bandura, A. (1997b). *Self-efficacy in changing societies*. New York: Cambridge University Press.

Bronfenbrenner, U. (1986). Ecology of the family as a context for human development: Research perspectives. *Developmental Psychology, 22*, 723–742.

Bronfenbrenner, U. (Ed.). (2005). *Making human beings human: Bioecological perspectives on human development*. Thousand Oaks, CA: Sage Publications.

Bronfenbrenner, U., McClelland, P. D., Ceci, S. J., Moen, P., & Wethington, E. (1996). *The state of Americans*. New York: Free Press.

Chess, S., & Thomas, A. (1995). *Temperament in clinical practice*. New York: Guilford Press.

Chess, S., & Thomas, A. (1996). *Temperament: Theory and practice*. Philadelphia: Brunner/Mazel Publishers.

Chess, S., & Thomas, A. (1999). *Goodness of fit: Clinical applications from infancy through adult life*. Philadelphia: Brunner/Mazel Publishers.

Cummings, E., & Henry, W. (1961). *Growing old: The process of disengagement*. New York: Basic Books.

Diego, M., et al. (2006). Maternal Psychological Distress, Prenatal Cortisol, and Fetal Weight. *Psychosomatic Medicine, 68*, 747–753.

Eaton, D. K., Kann, L., Kinchen, S., Ross, J., Hawkins, J., Harris, W. A., et al. (2006). Youth risk behavior surveillance—United States, 2005. *Morbidity and Mortality Weekly Report, 55*(SS05), 1–108.

Edwards, M. E. (2002). Attachment, mastery, and interdependence: A model of parenting processes. *Family Process, 41*(3), 389–404.

Erikson, E. (1963). *Childhood and society*. New York: W.W. Norton.

Erikson, E. (1968). *Identity: Youth and crisis*. New York: W.W. Norton.

Fowler, J., & Keen, S. (1985). *Life maps: Conversations in the journey of faith*. Waco, TX: Word Books.

Fowler, J. W., Streib, H., & Keller, B. (2004). *Manual for faith development research* (3rd ed.). Bielefeld, Germany: Research Center for Biographical Studies in Contemporary Religion; Atlanta: Center for Research in Faith and Moral Development, Emory University.

Dennis, C. L. (2006). Identifying predictors of breastfeeding self-efficacy in the immediate postpartum period. *Research in Nursing and Health, 28*, 256–268.

Garvey, C., Julion, W., Fogg, L., Kratovil, A., & Gross, D. (2006). Measuring participation in a prevention trial with parents of young children. *Research in Nursing & Health, 29*, 212–222.

Gilligan, C. (1982). *In a different voice: Psychological theory and women's development*. Cambridge, MA: Harvard University Press.

Gould, R. L. (1972). The phases of adult life: A study in developmental psychology. *American Journal of Psychiatry, 129*, 33–43.

Havighurst, R. J. (1972). *Developmental tasks and education* (3rd ed.). Boston: Allyn & Bacon.

Huizink, A. C., & Mulder, E. J. (2006). Maternal smoking, drinking, or cannabis use during pregnancy and neurobehavioral and cognitive functioning in human offspring. *Neuroscience and Biobehavior Review, 30*, 24–41.

Kohlberg, L. (1981). *Essays on moral development: Vol. 1. The philosophy of moral development*. San Francisco: Harper & Row.

Kohlberg, L. (1984). *Essays on moral development: Vol. 2. The psychology of moral development*. San Francisco: Harper & Row.

Malone, J. A. (1998). The resiliency model of family stress, adjustment, and adaptation. In B. Vaughan-Cole, M. A. Johnson, J. A. Malone, & B. L. Walker. *Family nursing practice* (pp. 49–60). Philadelphia: W.B. Saunders.

McCarter-Spaulding, D. E. (2005). Medications in pregnancy and lactation. *MCN. American Journal of Maternal Child Nursing, 30*, 10–17.

Murray, R. B., & Zentner, J. P. (2001). *Health promotion strategies through the life span* (7th ed.). Upper Saddle River, NJ: Prentice Hall.

Peck, R. (1968). Psychological developments in the second half of life. In B. L. Neugarten (Ed.), *Middle age and aging*. Chicago: University of Chicago Press.

Piaget, J. (1966). *Origins of intelligence in children*. New York: W.W. Norton.

Rew, L., Whittaker, T. A., Taylor-Seehafer, M. A., & Smith, L. R. (2005). Sexual health risks and protective resources in gay, lesbian, bisexual, and heterosexual homeless youth. *Journal of Specialists in Pediatric Nursing, 10*, 11–19.

Stewart, M., Reid, G., & Mangham, C. (1997). Fostering children's resilience. *Journal of Pediatric Nursing, 12*, 21–31.

Westerhoff, J. (1976). *Will our children have faith?* New York: Seabury Press.

Witt, C. (2003). Detecting developmental dysplasia of the hip. *Advances in Neonatal Care, 3*, 65–75.

Elimination

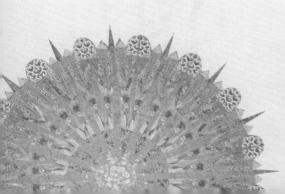

Concept at-a-Glance

Concept Learning Outcomes

After reading about this concept, you will be able to do the following:

1. Summarize the structure and physiologic processes of the renal and gastrointestinal systems related to elimination.

2. List factors affecting elimination.

3. Identify commonly occurring alterations in elimination and their related treatments.

4. Explain common physical assessment procedures used to evaluate bowel and urinary health of clients across the life span.

5. Outline diagnostic and laboratory tests and expected findings to determine the individual's elimination status.

6. Explain management of urinary and bowel health and prevention of urinary and bowel illness.

7. Demonstrate the nursing process in providing culturally competent care across the life span for individuals with common alterations in elimination.

8. Identify pharmacologic interventions in caring for individuals with alterations in urinary and bowel function.

Concept Key Terms

Anuria, *78*

Blood urea nitrogen (BUN), *78*

Borborygmus, *94*

Bruits, *94*

Calculi, *82*

Creatinine clearance, *83*

Defecation, *89*

Detrusor muscle, *73*

Dialysis, *78*

Diarrhea, *92*

Diuresis, *78*

Diuretics, *76*

Dysuria, *79*

Elimination, *71*

Enuresis, *76*

Feces, *89*

Flatulence, *93*

Flatus, *90*

Gastrocolic reflex, *91*

Glomerulus, *72*

Glycosuria, *75*

Hemodialysis, *78*

Hernia, *94*

Hyponatremia, *78*

Ileus, *92*

Laxatives, *92*

Meconium, *90*

Meatus, *73*

Micturition, *74*

Neurogenic bladder, *79*

Nocturia, *79*

Nocturnal enuresis, *76*

Nocturnal frequency, *76*

Occult blood, *97*

Oliguria, *78*

Peritoneal dialysis, *78*

Polydipsia, *78*

Polyuria, *78*

Reflux, *90*

Renal failure, *77*

Residual urine, *75*

Stool, *89*

Striae, *94*

Urgency, *79*

Urinary frequency, *79*

Urinary hesitancy, *79*

Urination, *74*

Voiding, *74*

About Elimination

This concept will discuss the process of urinary and gastrointestinal elimination. The term **elimination** refers to the secretion and excretion of body wastes from the kidneys and intestines and any alterations from normal of those processes. Using the nursing process, along with critical thinking and scientific rationales, to make decisions about the care of clients of all ages who are experiencing alterations in elimination, nurses can work with clients to optimize their health and well-being.

Elimination processes are intertwined in the physiology of the human body. Alterations in elimination often indicate alterations from normal in other physiologic areas, side effects from medications, or improper levels of hydration or nutrition. Because nurses frequently are the first health care professionals to determine that a client is experiencing problems with elimination, nurses must be familiar with the different alterations in elimination, their risk factors, and how these alterations affect other physiologic processes. ●

Urinary Elimination

Urinary elimination habits depend on social, cultural, personal, and physical factors. In North America, most people are accustomed to privacy and clean, even decorative, surroundings while they eliminate.

Personal habits regarding urinary elimination are affected by the social propriety of leaving to urinate, the availability of a private and clean facility, and initial training. Elimination is essential to health, and it can be postponed for only so long before the urge becomes too great to control.

NORMAL PRESENTATION

Urinary elimination depends on effective functioning of the upper urinary tract (kidneys and ureters) and the lower urinary tract (urinary bladder, urethra, and pelvic floor). Figure 4–1 ■ shows the anatomic structures of the urinary tract.

Kidneys

The paired kidneys are situated on either side of the spinal column, behind the peritoneal cavity. The right kidney is slightly lower than the left because of the position of the liver. The kidneys are the primary regulators of fluid and acid–base balance in the body. The functional units of the kidneys—the nephrons (Figure 4–2 ■)—filter the blood and remove metabolic wastes. In the average adult, 1,200 mL of blood, or approximately 21% of the cardiac output, passes through the kidneys every minute. Each kidney contains approximately 1 million nephrons. Each nephron has a **glomerulus**, a tuft of capillaries surrounded by the Bowman's capsule. The endothelium of glomerular capillaries is porous, allowing fluid and solutes to move readily across this membrane into the capsule. Plasma proteins and blood cells are too large to cross the membrane normally. Glomerular filtrate, which is made up of water, electrolytes, glucose, amino acids, and metabolic wastes, is similar in composition to plasma.

From the Bowman's capsule, the filtrate moves into the tubule of the nephron. In the proximal convoluted tubule, most of the water and electrolytes are reabsorbed. Solutes, such as glucose, are reabsorbed in the loop of Henle, proximal tubule, and collecting ducts; however, other substances also are secreted into the filtrate, concentrating the urine. In the distal convoluted tubule, additional water and sodium are reabsorbed under the control of hormones such as antidiuretic hormone

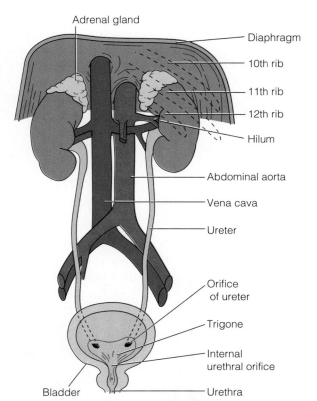

Figure 4–1 ■ Anatomic structures of the urinary tract.

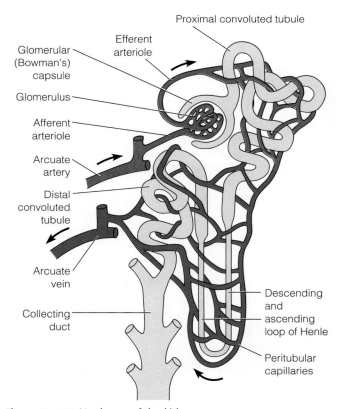

Figure 4–2 ■ Nephrons of the kidneys.

(ADH) and aldosterone. This controlled reabsorption allows fine regulation of fluid and electrolyte balance in the body. When fluid intake is low or the concentration of solutes in the blood is high, ADH is released from the anterior pituitary, more water is reabsorbed in the distal tubule, and less urine is excreted. By contrast, when fluid intake is high or the blood solute concentration is low, ADH is suppressed. Without ADH, the distal tubule becomes impermeable to water, and more urine is excreted. Aldosterone also affects the tubule. When aldosterone is released from the adrenal cortex, sodium and water are reabsorbed in greater quantities, increasing the blood volume and decreasing the urinary output.

Ureters

Once the urine is formed in the kidneys, it moves through the collecting ducts into the calyces of the renal pelvis and, from there, into the ureters. In the adult, the ureters are 25–30 cm (10–12 in.) in length and approximately 1.25 cm (0.5 in.) in diameter. The upper end of each ureter is funnel shaped as it enters the kidney. The lower ends of the ureters enter the bladder at the posterior corners of the floor of the bladder. At the junction between the ureter and the bladder, a flap-like fold of mucous membrane acts as a valve to prevent backflow of urine up the ureters.

Bladder

The urinary bladder (vesicle) is a hollow, muscular organ that serves as a reservoir for urine and as the organ of excretion. When empty, it lies behind the symphysis pubis. In men, the bladder lies in front of the rectum and above the prostate gland; in women, it lies in front of the uterus and vagina (Figures 4–3 ■ and 4–4 ■). The bladder wall is made up of four layers: (a) an inner mucous layer; (b) a connective tissue layer; (c) three layers of smooth muscle fibers, some of which extend lengthwise, some obliquely, and some more or less circularly; and (d) an outer serous layer. The smooth muscle layers are collectively called the **detrusor muscle** The detrusor muscle allows the bladder to expand as it fills with urine and to contract as it releases urine to the outside of the body during voiding (D'Amico & Barbarito,

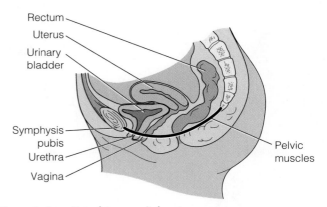

Figure 4–4 ■ Female urogenital system.

2007). At the base of the bladder is the trigone, a triangular area marked by the ureter openings at the posterior corners and the opening of the urethra at the anteroinferior corner.

The bladder is capable of considerable distention because of rugae (folds) in the mucous membrane lining and because of the elasticity of its walls. When full, the dome of the bladder may extend above the symphysis pubis; in extreme situations, it may extend as high as the umbilicus. Normal bladder capacity is between 300 and 600 mL of urine.

Urethra

The urethra extends from the bladder to the urinary **meatus** (opening). In the adult woman, the urethra lies directly behind the symphysis pubis, anterior to the vagina, and is between 3 and 4 cm (1.5 in.) in length (see Figure 4–4). The urethra serves only as a passageway for the elimination of urine. The urinary meatus is located between the labia minora, in front of the vagina and below the clitoris. The male urethra is approximately 20 cm (8 in.) in length and serves as a passageway for semen, as well as for urine (see Figure 4–3). In men, the meatus is located at the distal end of the penis.

In men and women both, the urethra has a mucous membrane lining that is continuous with the bladder and the ureters. Thus, an infection of the urethra can extend through the urinary tract to the kidneys. Women are particularly prone to urinary tract infections (UTIs) because of their short urethras and the proximity of the urinary meatus to the vagina and anus.

Pelvic Floor

The vagina, urethra, and rectum pass through the pelvic floor, which consists of sheets of muscles and ligaments that support the viscera of the pelvis (see Figures 4–3 and 4–4). The pelvic floor muscles are under voluntary control and are important in controlling urination. Specific sphincter muscles contribute to the continence mechanism (Figure 4–5 ■). These muscles can become weakened by pregnancy and childbirth, chronic constipation, decrease in estrogen (menopause), being overweight, aging, and lack of general fitness. The internal sphincter muscle situated in the proximal urethra and the bladder neck is composed of smooth muscle under involuntary control. It provides active tension

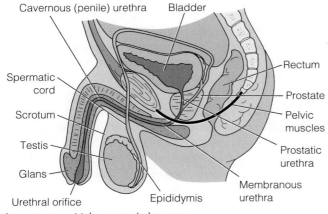

Figure 4–3 ■ Male urogenital system.

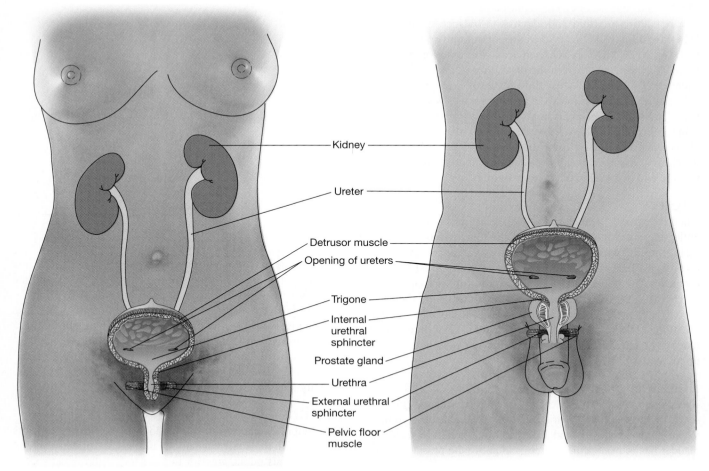

Figure 4–5 ■ Female and male urinary bladders and urethras, showing sphincter muscles.

Source: Custom Medical Stock Photo, Inc.

designed to close the urethral lumen. The external sphincter muscle is composed of skeletal muscle under voluntary control, allowing the individual to choose when urine is eliminated.

Urination

Micturition, **voiding**, and **urination** all refer to the process of emptying the urinary bladder. Urine collects in the bladder until pressure stimulates special sensory nerve endings, called stretch receptors, in the bladder wall. This stimulation occurs when the adult bladder contains between 250 and 450 mL of urine. In children, a considerably smaller volume (50–200 mL) stimulates these nerves.

The stretch receptors transmit impulses to the spinal cord—specifically to the voiding reflex center located at the level of the second to fourth sacral vertebrae, causing the internal sphincter to relax and stimulating the urge to void. If the time and place are appropriate for urination, the conscious portion of the brain relaxes the external urethral sphincter muscle, and urination takes place. If the time and place are inappropriate, the micturition reflex usually subsides until the bladder becomes more filled and the reflex is stimulated again.

Voluntary control of urination is possible only if the nerves supplying the bladder and urethra, the neural tracts of the cord and the brain, and the motor area of the cerebrum are all intact. The individual must be able to sense that the bladder is full. Injury to any of these parts of the nervous system—for example, by a cerebral hemorrhage or a spinal cord injury above the level of the sacral region—results in intermittent involuntary emptying of the bladder. Older adults whose cognition is impaired may not be aware of the need to urinate or be able to respond to this urge appropriately.

Although patterns of urination are highly individual, most people void about five or six times a day. People usually void when they first awaken in the morning, before they go to bed, and around mealtimes. Table 4–1 shows the average urinary output per day at different ages.

Pregnancy

During the first trimester of pregnancy, the enlarging uterus is still a pelvic organ and presses against the bladder, producing urinary frequency. This symptom decreases during the second trimester when the uterus becomes an abdominal organ and pressure against the bladder decreases. Urinary frequency reappears during the third trimester when the presenting part of the uterus descends into the pelvis and again presses on the bladder, thus reducing bladder capacity, contributing to hyperemia, and irritating the bladder. The ureters elongate and dilate above the pelvic brim; this is especially the case for the right ureter. The glomerular filtration rate (GFR) rises by as much as 50% beginning in the second trimester, and it remains elevated until birth. To compensate for this increase, renal tubular reabsorption also increases. However, **glycosuria** (excretion of carbohydrates into the urine) sometimes arises during pregnancy because of the kidneys' inability to reabsorb all the glucose filtered by the glomeruli. Glycosuria may be normal or may indicate gestational diabetes, so it always warrants further testing. Presence of protein, blood, or white cells is always considered to be abnormal and should be evaluated.

The postpartum woman has an increased bladder capacity, swelling and bruising of the tissue around the urethra, decreased sensitivity to fluid pressure, and decreased sensation of bladder filling. Consequently, the postpartum woman is at risk for overdistention, incomplete bladder emptying, and buildup of **residual urine** (urine that remains in the bladder after voiding). Women who have had an anesthetic block have inhibited neural functioning of the bladder and are more susceptible to bladder distention, difficulty with voiding, and bladder infections. In addition, immediate postpartum use of oxytocin (to facilitate uterine contractions following expulsion of the placenta) has an antidiuretic effect. After oxytocin is discontinued, the woman will experience rapid bladder filling (Cunningham et al., 2005).

Urinary output increases during the early postpartum period (first 12–24 hours) because of puerperal diuresis. The kidneys must eliminate an estimated 2,000–3,000 mL of extracellular fluid with a normal pregnancy, causing rapid filling of the bladder. As a result, adequate bladder elimination is an immediate concern. Women with preeclampsia, chronic hypertension, or diabetes experience greater fluid retention than other women do, and postpartum diuresis increases accordingly. If urine stasis exists, the chance for a UTI increases because of bacteriuria and the presence of dilated ureters and renal pelves, which persist for approximately 6 weeks after birth. A full bladder also may increase

the tendency of the uterus to relax by displacing the uterus and interfering with its contractility, increasing the risk for hemorrhage. In the absence of infection, the dilated ureters and renal pelves return to prepregnant size by the end of the sixth week.

Newborns

The GFR of the newborn's kidney is low compared to that of the adult. Because of this physiologic decrease in kidney glomerular filtration, the newborn's kidney is unable to dispose of water rapidly when necessary. Full-term newborns are less able to concentrate urine because the tubules are short and narrow. The limited tubular reabsorption of water and limited excretion of solutes (principally sodium, potassium, chloride, bicarbonate, urea, and phosphate) in the growing newborn also reduce the newborn's ability to concentrate urine, and because the newborn has difficulty concentrating urine, the effect of excessive insensible water loss or restricted fluid intake is unpredictable. The newborn kidney also is limited in dilutional capabilities. These limitations regarding concentration and dilution are important considerations in monitoring fluid therapy to prevent dehydration or overhydration. The newborn attains the ability to concentrate urine fully by 3 months of age.

Many newborns void immediately after birth, and the voiding frequently goes unnoticed. Among healthy newborns, 93% void by 24 hours after birth, and 100% void by 48 hours after birth (Thureen, Deacon, Hernandez, & Hall, 2005). A newborn who has not voided by 48 hours should be assessed for adequacy of fluid intake, bladder distention, restlessness, and symptoms of pain. If any of these signs are observed, the appropriate clinical personnel should be notified.

The initial bladder volume is 6–44 mL of urine. Unless edema is present, normal urinary output often is limited, and voiding is scanty until fluid intake increases. For the first 2 days after birth, the newborn voids from 2 to 6 times daily, with a urine output of 15 mL • kg^{-1} • day^{-1}. The newborn subsequently voids from 5 to 25 times every 24 hours, with a volume of 25 mL • kg^{-1} • day^{-1}.

After the first voiding episode, the newborn's urine frequently is cloudy (because of mucus content) and has a high specific gravity, which decreases as fluid intake increases. Occasionally, pink stains ("brick dust spots") appear on the diaper. These are caused by urates and are innocuous. During early infancy, normal urine is straw colored and almost odorless, although odor can occur when certain drugs are given, metabolic disorders exist, or infection is present.

FACTORS AFFECTING URINARY ELIMINATION

Numerous factors affect the volume and characteristics of the urine produced and the manner in which it is excreted.

Developmental Factors

Factors specific to infants, preschoolers, school-age children, and older adults can affect the elimination of urine.

TABLE 4–1 **Average Daily Urine Output by Age**

AGE	AMOUNT (mL)
1 to 2 days	15–60
3 to 10 days	100–300
10 days to 2 months	250–450
2 months to 1 year	400–500
1 to 3 years	500–600
3 to 5 years	600–700
5 to 8 years	700–1,000
8 to 14 years	800–1,400
14 years through adulthood	1,500
Older adulthood	1,500 or less

Source: Berman, A., Snyder, S. J., Kozier, B., & Erb, G. (2008). *Kozier & Erb's fundamentals of nursing: Concepts, process, and practice* (8th ed., p. 1290). Upper Saddle River, NJ: Pearson Education.

INFANTS Urine output varies according to fluid intake but gradually increases to between 250 and 500 mL a day during the first year. Infants are born without urinary control and may urinate as often as 25 times a day. Most will develop urinary control between 2 and 5 years of age. Control during the daytime normally precedes control during the nighttime.

PRESCHOOLERS A preschooler is able to take responsibility for independent toileting. Parents must realize that accidents occur; however, the child should never be punished or chastised for a toileting accident. Because children at this age often forget to wash their hands or flush the toilet, they require reminders and appropriate adult modeling. Young children also require instruction in wiping themselves. Girls should be taught to wipe from front to back to prevent contamination of the urinary tract by feces.

SCHOOL-AGE CHILDREN The school-age child's elimination system reaches maturity during this period. The kidneys double in size between 5 and 10 years of age. During this period, the child urinates six to eight times a day.

Enuresis which is defined as the involuntary passing of urine when control should be established (approximately 5 years of age), can be a problem for some school-age children. About 10% of all 6 year olds experience difficulty controlling the bladder.

Nocturnal enuresis, or bed-wetting, is the involuntary passing of urine during sleep. It has many causes but basically occurs because the child fails to awaken when the bladder empties (Nield & Kamat, 2004, p. 409). The incidence of nocturnal enuresis decreases as the child matures, and bed-wetting should not be considered a problem until after 6 years of age. Nocturnal enuresis may be referred to as primary when the child has never achieved nighttime urinary control. Secondary enuresis is that which appears after the child has achieved dryness for a period of 6 consecutive months. Often, it is related to another problem, such as constipation, stress, or illness, and may resolve when the cause is eliminated. Recent research indicates that primary and secondary nocturnal enuresis both may be related to poor daytime voiding habits, and children should be taught to be aware of the sensation of needing to void (Robson, Leung, & Van Howe, 2005).

OLDER ADULTS The excretory function of the kidneys diminishes as people age, but function usually does not diminish significantly below normal levels unless a disease process intervenes. Arteriosclerosis can reduce blood flow, impairing renal function. As a person ages, the number of functioning nephrons decreases to some degree, impairing the kidney's filtering abilities. Conditions that alter normal fluid intake and output, such as influenza or surgery, can compromise the kidney's ability to filter, maintain acid–base balance, and maintain electrolyte balance in older adults, and the amount of time necessary for these processes to return to normal functioning also increases as a person ages. The decrease in kidney function also places older adults at higher risk for toxicity from medications when excretion rates are longer.

The more noticeable changes as a person ages are related to the bladder. Reports of urinary urgency and urinary frequency are common. In men, these changes often are caused by an enlarged prostate gland; in women, they may be caused by weakened muscles supporting the bladder or by weakness of the urethral sphincter. The capacity of the bladder and its ability to empty both diminish as a person ages. This explains the need for older adults to awaken at night to void (**nocturnal frequency**) and the increase in retention of residual urine. The increased retention of residual urine predisposes the older adult to bladder infection. Table 4–2 shows a summary of the developmental changes that affect urinary output.

Psychosocial Factors

For many people, a set of conditions helps stimulate the micturition reflex. These conditions include privacy, normal position, sufficient time, and occasionally, running water. Circumstances that do not allow for the client's accustomed conditions may produce anxiety and muscle tension. When this happens, the person is unable to relax the abdominal and perineal muscles and the external urethral sphincter, and voiding is inhibited. People also may voluntarily suppress urination because of perceived time pressures; for example, nurses often ignore the urge to void until they are able to take a break. This behavior can increase the risk of UTIs.

Fluid and Food Intake

The healthy body maintains a balance between the amount of fluid ingested and the amount of fluid eliminated. When the amount of fluid intake increases, the output normally increases. Certain fluids, such as alcohol, increase fluid output by inhibiting the production of ADH. By contrast, food and fluids that are high in sodium can cause fluid retention so that the body will be able to maintain the normal concentration of electrolytes. Some foods and fluids can change the color of urine: Beets can cause urine to appear red; foods containing carotene can cause yellow discoloration of the urine.

Medications

Many medications, particularly those affecting the autonomic nervous system, interfere with the normal urination process and may cause retention (Box 4–1). **Diuretics** (e.g., chlorothiazide and furosemide) increase urine formation by preventing the reabsorption in the bloodstream of water and electrolytes from the tubules of the kidney. Some medications may alter the color of the urine.

Muscle Tone

Good muscle tone is important to maintain the elasticity and contractility of the detrusor muscle, allowing the bladder to fill adequately and empty completely. Clients who require long-term use of a retention catheter may develop poor bladder muscle tone because continuous drainage of urine prevents the bladder from filling and emptying normally. Pelvic muscle tone also contributes to the ability to store and empty urine.

Pathologic Conditions

Some diseases and conditions can affect the formation and excretion of urine. Diseases of the kidneys may affect the ability of the nephrons to produce urine. Abnormal amounts of protein or

TABLE 4–2 Changes in Urinary Elimination Through the Life Span

STAGE	VARIATIONS
Fetuses	The fetal kidney begins to excrete urine between the 11th and 12th weeks of development.
Infants	Ability to concentrate urine is minimal; therefore, urine appears light yellow. Because of neuromuscular immaturity, voluntary urinary control is absent.
Children	Kidney function reaches maturity between the first and second year of life; urine is concentrated effectively and appears a normal amber color. Between 18 and 24 months of age, the child starts to recognize bladder fullness and is able to hold urine beyond the urge to void. At approximately 2.5–3 years of age, the child can perceive bladder fullness, hold urine after the urge to void, and communicate the need to urinate. Full urinary control usually occurs at 4 or 5 years of age; daytime control is usually achieved by 3 years of age. The kidneys grow in proportion to overall body growth.
Adults	The kidneys reach maximum size between 35 and 40 years of age. After 50 years, the kidneys begin to diminish in size and function. Most shrinkage occurs in the cortex of the kidney as individual nephrons are lost.
Older adults	An estimated 30% of nephrons are lost by 80 years of age. Renal blood flow decreases because of vascular changes and a decrease in cardiac output. The ability to concentrate urine declines. Bladder muscle tone diminishes, causing increased frequency of urination and nocturia (voiding two or more times at night). Diminished bladder muscle tone and contractility may lead to residual urine in the bladder after voiding, increasing the risk of bacterial growth and infection. Urinary incontinence may occur because of mobility problems or neurologic impairments.

Source: Berman, A., Snyder, S. J., Kozier, B., & Erb, G. (2008). *Kozier & Erb's fundamentals of nursing: Concepts, process, and practice* (8th ed., p. 1289). Upper Saddle River, NJ: Pearson Education.

blood cells may be present in the urine, or the kidneys may virtually stop producing urine altogether, a condition known as **renal failure**. Heart and circulatory disorders, such as heart failure, shock, or hypertension, can affect blood flow to the kidneys, interfering with urine production. When abnormal amounts of fluid are lost through another route (e.g., vomiting or high fever), the kidneys retain water, and urinary output decreases.

Processes that interfere with the flow of urine from the kidneys to the urethra also affect urinary excretion. A urinary stone (calculus) may obstruct a ureter, blocking urine flow

from the kidney to the bladder. Hypertrophy of the prostate gland, a common condition affecting older men, may obstruct the urethra, impairing urination and bladder emptying.

Surgical and Diagnostic Procedures

Some surgical and diagnostic procedures affect the passage of urine and even the urine itself. The urethra may swell after cystoscopy (endoscopy of the urinary bladder), and surgical procedures on any part of the urinary tract may result in some postoperative bleeding, which can cause the urine to be tinged red or pink for a time.

Spinal anesthetics can affect the passage of urine because they decrease the client's awareness of the need to void. Swelling in the lower abdomen because of surgery on structures adjacent to the urinary tract (e.g., the uterus) also can affect voiding.

AGE-RELATED CHANGES IN THE URINARY SYSTEM

It is difficult to differentiate normal aging of the genitourinary system from changes related to common conditions found in older people. It is prudent, therefore, to keep an open mind when discussing age-related changes.

Renal function begins to decline around 40 years of age but does not create significant issues for an otherwise healthy individual until the ninth decade of life. At that time, decreases in GFR, renal blood flow, maximal urinary concentration, and response to sodium loss are marked. Renal function in an 85-year-old person is approximately 50% of

Box 4–1 Medications That May Cause Urinary Retention

- Anticholinergic and antispasmodic medications, such as atropine and papaverine
- Antidepressant and antipsychotic agents, such as phenothiazines and monoamine oxidase inhibitors
- Antihistamine preparations, especially those containing pseudoephedrine (e.g., Claritin-D and Sudafed)
- Antihypertensive agents, such as hydralazine (Apresoline) and methyldopa (Aldomet)
- Antiparkinsonism drugs, such as levodopa, trihexyphenidyl (Artane), and benztropine mesylate (Cogentin)
- Beta-adrenergic blockers, such as propranolol (Inderal)
- Opioids, such as hydrocodone (Vicodin)

Source: Berman, A., Snyder, S. J., Kozier, B., & Erb, G. (2008). *Kozier & Erb's fundamentals of nursing: Concepts, process, and practice* (8th ed., p. 1290). Upper Saddle River, NJ: Pearson Education.

that in a 30-year-old person (Timiras & Leary, 2007). Sclerosis may be found in as many as 40% of the remaining glomeruli, and fibrous changes in the interstitial tissues may be found in older persons without kidney disease (Bailey & Sands, 2003; Wiggins, 2003). Blood flow to the kidney decreases as a result of atrophy in the supplying blood vessels, particularly in the renal cortex. In addition, the proximal tubules decrease in number and length. Compared with a young adult, an older adult usually has a lower creatinine clearance, has urine that is more dilute (lower specific gravity), and typically excretes lower levels of glucose, acid, and potassium. As these changes progress, the serum creatinine level and the **blood urea nitrogen (BUN)** will increase (Esposito et al., 2007). In addition, the kidneys of older adults excrete more fluid and electrolytes during the night than during the day, and more urine is formed at night, potentially interrupting sleep patterns.

One very important consequence of these changes is impaired excretion of drugs and their metabolites, making older adults extremely susceptible to drug overdose and other adverse effects of medication (even when administered within a normal dose range). This is of particular concern for the older adult with multiple health impairments who requires several types of pharmacologic therapies. Another consequence of age-related changes is an increased probability of hyperkalemia, particularly when potassium-sparing diuretics, angiotensin-converting enzyme inhibitors, nonsteroidal anti-inflammatory drugs, or beta-blockers are used (Timiras & Luxenberg, 2007). The older adult's decreased ability to concentrate urine results in an increased susceptibility to dehydration, a problem that is further complicated by a deficit in the thirst response; therefore, the older person may not feel thirsty even when significantly dehydrated. In addition, an older adult who has concerns about incontinence may choose not to drink for fear of an incontinence accident. These changes also produce a decline in the ability of older adults to respond to a fluid overload by increasing urine production.

Changes in the bladder and urethra also occur with aging. The bladder becomes more fibrous, with a subsequent decrease in capacity and an increase in residual urine (Huether & McCance, 2005). Autonomic regulation of the bladder by the nervous system decreases as a person ages, affecting contraction of both the detrusor muscle and the external sphincter. The detrusor muscle becomes less contractile but also somewhat unstable. This means that the older adult is subject both to the inability to empty the bladder completely and to involuntary contractions of the bladder (Ouslander & Johnson, 2003). Age-related weakening also occurs in the voluntary pelvic floor muscles, which are important in controlling the release of urine from the urethra. These changes make older adults more likely to have difficulty delaying urination and predispose them to urinary incontinence and UTI. However, it is important for the nurse to remember that even though some anatomic and physiologic changes make incontinence more probable with increased age, urinary incontinence is not a normal part of aging.

Older adults tend to have higher basal levels of ADH than younger adults do, and the pituitary responds more vigorously to osmotic stimuli by secreting more ADH than in younger people (Timiras & Leary, 2007). Although ADH is released as a response to hypotension and hypovolemia (low blood volume), its action is blunted in older adults, requiring the release of more hormones to achieve the desired antidiuretic effect. In addition, the aging kidney is less responsive to circulating ADH, producing urine that is poorly concentrated and rich in sodium. This puts the older adult at increased risk of **hyponatremia**, an abnormally low concentration of sodium in the blood that can be magnified with the use of diuretics.

ALTERATIONS

A number of diseases and processes can interfere with the flow of blood to the kidneys or of urine from the kidneys, interfering with the production and elimination of urine.

Altered Urine Production

Polyuria (or **diuresis**) is the production of abnormally large amounts of urine by the kidneys—often several liters more than the client's usual daily output. Polyuria can occur after excessive fluid intake, a condition known as **polydipsia** or it may be associated with diseases such as diabetes mellitus, diabetes insipidus, and chronic nephritis. Polyuria can cause excessive fluid loss, leading to intense thirst, dehydration, and weight loss.

The terms "anuria" and "oliguria" are used to describe decreased urinary output. **Anuria** refers to an absence of urine production, whereas **oliguria** refers to a low urine output, usually less than 500 mL a day or 30 mL an hour for an adult. Although oliguria may occur as a result of abnormal fluid losses or a lack of fluid intake, it often indicates impaired blood flow to the kidneys or impending renal failure, and it should be reported promptly to the primary care provider. Rapid restoration of renal blood flow and urinary output can prevent renal failure and its complications.

Should the kidneys become unable to function adequately, some mechanism of filtering the blood is necessary to prevent illness and death. This filtering is done through renal **dialysis**, a technique by which fluids and molecules pass through a semipermeable membrane according to the rules of osmosis. The two most common methods of dialysis are hemodialysis and peritoneal dialysis. In **hemodialysis**, the client's blood flows through vascular catheters, passes by the dialysis solution in an external machine, and then returns to the client. In **peritoneal dialysis**, the dialysis solution is instilled into the abdominal cavity through a catheter, allowed to rest there while the fluid and molecules exchange, and then removed through the catheter. Both hemodialysis and peritoneal dialysis must be performed at frequent intervals until the client's kidneys can resume the filtering function.

Altered Urinary Elimination

Despite normal production of urine, a number of factors or conditions can affect its elimination. Urinary frequency, nocturia, urgency, and dysuria often are manifestations of underlying conditions such as a UTI. Enuresis, incontinence, retention, and neurogenic bladder may be either a manifestation of an underlying condition or the primary problem affecting elimination of urine. Selected factors associated with altered patterns of urinary elimination are identified in Table 4–3.

Urinary frequency is voiding at frequent intervals—that is, more than four to six times a day. An increased intake of fluid causes some increase in the frequency of voiding. Conditions such as UTI, stress, and pregnancy can cause frequent voiding of small quantities (50–100 mL) of urine. Total fluid intake and output may be normal. **Nocturia** usually is expressed in terms of the number of times the person gets out of bed to void—for example, "nocturia ×4."

Urgency is the sudden strong desire to void. Whether or not a great deal of urine is present in the bladder, the person feels a need to void immediately. Urgency often accompanies psychologic stress and irritation of the trigone and urethra. It also is common in people who have poor external sphincter control and unstable bladder contractions. It is not a normal finding.

Dysuria means voiding that is either painful or difficult. It can accompany a stricture (decrease in diameter) of the urethra, UTI, and injury to the bladder and urethra. Often, clients will say they have to push to void or that burning accompanies or follows voiding. The burning may be described as severe, like a hot poker, or more subdued, like sunburn. **Urinary hesitancy** (a delay and difficulty in initiating voiding) is associated often with dysuria.

Adults and children can experience enuresis. Diurnal (daytime) enuresis may be persistent and pathologic in origin. It affects women and girls more frequently than it does men and boys. The occurrence of enuresis after voluntary bladder control has been acquired successfully should be reported to the primary care provider.

Impaired neurologic function can interfere with the normal mechanisms of urinary elimination, resulting in a **neurogenic bladder**. The client with a neurogenic bladder does not perceive bladder fullness and is unable to control the urinary sphincters. The bladder may become flaccid and distended or spastic, with frequent involuntary urination. For additional details, see the Alterations and Treatments features.

TABLE 4–3 Selected Factors Associated With Altered Urinary Elimination

PATTERN	SELECTED ASSOCIATED FACTORS
Polyuria	Ingestion of fluids containing caffeine or alcohol Prescribed diuretic Presence of thirst, dehydration, and weight loss History of diabetes mellitus, diabetes insipidus, or kidney disease
Oliguria, anuria	Decrease in fluid intake Signs of dehydration Presence of hypotension, shock, or heart failure History of kidney disease Signs of renal failure, such as elevated BUN and serum creatinine Edema, hypertension
Frequency or nocturia	Pregnancy Increase in fluid intake UTI
Urgency	Presence of psychologic stress UTI
Dysuria	Urinary tract inflammation, infection, or injury Hesitancy, hematuria, pyuria (pus in the urine), and frequency
Enuresis	Family history of enuresis Difficult access to toilet facilities Home stresses
Incontinence	Bladder inflammation or other disease Difficulties in independent toileting (mobility impairment) Leakage when coughing, laughing, sneezing Cognitive impairment
Retention	Distended bladder on palpation and percussion Associated signs, such as pubic discomfort, restlessness, frequency, and small urine volume Recent anesthesia Recent perineal surgery Presence of perineal swelling Medications prescribed Lack of privacy or other factors inhibiting micturition

Source: Berman, A., Snyder, S. J., Kozier, B., & Erb, G. (2008). *Kozier & Erb's fundamentals of nursing: Concepts, process, and practice* (8th ed., p. 1291). Upper Saddle River, NJ: Pearson Education.

ALTERATIONS AND TREATMENTS Urinary Elimination Problems

Alteration	Description	Treatment
Urinary incontinence	Involuntary leakage of urine	■ Kegel exercises ■ Surgery ■ Bladder training
Urinary retention	Incomplete emptying or inability to empty bladder completely	■ Credé maneuver ■ Urinary catheter insertion
Prostatic hypertrophy	Enlargement of the prostate—may be benign or malignant	■ Surgical removal ■ Medications
Cancer of the urinary system	Abnormal cellular growth within the organs of the urinary tract	■ Surgery ■ Chemotherapy ■ Radiation therapy
Kidney stones	Formation of calculi within the calyx of the kidney, causing severe pain when moving through ureters	■ Administration of pain medication ■ Lithotripsy ■ Dietary alteration to reduce risk of recurrence ■ Increased fluid intake
Renal failure	Insufficient or absent kidney function	■ Administration of diuretics if some kidney function remains ■ Dialysis (hemodialysis or peritoneal dialysis) ■ Kidney transplantation
Infection of the urinary system	Pathogens within the sterile urinary system creating infection, which can occur in the bladder, ureter, or kidney	■ Administration of antibiotics if infection is caused by bacterium ■ Increased fluid intake ■ Cranberry juice to increase urine pH

PHYSICAL ASSESSMENT

Physical assessment, a health assessment interview that collects subjective data, and diagnostic tests are used to assess urinary system function. Box 4–2 shows sample documentation for an assessment of urinary system function, and the following Urinary Assessments feature provides additional information. Table 4–4 lists characteristics of normal and abnormal urine, and the following Assessment Interview feature gives further details regarding urinary elimination.

Box 4–2 Sample Documentation

Assessment of Urinary System Function

Home visit made to 66-year-old woman with end-stage chronic kidney failure. Skin pale and oral mucous membranes dry. 4+ edema in ankles and feet. Eyelids swollen. Skin tight and shiny over abdomen and bilateral lower extremities. Abdomen distended and tender on light palpation; further palpation deferred. Urinary bladder not palpable. Urine output for past 24 hours is 15 mL.

Urinary Assessment

Technique/Normal Findings	Abnormal Findings

Skin Assessment

Inspect the skin and mucous membranes, noting color, turgor, and excretions. *The color of skin and mucous membranes should be even and appropriate to the age and race of the client; skin should be dry with no visible excretions.*

- Pallor of the skin and mucous membranes may indicate kidney disease with resultant anemia.
- Decreased turgor of the skin may indicate dehydration.
- Edema (generalized or in the lower extremities) may indicate fluid volume excess. (Changes in skin turgor may indicate renal insufficiency with either excess fluid loss or retention.)
- An accumulation of uric acid crystals, called uremic frost, may be seen on the skin of the client with late-stage renal failure.

Abdominal Assessment

Inspect the abdomen, noting size, symmetry, masses or lumps, swelling, distention, glistening, or skin tightness. *The abdomen should be slightly concave, symmetric, without distention or masses.*

- Enlargements or asymmetry may indicate a hernia or superficial mass.
- If the urinary bladder is distended, it rises above the symphysis pubis as a rounded mass.
- Distention, glistening, or skin tightness may be associated with fluid retention.
- Ascites is an accumulation of fluid in the peritoneal cavity.

Urinary Assessment (continued)

Technique/Normal Findings	Abnormal Findings

Urinary Meatus Assessment

This technique is not part of a routine assessment, but it is an important component in clients with health problems of the urinary system.

For the male client: With the client in a sitting or standing position, compress the tip of the glans penis with your gloved hand to open the urinary meatus (Figure 4–6 ■).

For the female client: With the client in the dorsal lithotomy position, spread the labia with your gloved hand to expose the urinary meatus.

The urinary meatus should be midline and free of redness, lesions, or discharge.

- Increased redness, swelling, or discharge from the urinary meatus may indicate infection or sexually transmitted infection.
- Ulceration of the urinary meatus may indicate a sexually transmitted infection.
- Hypospadias is displacement of the urinary meatus to the ventral surface of the penis.
- Epispadias is displacement of the urinary meatus to the dorsal surface of the penis.

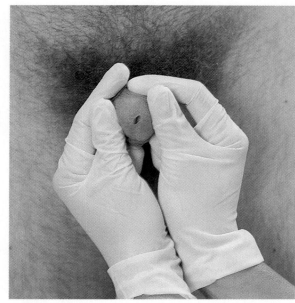

Figure 4–6 ■ Inspecting the urinary meatus of the male.

Kidney Assessment

Auscultate the renal arteries by placing the bell of the stethoscope lightly in the areas of the renal arteries, located in the left and right upper abdominal quadrants. *Bruits are not normally heard over the renal arteries.*

- Systolic bruits ("whooshing" sounds) may indicate renal artery stenosis.

Percuss the kidneys for tenderness or pain. *No tenderness or pain should be elicited.*

- Tenderness and pain on percussion of the costovertebral angle suggest glomerulonephritis or glomerulonephrosis.

Palpate the kidneys. The lower pole of the right kidney may be palpable with deep palpation; the remaining right kidney and the left kidney are normally not palpable. *If palpable, they should be nontender, bilaterally of appropriate size and density, without palpable masses.*

- A mass or lump may indicate a tumor or cyst.
- Tenderness or pain on palpation may suggest an inflammatory process.
- A soft kidney that feels spongy may indicate chronic renal disease.
- Bilaterally enlarged kidneys may suggest polycystic kidney disease.
- Unequal kidney size may indicate hydronephrosis.

Bladder Assessment

Percuss the bladder for tone and position. *The bladder should be midline without dullness.*

- A dull percussion tone over the bladder of a client who has just urinated may indicate urinary retention.

Palpate the bladder (over the symphysis pubis and abdomen) for distention. *The bladder is normally not palpable.*

- A distended bladder may be palpated at any point from the symphysis pubis to the umbilicus and is felt as a firm, rounded organ. It indicates urinary retention.

TABLE 4–4 **Characteristics of Normal and Abnormal Urine**

CHARACTERISTIC	NORMAL	ABNORMAL	NURSING CONSIDERATIONS
Amount in 24 hours (adult)	1,200–1,500 mL	1,200 mL A large amount over intake	Normally, urinary output is approximately equal to fluid intake. Output of less than 30 mL/hr may indicate decreased blood flow to the kidneys and should be reported immediately.
Color, clarity	Straw, amber Transparent	Dark amber Cloudy Dark orange Red or dark brown Mucous plugs, viscid, thick	Concentrated urine is darker in color. Dilute urine may appear almost clear, or very pale yellow. Some foods and drugs may color urine. Red blood cells in the urine (hematuria) may be evident as pink, bright red, or rusty brown urine. Menstrual bleeding also can color urine but should not be confused with hematuria. White blood cells, bacteria, pus, or contaminants (e.g., prostatic fluid, sperm, vaginal drainage) may cause cloudy urine.
Odor	Faint, aromatic	Offensive	Some foods (e.g., asparagus) cause a musty odor; infected urine can have a fetid odor; urine high in glucose has a sweet odor.
Sterility	No microorganisms present	Microorganisms present	Urine in the bladder is sterile. Urine specimens, however, may be contaminated by bacteria from the perineum during collection.
pH	4.5–8	8<4.5	Freshly voided urine is somewhat acidic. Alkaline urine may indicate a state of alkalosis, a UTI, or a diet high in fruits and vegetables. More acidic urine (low pH) is found in starvation, with diarrhea, or with a diet high in protein foods or cranberries.
Specific gravity	1.010–1.025	1.02<1.010	Concentrated urine has a higher specific gravity; diluted urine has a lower specific gravity.
Glucose	Not present	Present	Glucose in the urine indicates high blood glucose levels (>180 mg/dL) and may be indicative of undiagnosed or uncontrolled diabetes mellitus.
Ketone bodies (acetone)	Not present	Present	Ketones, the end product of the breakdown of fatty acids, are not normally present in the urine. They may be present in the urine of clients who have uncontrolled diabetes mellitus, who are in a state of starvation, or who have ingested excessive amounts of aspirin.
Blood	Not present	Occult (microscopic) Bright red	Blood may be present in the urine of clients who have a UTI, kidney disease, or bleeding from the urinary tract.

Note: Urine outputs below 30 mL/hr may indicate low blood volume or kidney malfunction. Nurses monitor urine output and should notify the primary provider if urine output averages less than 30 mL/hr over a 4-hour period of time.

Source: Berman, A., Snyder, S. J., Kozier, B., & Erb, G. (2008). *Kozier & Erb's fundamentals of nursing: Concepts, process, and practice* (8th ed., p. 1293). Upper Saddle River, NJ: Pearson Education.

DIAGNOSTIC TESTS

The results of diagnostic tests of urinary system function are used to support the diagnosis of a specific disease, to provide information to identify or modify the appropriate medication or therapy used to treat the disease, and to help nurses monitor the client's responses to treatment and nursing care interventions. Diagnostic tests to assess the structures and functions of the urinary system are described in the Diagnostic Tests feature and summarized in the bulleted list that follows.

- Urine may be tested for characteristics and components through routine analysis, a urine culture, a postvoiding residual urine, and a 24-hour collection for creatinine. Results of these tests include findings to serve as baseline data, to support the diagnosis of various health problems, to evaluate the ability to empty the bladder of urine, and to evaluate renal function.

- The ability to empty the bladder of urine may be evaluated by an ultrasonic bladder scan to examine for residual urine; uroflowmetry to measure the volume of urine voided per second; and cystometrography to evaluate bladder capacity, neuromuscular functions of the bladder, urethral pressures, and causes of bladder dysfunction.

- Radiologic examinations include intravenous pyelography (IVP), retrograde pyelography, and renal arteriography or angiography. These examinations are useful in visualizing (via radiographs) the urinary tract to identify abnormal size, shape, and function of the kidneys, kidney pelvis, and ureters, and to detect renal **calculi** (stones), tumors, or cysts.

Assessment Interview   Urinary Elimination

The assessment interview conducted by the nurse provides critical information about urinary function. The nurse should be direct but polite, recognizing that discussing urinary function can be embarrassing to many clients. Initially, the nurse should ask the client to describe the frequency of urination and any problems with urination. During the remainder of the interview, the nurse should use the vocabulary the client uses (to ensure understanding). In addition to recording the client's answers, the nurse should record any abnormalities that he or she observes in the client, such as swelling and changes in skin integrity.

VOIDING PATTERN

- How many times do you urinate during a 24-hour period?
- Has this pattern changed recently?
- Do you need to get out of bed to void at night? How often?

DESCRIPTION OF URINE AND ANY CHANGES

- How would you describe your urine in terms of color, clarity (clear, transparent, or cloudy), and odor (faint or strong)?

URINARY ELIMINATION PROBLEMS

What problems have you had or do you now have with passing your urine?

- Passage of small amounts of urine?
- Voiding at intervals that are more frequent?
- Trouble getting to the bathroom in time or feeling an urgent need to void?
- Painful voiding?
- Difficulty starting urine stream?

- Frequent dribbling of urine or a feeling of bladder fullness associated with voiding small amounts of urine?
- Reduced force of stream?
- Accidental leakage of urine? If so, when does this occur (e.g., when coughing, laughing, or sneezing; at night; during the day)?
- Past urinary tract illness, such as infection of the kidney, bladder, or urethra; urinary calculi; surgery of kidney, ureters, or bladder?

FACTORS INFLUENCING URINARY ELIMINATION

- *Medications.* Do you take any medications that could increase urinary output or cause urinary retention? Nurses should note the name and specific dosage of all medications because the individual may not be aware that a medication could influence elimination.
- *Fluid intake.* What amount and kind of fluid do you take each day (e.g., six glasses of water, two cups of coffee, three cola drinks with or without caffeine)?
- *Environmental factors.* Do you have any problems with toileting (mobility, removing clothing, toilet seat too low, facility without grab bar)?
- *Stress.* Are you experiencing any major stress? If so, what are the stressors? Do you think these affect your urinary pattern?
- *Disease.* Have you had or do you have any illnesses that may affect urinary function, such as hypertension, heart disease, neurologic disease, cancer, prostatic enlargement, or diabetes?
- *Diagnostic procedures and surgery.* Have you recently had a cystoscopy or anesthetic?

Source: Berman, A., Snyder, S. J., Kozier, B., & Erb, G. (2008). *Kozier & Erb's fundamentals of nursing: Concepts, process, and practice* (8th ed., p. 1293). Upper Saddle River, NJ: Pearson Education.

- A cystoscopy allows direct visualization of the bladder wall and urethra. During this procedure, small stones can be removed, a sample of tissue may be taken for biopsy, and retrograde pyelography may be done. If a contrast dye is instilled in the bladder, then fistulas, tumors, or ruptures can be identified.
- Noninvasive tests include renal ultrasound, computed tomography (CT), magnetic resonance imaging (MRI), and renal scan. These tests are used to identify and evaluate kidney size and structure as well as renal or perirenal masses and obstructions. In addition, a renal scan may be used to evaluate kidney blood flow, perfusion, and urine production.
- A kidney biopsy is done to obtain tissue for use in diagnosing or monitoring kidney disease.

Regardless of the type of diagnostic test, the nurse is responsible for explaining the procedure and any special preparations needed as well as assessing for medication use

that may affect the outcome of the tests. It is critical that the nurse ensures the client fully understands the conditions under which the test will be administered and which preparations the client may need to take in advance (e.g., fasting) for tests to be accurate and successful. The nurse also supports the client during the examination as necessary, documents the procedures as appropriate, and monitors the results of the tests.

Blood levels of two metabolically produced substances, urea and creatinine, are used routinely to evaluate renal function. Both substances normally are eliminated by the kidneys through filtration and tubular secretion. Urea, the end product of protein metabolism, is measured as BUN. Creatinine is produced in relatively constant quantities by the muscles. The **creatinine clearance** test uses 24-hour urine and serum creatinine levels to determine the GFR, a sensitive indicator of renal function. Other tests related to urinary functions include collection of a urine specimen, measurement of specific gravity, and visualization procedures.

DIAGNOSTIC TESTS Urinary System Disorders

NAME OF TEST Blood urea nitrogen (BUN)

PURPOSE AND DESCRIPTION This blood test measures urea, the end product of protein metabolism. Increased levels may result from dehydration, vomiting, diarrhea, digested blood, or prerenal/renal failure.

Normal values: 5–25 mg/dL

NURSING CONSIDERATIONS No special preparation is needed. If values are increased in a client who is dehydrated, he or she should return to normal with hydration. If not, this is an indicator of kidney disease.

Developmental Considerations Children and older adults are at higher risk for dehydration, which elevates BUN results.

NAME OF TEST Serum creatinine

PURPOSE AND DESCRIPTION This blood test is used to diagnose kidney dysfunction. Creatinine is a by-product of the breakdown of muscle and is excreted by the kidneys. When 50% or more of the nephrons are destroyed, serum creatinine levels rise.

Normal value: Serum: 0.5–1.5 mg/dL.

NURSING CONSIDERATIONS No special preparation is needed. Values may be increased by antibiotics, ascorbic acid, L-dopa, methyldopa, and lithium carbonate. Value is not affected by hydration status.

Developmental Considerations Older adults may have decreased values due to decreased muscle mass.

NAME OF TEST Routine urinalysis

PURPOSE AND DESCRIPTION This test examines the constituents of a urine sample to establish a baseline, to provide data for diagnosis, or to monitor results of treatment. Normal findings and abnormal findings with causes are outlined in Table 4–5.

RELATED NURSING CARE Provide a clean specimen cup for a sample of urine. Note if the client is menstruating. Assess medications, fluid status, and foods that might affect results.

Developmental Considerations Call the facility's lab to determine the minimum amount of urine required when collecting specimens from neonates or young infants. Most labs will require approximately 3–5 mL.

NAME OF TEST Urine culture (midstream, clean-catch)

PURPOSE AND DESCRIPTION A urine culture identifies the causative organism of a UTI.

Normal value: <10,000 organisms/mL (urine is sterile, but the urethra contains bacteria and a few white blood cells).

Values of more than 100,000 organisms/mL indicate UTI.

NURSING CONSIDERATIONS Provide the client with a sterile container. Ask women to separate labia with one hand and clean labia with the other hand, using sterile cotton sponges saturated with a cleansing solution and wiping three times front to back. Ask men to retract the foreskin and cleanse glans with three cotton sponges saturated with a cleansing solution, using a circular motion. After cleaning, tell the client to begin voiding and then collect the specimen in the container (initial voiding will contain urethral contaminants). If the client is unable to void, it may be necessary to obtain a specimen with a urinary catheterization.

Developmental Considerations A urine culture can be obtained from infants and toddlers by cleaning the perineum and placing a Pedi collection bag. If absolute sterility is required, the physician may prefer to perform a suprapubic puncture to collect urine from an infant, because the risk of injury and infection with this method is less than that from inserting a catheter.

NAME OF TEST Residual urine (postvoiding residual urine)

PURPOSE AND DESCRIPTION This test is conducted to measure the amount of urine left in the bladder after voiding.

Normal value: ≤50 mL.

NURSING CONSIDERATIONS Ask the client to void in a collection device and measure the amount. Immediately after voiding, catheterize using aseptic technique and a straight catheter. Drain the bladder completely. Document the time, amount voided, amount obtained on catheterization, color, clarity, odor, and any other significant data. Report the amount of residual urine if more than 100 mL. Document the voiding amount and the residual amount.

Developmental Considerations Bladder scanning technology may be used in older adults or young children with reduced immune response to avoid the risk of infection inherent in catheter insertion.

NAME OF TEST Portable ultrasonic bladder scan

PURPOSE AND DESCRIPTION This test is used to obtain information about residual urine. Warmed ultrasound gel is applied over the lower abdomen, and the ultrasound probe is placed just above the pubic bone. The scanner shows an outline of the bladder and displays the amount of urine in the bladder in milliliters. Obtain several readings. and record the largest (the most accurate). Print the information, place it on the client's chart, and document the amount of residual urine.

NURSING CONSIDERATIONS No special preparation is needed, but the test usually is not used for pregnant women. Report a residual amount of more than 100 mL.

Developmental Considerations Bladder scanning is best performed on neonates and infants when they are sleeping and less likely to squirm. Unwrap only the area required, and maintain swaddling on neonates.

DIAGNOSTIC TESTS   Urinary System Disorders (continued)

NAME OF TEST   Creatinine clearance

PURPOSE AND DESCRIPTION   This is a 24-hour urine test used to identify renal dysfunction and to monitor renal function.

Normal value: 85–135 mL/min.
Women and older adults may have slightly lower values.

NURSING CONSIDERATIONS   Assess medications: Phenacetin, steroids, and thiazides may decrease creatinine clearance; ascorbic acid, steroids, L-dopa, methyldopa (Aldomet), and cefoxitin may increase creatinine clearance. Levels of creatinine are elevated in hypothyroidism, hypertension, pregnancy, and during exercise. Obtain an appropriate specimen container. Ask the client to void and discard the first voiding. Instruct the client, family, and staff to then save all urine for a clearly designated 24-hour period, maintaining the specimen in the container either on ice or in the refrigerator.

Developmental Considerations   Collecting 24-hour specimens from infants and young children who do not have bladder control is challenging. The pediatric urine bag must be securely placed to last for 24 hours, and chemical compounds often are needed to increase adhesive contact with skin. Pediatric urine bags come with tubing that allows periodic removal of urine using a syringe to avoid spillover. If necessary, an indwelling catheter may be placed to collect all urine for 24 hours if other methods are unsuccessful.

NAME OF TEST   Uroflowmetry

PURPOSE AND DESCRIPTION   This test measures the volume of urine voided per second.

NURSING CONSIDERATIONS   Ask the client to increase fluid intake and refrain from voiding for several hours before the test to ensure a full bladder and a strong urge to void during testing. Tell the client he or she will be asked to urinate into a funnel.

Developmental Considerations   This test is not done on children or older adults who do not have bladder control.

NAME OF TEST   Cystometrography (voiding cystography)

PURPOSE AND DESCRIPTION

This test is conducted to evaluate bladder capacity and neuromuscular functions of the bladder, urethral pressures, and causes of bladder dysfunction. A measured quantity of fluid is instilled into the bladder, and the filling capacity and voiding pressures are measured.

Normal value: Urine stream strong and uninterrupted, normal filling pattern and sensation of fullness; bladder capacity: 300–600 mL; urge to void: >150 mL; fullness felt: 300 mL.

NURSING CONSIDERATIONS   Tell the client that the bladder will be filled and that during filling, he or she will be asked to describe the first urge to void and the sensation of being unable to delay urination any longer.

Developmental Considerations   This test is not normally performed on infants or neonates.

NAME OF TEST   Intravenous pyelography (IVP)

PURPOSE AND DESCRIPTION   This radiologic examination is done to visualize the entire urinary tract to identify abnormal size, shape, and function of the kidneys or to detect renal calculi (stones), tumors, or cysts. A radiopaque substance is injected intravenously and a series of radiographs taken.

CLIENT PREPARATION

- Assess knowledge and understanding of procedure, clarifying information as needed.
- Schedule IVP before any ordered barium test or gallbladder studies using contrast material.
- Ask about allergies to seafood, iodine, or radiologic contrast dye. Notify physician or radiologist if allergies are known.
- Verify the presence of a signed informed consent for the procedure.
- Assess renal and fluid status, including serum osmolality, creatinine, and BUN levels. Notify the physician of any abnormal values.
- Instruct the client to complete the ordered pretest bowel preparation, including prescribed laxative or cathartic the evening before the test and an enema (cleansing of the bowel with fluid) or suppository the morning of the test. Instruct the client to withhold food for 8 hours before the test (clear liquids are allowed).
- Obtain baseline vital signs and record.
- Monitor vital signs and urine output.

HEALTH EDUCATION FOR THE CLIENT AND FAMILY

- X-rays and a dye that is rapidly excreted in the urine are used to show the structures of the kidney, ureters, and bladder. The test takes approximately 30 minutes.
- A laxative, and possibly an enema or suppository, are used before the test to clear the bowel of feces and gas. Do not eat after the ordered time on the evening before the test; you may drink clear fluids, such as water, coffee, or tea (without creamer).
- As the dye is injected, you may feel a transient flushing or burning sensation, along with possible nausea and a metallic taste.
- Notify your doctor immediately if you develop a rash, difficulty breathing, rapid heart rate, or hives during or after the test.

After the Procedure

- Increase fluid intake after the test.
- Report manifestations of delayed reaction to the contrast media (e.g., dyspnea, tachycardia, itching, hives, or flushing).

NAME OF TEST   Retrograde pyelography

PURPOSE AND DESCRIPTION   This radiologic test is done to evaluate the structures of the ureters and kidney pelvis. It may be performed alone or in conjunction with a cystoscopy. A contrast dye is injected through a catheter into the ureters and kidney pelvis, and radiographs are obtained.

NURSING CONSIDERATIONS   Nursing care for the client undergoing retrograde pyelography is the same as that for clients undergoing IVP.

(continued)

DIAGNOSTIC TESTS Urinary System Disorders (continued)

NAME OF TEST   Renal arteriography or angiography

PURPOSE AND DESCRIPTION   This radiologic test is done to visualize renal blood vessels to detect renal artery stenosis, renal thrombosis or embolism, tumors, cysts, or aneurysm; to determine the causative factor for hypertension; and to evaluate renal circulation. A contrast medium is injected into the femoral artery.

NURSING CONSIDERATIONS   Assess for allergies to iodine, seafood, or other contrast dye from other radiographic procedures. A laxative or cleansing enema usually is given the night before, and the client should be NPO for 8–12 hours before the test. Anticoagulants should be discontinued. Results may be affected by feces, gas, and barium sulfate. After the test, monitor for bleeding from the femoral artery, restrict activity for a day, assess peripheral pulses, and monitor urine output.

NAME OF TEST   Cystoscopy (cystography), cystography

PURPOSE AND DESCRIPTION   Direct visualization of the bladder wall and urethra is accomplished using a cystoscope. During the procedure, small renal calculi can be removed from the ureter, bladder, or urethra, and tissue biopsy can be done. This test also permits determination of the cause of hematuria or UTI. A stent may be inserted during the procedure to facilitate urinary drainage past an obstruction. Retrograde pyelography also may be done during the cystoscopy. By instilling a contrast dye into the bladder (cystography), a neurogenic bladder, fistulas, tumors, or ruptures can be identified.

CLIENT PREPARATION

Assess knowledge and understanding of the procedure, clarifying information as needed.

- Verify the presence of a signed informed consent for the procedure.
- Instruct in pretest preparation as ordered, including prescribed laxatives the evening before the test and any ordered food or fluid restrictions.

- Administer sedation and other medications as ordered before the test.

HEALTH EDUCATION FOR THE CLIENT AND FAMILY

- Cystoscopy is performed using local or general anesthesia in a special cystoscopy room.
- You may feel some pressure or a need to urinate as the scope is inserted through the urethra into the bladder.
- The procedure takes approximately 30–45 minutes.
- Do not attempt to stand without assistance immediately after the procedure because you may feel dizzy or faint.
- Burning on urination for a day or two after the procedure is to be expected.
- Immediately notify the physician if your urine remains bloody for more than three voidings after the procedure or if you develop bright bleeding, low urine output, abdominal or flank pain, chills, or fever.
- Warm sitz baths, analgesic agents, and antispasmodic medications may relieve discomfort after the procedure.
- Increase fluid intake to decrease pain and difficulty voiding and to reduce the risk of infection.
- Laxatives may be ordered after the procedure to prevent constipation and straining, which may cause urinary tract bleeding.

NAME OF TEST   Renal ultrasound

PURPOSE AND DESCRIPTION   This noninvasive test is conducted to detect renal or perirenal masses, to identify obstructions, and to diagnose renal cysts and solid masses. A

conductive gel is applied to the skin, and a small external ultrasound probe is placed on the client's skin. Sound waves are recorded on a computer as they are reflected off tissues.

NURSING CONSIDERATIONS   No special preparation is indicated.

NAME OF TEST   CT of the kidneys

PURPOSE AND DESCRIPTION   CT allows evaluation of kidney size, tumors, abscesses, suprarenal masses, and obstructions. A contrast dye is injected intravenously, allowing greater visualization of the density of renal tissue and masses compared to an ultrasound.

NURSING CONSIDERATIONS   Assess the client for allergies to iodine, radiographic contrast dye, and seafood. Tell the client to remain NPO for 4 hours before the test, and laxatives or enemas may be ordered to remove gas or fecal material from the bowel.

Developmental Considerations   Pediatric clients may require sedation before testing to obtain cooperation.

NAME OF TEST   MRI of the kidneys

PURPOSE AND DESCRIPTION   MRI is used to visualize the kidneys by assessing computer-generated films of radiofrequency waves for changes in magnetic fields.

NURSING CONSIDERATIONS   Ask client to remove all metal objects. Assess for metal implants (test will not be conducted if present). Clients who are claustrophobic may require minimal sedation or "open" MRI.

Developmental Considerations   Pediatric clients may require sedation before testing to obtain cooperation.

NAME OF TEST   Renal scan

PURPOSE AND DESCRIPTION   This test is done to evaluate the blood flow, location, size, and shape of the kidneys and to assess kidney perfusion and urine production. Radioactive isotopes are injected intravenously, and radiation detector probes are placed over the kidneys to monitor activity in those organs. Radioisotope distribution in the kidneys is scanned and graphed.

Nonfunctioning tissue, such as in tumors and cysts, appears as cold spots.

NURSING CONSIDERATIONS   Ask client to drink several glasses of water before the test. Obtain the client's weight, and have the client void. After the procedure, have the client increase fluid intake.

Developmental Considerations   Pediatric clients may require sedation before testing to obtain cooperation.

DIAGNOSTIC TESTS Urinary System Disorders (continued)

NAME OF TEST Renal biopsy

PURPOSE AND DESCRIPTION A renal biopsy is done to obtain tissue to diagnose or monitor kidney disease. A needle usually is inserted through the skin into the lower lobe of the kidney. The test also can be done with CT or ultrasound guidance.

CLIENT PREPARATION

- Informed consent is required for a kidney biopsy. Answer questions and provide additional information as needed.
- Maintain NPO status from midnight before the procedure.
- Note hemoglobin and hematocrit before the procedure.
- If the procedure is to be performed at the bedside, obtain the biopsy tray and other necessary supplies.
- After the procedure, apply a pressure dressing, and place the patient in a supine position to help maintain pressure on the biopsy site.
- Monitor closely for bleeding during the first 24 hours after the procedure:
  a. Check vital signs frequently. Notify the physician of tachycardia, hypotension, or other signs of shock.
  b. Monitor biopsy site for bleeding.
  c. Check hemoglobin and hematocrit, comparing with preprocedure values.
  d. Observe for and report complaints of flank or back pain, shoulder pain (caused by diaphragmatic irritation if hemorrhage occurs), pallor, and light-headedness.
  e. Monitor urine output for quantity and hematuria. Initial hematuria should clear within 24 hours.
- Monitor for other potential complications, such as inadvertent penetration of the liver or bowel. Report abdominal pain, guarding, and decreased bowel sounds.
- Encourage fluids during the initial postprocedural period.

HEALTH EDUCATION FOR THE CLIENT AND FAMILY

- Local anesthesia is used at the injection site. The procedure may be uncomfortable but should not be painful.
- When the needle is inserted, the client will be instructed not to breathe to prevent kidney motion.
- The entire procedure takes approximately 10 minutes.

After the Procedure

- Avoid coughing during the first 24 hours after the procedure. Strenuous activity, such as heavy lifting, may be prohibited for approximately 2 weeks after the procedure.
- Report any manifestations of complications, such as hemorrhage or UTI, to the physician.

Source: LeMone, P., & Burke, K. (2008). *Medical-surgical nursing: Critical thinking in client care* (4th ed., pp. 835–838). Upper Saddle River, NJ: Pearson Education.

TABLE 4–5 Normal and Abnormal Findings: Urinalysis

CHARACTERISTIC OR COMPONENT	NORMAL RESULTS	ABNORMAL FINDING WITH POSSIBLE CAUSE
Color	Light straw to amber yellow	■ Red, dark, smoky color may be the result of blood in the urine (hematuria or menstrual blood). ■ Cloudy urine occurs from infection. ■ Colorless urine indicates very dilute urine, such as in overhydration, kidney disease, alcohol ingestion, or diabetes insipidus. ■ Very dark yellow urine indicates dehydration and/or fever. ■ Red or red brown urine may be caused by sulfisoxazole-phenazopyridine (Azo Gantrisin), phenytoin (Dilantin), cascara, chlorpromazine (Thorazine), docusate calcium and phenolphthalein (Doxidan); and by carrots, rhubarb, and food coloring. ■ Orange urine is caused by fever, urobilin, phenazopyridine (Pyridium), amidopyrine, nitrofurantoin, sulfonamides, carrots, beets, and food coloring. ■ Blue or green urine is caused by Pseudomonas, amitriptyline (Elavil), methylene blue, methocarbamol (Robaxin), and yeast concentrate. ■ Brown or black urine is caused by Lysol poisoning, melanin, bilirubin, methemoglobin, porphyrin, cascara, and injectable iron.
Appearance	Clear	■ Hazy or cloudy urine indicates bacteria, pus, RBCs, WBCs, phosphates, prostatic fluid spermatozoa, or urates. ■ Milky urine is the result of fats or pyuria. ■ Yellow foam results from bilirubin, bile, or severe cirrhosis of the liver. ■ A dark yellow to brownish color is seen with deficient fluid volume.

(continued)

TABLE 4–5 Normal and Abnormal Findings: Urinalysis (continued)

CHARACTERISTIC OR COMPONENT	NORMAL RESULTS	ABNORMAL FINDING WITH POSSIBLE CAUSE
Odor	Aromatic	■ Ammonia smell increases as urine stands outside the body. ■ Urinary tract infection (UTI) causes a foul or unpleasant odor, depending on the causative organism. ■ Asparagus causes a distinctive odor. ■ Mousy odors result from phenylketonuria. ■ Sweet or fruity odors occur in starvation and diabetic ketoacidosis.
pH	4.5–8.0	■ < 4.5: metabolic acidosis, respiratory acidosis, diet high in meat protein, ammonium chloride and mandelic acid. ■ > 8.0: bacteriuria, UTI, antibiotics (neomycin, kanamycin), sulfonamides, sodium bicarbonate, acetazolamide (Diamox), potassium citrate.
Specific gravity	1.005–1.030	■ < 1.005: diabetes insipidus, overhydration, renal disease, severe potassium deficit. ■ > 1.030: dehydration, fever, diabetes mellitus, vomiting, diarrhea, contrast media.
Protein	2–8 mg/dL	■ > 8 mg/dL: proteinuria, exercise, fever, stress, acute infection, kidney disease, lupus erythematosus, leukemia, multiple myeloma, cardiac disease, toxemia of pregnancy, septicemia, lead, mercury, neomycin, barbiturates, sulfonamides.
Glucose	Negative	■ > 15 mg/dL or +4: diabetes mellitus, stroke, Cushing's syndrome, anesthesia, glucose infusions, severe stress, infections, ascorbic acid, aspirin, cephalosporins, and epinephrine.
Ketones	Negative	■ +1 to +3: ketoacidosis, starvation, high-protein diet.
RBCs	Rare	■ > 2 per low-power field: kidney trauma, kidney diseases, renal calculi, cystitis, excess aspirin, anticoagulants, sulfonamides, menstrual contamination.
WBCs	3–4	■ > 4 per low-power field: UTI, fever, strenuous exercise, kidney diseases.
Casts	Occasional hyaline	■ Fever, kidney diseases, heart failure.

Source: LeMone, P., & Burke, K. (2008). *Medical-surgical nursing: Critical thinking in client care* (4th ed. p. 832). Upper Saddle River, NJ: Pearson Education.

THERAPEUTIC MANAGEMENT INTERVENTIONS FOR ALTERED URINARY ELIMINATION

Medical management of altered urinary output is based on the cause and severity of the problem. Clients with reduced urine output secondary to dehydration will require increased fluid intake. Poor kidney perfusion or function may require the addition of medications such as diuretics. If renal function is severely compromised or nonfunctional, the client may require dialysis (peritoneal or hemodialysis) or kidney transplantation.

CARING INTERVENTIONS

The primary purpose for performing nursing interventions associated with elimination of urine is to maintain the integrity of the urinary system, which eliminates excess fluid and wastes, thereby promoting homeostasis.

Aseptic technique is essential whenever performing procedures that could introduce bacteria into the urinary tract. Washing hands, using sterile gloves, and maintaining a closed urinary collection system decrease the incidence of ascending bladder contamination and subsequent UTI. Maintaining aseptic technique throughout dialysis procedures is necessary to prevent infection in grafts, fistulas, and catheters.

Consult your skills manual for step-by-step descriptions of the following caring interventions related to urinary elimination:

■ Measurement of intake and output
■ External urine collection systems
■ Urinary catheterization
■ Bladder irrigation
■ Suprapubic catheter care
■ Collecting specimens from a closed urinary system
■ Urinary diversions
■ Hemodialysis

PHARMACOLOGIC THERAPIES

Pharmacologic therapy for urinary elimination includes diuretics to increase the production of urine, anticholinergic medications to reduce urinary frequency and treat incontinence related to urgency, and cholinergic medications to stimulate bladder contractions and promote urination, especially in

MEDICATIONS Urinary Elimination

Drug classifications	Mechanism of action	Commonly prescribed drugs	Nursing considerations
Anticholinergic agents	These reduce urgency and frequency by blocking muscarinic receptors in the detrusor muscle of the bladder, thereby inhibiting contractions and increasing storage capacity. They can be useful in relieving symptoms associated with voiding in clients who have neurogenic bladder, reflex neurogenic bladder, or urge urinary incontinence.	Oxybutynin	■ Monitor for constipation, dry mouth, urinary retention, blurred vision, and (in older adults) mental confusion. Symptoms may be dose related. ■ Start with small doses for clients older than 75 years. ■ Oxybutynin is contraindicated in clients with urinary retention, gastrointestinal (GI) motility problems (partial or complete GI obstruction, paralytic ileus), or uncontrolled narrow-angle glaucoma.
Cholinergic agents or parasympathomimetics	These medications stimulate bladder contraction and facilitate voiding.	Bethanechol chloride (Urecholine)	■ Do not administer to clients with GI or urinary tract obstructions, asthma, bradycardia, hypotension, or Parkinson's disease. ■ May increase serum aspartate aminotransferase, amylase, and lipase levels. ■ Effect of medications is antagonized by angel's trumpet, jimson weed, or scopolia. ■ Overdose is treated with atropine sulfate.
Diuretics: loop, thiazide, potassium-sparing, and miscellaneous type	Each type of diuretic works in a specific place within the nephron to increase fluid excretion and prevent fluid reabsorption.		■ Monitor hydration and electrolyte balance. ■ Monitor vital signs, and be alert for signs of hypotension secondary to fluid loss. ■ Monitor serum BUN, creatinine, electrolyte, and other pertinent laboratory values. ■ Clients taking potassium-sparing diuretics should avoid salt substitutes.

clients with difficulty voiding. See the Medications feature for additional information.

There are four subclassifications of diuretics based on where and how they act in the kidney. Loop diuretics, as the name implies, work in the loop of Henle by blocking reabsorption of sodium and chloride. Thiazide diuretics act on the distal tubule to block sodium reabsorption and increase potassium and water excretion. Potassium-sparing diuretics work in the distal tubule allowing sodium to be excreted while restoring much of the potassium to the body, thereby avoiding the large potassium loss seen with other types of diuretics. Finally, diuretics that cannot be otherwise classified make up a miscellaneous group; this group includes carbonic anhydrase inhibitors and osmotic diuretics.

Bowel Elimination

Nurses frequently are consulted or involved in assisting clients with fecal elimination problems. These problems can be embarrassing to clients and can cause considerable discomfort. The elimination of feces is a prominent public topic in North America. For example, laxative advertisements, which describe feelings such as tiredness because of irregularity, keep the subject in the public consciousness. Some older adults are preoccupied with their bowels. People who have had a bowel movement once a day for 75 years can view missing one day as a serious problem.

NORMAL PRESENTATION

The excreted waste products from the bowel are referred to as **feces** or **stool**. Individuals (especially children) may use very different terms for a bowel movement. The nurse may need to try several common words before finding one the client understands.

Defecation is the expulsion of feces from the anus and rectum. It is also called a bowel movement. The frequency of defecation is highly individual, varying from several times a day to two or three times a week. The amount defecated also varies from person to person.

Normal feces are made up of approximately 75% water and 25% solid materials. They are soft but formed. If the feces are propelled very quickly along the large intestine, there is inadequate time for most of the water in the chyme to be reabsorbed, and the feces will be more fluid, containing perhaps 95% water. Normal feces require a normal fluid intake; feces that contain less water may be hard and difficult to expel. Feces normally are brown, chiefly because of the presence of stercobilin and urobilin, which are derived from bilirubin (a red pigment in bile). Another factor that affects fecal color is the action of bacteria, such as *Escherichia coli* or *Staphylococcus* sp., which normally are present in the large intestine. The action of microorganisms on the chyme also is responsible for the odor of feces.

An adult usually forms 7–10 L of **flatus** (gas) in the large intestine every 24 hours. The gases include carbon dioxide, methane, hydrogen, oxygen, and nitrogen. Some are swallowed with food and fluids taken by mouth. Others are formed through the action of bacteria on the chyme in the large intestine. Still other gas diffuses from the blood into the gastrointestinal tract.

Bowel Elimination and Pregnancy

During pregnancy, elevated progesterone levels cause smooth muscle relaxation, resulting in delayed gastric emptying and decreased peristalsis. As a result, the pregnant woman may complain of bloating and constipation. These symptoms are aggravated as the enlarging uterus displaces the stomach upward and the intestines are moved laterally and posteriorly. The cardiac sphincter also relaxes, and heartburn (pyrosis) may occur as a result of **reflux**, a backward flow of acidic secretions into the lower esophagus. Hemorrhoids frequently develop in late pregnancy from constipation and from pressure on vessels below the level of the uterus.

In the postpartum period, the bowels tend to be sluggish following birth because of the lingering effects of progesterone, decreased abdominal muscle tone, and bowel evacuation associated with the labor and birth process. A woman who has had an episiotomy, lacerations, or hemorrhoids may tend to delay elimination for fear of increasing her pain or because she believes her stitches will be torn if she bears down. In refusing or delaying the bowel movement, the woman may cause increased constipation and pain when bowel elimination finally occurs.

The woman who has had a cesarean birth may experience some initial discomfort from flatulence, which can be relieved by early ambulation and use of antiflatulent medications. Chamomile or peppermint tea also may be helpful in reducing discomfort from flatulence. It may take a few days for the bowel to regain its tone, especially if general anesthesia was used. The woman who has had a cesarean or a difficult birth may benefit from stool softeners.

FACTORS AFFECTING BOWEL ELIMINATION

Defecation patterns vary at different stages of life. Circumstances of diet, fluid intake and output, activity, psychologic factors, lifestyle, medications and medical procedures, and disease also affect defecation.

Developmental Factors

Newborns and infants, toddlers, children, and older adults are groups within which members have similarities in elimination patterns.

NEWBORNS AND INFANTS Term newborns usually pass meconium within 8–24 hours of life and almost always within 48 hours. **Meconium** is formed in utero from the amniotic fluid and its constituents, intestinal secretions, and shed mucosal cells. It is recognized by its thick, tarry black or dark green appearance. Transitional (thin brown to green) stools consisting of part meconium and part fecal material are passed for the next day or two, and then the stools become entirely fecal. Generally, the stools of a breast-fed newborn are pale yellow (but may be pasty green) and usually are more liquid and more frequent than those of formula-fed newborns, whose stools are paler (Figure 4–7 ■).

Frequency of bowel movement varies but ranges from one every 2 or 3 days to as many as 10 movements daily. Totally breast-fed infants often progress to stools that occur every 5–7 days. Mothers should be counseled that the newborn is not constipated as long as the bowel movement remains soft.

Infants pass stool frequently, often after each feeding. Because the intestine is immature, water is not well absorbed, and the stool is soft, liquid, and frequent. When the intestine matures, bacterial flora increase. After solid foods are introduced, the stool becomes firmer and less frequent.

TODDLERS Some control of defecation starts at between 1.5 and 2 years of age. By this time, children have learned to walk, and their nervous and muscular systems are sufficiently well developed to permit bowel control. A desire to control daytime bowel movements and to use the toilet generally starts when the child becomes aware of the discomfort caused by a soiled diaper and the sensation that indicates the need for a bowel movement. Daytime control typically is attained by 2.5 years of age, after a process of toilet training.

SCHOOL-AGE CHILDREN AND ADOLESCENTS School-age children and adolescents have bowel habits similar to those of adults. Patterns of defecation vary in frequency, quantity, and consistency. Some school-age children may delay defecation because of an activity such as play.

OLDER ADULTS Constipation is the most common bowel management problem in the older adult population (Mauk, 2005). This is caused, in part, by reduced activity levels, inadequate fluid and fiber intake, and muscle weakness. Many older people believe that "regularity" means a bowel movement every day. Those who do not meet this criterion often seek over-the-counter preparations to relieve what they believe to be constipation. Older adults should be advised that normal patterns of bowel elimination vary considerably. For some, a normal pattern may be every other day; for others, a normal pattern may be twice a day. Adequate roughage in the diet, adequate exercise, and six to eight glasses of fluid daily are essential preventive measures for constipation. A cup of hot water or tea at a regular time in the morning also

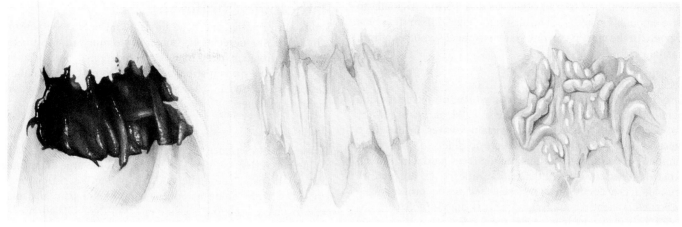

Figure 4–7 ■ Newborn stool samples.

is helpful for some. Responding to the **gastrocolic reflex** (increased peristalsis of the colon after food has entered the stomach) is an important consideration as well. For example, toileting is recommended 5–15 min after meals—especially after breakfast, when the gastrocolic reflex is strongest (Hinrichs & Huseboe, 2001, p. 23).

The older adult should be warned that consistent use of laxatives inhibits natural defecation reflexes and is thought to cause, rather than cure, constipation. The habitual user of laxatives eventually requires larger or stronger doses because the effect is progressively reduced with continual use. Laxatives also may interfere with the body's electrolyte balance and reduce the absorption of certain vitamins. The reasons for constipation can range from lifestyle habits (e.g., lack of exercise) to serious malignant disorders (e.g., colorectal cancer). The nurse should evaluate carefully any complaints of constipation. A change in bowel habits over several weeks with or without weight loss, pain, or fever should be referred to a primary care provider for a complete medical evaluation.

Diet

Sufficient bulk (cellulose, fiber) in the diet is necessary to provide fecal volume. Bland diets and low-fiber diets lack bulk and therefore create insufficient residue of waste products to stimulate the reflex for defecation. Low-residue foods, such as rice, eggs, and lean meats, move more slowly through the intestinal tract. Increasing fluid intake with such foods increases their rate of movement.

Certain foods are difficult, or even impossible, for some people to digest. This difficulty can result in digestive upsets and, in some instances, the passage of watery stools. Irregular eating also can impair regular defecation. Individuals who eat at the same times every day usually have a regularly timed, physiologic response to the food intake and a regular pattern of peristaltic activity in the colon.

Spicy foods can produce diarrhea and flatus in some individuals. Excessive sugar also can cause diarrhea. Other foods that may influence bowel elimination include the following:
- Gas-producing foods, such as cabbage, onions, cauliflower, bananas, and apples
- Laxative-producing foods, such as bran, prunes, figs, chocolate, and alcohol
- Constipation-producing foods, such as cheese, pasta, eggs, and lean meat

Fluid

Healthy fecal elimination usually requires a daily fluid intake of 2,000–3,000 mL, but even when fluid intake is inadequate or output (e.g., urine or vomitus) is excessive, the body continues to reabsorb fluid from the chyme as it passes along the colon. The chyme becomes drier than normal, however, resulting in hard feces. In addition, reduced fluid intake slows the passage of chyme along the intestines, further increasing the reabsorption of fluid from the chyme. If, on the other hand, chyme moves abnormally quickly through the large intestine, there is less time for fluid to be absorbed into the blood, and soft or even watery feces will result.

Activity

Activity stimulates peristalsis, facilitating the movement of chyme along the colon. Weak abdominal and pelvic muscles often are ineffective in increasing the intra-abdominal pressure during defecation or in controlling defecation. Weak muscles can result from lack of exercise, immobility, or impaired neurologic functioning. Clients confined to bed are often constipated.

Psychologic Factors

Some people who are anxious or angry experience increased peristaltic activity and subsequent nausea or diarrhea. In contrast, people who are depressed may experience slowed intestinal motility, resulting in constipation. How a person responds to these emotional states is the result of individual differences in the response of the enteric nervous system to vagal stimulation from the brain.

Defecation Habits

Early bowel training may establish the habit of defecating at a regular time. Many people defecate after breakfast, when the gastrocolic reflex causes mass peristaltic waves in the large intestine. If a person ignores the urge to defecate, then water continues to be reabsorbed, making the feces hard and difficult to expel. When the normal defecation reflexes are inhibited or ignored, these conditioned reflexes tend to be progressively weakened. When habitually ignored, the urge to defecate ultimately is lost. Adults may ignore these reflexes because of the pressures of time or work. Hospitalized clients may suppress the urge because of embarrassment about using a bedpan, because of lack of privacy, or because defecation is too uncomfortable.

Medications

Some drugs have side effects that can interfere with normal elimination. Large doses of certain tranquilizers and repeated administration of morphine or codeine cause constipation by decreasing gastrointestinal activity through their action on the central nervous system. Iron tablets, which have an astringent effect, act more locally on the bowel mucosa to cause constipation. A variety of other drugs cause diarrhea.

Some medications directly affect elimination. **Laxatives** are medications that stimulate bowel activity and assist in fecal elimination. Other medications soften stool, facilitating defecation. Certain medications suppress peristaltic activity and may be used to treat diarrhea.

Medications also affect the appearance of the feces. Any drug that causes gastrointestinal bleeding (e.g., aspirin products) can cause the stool to be red or black. Iron salts cause black stool because of the oxidation of the iron. Antibiotics may cause a gray-green discoloration. Antacids can cause a whitish discoloration or white specks in the stool. Pepto-Bismol, a common over-the-counter drug, causes stools to be black.

Diagnostic Procedures

Before certain diagnostic procedures, such as visualization of the colon (colonoscopy or sigmoidoscopy), the client is restricted from ingesting food or fluid. The client also may be given a cleansing enema before the examination. In these instances, normal defecation usually will not occur until eating resumes.

Anesthesia and Surgical Procedures

General anesthetics cause the normal colonic movements to cease or slow by blocking parasympathetic stimulation to the muscles of the colon. Clients who have regional or spinal anesthesia are less likely to experience this problem.

Surgery that involves direct handling of the intestines can cause temporary cessation of intestinal movement. This condition, called **ileus**, usually lasts from 24–48 hours. Listening for bowel sounds that reflect intestinal motility is an important nursing assessment following surgery.

Pathologic Conditions

Spinal cord injuries and head injuries can reduce the sensory stimulation for defecation. Impaired mobility may limit the client's ability to respond to the urge to defecate, and the client may experience constipation as a result. Alternatively, a client may experience fecal incontinence because of poorly functioning anal sphincters.

Pain

Clients who experience discomfort when defecating (e.g., following hemorrhoid surgery) often suppress the urge to defecate to avoid the pain. These clients can experience constipation as a result. Clients taking narcotic analgesics for pain also may experience constipation as a side effect of the medication.

ALTERATIONS

Four common problems are related to fecal elimination: diarrhea, flatulence, constipation, and bowel incontinence. Constipation and bowel incontinence will be discussed later in this concept. For more details, see the Alterations and Treatments feature.

Diarrhea

Diarrhea refers to the passage of liquid feces and an increased frequency of defecation. The opposite of constipation, it results from rapid movement of fecal contents through the large intestine. Rapid passage of chyme reduces the time available for the large intestine to reabsorb water and electrolytes. Some people pass stool with increased frequency, but diarrhea is not present unless the stool is relatively unformed and excessively liquid. The person with diarrhea finds it difficult or impossible to control the urge to defecate for very long. Often, spasmodic cramps are associated with diarrhea. Bowel sounds usually increase. With persistent diarrhea, irritation of the anal region, extending to the perineum and buttocks, generally results. Fatigue, weakness, malaise, and emaciation are the results of prolonged diarrhea.

Diarrhea is thought to be a protective flushing mechanism when caused by irritants in the intestinal tract. It can create serious fluid and electrolyte losses in the body, however, and these losses can develop within frighteningly short periods of time, particularly in infants, small children, and older adults. Table 4–6 lists some of the major causes of diarrhea and the physiologic responses of the body.

The irritating effects of diarrhea stool increase the risk for skin breakdown. The area around the anal region should be kept clean and dry and be protected with zinc oxide or other ointment. In addition, a fecal collector can be used.

Flatulence

There are three primary sources of flatus: action of bacteria on the chyme in the large intestine, swallowed air, and gas that diffuses between the bloodstream and the intestine.

Most gases that are swallowed are expelled through the mouth by eructation (belching). Large amounts of gas can

ALTERATIONS AND TREATMENTS   Bowel Elimination

Alteration	Description	Treatment
Constipation	Infrequent passage of hard stool	■ Increase fluid and fiber intake. ■ Increase activity level. ■ Administer enema. ■ May require medications (e.g., laxatives, stool softeners, cathartics). ■ Evaluate medication profile for gastrointestinal side effects.
Diarrhea	Passage of liquid stools	■ Increase fluid intake. ■ Administer antidiarrheal medications. ■ Assess for cause (medications, diet, bacterial infection).
Bowel incontinence	Inability to control release of feces	■ Administer bowel training. ■ Treat with surgery (sphincter repair and fecal diversion or colostomy).
Impaction	Mass or collection of hardened feces in the folds of the rectum	■ Digital removal may be necessary. ■ Administer enema as necessary. ■ Increase fluid and fiber intake to prevent recurrence. ■ Evaluate medication profile for gastrointestinal side effects. ■ Improve defecation habits, and reduce constipation.
Bowel cancer	Abnormal growth of cells in the bowel	■ Take preventive measures, and make an early diagnosis. ■ Remove surgically. ■ Administer chemotherapy or radiation therapy.
Obstruction	Blockage in the bowel preventing or reducing the passage of fecal material	■ Remove blockage surgically.

accumulate in the stomach, however, resulting in gastric distention. The gases formed in the large intestine are chiefly absorbed through the intestinal capillaries into the circulation. **Flatulence** is the presence of excessive flatus in the intestines and leads to stretching and inflation of the intestines (intestinal distention). Flatulence can occur in the colon from a variety of causes, including foods (e.g., cabbage and onions), abdominal surgery, or narcotics. If the gas is propelled by increased colon activity before it can be absorbed, it may be expelled through the anus. If excessive gas cannot be expelled through the anus, it may be necessary to insert a rectal tube to remove it.

PHYSICAL ASSESSMENT

Assessment of fecal elimination includes taking a nursing history; performing a physical examination of the abdomen, rectum, and anus; and inspecting the feces. The nurse also should review any data obtained from relevant diagnostic tests. For more details, see the Bowel Assessment and Assessment Interview features.

Nursing History

A nursing history for fecal elimination helps the nurse to identify the client's normal pattern. The nurse obtains a description of usual feces and any recent changes and collects

TABLE 4–6 **Major Causes of Diarrhea**

CAUSE	PHYSIOLOGIC EFFECT
Psychologic stress (e.g., anxiety)	Increased intestinal motility and secretion of mucus
Medications	Inflammation and infection of mucosa caused by overgrowth of pathogenic intestinal microorganisms
Antibiotics	Irritation of intestinal mucosa
Iron	Irritation of intestinal mucosa
Cathartics	Incomplete digestion of food or fluid
Allergy to food, fluid, drugs	Increased intestinal motility and secretion of mucus
Intolerance of food or fluid	Reduced absorption of fluids
Diseases of the colon (e.g., malabsorption syndrome, Crohn's disease)	Inflammation of the mucosa, often leading to ulcer formation

Source: Berman, A., Snyder, S. J., Kozier, B., Erb, G. (2008). *Kozier & Erb's fundamentals of nursing: Concepts, process, and practice* (8th ed., p. 1330). Upper Saddle River, NJ: Pearson Education.

Bowel Assessment

Technique/Normal Findings	Abnormal Findings

Abdominal Assessment

Inspect abdominal contour, skin integrity, venous pattern, and aortic pulsation. *Abdomen should be slightly concave with intact skin. There should not be distended veins or obvious aortic pulsations.*

- Generalized abdominal distention may be seen in gas retention or obesity.
- Lower abdominal distention is seen in bladder distention, pregnancy, or ovarian mass.
- General distention and an everted umbilicus are seen with ascites and/or tumors.
- A scaphoid (sunken) abdomen is seen in malnutrition or when fat is replaced with muscle.
- **Striae** (whitish-silver stretch marks) are seen in obesity and during or after pregnancy.
- Spider angiomas may be seen in liver disease.
- Dilated veins are prominent in cirrhosis of the liver, ascites, portal hypertension, or veno-caval obstruction.
- Pulsation is increased in aortic aneurysm.

Auscultate all four quadrants of the abdomen with the diaphragm of the stethoscope. Begin in the lower right quadrant, where bowel sounds are almost always present. *Normal bowel sounds (gurgling or clicking) occur every 5–15 seconds. Listen for at least 5 minutes in each of the four quadrants to confirm the absence of bowel sounds.*

- **Borborygmus** (hyperactive high-pitched, tinkling, rushing, or growling bowel sounds) is heard in diarrhea or at the onset of bowel obstruction.
- Bowel sounds may be absent later in bowel obstruction, with an inflamed peritoneum, and/or following surgery of the abdomen.

Auscultate the abdomen for vascular sounds with the bell of the stethoscope. *No sounds (bruits, venous hum, or friction rub) other than bowel sounds should be auscultated.*

- **Bruits** (blowing sound due to restriction of blood flow through vessels) may be heard over constricted arteries. A bruit over the liver may be heard in hepatic carcinoma.
- A venous hum (continuous medium-pitched sound) may be heard over a cirrhotic liver.
- Friction rubs (rough grating sounds) may be heard over an inflamed liver or spleen.

Percuss the abdomen in all four quadrants. *Normally, tympany is heard over the stomach and gas-filled bowels.*

- Dullness is heard when the bowel is displaced with fluid or tumors or filled with a fecal mass.

Palpate the abdomen in all four quadrants. Use a circular motion to move the abdominal wall over underlying structures. Feel for masses and note any tenderness or pain the client may have during this part of the exam. Palpate lightly at first (0.5–0.75 in.), then more deeply (1.5–2 in.) with caution. If a mass is palpated, ask the client to raise head and shoulders. *There should be no abdominal masses or pain on palpation.*

- A mass in the abdomen may become more promiznent when the head and shoulders are raised, as will a ventral abdominal wall hernia. If the mass is no longer palpable, it is deeper in the abdomen.

> ### PRACTICE ALERT
> Never use deep palpation in a client who has had a pulsatile abdominal mass, renal transplant, polycystic kidneys, or is at risk for hemorrhage.

- In cases of peritoneal inflammation, palpation causes abdominal pain and involuntary muscle spasms.
- Abnormal masses include aortic aneurysms, neoplastic tumors of the colon or uterus, and a distended bladder or distended bowel due to obstruction.
- A rigid, boardlike abdomen may be palpated when the client has a perforated duodenal ulcer.

Palpate for rebound tenderness. Press the fingers into the abdomen slowly and release the pressure quickly. *Releasing pressure should not cause or increase pain.*

- In peritoneal inflammation, pain occurs when the fingers are withdrawn.
- Right upper quadrant pain occurs with acute cholecystitis.
- Upper middle abdominal pain occurs with acute pancreatitis.
- Right lower quadrant pain at McBurney's point occurs with acute appendicitis.
- Left lower quadrant pain is seen in acute diverticulitis.

Inguinal Area Assessment

Inspect the inguinal area for bulges after asking the client to bear down. *The inguinal area is normally free of bulges.*

- Bulges that appear in the inguinal area when the client bears down may indicate a **hernia** (a defect in the abdominal wall that allows abdominal contents to protrude outward).

Bowel Assessment (continued)

Technique/Normal Findings	Abnormal Findings
Palpate the inguinal area with the gloved hand. Ask the client to shift weight to the left to palpate the right inguinal area and vice versa. Place your right index finger upward into the inguinal area and ask the client to bear down or cough. *Bulging or masses are normally not palpable.*	▪ A bulge or mass may indicate a hernia.

Perianal Assessment

Inspect the perianal area. Wearing gloves, spread the client's buttocks apart. Observe the area, and ask client to bear down as if trying to have a bowel movement. *The perianal area should be intact, without obvious lesions.*	▪ Swollen, painful, longitudinal breaks in the anal area may appear in clients with anal fissures. (These are caused by the passing of large, hard stools or by diarrhea.) ▪ Dilated anal veins appear with hemorrhoids. ▪ A red mass may appear with prolapsed internal hemorrhoids. ▪ Doughnut-shaped red tissue at the anal area may appear with a prolapsed rectum.
Palpate the anus and rectum. Lubricate the gloved index finger and ask the client to bear down. Touch the tip of your finger to the client's anal opening. Flex the index finger, and slowly insert it into the anus, pointing the finger toward the umbilicus (Figure 4–8 ▪). Rotate the finger in both directions to palpate any lesions or masses. *There should be no masses in the anus or rectum.*	▪ Movable, soft masses may be polyps. ▪ Hard, firm, irregular embedded masses may indicate carcinoma.

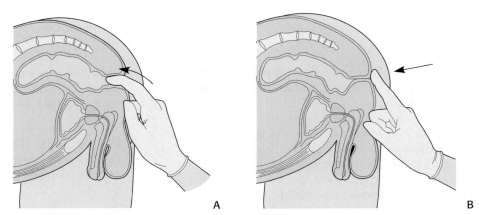

Figure 4–8 ▪ Digital examination of the *A*, rectum and *B*, anus.

Fecal Assessment

Inspect the client's feces. After palpating the rectum, withdraw your finger gently. Inspect any feces on the glove. Note color and/or presence of blood. Also use gloved fingers to note consistency. *Stool should be soft with no blood present, either on the stool or as occult blood.*	
Test the feces for occult blood. Use a testing kit such as Occultest or Hemoccult II. *There should be no blood in the feces.*	▪ A positive occult blood test requires further testing for colon cancer or gastrointestinal bleeding due to peptic ulcers, ulcerative colitis, or diverticulosis.
Note the odor of the feces. *No distinctly foul odors should be present.*	▪ Distinctly foul odors may be noted with stools containing blood or extra fat or in cases of colon cancer.

Source: LeMone, P., & Burke, K. (2008). *Medical-surgical nursing: Critical thinking in client care* (4th ed., pp. 748–750). Upper Saddle River, NJ: Pearson Education.

Assessment Interview   Fecal Elimination

DEFECATION PATTERN
- When do you usually have a bowel movement?
- Has this pattern changed recently?

DESCRIPTION OF FECES AND ANY CHANGES
- Have you noticed any changes in the color, texture (hard, soft, watery), shape, or odor of your stool recently?

FECAL ELIMINATION PROBLEMS
- What problems have you had or do you now have with your bowel movements (constipation, diarrhea, excessive flatulence, seepage, or incontinence)?
- When and how often do they occur?
- What do you think causes these problems (food, fluids, exercise, emotions, medications, disease, surgery)?
- What have you tried to solve the problems, and how effective was it?

FACTORS INFLUENCING ELIMINATION
- *Use of elimination aids.* What routines do you follow to maintain your usual defecation pattern? Do you use natural aids such as specific foods or fluids (e.g., a glass of hot lemon juice before breakfast), laxatives, or enemas to maintain elimination?

- *Diet.* What foods do you believe affect defecation? What foods do you typically eat? What foods do you avoid? Do you take meals at regular times?
- *Fluid.* What amount and kind of fluid do you take each day (e.g., six glasses of water, two cups of coffee)?
- *Exercise.* What is your usual daily exercise pattern? (Obtain specifics about exercise rather than asking whether it is sufficient; ideas of what is sufficient vary among individuals.)
- *Medications.* Have you taken any medications that could affect the intestinal tract (e.g., iron or antibiotics)? (Note the name and specific dosage of all medications because the client may not be aware what medications may affect elimination.)
- *Stress.* Are you experiencing any stress? Do you think this affects your defecation pattern? If so, how?

PRESENCE AND MANAGEMENT OF OSTOMY
- What is your usual routine with your colostomy/ileostomy?
- What type of appliance do you wear, and did you bring a spare with you?
- What problems, if any, do you have with it?
- How can the nurses help you manage your colostomy/ileostomy?

Source: Berman, A., Snyder, S. J., Kozier, B., & Erb, G. (2008). *Kozier & Erb's fundamentals of nursing: Concepts, process, and practice* (8th ed., p. 1334). Upper Saddle River, NJ: Pearson Education.

information about any past or current problems with elimination, presence of an ostomy, and factors influencing the elimination pattern.

Examples of questions to elicit this information can be found in the Assessment Interview. The number of questions to ask is adapted to the individual client, according to the client's responses in the first three categories listed.

When obtaining data about the client's defecation pattern, the nurse needs to understand that the time of defecation and the amount of feces expelled are as individual as the frequency of defecation. Often, the patterns that individuals follow depend largely on early training and convenience.

Physical Examination
Physical examination of the abdomen in relation to fecal elimination problems includes inspection, auscultation, percussion, and palpation with specific reference to the intestinal tract.

Auscultation precedes palpation, because palpation can alter peristalsis. Examination of the rectum and anus includes inspection and palpation.

Inspecting the Feces
Observe the client's stool for color, consistency, shape, amount, odor, and presence of abnormal constituents.

DIAGNOSTIC TESTS
Diagnostic studies of the gastrointestinal tract include direct visualization techniques, indirect visualization techniques, and laboratory tests for abnormal constituents within the stool, such as parasites, microorganisms, or products of incomplete digestion. For details, see the Diagnostic Tests feature that follows.

DIAGNOSTIC TESTS   Intestinal Disorders

NAME OF TEST   Stool specimen, stool culture

PURPOSE AND DESCRIPTION   A sample of stool is collected for gross and microscopic examination as well as for evaluation of form, consistency, and color. Gross examination includes volume and water content and the presence of any blood, pus, mucus, or excess fat. Microscopic examination identifies the presence of white blood cells, unabsorbed fat, and parasites. When an enteric pathogen is suspected, a stool culture is done.

RELATED NURSING CARE   Ask the client to provide a fresh stool sample. A sterile container should be used to collect a stool sample for a culture. Ask women of childbearing age if they are having their menstrual period; if so, note this on the laboratory request.

Developmental Considerations   Specimens can be collected from the diaper of an infant or young child using a sterile tongue blade and then placed in a sterile container. It is best to collect the sample as soon after defecation as possible.

DIAGNOSTIC TESTS Intestinal Disorders (continued)

NAME OF TEST Test for **occult blood** (hidden blood)

PURPOSE AND DESCRIPTION A stool specimen may be sent to the laboratory, or the test may be done with a commercial kit, such as Hemoccult II or Occultest.

RELATED NURSING CARE When testing for occult blood with a commercial kit following a rectal examination, place a smear of stool on the designated area, and drop the reagent on the area. A blue color that develops in response to the reagent indicates the presence of blood.

Developmental Considerations No special developmental considerations are needed.

NAME OF TEST Small bowel series

PURPOSE AND DESCRIPTION This radiologic examination is done to diagnose abnormalities of the small intestine. The client drinks a contrast medium, and radiographs are taken every 20 minutes until the medium reaches the terminal ileum. It also may be done in conjunction with an upper gastrointestinal GI series or barium swallow.

CLIENT PREPARATION

- Ensure the presence of a signed informed consent for the procedure.
- A low-residue diet may be ordered for 48 hours preceding the examination, and a tap-water enema or cathartic may be given the evening before the examination.
- Withhold all food for 8 hours and all water for 4 hours before the examination.
- Withhold medications affecting bowel motility for 24 hours before the examination if possible (unless prescribed as part of the preparation procedure).

HEALTH EDUCATION FOR THE CLIENT AND FAMILY

- Although the test is not uncomfortable, it requires several hours to complete. Bring along reading material, paperwork, or crafts to occupy time.
- For a small bowel exam, the barium may be administered orally or instilled through a weighted tube inserted into the small bowel or endoscopically.
- Increase fluid intake for at least 24 hours after the procedure to facilitate evacuation of the barium. A laxative or cathartic may be prescribed.
- Stool will be chalky white for up to 72 hours after the examination. Normal stool color will return on complete evacuation of the barium.

Developmental Considerations Contrast medium can be fed to infants through a bottle, or a nasogastric tube can be placed to introduce the contrast medium into the stomach if swallowing studies are not included with the test.

NAME OF TEST Barium enema

PURPOSE AND DESCRIPTION This fluoroscopic radiologic examination is done to identify structural abnormalities of the rectum and colon by administering a contrast medium rectally. Double-contrast or air-contrast studies are the examination of choice, with air being infused after the barium is evacuated.

CLIENT PREPARATION

- Ensure the presence of a signed informed consent for the procedure.
- Provide or instruct the client to follow a clear liquid diet for 24 hours before the test. All food and fluids may be withheld for 8 hours before the test.
- Administer or instruct the client to use laxatives, enemas, or suppositories on the evening before the procedure as ordered. Additional bowel preparation may be ordered for the morning just before the procedure.

HEALTH EDUCATION FOR THE CLIENT AND FAMILY

Before the Procedure

- The procedure takes approximately 1 hour.
- The barium will be instilled through a lubricated tube inserted into the rectum. The client will experience a sensation of fullness and may feel the need to defecate.
- He or she will be positioned on the left side, on the back, and prone during this procedure.
- A fluoroscope will be used to follow the progress of the barium, and radiographs will be obtained.
- The client will expel the barium in the bathroom.

After the Procedure

- Following the procedure, a laxative will be given.
- Stools may be white for the next 1–2 days.

Developmental Considerations Reduced volume of contrast medium is indicated for infants and young children. To gain the cooperation of a very young child, sedation may be required.

NAME OF TEST Abdominal ultrasound

PURPOSE AND DESCRIPTION This test is used to identify abdominal masses, ascites, and disorders of the appendix. A lubricant gel is applied to the skin, and a transducer is placed over the area of interest. High-frequency sound waves pass through the body structures and are recorded as they are reflected.

RELATED NURSING CARE Tell client not to eat or drink for 8–12 hours before the examination.

Developmental Considerations No special developmental considerations are necessary.

(continued)

DIAGNOSTIC TESTS Intestinal Disorders (continued)

NAME OF TEST Magnetic resonance imaging (MRI)

PURPOSE AND DESCRIPTION This test may be done to identify sources of gastrointestinal bleeding and to stage colon cancer.

RELATED NURSING CARE Ask whether the client is pregnant or has a metal implant (if so, the examination will be canceled).

Developmental Considerations To gain the cooperation of a very young child, sedation may be required. Swaddling the newborn or infant and using a pacifier may help to keep the child still during the procedure.

NAME OF TEST Sigmoidoscopy

PURPOSE AND DESCRIPTION This test allows visual examination of the anus, rectum, and sigmoid colon to identify tumors, polyps, infections, inflammations, hemorrhoids, and fissures. The test is done by using a flexible sigmoidoscope. Specimens are obtained and polyps removed during the procedure.

CLIENT PREPARATION

- Ensure the presence of a signed informed consent for the procedure.
- Generally, clear liquid or a light diet is ordered for the evening before the procedure.
- Instruct the client to take a laxative.
- Administer an enema or rectal suppository before the procedure as ordered.

HEALTH EDUCATION FOR THE CLIENT AND FAMILY

Before the Procedure

- The procedure takes approximately 15 minutes.

- A mild sedative or tranquilizer may be given during the procedure.
- The client may be positioned on his or her left side or in the knee-chest position.
- The scope will be inserted through the anus into the sigmoid colon.
- Feces may be suctioned.
- A biopsy may be performed. Polyps may be removed.
- Taking deep breaths when the client feels discomfort may help him or her to relax.

After the Procedure

- Sit up slowly to avoid dizziness or light-headedness.
- You may pass large amounts of flatus if air was instilled into the bowel.
- Report any abdominal pain, fever, chills, or rectal bleeding.
- If a polyp is removed, avoid heavy lifting for 7 days, and avoid high-fiber foods for 1–2 days.

Developmental Considerations A smaller sigmoidoscope is available for use in young children.

NAME OF TEST Colonoscopy

PURPOSE AND DESCRIPTION This test allows visual examination of the entire colon to the ileocecal valve to identify tumors, polyps, and inflammatory bowel disease and to dilate strictures. A flexible endoscope is inserted anally and advanced through the colon. Polyps are removed during the procedure to prevent them from becoming malignant.

CLIENT PREPARATION

- Ensure the presence of a signed informed consent for the procedure.
- A liquid diet may be prescribed for 2 days before the procedure, and the client usually is NPO for 8 hours just before the procedure.
- Administer or instruct the client in bowel preparation procedures, such as taking citrate of magnesia or polyethylene glycol the evening before the examination.
- Sedation usually is given during the procedure.

HEALTH EDUCATION FOR THE CLIENT AND FAMILY

Before the Procedure

- Explain dietary restrictions and their purpose.
- The procedure takes from 30 minutes to 1 hour.
- The scope is inserted through the anus and advanced to the cecum.
- A biopsy may be performed. Polyps may be removed.
- Discomfort is minimal.
- The client should arrange for transportation, because he or she may not be allowed to drive for 24 hours after the procedure.

After the Procedure

- The client may have increased flatus, because air is instilled into the bowel during the procedure.
- Report any abdominal pain, chills, fever, rectal bleeding, or mucopurulent discharge.
- If a polyp has been removed, the client should avoid heavy lifting for 7 days, and avoid high-fiber food for 1–2 days.

Developmental Considerations A smaller colonoscope is available for use in young children.

Source: LeMone, P., & Burke, K. (2008). *Medical-surgical nursing: Critical thinking in client care* (4th ed., p. 744–745). Upper Saddle River, NJ: Pearson Education.

CARING INTERVENTIONS

Medical management of altered bowel elimination is based on the diagnosed problem impacting elimination. Treatment for minor problems may include increasing the amount of fiber and fluid in the diet. Medications such as laxatives, antidiarrheal agents, or stool softeners may be indicated. Clients with more acute problems, such as obstruction, ulceration, perforation, or cancer, may require surgical resection of the bowel with or without creation of an ostomy. Medical management of obstructions may involve gut rest with placement of a nasogastric tube.

PHARMACOLOGIC THERAPIES

Medications for management of bowel elimination may be given to promote bowel movement, to promote absorption of excess fluid in the intestine, or to coalesce gas or reduce the production of gas. For details regarding medications, see the Medications feature that follows.

MEDICATIONS Bowel Elimination

Drug Classifications	Mechanism of Action	Commonly Prescribed Drugs	Nursing Considerations
Laxatives: bulk-forming agents, stool softeners, stimulants, saline or osmotic laxatives, herbal agents, and miscellaneous agents	Promote bowel movement	Psyllium hydrophilic mucilloid, methylcellulose, docusate sodium, senna, mineral oil, and Epsom salts	■ Contraindicated in clients with nausea, cramps, colic, vomiting, or undiagnosed abdominal pain. Also contraindicated in clients after abdominal surgery. ■ Should not be used continuously, because they weaken bowel's natural response to fecal distention. ■ Before administration, assess abdomen for distention, bowel sounds, and bowel patterns. ■ Teach clients preventive measures for constipation to avoid overdependence on laxatives.
Antidiarrheal agents	Slow motility of the intestines or promote absorption of excess fluid in the intestine	Diphenoxylate with atropine, camphorated opium tincture, difenoxin with atropine, loperamide, bismuth salts, and furazolidone	■ Monitor fluid and electrolyte status. ■ Contraindicated in clients with severe dehydration, electrolyte imbalance, liver and renal disorders, and glaucoma. ■ Teach clients to seek medical care if diarrhea does not subside in 2 days, fever develops, or dehydration occurs.
Antiflatulent agents	Coalesce gas bubbles and facilitate passage	Simethicone	■ Teach clients to seek medical care if symptoms persist or recur. ■ Side effects include bloating, constipation, diarrhea, gas, and heartburn.

4.1 BLADDER: INCONTINENCE AND RETENTION

KEY TERMS

BASIS FOR SELECTION OF EXEMPLAR

Institute of Medicine (IOM)

Chronic Disease Management

LEARNING OUTCOMES

After learning about this exemplar, you will be able to do the following:

1. Describe the pathophysiology, etiology, clinical manifestations, and direct and indirect causes of bladder incontinence and retention.

2. Identify risk factors associated with bladder incontinence and retention.

3. Illustrate the nursing process in providing culturally competent care across the life span for individuals with bladder incontinence and retention.

4. Formulate priority nursing diagnoses appropriate for an individual with bladder incontinence and retention.

5. Create a plan of care for an individual with bladder incontinence and retention that includes family members and caregivers.

6. Assess expected outcomes for an individual with bladder incontinence and retention.

7. Discuss therapies used in the collaborative care of an individual with bladder incontinence and retention.

8. Employ evidence-based caring interventions (or prevention) for an individual with bladder incontinence and retention.

OVERVIEW

When caring for clients with urinary tract disorders, it is important to consider the client's modesty in voiding, possible difficulty in discussing the genitals, embarrassment about being exposed for examination and testing, and fear of changes in body image or function. These psychosocial issues may interfere with the client's willingness to seek help, discuss treatment, and learn about preventive measures. Nursing interventions for clients with urinary tract disorders are directed toward primary prevention, early detection, and management of the disorder through health teaching and nursing care.

URINARY INCONTINENCE

Urinary incontinence or involuntary urination, is a symptom, not a disease. It is the most common manifestation of impaired bladder control. It can have a significant impact on the client's life, creating physical problems, such as skin breakdown, and it can lead to psychosocial problems, including embarrassment, isolation, and social withdrawal.

Incidence and Prevalence

Approximately 17 million people in the United States have some degree of urinary incontinence (Mason, Newman, & Palmer, 2003). The estimated annual cost of managing urinary incontinence is $10 billion. Although urinary incontinence is especially common among older clients, it is not a normal consequence of aging, and it can be treated. An estimated 30% or more of older women living in the community experience urinary incontinence. In long-term care, foster care, and home-bound populations, the incidence is approximately 50% (Mason et al., 2003; Tierney, McPhee, & Papadakis, 2005). Despite these statistics, the actual prevalence of urinary incontinence is nearly impossible to determine. Embarrassment and the availability of products to protect clothing and prevent detection contribute to clients not seeking evaluation and treatment of incontinence.

Etiology and Pathophysiology

Urinary continence requires a bladder that is able to expand and contract and sphincters that can maintain a urethral pressure higher than that of the bladder. Incontinence results when the pressure within the urinary bladder exceeds urethral resistance, allowing urine to escape. Any condition causing higher-than-normal bladder pressures or reduced urethral resistance can potentially result in incontinence. Relaxation of the pelvic musculature, disruption of cerebral and nervous system control, and disturbances of the bladder and its musculature are common contributing factors.

Incontinence may be an acute, self-limited disorder, or it may be chronic. The causes may be congenital or acquired, reversible or irreversible. Congenital disorders associated with incontinence include epispadias (absence of the upper wall of the urethra), and meningomyelocele (a neural tube defect in which a portion of the spinal cord and its surrounding meninges protrude through the vertebral column). Central nervous system or spinal cord trauma, stroke, and chronic neurologic disorders, such as multiple sclerosis and Parkinson's disease, are examples of acquired, irreversible causes of incontinence. Reversible causes include medications (e.g., diuretics and sedatives), prostatic enlargement, vaginal and urethral atrophy, UTI, and fecal impaction. Fecal impaction occurs when a mass of hard, dry stool will not void with a normal bowel movement. Vaginal childbirth also may contribute to urinary incontinence. In addition, acute confusion can cause incontinence that may or may not be reversible, depending on the underlying cause of the confusion.

Incontinence commonly is categorized as stress incontinence, urge incontinence (also known as overactive bladder), overflow incontinence, and functional incontinence. Table 4–7 summarizes each type with its physiologic cause and associated factors. Mixed incontinence (elements of both stress and urge incontinence) is common. Total incontinence is loss of all

TABLE 4–7 Types of Urinary Incontinence

	DESCRIPTION	PATHOPHYSIOLOGY	CONTRIBUTING FACTORS
Stress	Loss of urine associated with increased intra-abdominal pressure during sneezing, coughing, lifting. Quantity of urine lost usually is small	Relaxation of pelvic musculature and weakness of urethra and surrounding muscles and tissues leads to decreased urethral resistance	■ Multiple pregnancies ■ Decreased estrogen levels ■ Short urethra, change in angle between bladder and urethra ■ Abdominal wall weakness ■ Prostate surgery ■ Increased intra-abdominal pressure caused by tumor, ascites, obesity
Urge	Involuntary loss of urine associated with a strong urge to void	Hypertonic or overactive detrusor muscle leads to increased pressure within bladder and inability to inhibit voiding	■ Neurologic disorders, such as stroke, Parkinson's disease, multiple sclerosis; peripheral nervous system disorders ■ Detrusor muscle overactivity associated with bladder outlet obstruction, aging, or disorders such as diabetes
Overflow	Inability to empty bladder, resulting in overdistention and frequent loss of small amounts of urine	Outlet obstruction or lack of normal detrusor activity leads to overfilling of bladder and increased pressure	■ Spinal cord injuries below S_2 ■ Diabetic neuropathy ■ Prostatic hypertrophy ■ Fecal impaction ■ Drugs, especially those with anticholinergic effect
Functional	Incontinence resulting from physical, environmental, or psychosocial causes	Ability to respond to the need to urinate is impaired	■ Confusion or dementia ■ Physical disability or impaired mobility ■ Therapy or sedation ■ Depression ■ Regression

Source: LeMone, P., & Burke, K. (2008). *Medical-surgical nursing: Critical thinking in client care* (4th ed., p. 874). Upper Saddle River, NJ: Pearson Education.

voluntary control over urination, with urine loss occurring without stimulus and in all positions.

Common causes of incontinence include UTI, urethritis, pregnancy, hypercalcemia, volume overload, delirium, restricted mobility, stool impaction, and psychologic causes (Morantz, 2005, p. 175). Urinary incontinence can be broken into two categories: acute and chronic.

ACUTE INCONTINENCE Many factors can contribute to acute, or reversible, incontinence, including polyuria, exposure to irritants, infection, urinary retention, use of pharmaceuticals, stool impaction or constipation, atrophic urethritis or vaginitis, restricted mobility or dexterity, psychologic conditions, and delirium or acute confused state. Some of these factors are readily reversible, with a decrease in symptoms if not complete resolution of urinary incontinence.

CHRONIC INCONTINENCE There are different types of chronic incontinence, including stress, urge, reflex, retention with overflow, and functional incontinence. Each type of chronic incontinence has a different etiology.

Risk Factors

Women are much more susceptible than men to urinary incontinence. Smokers have a higher risk for urinary incontinence, as do older adults who are housebound or living in nursing homes (see the Developmental Considerations feature that follows). Obesity, diabetes, inactivity, depression, and neurological disorders (e.g., stroke) are all risk factors for urinary incontinence. Individuals who experience two or more UTIs per year also are at higher risk.

Certain medications can cause urinary incontinence. These include medications that affect the adrenergic system, diuretics, and calcium-channel blockers.

Clinical Manifestations and Therapies

Symptoms of urinary incontinence include the inability to avoid urinating until a bathroom can be found, inability to urinate, increased rate of urination, leakage, uncontrollable wetting, and frequent bladder infections. A number of medications and therapies are available to help individuals experiencing urinary incontinence.

MEDICATIONS Both stress and urge incontinence may improve with drug treatment. Drugs that contract the smooth muscles of the bladder neck may reduce episodes of mild stress incontinence. Imipramine (Tofranil), an antidepressant, is an effective preparation. It can make people drowsy, however, so it typically is taken at night. Adverse effects, such as dizziness and irregular heartbeat, and contraindications with a number of other medications may limit its use.

When incontinence is associated with postmenopausal atrophic vaginitis, estrogen therapy may be effective. Options include systemic estrogens and local creams. Clients with urge incontinence may be treated with preparations that increase bladder capacity. The primary drugs used to inhibit detrusor muscle contractions and increase bladder capacity include oxybutynin (Ditropan and the extended-release form, Ditropan XL), an anticholinergic drug, and tolterodine (Detrol and its longer-acting form, Detrol LA), a more specific antimuscarinic agent. These drugs can be taken once or twice a day and have fewer side effects than less-specific anticholinergic drugs. Drugs with anticholinergic effects are contraindicated for the client with acute glaucoma. Urinary retention is a potential side effect that must be considered when these drugs are used.

SURGERY Surgery may be used to treat stress incontinence associated with cystocele or urethrocele and overflow incontinence associated with an enlarged prostate gland. Suspension

---

DEVELOPMENTAL CONSIDERATIONS **The Institutionalized Older Adult and Self-Care Deficit**

Functional incontinence may be the predominant problem in an institutionalized older adult. Limited mobility, impaired vision, dementia, lack of access to facilities and privacy, and tight staffing patterns increase the risk for incontinence in previously continent residents. The primary problem in functional incontinence is an outside factor that interferes with the ability to respond normally to the urge to void. An immobilized client may wet the bed if a call light is not within reach; a client with Alzheimer's disease may perceive the urge to void but be unable to interpret its meaning or respond by seeking a bathroom. For these clients, self-care deficit in toileting is a primary problem.

To assist clients with self-care, the nurse should do the following:

- Assess physical and mental abilities and limitations, usual voiding pattern, and ability to assist with toileting. A thorough assessment allows planned interventions to address specific needs and promote independence.
- Provide assistive devices. such as raised toilet seats, grab bars, a bedside commode, or night lights, as needed to facilitate independence. Fostering independence in toileting bolsters self-concept and maintains a positive body image.

- Plan a toileting schedule based on the client's normal elimination patterns to achieve a urine output of approximately 300 mL with each voiding. Allowing the bladder to fill to a point at which the urge to void is experienced and then emptying it completely helps to maintain normal bladder capacity and bacteriostatic functions.
- Position for ease of voiding—sitting for females, standing for males—and provide privacy. Normal positioning, usual toileting facilities, and privacy all enhance the ability to void on schedule and empty the bladder completely.
- Adjust fluid intake so that the majority of fluids are consumed during times of the day when the client is most able to remain continent. Unless fluids are restricted, maintain a fluid intake of at least 1.5–2.0 L per day. An adequate fluid intake is vital to promote hydration and urinary function. Overly concentrated urine can irritate the bladder, increasing incontinence.
- Assist with clothing that is easily removed (e.g., elastic-waist pants or loose dresses). Velcro and zipper fasteners may be easier to use than snaps and buttons. Clothing that is difficult to remove can increase the risk of incontinence in clients with mobility problems or impaired dexterity.

Box 4–3 Nursing Care of the Client Undergoing Bladder Neck Suspension

PREOPERATIVE CARE

- Discuss the need to avoid straining and the use of the Valsalva maneuver postoperatively. *Straining and increased abdominal pressure during the Valsalva maneuver may place excessive stress on suture lines and interfere with healing.*
- Suggest measures such as increasing fluid and fiber intake and using a stool softener to prevent postoperative constipation.

POSTOPERATIVE CARE

- Monitor urine output, including quantity, color, and clarity. Expect urine to be pink initially, then to clear gradually. *Bright red urine, excessive vaginal drainage, or incisional bleeding may indicate hemorrhage. Instrumentation of the urinary tract increases the potential for UTI; cloudy urine may be an early sign.*
- Maintain stability and patency of suprapubic and/or urethral catheters. Secure catheters in position. *Maintaining bladder*

decompression eliminates pressure on suture lines. Preventing movement of or pulling on catheters reduces the risk for resultant pressure on surgical incisions.

- Carefully monitor urine output after catheter removal. Difficulty voiding is common following catheter removal. *Early intervention to prevent bladder distention is important to prevent pressure on suture lines.*
- If the urethral or suprapubic catheter will remain in place on discharge, teach proper care to the client and family members as needed. *Appropriate self-care and early recognition of problems reduce the risk for significant complications.*

Source: LeMone, P., & Burke, K. (2008). Medical-surgical nursing: Critical thinking in client care (4th ed. p. 876). Upper Saddle River, NJ: Pearson Education.

---

of the bladder neck (Box 4–3), a technique that brings the angle between the bladder and urethra closer to normal, is effective in treating stress incontinence associated with urethrocele in 80–95% of clients. A laparoscopic, vaginal, or abdominal approach may be used to perform this surgery.

Prostatectomy, using either the transurethral or suprapubic approach, is indicated for the client who is experiencing overflow incontinence as a result of an enlarged prostate gland and urethral obstruction.

Other surgical procedures of potential benefit in the treatment of incontinence include implantation of an artificial sphincter, formation of a urethral sling to elevate and compress the urethra, augmentation of the bladder with bowel segments

to increase bladder capacity, and injection of collagen along the urethra to narrow the urinary passageway and support more normal urethral positioning.

COMPLEMENTARY THERAPIES Biofeedback and relaxation techniques may help to reduce episodes of urinary incontinence. Biofeedback uses electronic monitors to teach conscious control over physiologic responses of which the individual is not normally aware. Developing an awareness of perceptible information allows the client to gain voluntary control over urination. Biofeedback is widely used to manage urinary incontinence.

For more information, see the Evidence-Based Practice feature.

EVIDENCE-BASED PRACTICE   Urinary Incontinence

An accurate diagnosis of stress urinary incontinence often is made based on clinical data, but motor urge incontinence generally is more difficult to diagnose accurately without urodynamic testing. This presents a difficulty for nurses and nurse practitioners in planning care for clients with incontinence when urologic testing is not feasible or readily available. A model developed by Gray, McClain, Peruggia, Patrie, and Steers (2001) may be useful in addressing this problem in adults whose cognitive abilities are intact. By comparing client data with urodynamic testing results, this team of researchers identified factors predictive of motor urge incontinence. These factors included age, gender, and three key symptoms: diurnal frequency (urinating more often than every 2 hours while awake), nocturia (awakening with the urge to urinate more than once per night if younger than 65 years and twice per night if older than age 65), and urge incontinence (urine loss associated with a strong desire to urinate). The presence of all three symptoms was more than 92% predictive of motor urge incontinence in study participants of all ages (range, 18–89 years; median, 61 years) and both genders.

Implications for Nursing

Asking specific questions about urinary tract symptoms can facilitate accurate identification of the nursing diagnosis *Urge Urinary Incontinence*. Accurate diagnosis is vital to planning care

implementing appropriate care measures and to achieving the desired outcome—namely, continence. Successful treatment promotes self-esteem and provides positive reinforcement for continuing planned strategies.

Critical Thinking in Client Care

1. What nursing care measures and client teaching will you provide for the client with stress incontinence that may not be appropriate or necessary for the client with urge incontinence? What nursing care measures and client teaching will you provide for the client with urge incontinence but not stress incontinence?

2. Identify circumstances in which it may not be possible or feasible to have the client undergo urodynamic testing to differentiate stress, urge, or mixed (stress and urge) incontinence.

3. The clients in the study by Gray et al. lived independently in the community with no known or visible cognitive impairment. Can the data in this study be generalized to clients residing in a long-term care facility? Can the results be applied to all types of incontinence? Why, or why not?

Source: Gray, M., McClain, R., Perrugia, M., Patrie, J., & Steers, W. D. (2001). A model for predicting motor urge urinary incontinence. Nursing Research, 50(2), 116–122.

HEALTH PROMOTION Although urinary incontinence rarely has serious physical effects, it frequently has significant psychosocial effects, and it can lead to lowered self-esteem, social isolation, and even institutionalization (Lauver, Gross, Ruff, & Wells, 2004). The nurse should get the word out—informing all clients that urinary incontinence is not a normal consequence of aging and that treatments are available. To reduce the incidence of urinary incontinence, the nurse should teach all women to perform pelvic floor muscle (Kegel) exercises (Box 4–4) to improve perineal muscle tone. Women should be urged to seek advice from their primary care practitioner about using topical or systemic hormone therapy during menopause to maintain perineal tissue integrity. Older men should be advised to have routine prostate examinations to prevent urethral obstruction and overflow incontinence. Pelvic floor muscle exercises also may benefit men who experience urinary incontinence following prostatectomy, but evidence supporting this is limited (Moore & Gray, 2004).

PRACTICE ALERT

Clients who have difficulty emptying the bladder completely should not to stop urine flow while voiding in order to identify the pelvic floor muscles. Repeated interruption of micturition can interfere with complete bladder emptying and increase the risk for UTI.

CLIENT TEACHING Client teaching is essential for clients who experience problems with urinary incontinence and for their family members. The nurse should discuss the following points with clients to help prevent UTI and urinary incontinence:

- Maintain a generous fluid intake (see the Practice Alert feature that follows). Reduce or eliminate fluid intake after the evening meal to reduce nocturia.
- Wear comfortable clothing that is easy to remove for toileting.
- Maintain good hygiene, but do not bathe more often than necessary. Frequent bathing and use of feminine hygiene sprays or douches may dry perineal tissues, increasing the risk of UTI or urinary incontinence.
- Perform pelvic muscle (Kegel) exercises several times a day to increase perineal muscle tone.
- Reduce consumption of caffeine-containing beverages (e.g., coffee, tea, and colas), citrus juices, and artificially sweetened beverages containing NutraSweet.

- Use behavioral techniques to reduce the frequency of incontinence. **Scheduled toileting** is toileting at regular intervals (e.g., every 2–4 hours). **Habit training** is toileting the client on a schedule that corresponds with the normal pattern. **Bladder training** gradually increases the bladder capacity by increasing the intervals between voidings and resisting the urge to void.
- See your primary care provider regularly for a pelvic or prostate examination.
- For women, discuss possible benefits and risks of hormone replacement therapy, physical therapy, or surgery to treat incontinence.
- Report any change in urine color, odor, or clarity or symptoms such as burning, frequency, or urgency to your primary care provider.

PRACTICE ALERT

Limiting total fluid intake to less than 1.5–2.0 L per day is not recommended for clients with urinary incontinence. Inadequate fluid increases urine concentration, leading to bladder wall irritation and possibly increasing problems of urge incontinence.

URINARY RETENTION

When bladder emptying is impaired, urine accumulates and the bladder becomes overdistended, a condition known as **urinary retention**. Overdistention of the bladder causes poor contractility of the detrusor muscle, further impairing urination. If the problem persists, more serious problems, such as **hydronephrosis** (distension or dilation of the kidneys) can result. Common causes of urinary retention include prostatic hypertrophy (enlargement), surgery, and some medications.

Clients with urinary retention may experience overflow voiding or incontinence, eliminating from 25–50 mL of urine at frequent intervals. The bladder is firm and distended on palpation and may be displaced to one side of midline.

Etiology and Pathophysiology

Either mechanical obstruction of the bladder outlet or a functional problem can cause urinary retention. Benign prostatic hypertrophy (BPH) is a common cause, with difficulty initiating and maintaining urine flow often being the presenting complaint in men. Acute inflammation associated with infection or trauma

---

Box 4–4 **Pelvic Floor Muscle (Kegel) Exercises**

- Identify the pelvic muscles with these techniques:
  a. Stop the flow of urine during voiding, and hold for a few seconds (see the Practice Alert feature that follows).
  b. Tighten the muscles at the vaginal entrance around a gloved finger or tampon.
  c. Tighten the muscles around the anus as though resisting defecation.
- Perform exercises by tightening pelvic muscles, holding for 10 seconds, and then relaxing for 10–15 seconds. Continue the sequence (tighten, hold, relax) for 10 repetitions.
- Keep abdominal muscles and breathing relaxed while performing exercises.

- Initially, exercises should be performed twice a day, working up to four times a day.
- Encourage exercising at a specific time each day or in conjunction with another daily activity (e.g., bathing or watching the news). Establish a routine, because these exercises should be continued for life.
- Assistive devices, such as vaginal cones, and biofeedback may be useful for clients who have difficulty identifying appropriate muscle groups.

Source: LeMone, P., & Burke, K. (2008). *Medical-surgical nursing: Critical thinking in client care* (4th ed., p. 877). Upper Saddle River, NJ: Pearson Education.

of the bladder, urethra, or perineal tissues also may interfere with micturition. Scarring caused by repeated UTIs can lead to urethral stricture and a mechanical obstruction. Bladder calculi also may obstruct the urethral opening from the bladder.

Risk Factors

A number of factors may increase an individual's risk for urinary retention. Surgery, particularly abdominal or pelvic surgery, may disrupt function of the detrusor muscle, leading to retention of urine.

Drugs also may interfere with detrusor muscle function. Anticholinergic medications, such as atropine, glycopyrrolate (Robinul), propantheline bromide (Pro-Banthine), and scopolamine hydrochloride (Transderm-Scop), can lead to acute urinary retention and bladder distention. Many other drug groups have anticholinergic side effects and may cause urinary retention. Among these are antianxiety agents, such as diazepam (Valium); antidepressant and tricyclic drugs, such as imipramine (Tofranil); antiparkinsonian drugs (L-dopa); antipsychotic agents; and some sedative/hypnotic drugs. In addition, antihistamines, which are common in over-the-counter cough, cold, allergy, and sleep-promoting drugs, have anticholinergic effects and may interfere with bladder emptying. Diphenhydramine (Benadryl) is an example of a nonprescription antihistamine.

Voluntary urinary retention (particularly common among nurses!) may lead to overfilling of the bladder and a loss of detrusor muscle tone. Accidents to or infections of the brain or spinal cord can increase a client's risk for urinary retention. Diabetes, stroke, pelvic trauma, multiple sclerosis, and BPH all increase the risk for urinary retention.

Clinical Manifestations and Therapies

The client with urinary retention is unable to empty the bladder completely and may feel discomfort because of this inability. The client may have difficulty starting urination and may be able to produce only a weak flow. Overflow voiding or incontinence may occur, with 25–50 mL of urine eliminated at frequent intervals. Assessment reveals a firm, distended bladder that may be displaced to one side of midline. Percussion of the lower abdomen reveals a dull tone, reflective of fluid in the bladder. Urinary retention is confirmed using a bladder scan or by inserting a urinary catheter (if possible) and measuring the urine output. Use of a bladder scan is preferred to reduce the risk of UTI (Teng, Huang, Kuo, & Bih, 2005).

Severe urinary retention with resulting bladder distention impairs the ability of the vesicoureteral junction to prevent backflow of urine into the ureters (Figure 4–9 ■). Reflux of urine from the distended bladder distends the ureters (hydroureter) and kidneys (hydronephrosis). Hydronephrosis impairs renal function, and acute renal failure can result.

MEDICATIONS Cholinergic medications, such as bethanechol chloride (Urecholine), that promote contraction of the detrusor muscle and emptying of the bladder may be used. A medication with no anticholinergic side effects may be substituted when urinary retention is related to drug therapy.

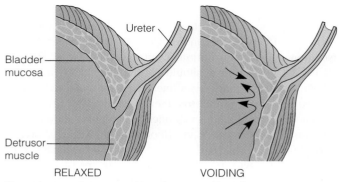

Figure 4–9 ■ A competent vesicoureteral junction.

SURGERIES AND PROCEDURES An indwelling urinary catheter or intermittent straight catheterization can prevent urinary retention and overdistention of the bladder. Mechanical obstructions are treated by removing or repairing the obstruction when possible. Resection of the prostate gland may be done for urinary retention related to BPH. Bladder calculi are removed, and measures to prevent their formation are instituted.

 NURSING PROCESS

Assessment

The preliminary assessment and identification of the symptoms of urinary incontinence and retention are truly within the scope of nursing practice. All clients should be asked about their voiding patterns. Clients with mild symptoms may not even realize that they are experiencing a problem. Older adults who are incontinent while in their home or who manage to contain or conceal their incontinence from others do not consider themselves to be incontinent. Therefore, if these older adults are asked whether they are incontinent, they may deny it. However, asking if they lose urine when they don't want to may provide more accurate information (Palmer & Newman, 2006). If incontinence is described, a thorough history and assessment is indicated.

A complete assessment of a client's urinary function includes the following:

- *Health history.* Voiding diary; frequency of urination, amount of urine loss, and activities associated with incontinence; methods used to deal with incontinence; use of Kegel exercises or medications; any chronic diseases, medications, or alternative health therapies, related surgeries, and so on; effects of incontinence or retention on usual activities, including social activities.
- *Physical examination.* Physical and mental status, including any physical limitations or impaired cognition; inspection, palpation, and percussion of abdomen for bladder distention; inspection of perineal tissues for redness, irritation, or tissue breakdown; observation for bulging of bladder into vagina when bearing down; assessment of pelvic muscle tone as indicated; assessment hydration status, and examination of urine.

Diagnosis

NANDA International (2007) includes one general diagnostic label for urinary elimination problems: Impaired Urinary Elimination, dysfunctional in urine elimination. other, more specific NANDA nursing diagnoses related to urinary elimination are subcategories of this diagnosis:

- Functional Urinary Incontinence
- Reflex Urinary Incontinence
- Stress Urinary Incontinence
- Total Urinary Incontinence
- Urge Urinary Incontinence
- Overflow Urinary Incontinence
- Urinary Retention

Box 4–5 lists definitions of NANDA diagnoses related to incontinence. Box 4–6 lists clinical examples of assessment data clusters and related nursing diagnoses, outcomes, and interventions.

Problems of urinary elimination also may become the etiology for other problems the client experiences. Examples include the following:

- Urinary retention and invasive procedures, such as catheterization or cystoscopic examination, can put a client at risk for infection.
- Incontinence is a risk factor for low self-esteem and social isolation because it is considered to be socially unacceptable and therefore can be physically and emotionally distressing to clients. Often, the client is embarrassed about dribbling or having an accident and may restrict normal activities for this reason.
- Incontinence increases risk for impaired skin integrity. Bed linens and clothes saturated with urine irritate and macerate the skin. Prolonged skin dampness leads to dermatitis (inflammation of the skin) and subsequent formation of dermal ulcers.
- Functional incontinence is a risk factor for self-care deficits in toileting.
- Impaired urinary function associated with a disease process may put a client at risk for deficient or excess fluid volume.

Box 4–5 Definitions of NANDA Incontinence Diagnoses

- Functional Urinary Incontinence: inability of usually continent person to reach toilet in time to avoid unintentional loss of urine
- Reflex Urinary Incontinence: involuntary loss of urine at somewhat predictable intervals when a specific bladder volume is reached
- Stress Urinary Incontinence: sudden leakage of urine occurring with activities that increase abdominal pressure
- Total Urinary Incontinence: continuous and unpredictable passage of urine
- Urge Urinary Incontinence: involuntary passage of urine occurring soon after a strong sense of urgency to void

Source: Adapted from Moorhead, S., Johnson, M., & Meridean M. (2004). *Nursing outcomes classification (NOC)* (3rd ed.). Copyright © 2004 with permission from Elsevier.

- A client who has a urinary diversion ostomy may develop a disturbed body image.
- Clients who require new self-care skills to manage (e.g., a new urinary diversion ostomy) may be at risk of deficient knowledge regarding management of their care.
- An incontinent client who is being cared for by a family member for extended periods may be at risk for caregiver role strain as well as for deteriorating family relationships as a result of that strain.

Planning

Goals established for a client will depend on the diagnosis and defining characteristics. Examples of overall goals for clients with urinary elimination problems may include the following:

- Maintain or restore a normal voiding pattern.
- Regain normal urine output.
- Prevent associated risks, such as infection, skin breakdown, fluid and electrolyte imbalance, and lowered self-esteem.
- Perform toilet activities independently, with or without assistive devices.
- Contain urine with the appropriate device, catheter, ostomy appliance, or absorbent product.

Appropriate preventive and corrective nursing interventions that relate to these goals must be identified. Specific nursing activities associated with each of these interventions can be selected to meet the client's individual needs. Box 4–6 and the Nursing Care Plan feature at the end of this exemplar show examples of clinical applications of these using NANDA, NIC, and NOC designations.

Planning for Home Care

To provide for continuity of care, the nurse must consider the client's needs for teaching and assistance with care in the home. Discharge planning includes assessment of client and family resources and abilities for self-care, available financial resources, and need for referrals and home health services. The Care Settings feature on urinary elimination outlines an assessment of home care capabilities related to urinary elimination problems and needs. The Client Teaching feature addresses the learning needs of the client and family.

Implementation

Independent nursing interventions for clients with urinary incontinence who are returning to their home or a residential facility include (a) a behavior-oriented continence training program that may consist of bladder training, habit training, prompted voiding, pelvic muscle exercises, and positive reinforcement; (b) meticulous skin care; and (c) for male clients, application of an external drainage device (condom-type catheter device). Other interventions include promoting adequate fluid intake, maintaining normal voiding habits, and assisting with toileting; also, see the following Practice Alert feature. Clients must be alert and physically able or have caregivers who can assist with implementing the plan of care so that the plan can be followed.

Box 4–6 Identifying Nursing Diagnoses, Outcomes, and Interventions: Clients With Urinary Elimination Disorders

Data Cluster: Mrs. Amy Brown, 75, reports accidental loss of urine before she is able to reach the toilet. She is aware of the urge to void but states, "Because of my stroke I sometimes can't get there soon enough."

Nursing diagnosis/ definition	Sample desired outcomes/ definition	Indicators	Selected interventions/ definition	Sample NIC activities
Functional Urinary Incontinence: Inability of usually continent person to reach toilet in time to avoid unintentional loss of urine	Urinary Continence [0502]: *Control of the elimination of urine from the bladder*	Consistently demonstrated: ■ Responds to urge in timely manner ■ Gets to toilet between urge and passage of urine ■ Voids >150 mL each time	Prompted Voiding [0640]: *Promotion of urinary continence through the use of timed verbal toileting reminders and positive social feedback for successful toileting*	■ Determine client awareness of continence status by asking if wet or dry. ■ Prompt up to three times to use toilet or substitute, regardless of continence status. ■ Give positive feedback by praising desired toileting behavior. ■ Document outcomes of toileting session.

Data Cluster: Anthony Cherry, a teenager with a spinal cord injury, has no awareness of bladder filling, the urge to void, or feelings of bladder fullness. He reports loss of urine at fairly regular intervals.

Reflex Urinary Incontinence: Involuntary loss of urine at somewhat predictable intervals when a specific bladder volume is reached	Urinary Elimination [0503]: *Collection and discharge of urine*	Not compromised: ■ Elimination pattern ■ Complete bladder emptying ■ Urine amount ■ Urine clarity	Urinary Catheterization: Intermittent [0582]: *Regular periodic use of a catheter to empty the bladder*	■ Teach client/family purpose, supplies, method, and rationale of intermittent catheterization. ■ Demonstrate procedure, and have a return demonstration. ■ Determine catheterization schedule based on a comprehensive assessment.

Data Cluster: Tammy Tyndale reports dribbling whenever she laughs, coughs, or sneezes. She is 8 months pregnant.

Stress Urinary Incontinence: Sudden loss of urine occurring with activities that increase abdominal pressure	Symptom Control [1608]: *Personal actions to minimize perceived adverse changes in physical and emotional functioning*	Consistently demonstrated: ■ Use of preventive measures ■ Use of available resources	Pelvic Muscle Exercise [0560]: *Strengthening and training the levator ani and urogenital muscles through voluntary repetitive contraction to decrease stress, urge, or mixed types of urinary incontinence*	■ Instruct client to tighten, then relax the ring of muscle around urethra and anus, as if trying to prevent urination or bowel movement. ■ Provide positive feedback for doing exercises as prescribed.

Data Cluster: Mrs. Gail Brady reports urinary urgency, difficulty in getting to the bathroom in time, frequency (more often than every 2 hours), and leakage of urine when unable to reach the toilet in time.

Urge Urinary Incontinence: *Involuntary passage of urine occurring soon after a strong sense of urgency to void*	Tissue Integrity: Skin and Mucous Membranes [1101]: *Structural intactness and normal physiological function of skin and mucous membranes*	Not compromised: ■ Skin integrity	Urinary Bladder Training [0570]: *Improving bladder function for those with urge incontinence by increasing the bladder's ability to hold urine and the client's ability to suppress urination*	■ Keep a continence record for 3 days to establish voiding pattern. ■ Establish interval for toileting, preferably more than 2 hours. ■ Reduce toileting interval by 30 minutes if more than three incontinence episodes in 24 hours. ■ Increase interval by 30 minutes if no incontinence episodes for 3 days until optimal 4-hour interval is reached.

Note: The NOC numbers for desired outcomes and the NIC numbers for nursing interventions are listed in brackets following the appropriate outcome or intervention. Outcomes, indicators, interventions, and activities selected are only a sample of those suggested by NOC and NIC and should be further individualized for each client.

Source: Berman, A., Snyder, S. J., Kozier, B., & Erb, G. (2008). *Kozier & Erb's fundamentals of nursing: Concepts, process, and practice* (8th ed., p. 1297). Upper Saddle River, NJ: Pearson Education.

CARE SETTINGS Urinary Elimination

CLIENT AND ENVIRONMENT
- Self-care abilities: Ability to consume adequate fluids, to perceive bladder fullness, to ambulate and get to the toilet, to manipulate clothing for toileting, and to perform hygiene measures after toileting
- Current level of knowledge: Fluid and dietary intake modifications to promote normal patterns of urinary elimination, bladder training methods, and specific techniques to promote voiding care for indwelling catheter or ostomy (if appropriate)
- Assistive devices required: Ambulatory aids such as walker, cane, or wheelchair; safety devices such as grab bars; toileting aids such as raised toilet seat, urinal, commode, or bedpan; presence of a urinary catheter
- Physical layout of the toileting facilities: Presence of mobility aids; toilet at correct height to enable elders to get up after voiding
- Home environment factors that interfere with toileting: Distance to the bathroom from living areas or bedrooms; barriers such as stairways, scatter rugs, clutter, or narrow doorways that interfere with bathroom access; lighting (including night lighting)
- Urinary elimination problems: Type of incontinence and precipitating factors; manifestations of urinary tract infection such as dysuria, frequency, urgency; evidence of prostatic hypertrophy and effect on urination; ability to perform self-catheterization

and care for other urinary elimination devices such as indwelling catheter, urinary diversion ostomy, or condom drainage

FAMILY
- Caregiver availability, skills, and responses: Ability and willingness to assume responsibilities for care, including assisting with toileting, intermittent catheterization, indwelling catheter care, urinary drainage devices or ostomy care; ready access to laundry facilities; access to and willingness to use respite or relief caregivers
- Family role changes and coping: Effect on spousal and family roles, sleep/rest patterns, sexuality, and social interactions
- Financial resources: Ability to purchase protective pads and garments, supplies for catheterization or ostomy care

COMMUNITY
- Environment: Access to public restrooms and sanitary facilities
- Current knowledge of and experience with community resources: Medical and assistive equipment and supply companies, home health agencies, local pharmacies, available financial assistance, support and educational organizations

Source: Berman, A., Snyder, S. J., Kozier, B., & Erb, G. (2008). *Kozier & Erb's fundamentals of nursing: Concepts, process, and practice* (8th ed., p. 1287). Upper Saddle River, NJ: Pearson Education.

PRACTICE ALERT
Stress incontinence in women may be successfully treated by insertion (under local anesthesia) of a transvaginal tape sling to support the urethra.

Successful home care for a client will involve a combination of the following strategies:
- *Education*, which involves the client, family and any non-family caregivers, including private nursing providers and respite caregivers.
- *Bladder training*, which requires that the client postpone voiding, resist or inhibit the sensation of urgency, and void according to a timetable rather than according to the urge to void. The goals are to gradually lengthen the intervals between urination to correct the client's frequent urination, to stabilize the bladder, and to diminish urgency. This form of training may be used for clients who have bladder instability and urge incontinence. Delayed voiding provides larger voided volumes and longer intervals between voiding. Initially, voiding may be encouraged every 2–3 hours except during sleep, and then every 4–6 hours. A vital component of bladder training is inhibiting the urge-to-void sensation. To do this, instruct the client to practice deep, slow breathing until the urge diminishes or disappears. This is performed every time the client has a premature urge to void.
- *Habit training*, also referred to as timed voiding or scheduled toileting, which attempts to keep clients dry by having them void at regular intervals. With habit training, no attempt is made to motivate the client to delay voiding if the urge occurs. This approach can be effective in children

who are experiencing urinary dysfunction. Biofeedback therapy, in which the child is taught to relax the pelvic floor, also can decrease incidents of wetting (Shei Dei Yang & Cheng Wang, 2005).
- *Prompted voiding*, which supplements habit training by encouraging the client to use the toilet (prompting) and reminding the client when to void.
- *Pelvic muscle exercises*, which includes the following technique: Ask the client to think of the perineal muscles as an elevator. When the client relaxes, the elevator is on the first floor. To perform the exercise, contract the perineal muscles, bringing the elevator to the second, third, and fourth floors. Keep the elevator on the fourth floor for a few seconds, and then gradually relax the area. When the exercise is properly performed, contraction of the muscles of the buttocks and thighs is avoided. Pelvic muscle exercises can be performed anytime, anywhere, sitting or standing—even when voiding. Specific client instructions for performing these exercises are summarized in the Client Teaching feature.

Maintaining Skin Integrity
Skin that is continually moist becomes macerated (softened). Urine that accumulates on the skin is converted to ammonia, which is very irritating to the skin. Because both skin irritation and maceration predispose the client to skin breakdown and ulceration, the incontinent person requires meticulous skin care. To maintain skin integrity, the nurse washes the client's perineal area with mild soap and water or a commercially prepared no-rinse cleanser after episodes of incontinence, rinses it thoroughly if soap and water were used, dries it gently and thoroughly, and provides clean, dry clothing or bed linen. The

CLIENT TEACHING **Urinary Elimination in the Home Setting**

FACILITATING URINARY ELIMINATION SELF-CARE

- Teach the client and family to maintain easy access to toilet facilities, including removing scatter rugs and ensuring that halls and doorways are free of clutter.
- Suggest graduated lighting for nighttime voiding: a dim night-light in the bedroom and low-wattage hallway lighting.
- Advise the client and family to install grab bars and elevated toilet seats as needed.
- Provide for instruction in safe transfer techniques. Contact physical therapy to provide training as needed.
- Suggest clothing that is easily removed for toileting, such as elastic waist pants or Velcro closures.

PROMOTING URINARY ELIMINATION

- Instruct the client to respond to the urge to void as soon as possible; avoid voluntary urinary retention.
- Teach the client to empty the bladder completely at each voiding.
- Emphasize the importance of drinking eight to ten 8-ounce glasses of water daily.
- Teach female clients about pelvic muscle exercises to strengthen perineal muscles.
- Inform the client about the relationship between tobacco use and bladder cancer and provide information about smoking cessation programs as indicated.
- Teach the client to promptly report any of the following to the primary care provider: pain or burning on urination, changes in urine color or clarity, malodorous urine, or changes in voiding patterns (e.g., nocturia, frequency, dribbling).

ASEPSIS

- Teach the client to maintain perineal-genital cleanliness, washing with soap and water daily and cleansing the anal and perineal area after defecating.
- Instruct female clients to wipe from front to back (from the urinary meatus toward the anus) after voiding, and to discard toilet paper after each swipe.
- Provide information about products to protect the skin, clothing, and furniture for clients who are incontinent. Emphasize the importance of cleaning and drying the perineal area after incontinence episodes. Instruct in the use of protective skin barrier products as needed.
- Teach clients with an indwelling catheter and their family about care measures such as cleaning the urinary meatus, managing and emptying the collection device, maintaining a closed system, and bladder irrigation or flushing if ordered.
- For clients with a urinary diversion, teach about care of the stoma, drainage devices, and surrounding skin. For continent diversions, teach the client how to catheterize the stoma to drain urine.
- For clients with an indwelling catheter or urinary diversion, emphasize the importance of maintaining a generous fluid intake (2.5–3 quarts daily) and of promptly reporting changes in urinary output, signs of urinary retention such as abdominal pain, and manifestations of urinary tract infection such as malodorous urine, abdominal discomfort, fever, or confusion.

MEDICATIONS

- Emphasize the importance of taking medications as prescribed. Instruct the client to take the full course of antibiotics ordered to treat a urinary tract infection, even though symptoms are relieved.
- Inform the client and family about any expected changes in urine color or odor associated with prescribed medications.
- For clients with urinary retention, emphasize the need to contact the primary care provider before taking any medication (even over-the-counter medications such as antihistamines) that may exacerbate symptoms.
- For clients taking medications that may damage the kidneys (e.g., aminoglycoside antibiotics), stress the importance of maintaining a generous fluid intake while taking the medication.
- Suggest measures to reduce anticipated side effects of prescribed medications, such as increasing intake of potassium-rich foods when taking a potassium-depleting diuretic such as furosemide.

DIETARY ALTERATIONS

- Teach the client about dietary changes to promote urinary function, such as consuming cranberry juice and foods that acidify the urine to reduce the risk of repeated urinary tract infections or forming calcium-based urinary stones.
- Instruct clients with stress or urge incontinence to limit their intake of caffeine, alcohol, citrus juices, and artificial sweeteners because these are bladder irritants that may increase incontinence. Also, teach clients to limit their evening fluid intake to reduce the risk of nighttime incontinence episodes.

MEASURES SPECIFIC TO URINARY PROBLEMS

- Provide instructions for clients with specific urinary problems or treatments such as
  a. timed urine specimens.
  b. urinary incontinence.
  c. urinary retention.
  d. retention catheters.

REFERRALS

- Make appropriate referrals to home health agencies, community agencies, or social services for assistance with resources such as grab bars and raised toilet seats, providing wheelchair access to bathrooms, obtaining toileting aids such as commodes, urinals, or bedpans, and services such as home health aides for assistance with activities of daily living.

COMMUNITY AGENCIES AND OTHER RESOURCES

- Provide information about resources for durable medical equipment such as commodes or raised toilet seats, possible financial assistance, and medical supplies such as drainage bags, incontinence briefs, or protective pads.
- Suggest additional sources of information and help such as the National Council of Independent Living, United Ostomy Association, National Association for Continence, and Simon Foundation for Continence.

Source: Berman, A., Snyder, S. J., Kozier, B., & Erb, G. (2008). *Kozier & Erb's fundamentals of nursing: Concepts, process, and practice* (8th ed., 1298). Upper Saddle River, NJ: Pearson Education.

nurse applies barrier ointments or creams to protect the skin from contact with urine. If it is necessary to pad the client's clothes for protection, the nurse should use products that absorb wetness and leave a dry surface in contact with the skin.

Clients returning home or to a care facility should be instructed in techniques for maintaining skin integrity.

Specially designed incontinence draw sheets, which provide significant advantages over standard draw sheets, may be used for incontinent clients confined to bed. These sheets are like a standard draw sheet but are double layered, with a quilted upper nylon or polyester surface and an absorbent viscose rayon layer below. The rayon soaker layer generally has a waterproof backing on its underside. Fluid (i.e., urine) passes through the upper quilted layer and is absorbed and dispersed by the viscose rayon, leaving the quilted surface dry to the touch. This absorbent sheet helps maintain skin integrity; it does not stick to the skin when wet, decreases the risk of bedsores, and reduces odor.

Maintaining Normal Voiding Habits

Prescribed medical therapies often interfere with a client's normal voiding habits. When a client's urinary elimination pattern is adequate, the nurse helps the client adhere to normal voiding habits as much as possible (Box 4–7).

Promoting Urination

Nursing measures to promote urination include placing the client in normal voiding position and providing for privacy. Additional measures include running water, placing the client's hands in warm water, pouring warm water over the perineum, and taking a warm sitz bath.

In acute urinary retention, catheterization may be necessary to relieve bladder distention and prevent hydronephrosis. Use a relatively small catheter (16 French for a man, 14 French for a woman). A coudé-tipped catheter is passed more easily in the older man with an enlarged prostate. Using 2% lidocaine gel (10 mL injected into the male urethra, or 6 mL injected into the female urethra) reduces discomfort during catheterization and the risk of catheter-associated infection, and it promotes pelvic muscle relaxation (Bardsley, 2005). Carefully observe the client as the distended bladder drains. See the following Practice Alert feature for additional information.

PRACTICE ALERT

Some clients may experience a vasovagal response, becoming pale, sweaty, and hypotensive if the bladder is rapidly drained. Draining urine in 500-mL increments and clamping the catheter for 5–10 minutes between increments may prevent this response. Hematuria, the presence of blood in the urine, also may occur with rapid bladder decompression. Promptly notify the physician if hematuria develops.

Home care for the client with urinary retention varies depending on the cause. Some clients may be taught intermittent self-catheterization. Nurses should instruct all clients who have experienced urinary retention to avoid over-the-counter drugs that affect micturition, especially those with an anticholinergic effect (allergy and cold medications, many nonprescription sleep aids). Other home care measures include double-voiding (urinate, remain on the toilet for 2–5 min, and then urinate again); scheduled voiding; or when other measures fail, an indwelling catheter. When an indwelling catheter is necessary, teach the client and family to use clean technique when changing from an overnight bag to a leg bag, and to report promptly any signs of UTI to the primary care provider.

Box 4–7 Maintaining Normal Voiding Habits

POSITIONING

- Assist the client to a normal position for voiding: standing for male clients; for female clients, squatting or leaning slightly forward when sitting. These positions enhance movement of urine through the tract by gravity.
- If the client is unable to ambulate to the lavatory, use a bedside commode for females and a urinal for males standing at the bedside.
- If necessary, encourage the client to push over the pubic area with the hands or to lean forward to increase intra-abdominal pressure and external pressure on the bladder.

RELAXATION

- Provide privacy for the client. Many people cannot void in the presence of another person.
- Allow the client sufficient time to void.
- Suggest the client read or listen to music.
- Provide sensory stimuli that may help the client relax. Pour warm water over the perineum of a female or have the client sit in a warm bath to promote muscle relaxation. Applying a hot water bottle to the lower abdomen of both men and women may also foster muscle relaxation.
- Turn on running water within hearing distance of the client to stimulate the voiding reflex and to mask the sound of voiding for people who find this embarrassing.

- Provide ordered analgesics and emotional support to relieve physical and emotional discomfort to decrease muscle tension.

TIMING

- Assist clients who have the urge to void immediately. Delays only increase the difficulty in starting to void, and the desire to void may pass.
- Offer toileting assistance to the client at usual times of voiding, for example, on awakening, before or after meals, and at bedtime.

FOR CLIENTS WHO ARE CONFINED TO BED

- Warm the bedpan. A cold bedpan may prompt contraction of the perineal muscles and inhibit voiding.
- Elevate the head of the client's bed to Fowler's position, place a small pillow or rolled towel at the small of the back to increase physical support and comfort, and have the client flex the hips and knees. This position simulates the normal voiding position as closely as possible.

Source: Berman, A., Snyder, S. J., Kozier, B., & Erb, G. (2008). *Kozier & Erb's fundamentals of nursing: Concepts, process, and practice* (8th ed., p. 1299). Upper Saddle River, NJ: Pearson Education.

NURSING CARE PLAN Urinary Elimination

ASSESSMENT DATA

Nursing Assessment

Mr. John Baker is a 68-year-old shopkeeper who is admitted to the hospital with urinary retention, hematuria, and fever. The admitting nurse gathers the following information when taking a nursing history: Mr. Baker states he has noticed urinary frequency during the day for the past 2 weeks and that he doesn't feel he has emptied his bladder after urinating. He also has to get up two or three times during the night to urinate. During the past few days, he has had difficulty starting urination and dribbles afterward. He verbalizes the embarrassment his urinary problems cause in his dealings with the public. Mr. Baker is concerned about the cause of this urinary problem. He is diagnosed with BPH and is referred to a urologist who suggests a transurethral resection of the prostate (TURP) in several months. He is placed on antibiotic therapy.

Physical examination

Height: 185.4 cm (6'2")
Weight: 85.7 kg (189 lb)
Temperature: 38.1°C (100.6°F)
Pulse: 88 beats/min
Respirations: 20 breaths/min
Blood pressure: 146/86 mmHg

Catheterization for urinary retention yielded 300 mL of amber urine, Foley left in place for 2 days

Diagnostic data

CBC normal; urinalysis: amber, clear, pH 6.5, specific gravity 1.025, negative for glucose, protein, ketone, RBCs, and bacteria; IVP: evidence of enlarged prostate gland

NURSING DIAGNOSIS

Impaired Urinary Elimination (retention and overflow incontinence) related to bladder neck obstruction by enlarged prostate gland (as evidenced by dysuria, frequency, nocturia, dribbling, hesitancy, and bladder distention)

DESIRED OUTCOMES

Urinary Continence [0502] as evidenced by the following:
- Able to start and stop stream
- Empties bladder completely

Knowledge: Treatment Regimen [1813] as evidenced by substantial
- description of self-care responsibilities for ongoing care.
- description of self-monitoring techniques.

NURSING INTERVENTIONS/SELECTED ACTIVITIES

Urinary Incontinence Care [0610]

NURSING INTERVENTIONS/SELECTED ACTIVITIES	RATIONALE
Monitor urinary elimination, including consistency, odor, volume, and color.	These parameters help determine adequacy of urinary tract function.
Help the client select appropriate incontinence garment or pad for short-term management while more definitive treatment is designed.	Appropriate undergarments can help diminish the embarrassing aspects of urinary incontinence.
Instruct Mr. Baker to limit fluids for 2–3 hours before bedtime.	Decreased fluid intake several hours before bedtime will decrease the incidence of urinary retention and overflow incontinence, and promote rest.
Instruct Mr. Baker to drink a minimum of 1,500 mL (six 8-oz glasses) fluids per day.	Increased fluids during the day will increase urinary output and discourage bacterial growth.
Limit ingestion of bladder irritants (e.g., colas, coffee, tea, chocolate).	Alcohol, coffee, and tea have a natural diuretic effect and are bladder irritants.

Urinary Retention Care [0620]

Instruct Mr. Baker or a family member to measure and record urinary output.	This serves as an indicator of urinary tract and renal function and of fluid balance.
Catheterize for residual urine as appropriate.	An enlarged prostate compresses the urethra so that urine is retained. Checking for residual urine provides information about bladder emptying.
Implement intermittent catheterization as appropriate.	This helps to maintain tonicity of the bladder muscle by preventing overdistention and providing for complete emptying.

NURSING CARE PLAN Urinary Elimination (continued)

Provide enough time for bladder emptying (10 minutes).	*In addition to the effect of an enlarged prostate on the bladder, stress or anxiety can inhibit relaxation of the urinary sphincter. Sufficient time should be allowed for micturition.*
Instruct the client in ways to avoid constipation or stool impaction.	*Impacted stool may place pressure on the bladder outlet, causing urinary retention.*

Teaching: Disease Process [5602]

Appraise Mr. Baker's current level of knowledge about BPH.	*Assessing the client's knowledge will provide a foundation for building a teaching plan based on his present understanding of his condition.*
Explain the pathophysiology of the disease and how it relates to urinary anatomy and function.	*In this case, urinary retention and overflow incontinence are caused by obstruction of the bladder neck by an enlarged prostate gland.*
Describe the rationale behind management, therapy, and treatment recommendations.	*Adequate information about treatment options is important to diminish anxiety, promote compliance, and enhance decision making.*
Instruct Mr. Baker on which signs and symptoms to report to the health care provider (e.g., burning on urination, hematuria, oliguria).	*In the individual with prostatic hypertrophy, urinary retention and an overdistended bladder reduce blood flow to the bladder wall, making it more susceptible to infection from bacterial growth. Monitoring for these manifestations of UTI is essential to prevent urosepsis.*

EVALUATION

Outcomes partially met. Following removal of the Foley catheter, Mr. Baker reported continued difficulty initiating a urinary stream but experienced less dribbling and nocturia. He and his wife selected an undergarment that was acceptable to Mr. Baker, and he reports that he feels more confident. Intermittent catheterization is not indicated. Intake is approximately 200 mL in excess of output. He is able to discuss the correlation between his enlarged prostate and urinary difficulties. A TURP is scheduled in 2 weeks.

The NOC numbers for desired outcomes and the NIC numbers for nursing interventions are listed in brackets following the appropriate outcome or intervention. Outcomes, interventions, and activities selected are only a sample of those suggested by NOC and NIC and should be further individualized for each client.

APPLYING CRITICAL THINKING

1. Considering Mr. Baker's history and assessment data, what other physical conditions could explain his symptoms?
2. The primary care provider has recommended surgery. What assumptions will the nurse need to validate in helping to prepare Mr. and Mrs. Baker for this surgery?
3. It does not appear that other alternatives have been considered. Why might this be so?
4. Incontinence can lead to client decisions to limit social interactions. What would be an appropriate response if Mr. Baker states that he will just stay home until he has his surgery?

Source: Berman, A., Snyder, S. J., Kozier, B., & Erb, G. (2008). *Kozier & Erb's fundamentals of nursing: Concepts, process, and practice* (8th ed., pp. 1316–1317). Upper Saddle River, NJ: Pearson Education.

Assisting With Toileting

Clients who are weakened by a disease process or impaired physically may require assistance with toileting. The nurse should assist these clients to the bathroom and remain with them if they are at risk for falling. The bathroom should contain an easily accessible call signal to summon help if needed. Clients also must be encouraged to use handrails placed near the toilet. For clients who are unable to use bathroom facilities, provide urinary equipment close to the bedside (e.g., urinal, bedpan, or commode) and the necessary assistance to use them.

Coping With Social Isolation

Urinary incontinence increases the risk for social isolation because of embarrassment, fear of not having ready access to a bathroom, body odor, or other factors. In turn, social isolation can increase problems of incontinence because normal cues and relationships are lost and the need to remain dry becomes less of a concern. To assist clients in the area of social isolation, the nurse should do the following:

- Assess for reasons and extent of social isolation. Verify the degree of social isolation with the client or significant other. Do not assume that social isolation is related only to urinary incontinence. Other problems frequently associated with aging (e.g., a hearing deficit) may be primary or contributing factors.

- Refer the client for urologic examination and incontinence evaluation. Clients who assume that urinary incontinence is a normal part of the aging process may not be aware of treatment options.
- Explore alternative coping strategies with the client, significant other, staff, and other health care team members. Protective pads or shields, good perineal hygiene, scheduled voiding, and clothing that does not interfere with toileting can enhance continence.

Community-Based Care

Because urinary incontinence is a contributing factor to the institutionalization of many older people, client and family teaching can have a significant impact on a client maintaining independence and residence in the community. Address possible causes of incontinence and appropriate treatment measures. Refer for urologic examination if one has not already completed. Discuss fluid intake management, perineal care, and products for clothing protection.

Evaluation

Using the overall goals and desired outcomes identified in the planning stage, the nurse collects data to evaluate the effectiveness of nursing activities. The Nursing Care Plan feature on urinary elimination lists examples of desired outcomes for the identified goals.

If the desired outcomes are not achieved, the nurse should explore the reasons before modifying the care plan. For example, the following are examples of questions that must be considered if the outcome "Remains dry between voidings and at night" is not met:

- What is the client's perception of the problem?
- Does the client understand and comply with the health care instructions provided?
- Is access to toilet facilities a problem?
- Can the client manipulate clothing for toileting? Are there adjustments that can be made to allow easier disrobing?
- Are scheduled toileting times appropriate?
- Is there adequate lighting for nighttime toileting?
- Are mobility aids (e.g., walker, elevated toilet seat, or grab bar) needed? If these aids are currently used, are they appropriate or adequate? If assistance from a family member or caregiver is needed, is that available and appropriate?
- Is the client performing pelvic floor muscle exercises appropriately as scheduled?
- Is the client's fluid intake adequate? Does the timing of fluid intake require adjustment (e.g., restricted after dinner)?
- Is the client restricting caffeine, citrus juice, carbonated beverages, and artificial sweetener intake?
- Is the client taking a diuretic? If so, when is the medication taken? Do the times require adjustment (e.g., taking second dose no later than 4 p.m.)?
- Should continence aids (e.g., a condom catheter or absorbent pads) be considered or used?

REVIEW Bladder: Incontinence and Retention

RELATE: LINK THE CONCEPTS

The nurse admits an 83-year-old client with medical diagnosis of congestive heart failure, chronic renal failure, and diabetes mellitus. While the nursing history is being taken, the client says she takes her diuretic in the morning and then spends the next few hours in the bathroom, because if she goes too far away, she ends up "wetting her pants" and then has to "clean up the mess." She says she gets so thirsty in the afternoon that she drinks several glasses of water but stops drinking fluids after 6 p.m. to avoid "wetting the bed." The client's skin turgor is poor, and assessment reveals possible dehydration.

Linking the concept of Fluids and Electrolytes with the concept of Elimination:

1. What recommendations and client teaching should the nurse provide this client to prevent further dehydration?
2. What lab values should the nurse review to confirm potential dehydration?
3. What questions should the nurse ask this client to assess for frequency and severity of urinary incontinence?
4. What nursing diagnosis would you choose for this client?

READY: GO TO COMPANION SKILLS MANUAL

1. Applying an external (condom) catheter
2. Inserting a retention or straight urinary catheter
3. Collecting a 24-hour urine specimen
4. Collecting a urine specimen from an infant

5. Teaching clients to test for urine ketone bodies
6. Recording intake and output
7. Using a bladder scanner
8. Providing catheter care
9. Removing a retention catheter
10. Irrigating the bladder using a closed or continuous irrigation system
11. Administering suprapubic catheter care
12. Obtaining urine specimens from an indwelling catheter system
13. Applying a urinary diversion pouch
14. Providing and terminating hemodialysis

REFLECT: CASE STUDY

Mr. Justin Gardner is a 26-year-old man who fractured his third thoracic vertebra when he fell while rock climbing. In preparation for transfer to a rehabilitation center, the doctor orders discontinuation of the client's indwelling urinary catheter and PRN straight catheterization to reduce urinary retention.

1. What assessment data will the nurse collect to determine the presence of urinary retention?
2. What signs and symptoms would the nurse recognize as indicative of the need for straight catheterization?
3. What nursing diagnosis would be appropriate for this client?
4. What client teaching will this client require, related to urinary retention, before discharge if he is to provide safe home care for himself?

4.2 BOWEL: INCONTINENCE, CONSTIPATION, AND IMPACTION

KEY TERMS

Constipation, *113*
Encopresis, *117*
Fecal impaction, *117*
Fecal incontinence, *118*
Ulcerative colitis, *114*

BASIS FOR SELECTION OF EXEMPLAR

Institute of Medicine (IOM)

Chronic Disease Managment

Standards of Nursing Practice

LEARNING OUTCOMES

After learning about this exemplar, you will be able to do the following:

1. Describe the pathophysiology and etiology of incontinence, constipation, and impaction.

2. Identify risk factors associated with incontinence, constipation, and impaction.

3. Illustrate the nursing process in providing culturally competent care across the life span for individuals with incontinence, constipation, and impaction.

4. Formulate priority nursing diagnoses appropriate for an individual with incontinence, constipation, and impaction.

5. Create a plan of care for an individual with incontinence, constipation, and impaction that includes family members and caregivers.

6. Assess expected outcomes for an individual with incontinence, constipation, and impaction.

7. Discuss therapies used in the collaborative care of an individual with incontinence, constipation, and impaction.

8. Employ evidence-based care (or prevention) for an individual with incontinence, constipation, impaction, clinical manifestations, direct and indirect causes.

OVERVIEW

Disorders of intestinal absorption and bowel elimination can affect not only functional elimination status but also other functional health patterns including, but not limited to, health perception and management, nutritional and metabolic, activity and exercise, self-perception and self-concept, and sexuality and reproductive health patterns. Bowel function can be affected by inflammations, infections, tumors, obstructions, or changes in structure.

Clients with intestinal disorders often face extensive diagnostic testing, surgery, and permanent changes in physical appearance and lifestyle. Nursing care is directed toward returning to or maintaining homeostasis, meeting the client's physiologic needs, providing emotional support, and educating the client to adapt to changes in lifestyle.

Few body functions respond as readily to internal and external influences as the process of defecation. Factors affecting the gastrointestinal tract directly, such as food intake and bacterial population, affect the number and consistency of stools. Indirect factors, such as psychologic stress or voluntary postponement of defecation, also affect elimination. It is important to evaluate each client's bowel elimination against his or her own normal pattern.

CONSTIPATION

Constipation may be defined as fewer than three bowel movements per week or difficult passage of stools. This infers either the passage of dry, hard stool or the passage of no stool. It occurs when the movement of feces through the large intestine is slow, allowing time for additional reabsorption of fluid from the large intestine. Difficult evacuation of stool and increased effort or straining of the voluntary muscles of defecation are associated with constipation. The individual also may have a feeling of incomplete stool evacuation after defecation. Careful

assessment of a client's habits is necessary before a diagnosis of constipation is made. Box 4–8 lists the frequent defining characteristics of constipation.

Constipation affects older adults more frequently than younger people. Recent studies indicate that approximately 20–35% of people older than 65 years report recurrent constipation and laxative use. Although fecal transit in the large intestine slows with aging, the increased incidence of constipation in older adults is thought to relate more to impaired general health status, increased medication use, and decreased physical activity.

The loss of teeth makes chewing and swallowing food difficult. Ill-fitting, broken, or lost dentures also alter nutritional status. Periodontal disease with subsequent loss of natural teeth is one such factor, because the accompanying inability to chew foods results in a diet of soft, nonfibrous foods. Lack of fresh fruits and vegetables or other sources of bulk or fiber contributes to the pattern of constipation. The older adult may self-limit daily fluid intake, especially water, to decrease frequency of urination, unintentionally increasing the potential for constipation.

Box 4–8 Sample Defining Characteristics of Constipation

- Decreased frequency of defecation
- Hard, dry, formed stools
- Straining at stool; painful defecation
- Reports of rectal fullness or pressure or of incomplete bowel evacuation
- Abdominal pain, cramps, or distention
- Diminished appetite, nausea
- Headache

Source: Berman, A., Snyder, S. J., Kozier, B., & Erb, G. (2008). *Kozier & Erb's fundamentals of nursing: Concepts, process, and practice* (8th ed., p. 1328). Upper Saddle River, NJ: Pearson Education.

Constipation is a common complaint of pregnant women. In pregnancy, mechanical pressure from the growing uterus contributes to displacement of the small intestine and reduces motility. The increased secretion of progesterone further reduces motility because of decreased gastric tone and increased smooth muscle relaxation; thus, the emptying time of the stomach and bowel is prolonged. Hemorrhoids (swollen and inflamed veins in the anus and rectum) frequently develop in late pregnancy from constipation and from pressure on vessels below the level of the uterus, causing the pregnant woman further discomfort.

Risk Factors

Many causes and factors contribute to constipation, including the following:

- Insufficient fiber intake
- Insufficient fluid intake
- Insufficient activity or immobility
- Irregular defecation habits
- Change in daily routine
- Lack of privacy
- Chronic use of laxatives or enemas
- Irritable bowel syndrome
- Pelvic floor dysfunction or muscle damage
- Poor motility or slow transit
- Neurologic conditions (e.g., Parkinson's disease), stroke, or paralysis
- Emotional disturbances (e.g., depression or mental confusion)
- Medications (e.g., opioids, iron supplements, antihistamines, antacids, and antidepressants)

Constipation itself can cause health problems for some clients. In children, it often is associated with a UTI. Straining associated with constipation often is accompanied by holding the breath, and this can present serious problems for people with heart disease, brain injuries, or respiratory disease: Holding one's breath while bearing down increases intrathoracic pressure and vagal tone, slowing the pulse rate (LeMone & Burke, 2008).

Pathophysiology

Constipation may be a primary problem or a manifestation of another disease or condition. Acute constipation, a definite change in the bowel elimination pattern, often is caused by an organic process. A change in bowel patterns that persists or becomes more frequent or severe may be caused by a tumor or other partial bowel obstruction. With chronic constipation, functional causes that impair storage, transport, and evacuation mechanisms impede the normal passage of stools.

Psychogenic factors are the most common causes of chronic constipation. These factors include postponing defecation when the urge is felt and the perception of satisfaction with defecation. Clients often use laxatives and enemas to stimulate a bowel movement when constipation is perceived. Overuse of these measures can lead to real intestinal problems which further aggravate the condition. For example, cathartic colon (impaired colonic motility and changes in bowel structure) mimics **ulcerative colitis** (a disease that causes sores in the lining of the rectum and colon) in that the normal pouch-like or saccular appearance of the colon is lost. Melanosis coli is a brownish-black discoloration of the colon mucosa. Both cathartic colon and melanosis coli may be caused by long-term laxative use. Table 4–8 lists selected causes of constipation.

Clinical Manifestations and Therapies

The manifestations of constipation include having bowel movements less often than the usual pattern, frequent flatus, abdominal discomfort, diminished appetite, straining to have a bowel movement, and the passage of hard, dry stools.

With significant constipation or long-term dependence on laxatives or enemas, fecal impaction may develop. Impaction may also occur after barium administration for radiologic examination. Fecal impaction is felt as a rock-hard or putty-like mass of feces in the rectum. Abdominal cramping and a full sensation in the rectal area may be manifestations of impaction. Watery mucus or foul-smelling liquid stool may be passed around the impaction, causing the client to complain of diarrhea.

Manifestations of constipation that may appear on examination include an abdomen that may appear somewhat distended

---

TABLE 4–8 Selected Causes of Constipation

FACTOR	RELATED CAUSE
Activity	Lack of exercise; bed rest
Dietary	Highly refined, low-fiber foods; inadequate fluid intake
Drugs	Antacids containing aluminum or calcium salts; narcotic analgesics; anticholinergic agents; many antidepressants, tranquilizers, and sedatives; antihypertensive agents, such as ganglionic blockers, calcium-channel blockers, beta-adrenergic blockers, and diuretics; iron salts
Large bowel	Diverticular disease, inflammatory disease, tumor, obstruction; changes in rectal or anal structure or function
Psychogenic	Voluntary suppression of urge; perceived need to defecate on schedule; depression
Systemic	Advanced age; pregnancy; neurologic conditions (e.g., trauma, multiple sclerosis, tumors, cerebrovascular accident, parkinsonism); endocrine and metabolic disorders (e.g., hypothyroidism, hypercalcemia, uremia, porphyria)
Other	Chronic laxative or enema use

Source: LeMone, P., & Burke, K. (2008). *Medical-surgical nursing: Critical thinking in client care* (4th ed., p. 758). Upper Saddle River, NJ: Pearson Education.

as well as reduced bowel sounds. If an impaction is present, digital examination of the rectum reveals a palpable, hard or putty-like fecal mass.

Simple or chronic constipation is treated with education (a daily bowel movement is not necessary for health), modification of diet, and exercise routines. If the problem is acute or does not resolve, further diagnostic examination may be ordered. This may include a barium enema to identify bowel structure, tumors, or diverticula. If the problem is acute, a sigmoidoscopy or colonoscopy may be used for evaluation and biopsy. For more information, see Box 4–9.

MEDICATIONS Laxative and cathartic preparations are used to promote stool evacuation. Milder preparations generally are known as laxatives; those known as cathartics have a stronger effect. Most laxatives are appropriate only for short-term use. Cathartics and enemas interfere with normal bowel reflexes and should not be used for simple constipation. Laxatives should never be given if an intestinal obstruction, abdominal pain, fecal impaction, rectal fissures, ulcerated hemorrhoids, Crohn's disease, ulcerative colitis, or chronic inflammatory bowel disease are suspected (Peate, 2003). When the bowel is obstructed, laxatives or cathartics may cause serious mechanical damage and perforate the bowel.

The only laxatives that are appropriate and safe for long-term use are bulking agents, such as psyllium seed, calcium polycarbophil, and methylcellulose. These agents act by increasing the bulk of the feces and drawing water into the bowel to soften it.

Pharmacologic management of severe constipation usually occurs in two stages. The first stage involves softening the stool with medications such as lactulose, and the second stage involves evacuation of stool with a laxative. The evacuation phase is the most difficult for the client and for caregivers who may be managing the constipation of a child or older adult (Clayden & Keshtgar, 2003).

Once a stool softener has been administered, the most effective means to evacuate the stool while causing the least amount of stress and anxiety to the client is considered. Suppositories and enemas can cause fear in children. Polyethylene glycol electrolyte solution (GoLYTELY) can be administered orally or instilled via a nasogastric tube to promote stool evacuation (Biggs & Dery, 2006). More recently, electrolyte-free polyethylene glycol (MiraLAX) has been used

effectively (Kinservik & Friedhoff, 2004). Once the stool has been evacuated, a routine stimulant laxative is given to prevent reaccumulation of stool in the bowel. The stimulant laxative of choice usually is Senokot or Bisacodyl (Biggs & Dery, 2006).

NUTRITION Foods are recommended for clients experiencing constipation. Vegetable fiber is largely indigestible and cannot be absorbed, so it increases stool bulk. Fiber also helps to draw water into the fecal mass, softening the stool and making defecation easier. Raw fruits and vegetables are good sources of dietary fiber, as is cereal bran. Use two to three teaspoons of unprocessed bran with meals (sprinkled on fruit or cereal), or up to one-quarter cup daily, to supply adequate fiber.

Fluids also are important to maintain bowel motility and soft stools. The client should drink six to eight glasses of fluid per day. It is important to advise the client to increase fluid intake when dietary fiber is initially increased to decrease flatus and help maintain softer stools.

ENEMAS Significant or chronic constipation or fecal impaction may require administration of an enema. As a general rule, enemas should be used only in acute situations and only on a short-term basis. They also may be ordered to prepare the bowel for diagnostic testing or examination.

DEVELOPMENTAL CONSIDERATIONS Constipation is a common complaint in the pediatric population and accounts for approximately 25% of referrals made to pediatric gastroenterologists (Coughlin, 2003). Because defecation patterns vary among children, identification of an abnormal pattern is sometimes difficult. Infants usually have several bowel movements a day. Breast-fed infants may have bowel movements as frequently as every feeding or just one bowel movement every several days. Because of differences in fat digestion and absorption, bottle-fed infants are more prone to hard stools (Coughlin, 2003). For a young child, one bowel movement a day may be normal. As the child grows, however, three to four bowel movements a week may be a normal pattern. Constipation is characterized by "pebble-like, hard stools for a majority of bowel movements for at least 2 weeks, firm stools ≤2 times per week for at least 2 weeks, and no evidence of structural, endocrine, or metabolic disease" (Lembo & Camilleri, 2003). Constipation in children can be influenced by a variety of factors. Refer to Table 4–9 for further information.

Box 4–9 **Constipation and the Older Adult**

Constipation and perceived constipation are common problems in older adults. Although constipation is not a normal consequence of aging, factors such as slowed peristalsis, lowered activity levels, reduced food and fluid intake, and decreased sensory perception contribute to the higher incidence of constipation seen in older adults. Chronic diseases such as diabetes, mobility problems, and medications also increase the risk of constipation in older adults.

Cultural influences and advertising lead many older adults to believe that a daily bowel movement is important for health. This belief contributes to an increased incidence of perceived constipation in older adults. Because of this perception, the older adult may come to rely on laxatives, suppositories, or enemas to facilitate regular bowel movements. These external aids to defecation can further impair the ability to maintain "normal" bowel habits (a movement of soft stool every 2–3 days).

Source: LeMone, P., & Burke, K. (2008). Medical-surgical nursing: Critical thinking in client care (4th ed., p. 761). Upper Saddle River, NJ: Pearson Education.

TABLE 4–9 Influential Factors In Childhood Constipation

PHYSICAL FACTORS IN INFANCY	PHYSICAL FACTORS IN CHILDREN	PSYCHOLOGICAL FACTORS IN CHILDREN
Familial stool patterns High milk and low fiber intake Cow's milk allergy	Hypertrophied rectum Residual stool blockage (fecalith) Overflow fecal soiling around a solid stool	Embarrassment/shame related to soiling resulting from early or coercive toilet training, or lack of privacy
Hard stools	Poor rectal sensation	Fear of pain from hard stool
Dehydration Perianal group A streptococcal infection Medications (e.g., diuretics) and analgesia	Diseases that influence gastrointestinal or neurologic systems (e.g., celiac disease, cerebral palsy)	Being too busy to use the bathroom Parental blame/anger related to soiling and toileting refusal
Intestinal or anal conditions (e.g., Hirschsprung disease), cystic fibrosis, anorectal malformations		Teasing and bullying related to incontinence Decreased mobility/activity

Source: Adapted from Clayden, G., & Keshtgar, A. S. (2003). Management of childhood constipation. *Postgraduate Medical Journal, 79,* 616–621. Used with permission.

Constipation during infancy is rare, and most often, it is caused by mismanagement of diet. The transition from formula to cow's milk may cause a transient constipation, because the bowel must adjust to the increased protein content of cow's milk.

Constipation occurs most frequently in toddlers and preschoolers. This increased incidence often is associated with learning to control body functions. Many children do not like the sensations of a bowel movement and may begin withholding stool, which accumulates in and dilates the rectum until the next urge to defecate. The increasingly hard and painful bowel movement reinforces the child's behavior, and a pattern develops (Clayden & Keshtgar, 2003). For information about constipation and stool toileting refusal, see Box 4–10.

Constipation in the school-age child and adolescent usually results in overflow fecal incontinence. Some children with constipation are discovered during their school years after being evaluated for recurrent UTIs or enuresis (Clayden & Keshtgar, 2003).

Constipation may occur as a result of limited time for toileting. Busy school-age children may delay toileting, and adolescents participating in sports or other extracurricular activities may have limited time for toileting. Children also may be hesitant to use an unfamiliar bathroom. Encouragement from parents and relaxation of bathroom privileges at school promote regularity and return of previous bowel patterns within a short time. Children and adolescents may need to get up earlier to have breakfast and time for toileting before going to school.

Constipation may follow surgery, especially in children who are immobilized, such as by traction or a body cast. Stool softeners and a diet high in fiber and fluids are given to prevent and treat constipation.

CLINICAL THERAPY Dietary management is the treatment of choice for constipation that has no underlying pathologic cause. Constipation in young infants usually can be corrected by increasing the amount of fluids or adding 2 ounces of pear or apple juice to daily intake. Increasing physical activity and fluid intake may be effective for some children.

Removing constipating foods (e.g., bananas, rice, and cheese) from the child's diet often reduces the constipation. Increasing the child's intake of high-fiber foods (whole-grain breads, raw fruits, and vegetables) and fluids also promotes bowel elimination. A single glycerin suppository or enema may be needed to remove hard stool, followed by dietary and fluid management.

BEHAVIOR MANAGEMENT Behavior modification may prove beneficial to managing constipation. For younger children, providing rewards for overcoming the fear of toilets or for toileting at routinely scheduled times can be effective. Older children also respond to rewards (Clayden & Keshtgar, 2003). These rewards can be simple items, such as an afternoon spent with the parent playing a game. For children with psychological issues, child and family psychotherapy may be necessary. In these cases, the family is referred to a child and family counselor.

Box 4–10 Bowel Elimination and STR

A recent study was conducted to determine whether constipation and painful bowel elimination occur as a result of or before stool toileting refusal (STR). In this prospective longitudinal study of toilet training, 380 children between the ages of 17 and 19 months were followed (Blum, Taubman, & Nemeth, 2004). Researchers found that when hard or painful bowel movements or painful bowel elimination were associated with STR, the first episode of constipation generally occurred before the STR (Blum et al., 2004). This suggests that constipation is a chronic problem for many children and that it is not being treated effectively. Thus, painful bowel elimination associated with hard bowel movements contribute to, rather than result from, STR (Blum et al., 2004).

Source: Ball, J. W., Bindler, R. M. W., & Cowen, K. J. (2010). *Child health nursing: Partnering with children and families* (2nd ed.). Upper Saddle River, NJ: Pearson Education.

> ### ALTERNATIVE THERAPIES Herbal Laxatives
>
> Herbal laxatives are used by some cultures as complementary therapies. The safety and effectiveness of many of these laxatives have not been established in children. Psyllium, for example, has been approved for use as an ingredient in bulk-forming laxatives, but no studies have evaluated its safety or effectiveness in treating constipation in children. Cascara sagrada and senna are stimulant laxatives that have been approved by the U.S. Food and Drug Administration for use in children older than 2 years to treat constipation. Stimulant laxatives should be used with caution in children, however, because they can lead to dependency as well as to abdominal pain. Senna also has been associated with skin problems in children, including diaper rash and blistering (Gardiner & Kemper, 2005).
>
> *Source:* Ball, J. W., Bindler, R. M. W., & Cowen, K. J. (2010). *Child health nursing: Partnering with children and families* (2nd ed.). Upper Saddle River, NJ: Pearson Education.

ENCOPRESIS

Encopresis is an abnormal elimination pattern characterized by recurrent soiling or passage of stool at inappropriate times by a child who should have achieved bowel continence. Encopresis is reported to occur in 55% of boys and 35% of girls with constipation (Biggs & Dery, 2006). Children with primary encopresis have never achieved bowel control. Children with secondary encopresis have had bowel continence for several months.

Encopresis usually is associated with voluntary or involuntary retention of stool in the lower bowel and rectum. This leads to constipation, dilation of the lower bowel, and incompetence of the inner sphincter. The retention of stool usually is a result of being "too busy"—the child puts off going to the bathroom because activities are occurring and leaving would be an inconvenience. The retention of stool leads to constipation that is untreated and chronic. Loose stool leaks around the hard feces, and the child becomes unaware of a need to eliminate. Soiling may occur during the day or night. Bowel movements are irregular, painful, small, and hard. The child may be ridiculed by peers because of his or her offensive body odor. This rejection leads to withdrawal and behavioral problems, often resulting in altered school performance and attendance. The child continues to hold stool because the passage has become painful. Parents commonly seek health care, believing that the child has diarrhea or constipation.

The underlying constipation that leads to encopresis may be caused by the stress of environmental changes (e.g., birth of a sibling, moving to a new house, attending a new school), issues of anger and control related to bowel training, diet, a full schedule of activities, or a genetic predisposition.

A thorough history, physical examination, and diagnostic studies (possibly including barium enema) are necessary to rule out organic causes and anatomic abnormalities. Examination of mental health and cognitive functioning may be indicated. Information about the child's toilet-training habits and parents' attitudes concerning those habits is obtained. A dietary history, including eating habits and types of foods eaten, often is helpful as well. Physical examination sometimes reveals a nontender mass in the lower abdomen.

Treatment may include behavior modification techniques, dietary changes, use of lubricants to clear the bowel of impacted stool and encourage normal defecation, and psychotherapy. Behavior modification programs that reward and reinforce appropriate toileting habits can be successful. Dietary changes include incorporating high-fiber foods, such as fruits, vegetables, and whole-grain cereals, into the diet. Limiting intake of refined and highly processed foods and dairy products also may be helpful. Drugs, such as mineral oil, bulk-forming laxatives, and stool softeners, are used temporarily to empty the bowel. The child should sit on the toilet for several minutes after the morning and evening meals. It takes several months for the bowel to be retrained to respond to sphincter stimulation. Psychotherapy involving the child and family may be indicated in instances of dysfunctional parent–child relationships.

Nursing Management

Prevention of encopresis is the nursing goal. Nurses should partner with parents to teach toilet-training techniques, emphasizing the child's developmental readiness. Encourage parents to praise the child for successes and to avoid punishment and power struggles. Encourage high-fiber diets and regular times for elimination.

Nursing care centers on educating the child and parents about the disorder and its treatment and on providing emotional support. Explain the treatment plan, including dietary changes and use of laxatives or stool softeners. Reassure the child that he or she has a healthy body and, with treatment, will achieve normal functioning. Nurses should monitor the child for at least 6 months to be certain new patterns become established.

FECAL IMPACTION

Fecal impaction is a mass or collection of hardened feces in the folds of the rectum. Impaction results from prolonged retention and accumulation of fecal material. In severe impactions, the feces accumulate and extend well up into the sigmoid colon and beyond. Fecal impaction can be recognized by the passage of liquid fecal seepage (diarrhea) without normal stool, as the liquid portion of the feces seeps out around the impacted mass. Impaction also can be assessed by digital examination of the rectum, during which the hardened mass often can be palpated.

Along with fecal seepage and constipation, symptoms include rectal pain and a frequent but nonproductive desire to defecate. A generalized feeling of illness results: The client becomes anorexic, the abdomen becomes distended, and nausea and vomiting may occur.

The causes of fecal impaction usually are poor defecation habits and constipation. Barium used in radiologic examinations of the upper and lower gastrointestinal tracts also can be a causative factor. After these examinations, laxatives or enemas usually are taken to ensure removal of the barium.

Digital examination of the impaction through the rectum should be done gently and carefully. Although digital rectal examination is within the scope of nursing practice, some agency policies require a primary care provider's order for digital manipulation and removal of a fecal impaction.

Although fecal impaction generally can be prevented, treatment of impacted feces sometimes is necessary. When fecal impaction is suspected, the client often is given an oil retention enema, a cleansing enema 2–4 hours later, and daily additional cleansing enemas, suppositories, or stool softeners. If these measures fail, manual removal may be necessary.

FECAL INCONTINENCE

Fecal incontinence, also called bowel incontinence, refers to the loss of voluntary ability to control fecal and gaseous discharges through the anal sphincter. It occurs less frequently than urinary incontinence but is no less distressing to the client. The incontinence may occur at specific times, such as after meals, or it may occur irregularly. Two types of bowel incontinence are described: partial and major. Partial incontinence is the inability to control flatus or to prevent minor soiling. Major incontinence is the inability to control feces of normal consistency.

Fecal incontinence generally is associated with impaired functioning of the anal sphincter or its nerve supply, such as in some neuromuscular diseases, spinal cord trauma, and tumors of the external anal sphincter muscle. Multiple factors contribute to fecal incontinence, including both physiologic and psychologic conditions (Box 4–11). Bowel incontinence usually is considered to be a manifestation of a disorder rather than a disorder unto itself. Clients often do not reveal fecal incontinence in discussing health concerns. Little information is available about its incidence and prevalence. Because many of the etiologic factors are more prevalent in the older adult, older clients are more often affected (see Evidence-Based Practice feature).

The rate of fecal incontinence among older adults living in the community has been reported to be 4–17%, compared with 2% in the general community population and 20 to 54% in older nursing home residents (Bliss, Fischer, & Savik, 2005, p. 36). Fecal incontinence is an emotionally distressing problem that ultimately can lead to social isolation. Afflicted persons withdraw into their homes or, if in the hospital, the confines of their room to minimize the embarrassment associated with soiling.

Several surgical procedures are used for the treatment of fecal incontinence. These include repair of the sphincter and fecal diversion or colostomy.

Pathophysiology

The most common causes of fecal incontinence are those that interfere with either sensory or motor control of the rectum and anal sphincters. If the external sphincter is paralyzed as a result of spinal cord injury or disease, defecation occurs automatically when the internal sphincter relaxes with the defecation reflex. If sphincter muscles have been damaged or excessive pelvic floor relaxation has occurred, it may not be possible to override the defecation reflex with voluntary control.

Box 4–11 **Selected Causes of Fecal Incontinence**

NEUROLOGIC CAUSES
- Spinal cord injury or disease
- Head injury, stroke, or brain tumor
- Degenerative neurologic disease, such as multiple sclerosis, amyotrophic lateral sclerosis, dementia
- Diabetic neuropathy

LOCAL TRAUMA
- Obstetric tears
- Anorectal injury
- Anorectal surgery with sphincter damage

INFLAMMATORY PROCESSES
- Infection
- Radiation

OTHER PHYSIOLOGIC CAUSES
- Diarrhea
- Stool impaction
- Pelvic floor relaxation or loss of sphincter tone
- Tumors

PSYCHOLOGIC CAUSES
- Depression
- Confusion and disorientation

Source: LeMone, P., & Burke, K. (2008). *Medical-surgical nursing: Critical thinking in client care* (4th ed., p. 758). Upper Saddle River, NJ: Pearson Education.

Age-related changes in anal sphincter tone and response to rectal distention increase the risk for fecal incontinence in older adults. Resting and maximal anal sphincter pressures are decreased, particularly in older women. In addition, less rectal distension is needed to produce sustained relaxation of the anal sphincter in older women.

Clinical Manifestations and Therapies

The diagnosis of fecal incontinence includes client history and physical examination of the pelvic floor and anus to evaluate muscle tone and rule out a fecal impaction. Impaired sphincter muscles may be palpable on digital examination. Anorectal manometry or a rectal motility test may be used to evaluate the functional ability of the sphincter muscles. In this test, a small, flexible balloon catheter is introduced into the rectum, and pressures are measured in the rectum and internal and external sphincters. Normally, rectal dilation causes the internal sphincter to relax and the external sphincter to contract. Sigmoidoscopy also may be used to examine the rectum and anal canal.

Management of fecal incontinence is directed toward the identified cause. Medications to relieve diarrhea or constipation may be prescribed. A high-fiber diet, ample fluids, and regular exercise are helpful for many clients. Exercises to improve sphincter and pelvic floor muscle tone (Kegel exercises) may be of long-term benefit. Clients also may benefit from using loperamide before meals and prophylactically before running errands or leaving the house (Tierney et al., 2005). Biofeedback therapy may be used for mentally alert clients with intact sphincter muscles but low

EVIDENCE-BASED PRACTICE What Self-Care Practices Do Older Adults Use for Fecal Incontinence?

Researchers conducted the first systematic investigation of self-care for fecal incontinence (FI) among older adults living in the community. The purpose of the study was to describe the self-care practices used and to examine factors associated with the number of self-care practices and willingness to report FI to a health care practitioner. FI was described as accidental leakage of stool during the past 12 months. A 51-item survey was distributed at four HMO primary care clinics in the Midwest. The clinic staff offered surveys to individuals 65 years or older who lived in the community. More than 1,300 surveys were received, primarily from women.

The results indicated that the most common self-care practices for managing FI were changing diet (e.g., avoiding certain foods); wearing a sanitary panty liner, pad, or brief; and reducing activity or exercise. A significant difference was found in the number and types of self-care practices between men and women. Fifty-two percent of men, compared with 19% of women, did not use any self-care practices to manage FI. Only 43% of the respondents discussed their FI with a health care practitioner, with no significant difference between men and women. More of those who had a health problem or disability that caused FI or who were not sure about the cause of FI consulted with a health professional.

The study has some limitations in that it was based on self-report rather than a more rigorous method, such as observation. Also, the population included older adults who visited HMO clinics, and as a result, generalization for the population at large is limited.

The findings indicate that nurses who care for older adults living in the community must inquire routinely about FI. Discussing FI, and especially new-onset FI, with a client allows the health care practitioner to provide appropriate follow-up to ascertain if the FI is a symptom of a health problem. Some older adults believe that FI is a normal part of aging and therefore may minimize its significance. If the FI is not health related, the nurse needs to assess the self-care practices of the older adult and if those practices are effective. The authors also suggest future research be conducted to investigate the reasons for the differences between men and women regarding self-care practices for FI.

Source: Bliss, D., Fischer, L., & Savik, K. (2005). Managing fecal incontinence: self-care practices of older adults. *Journal of Gerontological Nursing,* Copyright © 2005 SLACK, Inc. Reprinted with permission.

---

muscle tone. With motivation and reinforcement, clients achieve improved sphincter control in response to a stimulus. The goal of biofeedback is to improve sensation, coordination, and strength of the sphincter muscle (Halverson, 2005).

When damage to the sphincter or rectal prolapse (protrusion of rectal mucous membrane through the anus) is the cause of fecal incontinence, surgical repair is the treatment of choice. Surgery also may be indicated when conservative measures have not been effective. Permanent colostomy (the creation of an opening from the large bowel on the abdominal wall) is a last-choice option for some clients, but it can control fecal output when other measures fail.

RISK FOR IMPAIRED SKIN INTEGRITY Good skin care is vital for the client with fecal incontinence. Stool contains enzymes and other irritating substances that promote skin breakdown when they are not promptly removed. This can lead to pressure ulcers, particularly when a neurologic disorder (e.g., spinal cord injury, dementia, or stroke) impairs mobility.

Good skin care includes the following:

- Clean the skin thoroughly with mild soap and water after each bowel movement. Toilet tissue may be more irritating to the skin and less effective in removing fecal material.
- Apply a skin barrier cream or ointment after each bowel movement. These help protect the skin from irritating substances in the feces.
- If incontinence pads or briefs are used, check frequently for soiling and change when feces is noted. Although these help to protect bedding and clothing from soiling, they can contribute to skin breakdown if they are not checked and changed frequently.

COMMUNITY-BASED CARE Managing fecal incontinence is a challenging problem for the client, family, and caregivers. For the client with intact cognition, it can be psychologically devastating. The client may become socially isolated from fear of odor or soiling clothing. The client's self-esteem may suffer from a sense of lost control over body functions and the inability to provide self-care. It is important to stress that incontinence is never normal (i.e., aging alone is not a cause of incontinence) and often is treatable. Encourage the client to seek medical evaluation of the problem.

Topics for client and family education include the following:

- Recommended dietary measures, such as consuming a high-fiber diet and ample fluids to maintain soft, formed stool or maintaining a low-residue diet to reduce the number of stools
- Suggestions for regular exercise to stimulate bowel peristalsis and regular evacuation
- Use of bulk-forming laxatives, such as psyllium seed (Metamucil), to provide stool bulk and reduce the number of small, liquid stools
- Prescribed medications (e.g., loperamide to reduce the number of stools), their appropriate use, and management of adverse effects (e.g., constipation)
- Bowel training program, including techniques for digital anal stimulation, inserting suppositories, or administering enemas as recommended (For digital anal simulation, teach the client to insert a lubricated, gloved finger through the anal sphincter into the rectum 1.5–2 in. while seated on the toilet or commode and then use a circular, side-to-side movement to gently stretch the rectal wall until the internal sphincter relaxes.)
- The importance of good skin care, particularly if neurologic impairment is present
- The potential benefits and associated risks of biofeedback and surgical treatment, if recommended
- Referrals for home care or community health services as indicated

NURSING PROCESS

Assessment

- *Health history.* The nurse and client discuss the extent, onset, and duration of incontinence; identified contributing factors; history of spinal cord or anorectal injury or surgery; chronic diseases, such as diabetes, multiple sclerosis, or other neurologic disorders; medications and use of alternative therapies; nutrition; and hydration patterns.
- *Physical examination.* The nurse palpates and assesses the abdomen for firmness or tenderness as well as for the presence of any mass (retained stool). Bowel sounds should be assessed. If a digital rectal examination is performed, the nurse assesses for the presence of stool in the rectum. The nurse also assesses for hemorrhoids, anal fissures, or other abnormalities of the abdomen or perineum.

Diagnoses

NANDA International (2007) includes the following diagnostic labels for fecal elimination problems:

- Bowel Incontinence
- Constipation
- Risk for Constipation
- Perceived Constipation
- Diarrhea

Clinical application of selected diagnoses is shown in Box 4–12 and at the end of the exemplar in the Nursing Care Plan.

Fecal elimination problems may affect many other areas of human functioning and, as a consequence, may be the etiology of other NANDA diagnoses. Examples include the following:

- Risk for Impaired Skin Integrity, related to
  a. bowel incontinence
  b. prolonged diarrhea
- Low Self-Esteem, related to
  a. fecal incontinence
  b. need for assistance with toileting
- Disturbed Body Image, related to bowel incontinence
- Deficient Knowledge (Bowel Training), related to lack of previous experience
- Anxiety, related to
  a. lack of control of fecal elimination
  b. response of others to fecal incontinence

Planning

The major goals for clients with fecal elimination problems include the following:

- Maintaining or restoring normal bowel elimination pattern
- Maintaining or regaining normal stool consistency
- Preventing associated risks, such as fluid and electrolyte imbalance, skin breakdown, abdominal distention, and pain

Implementation

Caring interventions include promoting regular defecation, digital removal of fecal impaction, bowel training programs, and use of a fecal incontinence pouch. The two Client

---

Box 4–12 **Clients With Fecal Elimination Problems**

Data Cluster: Mary Kuoko has had involuntary leakage of stool. She states her clothing is soiled several times a day, and says she is too embarrassed to go out with her friends because of the fecal odor. Her last bowel movement was more than 3 days ago. Digital examination reveals impaction.

Nursing diagnosis/ definition	Sample desired outcomes/ definition	Indicators	Selected interventions/ definition	Sample NIC activities
Bowel Incontinence: Change in normal bowel habits, characterized by involuntary passage of stool	Bowel Continence [0500]: *Control of passage of stool from the bowel*	Consistently demonstrated ■ Evacuates stool at least every 3 days ■ Responds to urge in a timely manner ■ Describes relationship of food intake to stool consistency	Bowel Management [0430]: *Establishment and maintenance of a regular pattern of bowel elimination* Bowel Incontinence Care [0410]: *Promotion of bowel continence and maintenance of perianal skin integrity*	■ Instruct on foods high in fiber as appropriate. ■ Give warm liquids after meals as appropriate. ■ Initiate a bowel training program as appropriate. ■ Wash perianal area with soap and water, and dry it thoroughly after each stool. ■ Monitor for adequate bowel evacuation. ■ Monitor diet and fluid requirements.

Note: The NOC numbers for desired outcomes and the NIC numbers for nursing interventions are listed in brackets following the appropriate outcome or intervention. The outcomes, indicators, interventions, and activities selected are only a sample of those suggested by NOC and NIC.

Source: Berman, A., Snyder, S. J., Kozier, B., & Erb, G. (2008). *Kozier & Erb's fundamentals of nursing: Concepts, process, and practice* (8th ed., p. 1335). Upper Saddle River, NJ: Pearson Education.

Teaching features also address aspects of fecal elimination and healthy defecation.

Promoting Regular Defecation

The nurse can help clients to achieve regular defecation by attending to (a) the provision of privacy, (b) timing, (c) nutrition and fluids, (d) exercise, and (e) positioning.

PRIVACY Privacy during defecation is extremely important to most people. The nurse should provide as much privacy as possible for such clients but may need to stay with those who are too weak to be left alone. Some clients also prefer to wipe, wash, and dry themselves after defecating. A nurse may need to provide water, a washcloth, and a towel for this purpose.

TIMING A client should be encouraged to defecate when the urge is recognized. To establish regular bowel elimination, the client and nurse can discuss when mass peristalsis normally occurs and provide time for defecation. Many people have well-established routines. Other activities, such as bathing and ambulating, should not interfere with the defecation time.

NUTRITION AND FLUIDS The diet a client needs for regular, normal elimination varies depending on the kind of feces the client currently has, the frequency of defecation, and the types of foods that the client finds assist with normal defecation.

For constipation, increase the daily fluid intake, and instruct the client to drink hot liquids and fruit juices, especially prune juice. Include fiber in the diet—that is, foods such as raw fruit, bran products, and whole-grain cereals and bread.

For flatulence, limit carbonated beverages, the use of drinking straws, and chewing gum—all of which increase the ingestion of air. Gas-forming foods, such as cabbage, beans, onions, and cauliflower, should be avoided as well.

EXERCISE Regular exercise helps clients to develop a regular defecation pattern. A client with weak abdominal and pelvic muscles, which impede normal defecation, may be able to strengthen them with the following isometric exercises:
- In a supine position, the client tightens the abdominal muscles as though pulling them inward, holding them for about 10 seconds and then relaxing them. This should be repeated 5–10 times each session and four times a day, depending on the client's health.
- Again in a supine position, the client can contract the thigh muscles and hold them contracted for about 10 seconds, repeating the exercise 5–10 times each session and four times a day. This helps the client confined to bed gain strength in the thigh muscles, thereby making it easier to use a bedpan.

POSITIONING Although the squatting position best facilitates defecation, the best position on a toilet seat for most people seems to be leaning forward.

For clients who have difficulty sitting down and getting up from the toilet, an elevated toilet seat can be attached to a regular toilet. Clients then do not have to lower themselves as far onto the seat or lift themselves as far off the seat. Elevated toilet seats can be purchased for use in the home.

CLIENT TEACHING Fecal Elimination

FACILITATING TOILETING
To facilitate successful client toileting, nurses should do the following:
- Ensure safe and easy access to the toilet. Make sure lighting is appropriate, scatter rugs are removed or securely fastened, and so on.
- Facilitate instruction as needed about transfer techniques.
- Suggest ways that garments can be adjusted to make disrobing easier for toileting (e.g., Velcro closing on clothing).

MONITORING BOWEL ELIMINATION PATTERN
- Nurses should instruct the client, if appropriate, to keep a record of time and frequency of stool passage, any associated pain, and color and consistency of the stool.

DIETARY ALTERATIONS
- Nurses should provide clients with information about required food and fluid alterations to promote defecation or manage diarrhea.

MEDICATIONS
- Medications should be discussed with the client at each health care interaction. Discussions should address problems associated with overuse of laxatives, if appropriate, and the use of alternatives to laxatives, suppositories, and enemas. Nurses also should discuss the addition of a fiber supplement if the client is taking a constipating medication.
- Discuss the addition of a fiber supplement if the client is taking a constipating medication.

MEASURES SPECIFIC TO ELIMINATION PROBLEM
- Nurses should provide instructions associated with specific elimination problems and treatment, including
  a. constipation,
  b. diarrhea, and
  c. ostomy care.

COMMUNITY AGENCIES AND OTHER SOURCES OF HELP
A number of agencies and resources are available to clients who need assistance. Nurses should be informed about what is available in their community and provide the following:
- Appropriate referrals to home care or community care for assistance with resources such as installation of grab bars and raised toilet seats, structural alterations for wheelchair access, homemaker or home health aide services to assist with activities of daily living, and enterostomal therapy nurse for assistance with stoma care and selection of ostomy appliances.
- Information about companies from which durable medical equipment (e.g., raised toilet seats, commodes, bedpans, and urinals) can be purchased, rented, or obtained free of charge and supplies (e.g., incontinence pads or ostomy irrigating supplies and appliances) can be obtained.
- Additional sources of information and help, such as ostomy self-help and support groups or clubs.

Source: Berman, A., Snyder, S. J., Kozier, B., & Erb, G. (2008). *Kozier & Erb's fundamentals of nursing: Concepts, process, and practice* (8th ed., p. 1336). Upper Saddle River, NJ: Pearson Education.

CLIENT TEACHING Healthy Defecation

SOME TEACHING POINTS FOR HEALTHY DEFECATION

- Establish a regular exercise regimen.
- Include high-fiber foods, such as vegetables, fruits, and whole grains, in the diet.
- Maintain fluid intake of 2,000–3,000 mL a day.
- Do not ignore the urge to defecate.
- Allow time to defecate, preferably at the same time each day.
- Avoid over-the-counter medications to treat constipation and diarrhea.

Source: Berman, A., Snyder, S. J., Kozier, B., & Erb, G. (2008). *Kozier & Erb's fundamentals of nursing: Concepts, process, and practice* (8th ed., p. 1337). Upper Saddle River, NJ: Pearson Education.

An enema is a solution introduced into the rectum and large intestine. The action of an enema is to distend the intestine and, sometimes, to irritate the intestinal mucosa, increasing peristalsis and the excretion of feces and flatus.

Digital Removal of a Fecal Impaction

Digital removal involves breaking up the fecal mass with a finger in the rectum and then removing the mass in portions. Because the bowel mucosa can be injured during this procedure, some agencies restrict and specify the personnel who are permitted to conduct digital disimpaction. Rectal stimulation also is contraindicated for some people because it may cause an excessive vagal response, resulting in cardiac arrhythmia. Before disimpaction is performed, an oil retention enema should be given and held for 30 minutes. After a disimpaction, the nurse can use various interventions to remove any remaining feces, such as a cleansing enema or insertion of a suppository.

Because manual removal of an impaction can be painful, the nurse may use, if the agency permits, 1–2 mL of lidocaine (Xylocaine) gel on a gloved finger inserted into the anal canal as far as the nurse can reach. The lidocaine will anesthetize the anal canal and rectum and should be inserted 5 minutes before the disimpaction.

Digital removal of a fecal impaction is performed as follows:

1. If indicated, obtain assistance from a second person who can comfort the client during the procedure.
2. Ask the client to assume a left-side-lying position with the knees flexed and the back toward the nurse.
3. Place a bed pad under the client's buttocks and a bedpan nearby to receive stool.
4. Drape the client for comfort and to avoid unnecessary exposure of the body.
5. Put on a pair of clean gloves, and liberally lubricate the index finger to be inserted.
6. Gently insert the index finger into the rectum, and move the finger along the length of the rectum.
7. Loosen and dislodge stool by gently massaging around it. Break up stool by working the finger into the hardened mass, taking care to avoid injury to the mucosa of the rectum.

8. Carefully work stool downward to the end of the rectum and remove it in small pieces. Continue to remove as much fecal material as possible. Periodically assess the client for signs of fatigue, such as facial pallor, diaphoresis, or change in pulse rate. Manual stimulation should be minimal.
9. Following disimpaction, assist the client to clean the anal area and buttocks. Then, assist the client onto a bedpan or commode for a short time, because digital stimulation of the rectum often induces the urge to defecate.

Bowel Training Programs

For clients who have chronic constipation, frequent impactions, or fecal incontinence, bowel training programs may be helpful. The program is based on factors within the client's control and is designed to help the client establish normal defecation. Such matters as food and fluid intake, exercise, and defecation habits are all considered. Before beginning such a program, clients must understand it and want to be involved. The major phases of the program are as follows:

- Determine the client's usual bowel habits and factors that help and hinder normal defecation.
- Design a plan with the client that includes the following:
  a. Fluid intake of approximately 2,500–3,000 mL per day
  b. Increase in fiber in the diet
  c. Intake of hot drinks, especially just before the usual defecation time
  d. Increase in exercise
- Maintain the following daily routine for 2–3 weeks:
  a. To stimulate peristalsis, administer a cathartic suppository (e.g., Dulcolax) 30 minutes before the client's defecation time to stimulate peristalsis.
  b. When the client experiences the urge to defecate, assist the client to the toilet or commode or onto a bedpan. Note the length of time between the insertion of the suppository and the urge to defecate.
  c. Provide the client with privacy for defecation and a time limit (30–40 minutes usually is sufficient).
  d. Teach the client to lean forward at the hips, to apply pressure on the abdomen with the hands, and to bear down for defecation. These measures increase pressure on the colon. Straining should be avoided because it can cause hemorrhoids.
- Provide positive feedback when the client successfully defecates. Refrain from negative feedback if the client fails to defecate.
- Offer encouragement to the client, and convey that patience often is required. Many clients require weeks or months of training to achieve success.

PRACTICE ALERT

Provide room odor control with deodorizer tablets, sprays, or other devices. Controlling odor is important to preserve the client's self-esteem.

NURSING CARE PLAN   Altered Bowel Elimination

ASSESSMENT DATA	NURSING DIAGNOSIS	DESIRED OUTCOMES
Nursing Assessment Mrs. Emma Brown is a 78-year-old who has been a widow for 9 months. She lives alone in a low-income housing complex for older adults. Her two children live with their families approximately 150 miles away. She has always enjoyed cooking for her family; however, now that she is alone, she does not cook for herself. As a result, she has developed irregular eating patterns and tends to prepare soup-and-toast meals. She gets little exercise and has had bouts of insomnia since her husband's death. For the past month, Mrs. Brown has been having a problem with constipation. She states she has a bowel movement about every 3–4 days and that her stools are hard and painful to excrete. Mrs. Brown decides to attend the health fair sponsored by the housing complex and seeks assistance from the county public health nurse. **Physical Examination** Height: 162 cm (5′4″) Weight: 65 kg (143 lb) Temperature: 36.2°C (97.2°F) Pulse: 82 beats/min Respirations: 20 breaths/min Blood pressure: 128/74 mmHg Active bowel sounds, abdomen slightly distended **Diagnostic Data** CBC: Hgb 10.8 Urinalysis negative	Constipation related to low-fiber diet and inactivity (as evidenced by infrequent, hard stools; painful defecation; abdominal distention)	Bowel Elimination [0501], as evidenced by the following: ■ Comfort of stool passage ■ Soft and formed stool ■ Passage of stool without aids

NURSING INTERVENTIONS/SELECTED ACTIVITIES	RATIONALE
Constipation/Impaction Management [0450]	
Identify factors (e.g., medications, bed rest, diet) that may cause or contribute to constipation.	*Assessing causative factors is an essential first step in teaching and planning for improved bowel elimination.*
Encourage increased fluid intake unless contraindicated.	*Sufficient fluid intake is necessary for the bowel to absorb sufficient amounts of liquid to promote proper stool consistency.*
Evaluate medication profile for gastrointestinal side effects.	*Constipation is a common side effect of many drugs including narcotics and antacids.*
Teach Mrs. Brown how to keep a food diary.	*An appraisal of food intake will help identify if Mrs. Brown is eating a well-balanced diet and consuming adequate amounts of fluid and fiber. Excessive meat or refined food intake will produce small, hard stools.*
Instruct Mrs. Brown on a high-fiber diet as appropriate.	*Fiber absorbs water, which adds bulk and softness to the stool and speeds up passage through the intestines.*
Instruct her on the relationship of diet, exercise, and fluid intake to constipation and impaction.	*Fiber without adequate fluid can aggravate, not facilitate, bowel function.*
Exercise Promotion [0200]	
Encourage verbalization of feelings about exercise or need for exercise.	*Perceptions of the need for exercise may be influenced by misconceptions, cultural and social beliefs, fears, or age.*
Determine her motivation to begin/continue an exercise program.	*Individuals who have been successful in an exercise program can assist Mrs. Brown by providing incentive and enhancing motivation. For example, a walking partner may be beneficial.*
Inform Mrs. Brown about the health benefits and physiologic effects of exercise.	*Activity influences bowel elimination by improving muscle tone and stimulating peristalsis.*

(continued)

NURSING CARE PLAN   Altered Bowel Elimination (continued)

In collaboration with a primary care provider, instruct her about appropriate types of exercise for her level of health.	*Any individual beginning an exercise program should consult a primary care provider (essentially for a cardiac evaluation). Mrs. Brown's age and lack of activity should be considered in planning the level of activity.*
Assist Mrs. Brown in setting short-term and long-term goals for the exercise program.	*Realistic goal setting provides direction and motivation.*

EVALUATION

Outcome not met. Mrs. Brown has kept a food diary and is able to identify the need for more fluid and fiber but has not consistently included fiber in her diet. She has started a walking program with a neighbor but is able to walk for only 10 minutes at a time twice a week. She states her last bowel movement was 3 days ago.

The NOC numbers for desired outcomes and the NIC numbers for nursing interventions are listed in brackets following the appropriate outcome or intervention. Outcomes, interventions, and activities selected are only a sample of those suggested by NOC and NIC and should be further individualized for each client.

APPLYING CRITICAL THINKING

1. You learn that Mrs. Brown's stools have been liquid, in very small amounts, and occurring at infrequent intervals, generally when she feels the urge to defecate. What additional data are important to obtain from her?
2. What nursing intervention is most appropriate before making suggestions to correct or prevent the problem Mrs. Brown is experiencing?
3. What suggestions can you give Mrs. Brown about maintaining a regular bowel pattern?
4. Explain why cathartics and laxatives generally are contraindicated for people in Mrs. Brown's situation.

Source: Berman, A., Snyder, S. J., Kozier, B., & Erb, G. (2008). *Kozier & Erb's fundamentals of nursing: Concepts, process, and practice* (8th ed., pp. 1350–1351). Upper Saddle River, NJ: Pearson Education.

Fecal Incontinence Pouch

To collect and contain large volumes of liquid feces, the nurse may place a fecal incontinence collector pouch around the anal area. The purpose of the pouch is to prevent progressive perianal skin irritation and breakdown as well as frequent linen changes necessitated by incontinence. In many agencies, the pouch is replacing the more traditional approach of inserting a large Foley catheter into the client's rectum and inflating the balloon to keep it in place—a practice that may damage the rectal sphincter and rectal mucosa. A rectal catheter also increases peristalsis and incontinence by stimulating sensory nerve fibers in the rectum.

A fecal collector is secured around the anal opening and may or may not be attached to drainage. Pouches are best applied before the perianal skin becomes excoriated. If perianal skin excoriation is present, the nurse either (a) applies a dimethicone-based moisture-barrier cream or alcohol-free barrier film to the skin to protect it from feces until it heals and then applies the pouch or (b) applies a skin barrier or hydrocolloid barrier underneath the pouch to achieve the best possible seal.

Nursing responsibilities for clients with a rectal pouch include (a) regular assessment and documentation of the perianal skin status, (b) changing the bag every 72 hours or sooner if leakage occurs, (c) maintaining the drainage system, and (d) providing explanations and support to the client and support people.

Some clients (e.g., those who are quadriplegic or paraplegic, or after trauma or stroke) may be treated for fecal incontinence by surgical repair of a damaged sphincter or an artificial bowel sphincter. The artificial sphincter consists of three parts: a cuff around the anal canal, a pressure-regulating balloon, and a pump that inflates the cuff. The cuff is inflated to close the sphincter, maintaining continence. To have a bowel movement, the client deflates the cuff. The cuff automatically reinflates in 10 minutes. Management of this device usually is specific to the model being used; contact the manufacturing company for details. Administering enemas and rectal medications may be harmful with this device in place.

Evaluation

The goals established during the planning phase are evaluated according to specific desired outcomes that are also established during that phase. Examples of these were shown previously in Box 4–12. Other examples are shown in the Nursing Care Plan feature for this exemplar.

If the desired outcomes are not achieved, the nurse should explore the reasons. The nurse might consider some or all of the following questions:

- Were the client's fluid intake and diet appropriate?
- Was the client's activity level appropriate?
- Are prescribed medications or other factors affecting the gastrointestinal function?
- Do the client and family understand the provided instructions well enough to comply with the required therapy?
- Were sufficient physical support and emotional support provided?

COLLABORATION

Collaboration for the client with bowel elimination issues frequently will involve a nutritionist who can help support the client making any needed changes in diet or dietary patterns. Nurses also may want to consult with the client's pharmacist, who may be able to provide additional information regarding medications and supplements being taken and any related side

effects. Physical therapists may offer important points on exercise within the client's range of motion that can promote bowel health and management. Nurses working with children who have problems with bowel elimination should encourage parents to work with teachers and school dieticians to support the child in improving dietary habits that support healthy bowel elimination.

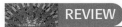 **REVIEW** **Bowel: Incontinence, Constipation, and Impaction**

RELATE: **LINK THE CONCEPTS**

Linking the concepts of Mobility, Intracranial Regulation, and Metabolism with the concept of Elimination:

1. What impact does the concept of mobility have on elimination?
2. When caring for a client with deficient fluid volume secondary to mannitol administration to lower intracranial pressure, what special precautions must the nurse implement related to bowel elimination?
3. When caring for a client with a slow metabolic rate secondary to inadequate thyroid hormone production, what impact would the nurse anticipate for the client's bowel elimination pattern?

READY: **GO TO COMPANION SKILLS MANUAL**

1. Collecting a stool specimen for ova and parasites or culture
2. Collecting an infant stool specimen
3. Testing the stool for occult blood
4. Teaching parents to test for pinworms
5. Providing assistive digital evacuation
6. Providing digital stimulation
7. Developing a regular bowel routine

8. Administering a suppository
9. Implementing the Zassi bowel management system
10. Administering an enema (large-volume, pediatric, small-volume, retention, return flow)
11. Applying a fecal ostomy pouch

REFLECT: **CASE STUDY**

Mr. Justin Gardner is a 26-year-old man who fractured his third thoracic vertebrae when he fell while rock climbing. The client is incontinent of feces secondary to sensory loss and the inability to feel the need to defecate.

1. Is there anything that can be implemented to return bowel continence to this client? Explain your answer.
2. What skin care precautions will the nurse implement to maintain skin integrity?
3. What nursing diagnosis would be appropriate for this client?
4. What client teaching will this client require, related to bowel continence, before discharge if he is to provide effective home care for himself?

REFERENCES

Bailey, J. L., & Sands, J. M. (2003). Renal disease. In W. R. Hazzard, J. P. Blass, J. B. Halter, J. G. Ouslander, & M. E. Tinetti (Eds.), Principles of geriatric medicine and gerontology (5th ed., pp. 551–568). New York: McGraw-Hill.

Bardsley, A. (2005). Use of lubricant gels in urinary catheterization. Nursing Standard, 20(8), 41–46.

Biggs, W. S., & Dery W. H. (2006). Evaluation and treatment of constipation in infants and children. American Family Physician, 73(3), 469–477.

Bliss, D. Z., Fischer, L., & Savik, K. (2005). Managing fecal incontinence: Self-care practices of older adults. Journal of Gerontological Nursing, 31(7), 35–44.

Blum, J., Taubman, B., & Nemeth, N. (2004). During toilet training, constipation occurs before stool toileting refusal. Pediatrics, 113, 1791–1792.

Clayden, G., & Keshtgar, A. S. (2003). Management of childhood constipation. Postgraduate Medical Journal, 79, 616–621.

Coughlin, E. C. (2003). Assessment and management of pediatric constipation in primary care. Pediatric Nursing, 29, 296–302.

Cunningham, F. G., Leveno, K. J., Bloom, S. L., Hauth, J. C., Gilstrap III, L. C., & Wenstrom, K. D. (2005). Williams obstetrics (22nd ed.). New York: McGraw-Hill.

D'Amico, D., & Barbarito, C. (2007). Health & physical assessment in nursing. Upper Saddle River, NJ: Pearson Education.

Esposito, C., Plati, A., Mazzullo, T., Fasoli, G., De Mauri, A., Grosjean, D., et al. (2007). Renal function and functional reserve in healthy elderly individuals. Journal of Nephrology, 20, 617–625.

Gardiner, P., & Kemper, K. J. (2005). Which herbs and supplements spell relief? Contemporary Pediatrics, 22(8), 50–55.

Gray, M., McClain, R., Peruggia, M., Patrie, J., & Steers, W. D. (2001). A model for predicting motor urge urinary incontinence. Nursing Research, 50(2), 116–122.

Halverson, A. L. (2005). Nonoperative management of fecal incontinence. Clinics in Colon and Rectal Surgery, 16(1), 17–20.

Hinrichs, M., & Huseboe, J. (2001). Research-based protocol: Management of constipation. Journal of Gerontological Nursing, 27(2), 17–28.

Huether, S., & McCance, K. (2005). Understanding pathophysiology. St. Louis, MO: Mosby.

Kinservik, M. A., & Friedhoff, M. M. (2004). The efficacy and safety of Polyethylene Glycol 3350 in the treatment of constipation in children. Pediatric Nursing, 30 (3), 232–237.

Lauver, D. R., Gross, J., Ruff, C., & Wells, T. J. (2004). Patient-centered interventions: Implications for incontinence. Nursing Research, 53(6S), S30–S35.

Lembo, A., & Camilleri, M. (2003). Chronic constipation. New England Journal of Medicine, 349, 1360.

LeMone, P., & Burke, K. (2008). Medical-surgical nursing: Critical thinking in client care (4th ed.). Upper Saddle River, NJ: Pearson Prentice Hall.

Mason, D. J., Newman, D. K., & Palmer, M. H. (2003). Changing UI practice. American Journal of Nursing, 103(3; Suppl.), 2–3.

Mauk, K. L. (2005). Preventing constipation in older adults. Nursing, 35(6), 22–23.

Moore, K. N., & Gray, M. (2004). Urinary incontinence in men. Nursing Research, 53(6S), S36–S41.

Moorhead, S., Johnson, M., & Maas, M. (2004). Nursing outcomes classification (NOC) (3rd ed.). St. Louis, MO: Mosby.

Morantz, C. A. (2005). ACOG guidelines on urinary incontinence in women. American Family Physician, 72(1), 175–178.

NANDA International. (2007). NANDA nursing diagnoses: Definitions and classification 2007–2008. Philadelphia: NANDA.

Nield, L. S., & Kamat, D. (2004). Enuresis: How to evaluate and treat. Clinical Pediatrics, 43(5), 409–415.

Ouslander, J. G., & Johnson, T. M. (2003). Incontinence. In W. R. Hazzard, J. P. Blass, J. B. Halter, J. G. Ouslander, & M. E. Tinetti (Eds.), Principles of geriatric medicine and gerontology (5th ed., pp. 1571–1586). New York: McGraw-Hill.

Palmer, M. H., & Newman, D. K. (2004). Urinary incontinence in nursing homes: Two studies show the inadequacy of care. American Journal of Nursing, 104(11), 57–59.

Palmer, M. H., & Newman, D. K. (2006). Bladder control: Educational needs of older adults. Journal of Gerontological Nursing, 32(1), 28–32.

Peate, I. (2003). Nursing role in the management of constipation: Use of laxatives. British Journal of Nursing, 12(19), 1130–1136.

Robson, W. L. M., Leung, A. K. C., & Van Howe, R. (2005). Primary and secondary nocturnal enuresis: Similarities in presentation. Pediatrics, 115, 956–959.

Shei Dei Yang, S., & Cheng Wang, C. (2005). Outpatient biofeedback relaxation of the pelvic floor in treating pediatric dysfunctional voiding: A short-course program is effective. Urologia Internationalis, 74(2), 118–122.

Teng, C. H., Huang, Y. H., Kuo, B. J., & Bih, L. I. (2005). Application of portable ultrasound scanners in the measurement of post-void residual urine. *Journal of Nursing Research, 13*(3), 216–223.

Thureen, P. J., Deacon, J., Hernandez, J., & Hall, D. M. (2005). *Assessment and care of the well newborn* (2nd ed.). St. Louis, MO: Elsevier Saunders.

Tierney, L. M., Jr., McPhee, S. J., & Papadakis, M. A. (Eds.). (2005). *Current medical diagnosis & treatment* (44th ed.). New York: McGraw-Hill.

Timiras, M. L., & Leary, J. (2007). The kidney, lower urinary tract, body fluids, and the prostate. In P. S. Timiras (Ed.), *Physiological basis of aging and geriatrics* (4th ed., pp. 297–313). New York: Informa Healthcare.

Timiras, M. L., & Luxenberg, J. S. (2007). Pharmacology and drug management in the elderly. In P. S. Timiras (Ed.), *Physiological basis of aging and geriatrics* (4th ed., pp. 355–361). New York: Informa Healthcare.

Wiggins, J. (2003). Changes in renal function. In W. R. Hazzard, J. P. Blass, J. B. Halter, J. G. Ouslander, & M. E. Tinetti (Eds.), *Principles of geriatric medicine and gerontology* (5th ed., pp. 543–549). New York: McGraw-Hill.

Family

5

Concept at-a-Glance

Concept Learning Outcomes

After reading about this concept, you will be able to do the following:

1. Describe the roles and functions of the family.
2. Outline the elements of the family system.
3. Describe characteristics of different types of families.
4. Identify the components of a family health assessment.
5. Identify four parenting styles and analyze their impact on child personality development.
6. Describe the effect of major family changes on children, including divorce, gaining a stepparent, being placed in foster care, and adoption.

Concept Key Terms

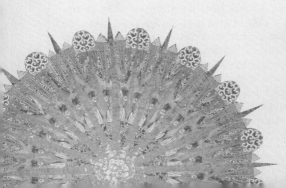

About Family

Do you ever find yourself sounding like your mother or father? Do you find yourself providing first aid for a minor problem at home and realize you are doing what you saw your grandparents do instead of what you learned in class? How big an influence does/did your family have on who you are today? If you suddenly became ill and needed to be admitted to the hospital, would your first call be to your family?

This concept will study the role of the family in development, childrearing, health promotion, and response to alterations in health status. Nurses assess and plan health care for three types of clients: the individual, the family, and the community. The beliefs and values of each person and the support he or she receives come, in large part, from the family and are reinforced by the community. Thus, an understanding of family dynamics and the context of the community assists the nurse in planning care. When a family is the client, the nurse determines the health status of the family and its individual members, the level of family functioning, family interaction patterns, and family strengths and weaknesses. ●

NORMAL PRESENTATION

The family is a basic unit of society. It consists of those individuals, male or female, youth or adult, legally or not legally related, genetically or not genetically related, whom the others consider to be their significant persons. The U.S. Bureau of the Census (2006) defines a **family** as individuals who are joined together by marriage, blood, adoption, or residence in the same household. More broadly, however, families are generally characterized by bonds of emotional closeness, sharing, and support. A family may be a self-identified group of two or more persons joined together by sharing resources and emotional closeness. Family members can also include "honorary relatives" of the family, whether or not they are related by blood, marriage, or adoption, or even living in the same household. The family as defined by its members is likely to be dynamic because membership changes over time. In today's world it is even more likely that extended family members will live in different cities, states, or even countries. So, there is no *typical* family.

Within families, members are guided by a common set of values that bind them together. These family values are greatly influenced by external factors including cultural background, social norms, education, environmental influences, and socioeconomic status, as well as beliefs held by peers, coworkers, political and community leaders, and other individuals outside the family unit. Because of the influence of these external factors, a family's values may change considerably over the years.

A family is generally understood to be a safe haven for its members as they learn group values, norms, and acceptable behaviors. However, child abuse and neglect is a significant problem and can occur within any family configuration.

Roles of the family include the following:

■ Caring, nurturing, and educating children; teaching children how to get along in the world
■ Maintaining the continuity of society by transmitting the family's knowledge, customs and traditions, values, and beliefs to children
■ Receiving and giving love
■ Preparing children to become productive members of society
■ Meeting the needs of its members, including protection and economic support
■ Serving as a buffer between its members and environmental and societal demands while advocating or addressing the interests and needs of the individual family members

Individual family members take on certain social and gender roles and hold a designated status within the family based on the values and beliefs that bind the family together. These values and beliefs may evolve from the family's religious or cultural values and practices, social norms, education, and other influences to which parents were exposed during childhood, adolescence, and early adult years. Parental roles, including childrearing practices and beliefs, are usually learned through a socialization process during childhood and adolescence.

Parents have important roles that involve childrearing and the long-term care of children until they reach adulthood. Depending on their other roles in society, parents work to nurture and rear children, helping them meet role expectations. Parents must also meet the needs of and provide economic support for the family. Children also learn specific roles through a socialization process. Parents set expectations of behavior with discipline and modeling of appropriate behavior.

Ideally, the family is a child's source of strength and support, the major constant in the child's life. Families are intimately involved in their children's physical and psychological well-being, and they play a vital role in the health promotion and health maintenance of their children. By respecting the family's role, strengths, and experiences with the health care system, nurses have an opportunity to develop an effective partnership with the child and family as they make health care decisions that promote the child's health. This partnership between nurses and families is known as **family-centered care**.

In the nursing profession, interest in the family unit and its impact on the health, values, and productivity of individual family members is expressed by **family-centered nursing**, nursing that considers the health of the family as a unit in addition to the health of individual family members.

Functions of the Family

The economic resources the family needs are secured by adult members. The family protects the physical health of its members by providing adequate nutrition and health care services. Family

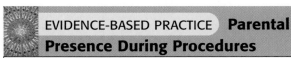

EVIDENCE-BASED PRACTICE Parental Presence During Procedures

Increasingly, parents are permitted to be present during medical procedures performed on their children. Previous resistance to parental presence has been based on the fear that parents would delay or interfere with the procedure, distract or increase the anxiety of the health professionals performing the procedure, or experience heightened anxiety of their own. Studies have investigated parental presence in various situations involving medical procedures such as anesthesia induction, intravenous (IV) starts, and resuscitation (Meyers, Eichhorn, & Guzzetta, 1998; Munro & D'Errico, 2000; Powers & Rubenstein, 1999). In most cases, parents are less anxious if they are able to be present when their child has a procedure, and the ability of health professionals to perform procedures is not affected (Lewandowski & Tesler, 2003; Sacchetti, Paston, & Carraccio, 2005).

nutritional and lifestyle practices directly affect the developing health attitudes and lifestyle practices of the children.

In addition to providing an environment conducive to physical growth and health, the family creates an atmosphere that influences the cognitive and the psychosocial growth of its members. Children and adults in healthy, functional families receive support, understanding, and encouragement as they progress through predictable developmental stages, as they move in or out of the family unit, and as they establish new family units. In families where members are physically and emotionally nurtured, individuals are encouraged to achieve their potential in the family unit. As individual needs are met, family members are able to reach out to others in the family, the community, and the larger society.

Families from different cultures are an integral part of North America's rich heritage. Each family has values and beliefs that are unique to its culture of origin and shape the family's structure, methods of interaction, health care practices, and coping mechanisms. These factors interact to influence the health of families. Families of a particular culture may cluster to form mutual support systems and to preserve their heritage; however, this practice may isolate them from the larger society (Figure 5–1 ■).

Although every family is unique, all families have certain structural and functional features in common. Family structure (family roles and relationships) and family function (interactions among family members and with the community) provide the following:

- *Interdependence:* The behaviors and level of development of individual family members constantly influence and are influenced by the behaviors and level of development of all other members of the family.

- *Maintaining boundaries:* The family creates boundaries that guide its members, providing a distinct and unique family culture. This culture, in turn, provides values.
- *Adapting to change:* The family changes as new members are added, current members leave, and the development of each member progresses.
- *Performing family tasks:* Essential tasks maintain the stability and continuity of the family. These tasks include physical maintenance of the home and the people in the home, the production and socialization of family members, and the maintenance of the psychological well-being of members.

Types of Families in Today's Society

Families consist of persons (structure) and their responsibilities within the family (roles). Governmental data are grouped by types of *households*: married couples with children, married couples without children, other family households (single-parent families), men living alone, women living alone, and other nonfamily households. Some families live in houses, some in apartments; some live in urban areas, some in rural towns, and some are homeless. Various types of families exist in contemporary American society.

NUCLEAR FAMILY   A family structure of parents and their offspring is known as the **nuclear family**. The nuclear family consists of a husband, a wife, and their shared biological children. Although the nuclear family was once the norm in the United States, it is no longer the most common type of family.

EXTENDED FAMILY   The relatives of nuclear families, such as grandparents or aunts and uncles, compose the **extended family**. In some families, members of the extended family live with the family. Although members of the extended family may live in different areas, they may be a source of emotional or financial support for the family. An extended family may share household and childrearing responsibilities with parents, siblings, or other relatives. According to the U.S. Bureau of the Census, 4.1 million children live in an extended family with at least one parent and usually a grandparent (U.S. Census Bureau, 2002). Grandparents may raise children because the parents are unable to care for them. Grandparents endure emotional, physical, and financial stresses when taking on the child-rearing role of one or more grandchildren.

EXTENDED-KIN NETWORK FAMILY   Another example of an extended family is the **extended-kin network family**. This is a specific form of an extended family in which two nuclear families of primary or unmarried kin live in close proximity to each other. The family shares a social support network, chores, goods, and services. This type of family model is common in the Latino community. Multigenerational arrangements of this sort are more common in non-U.S. cultures and working-class families.

TRADITIONAL FAMILY   The **traditional family** is viewed as an autonomous unit in which both parents reside in the home with their children, the mother often assuming the nurturing role and the father providing the necessary economic resources. In today's society both men and women are less bound to traditional role patterns. For example, fathers are

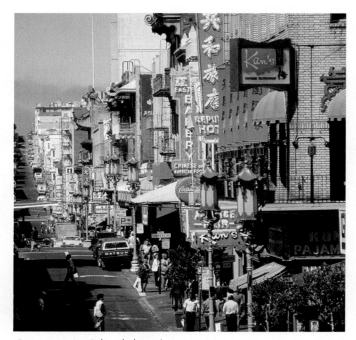

Figure 5–1 ■ Cultural clustering.

Courtesy of Morton Beebe/Corbis

more likely to be involved with the household chores, their children, and family life (Figure 5–2 ■). In 2004, the U.S. Bureau of the Census reported 26.5 million fathers in married-couple families, 98,000 of whom were stay-at-home fathers (caring for 336,000 children). This was the first time the number of stay-at-home parents was analyzed in the census. Of all the families with children, the percentage consisting of married couples decreased between 1980 and 1996 and has since remained constant at about 68% (Fields, 2003).

TWO-CAREER FAMILY   In **two-career families** (or dual-career families), both partners are employed by choice or by necessity. They may or may not have children. Two-career families have steadily increased since the 1960s because of increased career opportunities for women, a desire to increase the family's standard of living, and economic necessity. Today, two-thirds of all two-parent families are this type. Dual-career families have to address issues related to child care, household chores, and spending time together. The need to find good quality, affordable child care is one of the greatest stresses working parents face.

SINGLE-PARENT FAMILY   Of all types of households, about 9% (12 million) are **single-parent families** and the number continues to increase (Fields, 2003). Several reasons for the increasing rate of single-parent families are as follows (Friedman, Bowden, & Jones, 2003):
- High rates of divorce
- Large amount of financial aid available to one-parent families with dependent children
- Loss of stigma associated with unwed motherhood
- Growth in number of births to never-married mothers

Of these families, 10 million are headed by women and 2 million by men. In 2000, 26.7% of children under 18 years of age lived with a single parent, and almost 1 in 10 children lived with a

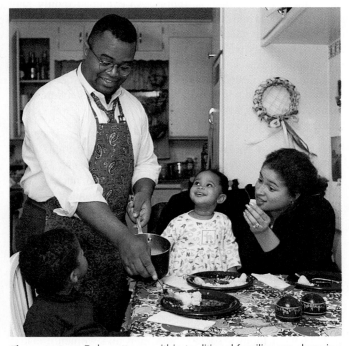

Figure 5–2 ■ Role patterns within traditional families are changing.

never-married parent (Lugaila & Overturf, 2004; U.S. Department of Health and Human Services, 2001). There are many reasons for single parenthood, including death of a spouse, separation, divorce, birth of a child to an unmarried woman (whether the pregnancy was planned), or adoption of a child by a single man or woman. The stresses of single parenthood are many: child care concerns, financial concerns, role overload and fatigue from managing daily tasks, and social isolation. Single-parent families often face difficulties because the sole parent may lack social and emotional support, need assistance with childrearing issues, or face financial strain. Single-parent families experience higher rates of poverty, which has important implications for the children (Denham, 2005). Depending on social support and family resources, the single parent may be stressed from working to support the family, maintaining household responsibilities, serving as both mother and father, and attempting to have a personal life. Single mothers are often at risk for poverty due to lack of child support, unequal pay for work performed, work skill deficiencies, and cutbacks in social welfare programs. An important nursing consideration for working with single parents is assessing their strengths and needs in providing care to the child, such as after-school and back-up child care arrangements that enable the parent to fulfill work commitments. Nurses working with a single-parent family should determine if the family has access to all resources available to support growth and development, such as school breakfast and lunch programs that provide nutritional support.

ADOLESCENT FAMILY   The birth rate among teenagers peaked in 1991 and has decreased progressively since then to 47.7 births per 1,000 women aged 15–19 in 2000 (Alan Guttmacher Institute, 2004). Rates are highest among Black teens, followed by Latina females, and then White women. These young parents are often developmentally, physically, emotionally, and financially ill prepared to undertake the responsibility of parenthood. Adolescent pregnancies frequently interrupt or stop formal education. Children born to adolescents are often at greater risk for health and social problems, and they have few role models to assist them in breaking out of the cycle of poverty.

FOSTER FAMILY   Children who can no longer live with their birth parents may require placement with a family that has agreed to include them temporarily. The legal agreement between the **foster family** and the court to care for the child includes the expectations of the foster parents and the financial compensation they will receive. A family (with or without its own children) may house more than one foster child at a time or different children over many years. Hopefully, at some time the fostered child can return to the birth parent(s) or be legally and permanently adopted by other parents.

CHILDLESS FAMILY   **Childless families** (also known as child-free families) are a growing trend. In some cases a family is child-free by choice; in other cases, a family is childless because of issues related to infertility or other medical conditions that present risks to the woman or fetus should the woman become pregnant.

STEPFAMILY   A **stepfamily** consists of a biologic parent with children and a new spouse who may or may not have children. This family structure has become increasingly common in the

United States because of high rates of divorce and remarriage. These families are also known as remarried, reconstituted, or blended families. There are no official statistics on the number of blended families, but a commonly accepted view is that about one of every three Americans is a member of a stepfamily.

Stepfamily models have both strengths and challenges. Stepfamilies may have fewer financial issues and may offer a child a new support person and role model. Remarriage also provides a new opportunity for a successful relationship for the parents; however, the relationship between stepparents and stepchildren can be strained. Stresses occur as blended families get acquainted with each other, respect differences, and establish new patterns of behavior. These stresses can include discipline issues, adjustment problems, role ambiguity, strain with the other biologic parent, and communication issues. When **blended families** with children form after the divorce or death of a parent, adjustment can be particularly challenged by the normal processes of grief and loss. Important nursing considerations include directing families to resources that may help reduce the potential conflicts associated with different parenting styles, discipline, and manipulative behaviors of children that can develop with the blended family.

PRACTICE ALERT

Children have the best emotional, behavioral, and educational outcomes when they live with two mutually committed parents who collaborate on childrearing and who have adequate social and financial resources (American Academy of Pediatrics Task Force on the Family, 2003).

BINUCLEAR FAMILY A **binuclear family** is a postdivorce family in which the biologic children are members of two nuclear households, both that of the father and that of the mother. The children alternate between the two homes. This is also called coparenting and involves joint custody. In **joint custody**, both parents have equal responsibility and legal rights, regardless of where the children live. The binuclear family model enables both parents to be involved. It is a model for effective communication. It enables both biological parents to be involved in a child's upbringing and provides additional support and role models from extended family members. Special nursing considerations in this family type involve ensuring that health promotion guidance and education for care of the child with an acute or chronic condition are communicated effectively to both biological parents.

INTRAGENERATIONAL FAMILY In some cultures, and as people live longer, more than two generations may live together. Children may continue to live with their parents even after having their own children, or the grandparents may move in with their grown children's families after some years of living apart. In other situations, a generation is skipped or missing; that is, grandparents live with and care for their grandchildren, but the children's parents are not a part of this family. Many life events and choices can lead to this type of family.

HETEROSEXUAL COHABITING FAMILY Cohabiting (or communal) families consist of unrelated individuals or families who live under one roof. This may include never-married individuals as well as divorced or widowed persons. According to the 2000 U.S. Census, approximately 2.9 million children under 18 years of age live with a parent and unmarried partner (Peterson, 2003). Biological children may result from the relationship, or in some cases children of one parent are present and help form a blended cohabitating family. Special concerns exist regarding the increased likelihood of the couple separating—approximately 50% in 5 years versus 20% for married couples (Peterson, 2003). Reasons for cohabiting may be a need for companionship, a desire to achieve a sense of family, testing a relationship or commitment, or sharing expenses and household management. Cohabiting families illustrate the flexibility and creativity of the family unit in adapting to individual challenges and changing societal needs. These families are less stable for the children because of the disruption associated with separation (American Academy of Pediatrics Task Force on the Family, 2003).

An important nursing consideration for children who live in informal cohabiting families is that the nonbiological parent has no legal authority to seek emergency medical care for the child. However, in the case of a true emergency that could result in loss of life or diminished functioning, health professionals are obligated to provide care and obtain consent as soon as possible afterwards. The nonbiological parent also may not have any knowledge of the child's medical history.

GAY AND LESBIAN FAMILIES Gay and lesbian families include those in which two or more people who share a same-sex orientation live together (with or without children), and those in which a gay or lesbian single parent rears a child. Children in these families may be from a previous heterosexual union, or be born to or adopted by one or both member(s) of the same-sex couple. For example, a biological child may be born to one of the partners through artificial insemination or through a surrogate mother. According to the 2000 U.S. Census, 96% of all U.S. counties have at least one gay or lesbian couple with children under 18 years in the household (Urban Institute, 2003). Small studies that have evaluated children reared by gay and lesbian couples found that the children show no significant differences from children reared in other types of families. Lesbian and gay couples function much like heterosexual couples, and children who are adopted or born into the family are highly valued. Children raised in gay and lesbian families may face unique issues in interacting with peers and in revealing their parents' sexual orientation. Homosexual adults form gay and lesbian families based on the same goals of caring and commitment seen in heterosexual relationships. In addition, the structure of gay and lesbian families is as diverse as that of heterosexual families—including stepfamilies and single-parent families. Children raised in these family units develop sex role orientations and behaviors similar to children in the general population. These children have been found to have the same advantages and expectations for health, adjustment, and development as children born into heterosexual families (American Academy of Pediatrics, 2002). Lesbian and gay parents are believed to be as effective as heterosexual couples in providing a supportive and healthy environment for their children (American Psychological Association, 2004).

> **PRACTICE ALERT**
> It is important to identify the biological or adoptive parent, or a caregiver's legal documentation proving the right to medical decision making, when obtaining consent for the child's health care.

Children in these families typically have only one biological or adoptive legal parent. The other partner is the coparent and has no legal parental status in the majority of states. Only seven states (California, Connecticut, Massachusetts, New Jersey, New York, Pennsylvania, Vermont) and the District of Columbia have considered legislative actions to ensure the security of children whose parents are gay or lesbian by guaranteeing access to the second parent of joint adoption rights (Urban Institute, 2003). Coparent adoption would help maintain the child's rights to a continuing relationship if the legal parent dies or becomes incapacitated, or if the parents separate. Either parent could then provide consent for health care and make other important decisions on behalf of the child. Financial support of the child also would be more assured if one parent dies or parents separate. Nursing considerations in this type of family involve respect for the relationship between partners and recognition of the nurturing capacity in these families.

Legal issues for same-sex couples are significant and constantly changing. Domestic partner policies extend the same rights and privileges to the partner of a nonmarried employee of the same or opposite gender as would be offered to spouses. California Family Code Section 297–297.5 defines domestic partners as "two adults who have chosen to share one another's lives in an intimate and committed relationship of mutual caring." Numerous state and federal laws have been introduced in the United States to allow or prohibit same-sex marriages or civil unions. It can be a challenge for the nurse to keep current on how such legislation affects health care issues such as insurance coverage and the right to consent for health care.

SINGLE ADULTS LIVING ALONE Individuals who live by themselves represent a significant portion of today's society. Of younger adults 18–34 years of age, about 10% live alone, with little variation between males and females. However, among adults 65 years and older, about 20% of men live alone, whereas about 40% of women live alone (Fields, 2003). Singles include young self-supporting adults who have recently left the nuclear family as well as older adults living alone. Young adults typically move in and out of living situations and may have membership in family, nonfamily household, and living alone categories at different times. Older adults may find themselves single through divorce, separation, or the death of a spouse, but generally remain living alone for the remainder of their lives.

Family Development Frameworks

Family development refers to the dynamics or changes that a family experiences over time, including changes in relationships, communication patterns, roles, and interactions. Although each family is unique, the members go through a set of fairly predictable changes. (See Box 5–1 for a new family dynamic.) For example, Duvall (1977) developed an eight-stage family life cycle that describes the developmental process each family encounters. This model is based on the nuclear family (Table 5–1). The oldest child serves as a marker for the family's developmental stages except in the last two stages, when children are no longer present. Couples with more than one child may find themselves in overlapping stages, with developmental advances occurring simultaneously. Other family development models have been developed to address the stages and developmental tasks facing the unattached young adult, the gay and lesbian family, those who divorce, and those who remarry.

FAMILY FUNCTIONING
Transition to Parenthood

Choosing to become a parent is a major life change for adults. From the time of a child's birth, the parents experience stresses and challenges along with feelings of pride and excitement.

Box 5–1 **The "Sandwich Generation"**

Adults who care for their own children and one or more of their own parents belong to a group that has come to be known as the "Sandwich Generation." This group of adults faces an incredible amount of stress trying to meet the diverse needs of young children and adolescents as well as aging parents. One of the chief sources of stress for these families is financial insecurity. A family with limited financial resources may face taking the aging parent into their own home or placing an aging parent who is no longer independent into a senior care facility that is below standard. If a family has very young children, taking an aging parent with dementia into the home can present either real or perceived hazards to the young children, increasing the stress level of the entire family. In addition, a member of the sandwich generation often faces additional stress addressing the elder parent's needs while still trying to get his or her own children off to school and to extracurricular activities and maintain his or her

own full-time job. End-of-life issues can be a great source of stress and conflict for these families.

A nurse who is assessing an adult who cares for both his or her own children and his or her aging parents may diagnose any one of several conditions including, but not limited to, the following: Ineffective Self Health Management, Sleep Deprivation or Disturbed Sleep Pattern, Risk for Situational Low Self-Esteem, Interrupted Family Processes, and Compromised Family Coping.

Critical Thinking
In small groups, discuss what assessment questions would be appropriate when working with a client who is a member of the "sandwich generation." Discuss what caring interventions might be appropriate, and what outcomes could be developed in collaboration with the client.

TABLE 5–1 The Eight-Stage Family Life Cycle

STAGE I	Beginning families	Marriage between partners, identification as partners, establishing goals for future, and interaction and building relationships with kin
STAGE II	Childbearing families	Birth of first child, new role as parents, integrating new family member into existing family
STAGE III	Families with preschool children	Establishing family network, socialization of children, reinforcing independence in children when separating from parents
STAGE IV	Families with school-age children	Facilitating peer relationships while maintaining family dynamics and adjusting to outside influences
STAGE V	Families with teenagers	Increase in children's independence and autonomy; parents' concerns shift to aging parents, careers, and marital relationship
STAGE VI	Families launching young adults	Readjustment of marital relationship; parents and children establish separate identities outside the family unit
STAGE VII	Middle-aged parents	Renewed marital relationship, new outside interests, fewer family responsibilities, new roles as grandparents and as in-laws, increased concern for aging parents, death, and disability of older generation
STAGE VIII	Retirement and old age	End of career, shift to retirement, maintain functioning during the aging process, maintain marital relationship, adjust to potential loss of spouse, friends, and siblings, prepare for eventual death

Source: Adapted from Duvall, Elizabeth M. *Marriage and family development* (5th ed.). Published by Allyn and Bacon, Boston, MA. Copyright © 1977 by Pearson Education. Adapted by permission of the publisher; and Friedman, M. M. (1998). *Family nursing: Research, theory, and practice* (4th ed., p. 113). Reprinted by permission of Pearson Education, Upper Saddle River, NJ.

Mothers and fathers both adjust their lifestyles to give priority to parenting. The baby is dependent for total care 24 hours a day, and this often results in sleep deprivation, irritability, less personal time, and less time for the couple's relationship. In addition, the family with a new baby often experiences a change in financial status.

Several factors influence how well the parents adjust to their new role. Social support provided to the mother, especially by the father, is important for the mother's adjustment. Marital happiness during pregnancy is an important factor for the adjustment of both parents. Infants with significant health conditions or those with difficult temperaments can cause parents extra stress and affect their adjustment to the parenting role.

With the birth of the first child, mothers and fathers both have challenges related to renegotiating their employment to accommodate family and child care time (Box 5–2). Fathers are sometimes additionally challenged to develop closeness with the infant and learn how to care for the infant, especially when they may not have had role models or any previous child care experience. Most parents find that caring for infants and children takes more time than anticipated.

Nurses can help parents through this important transition by listening to the challenges the parents describe during the infant's first health visits. Encourage fathers as well as mothers to attend and participate in health promotion visits with the health care provider. Answer questions and offer ideas to address described problems that the parents may be too tired to solve on their own. Help parents recognize that their frustrations and feelings regarding the challenges of infant care are normal. Encourage both parents to become active in caring for the infant and to gain comfort in that care. Help both parents find activities that they enjoy with regard to infant care that will encourage interaction and bonding with the infant.

Parental Influences on the Child

The qualities of family relationships and behaviors are important aspects of family strengths and functioning. Positive family relationships are characterized by parent–child warmth and supportiveness. Warm parent–child relationships can buffer children from stress and promote positive cognitive and social outcomes. Parents who are warm and place high demands on their children for appropriate behavior have children who tend to be content, self-reliant, self-controlled, and open to learning in school.

Mothers and fathers both contribute to the psychological, emotional, and social health and development of their children. Both parents provide affection, nurturing, and comfort. They teach children life skills and healthy lifestyles. Fathers play an important role in the sexual identity and gender role

Box 5–2 Medical and Family Leave Act

Eligible parents of newborns and adopted children are entitled to 12 weeks of unpaid leave during any 12-month period initially authorized under the federal Medical and Family Leave Act of 1993. Vacation or sick leave may be used to pay for time away from work, depending on the employer's leave policies. This act also applies if a child, spouse, or parent of the employee develops a serious health condition. The employee is entitled to return to the previous position or an equivalent position with all the same pay, benefits, and other conditions. The Act carries some additional conditions and requirements, including that employees are only eligible if they have worked for a covered employer for 1,250 hours over the previous 12 months. More information on the Act can be found at www.dol.gov.

Source: Family and Medical Leave, Public Law 103-3, February 5, 1999. 5 U.S.C. 6381–6387; 5 CFR part 630, subpart L. Adapted with permission.

development of both male and female children. Both mothers and fathers promote the social competence, academic achievement, and problem-solving abilities of their children (American Academy of Pediatrics, 2004).

Family Size

The size of the family influences the amount of attention children get. In small families parents often have more time to give attention to the children, encourage achievement, meet family expectations, and support involvement in community activities. Children in larger families are encouraged to be cooperative to support family functioning. The children usually receive less personal attention from the parents and often turn to others in the family for needed support. Family finances may be more limited. Children may adopt a specialized family role to gain recognition, such as the "responsible one," "the clown," or "the black sheep."

Sibling Relationships

Siblings are a child's first peers and often have a lifelong relationship. Siblings, especially those of the same gender or who are close in age, tend to have a closer relationship because they often share many common experiences through childhood and adolescence. In general, the parents have greater influence than siblings on children who are more widely spaced in age. However, the older sibling may be a very strong role model for younger siblings.

Sibling rivalry between children exists at times in all families. Within the family children learn to share, compete, and compromise with siblings. Some siblings take on roles such as protector, problem solver, friend, and supporter for dealing with issues in the family and in the environment. Some siblings learn to work well together to maintain privacy or to form a coalition for negotiating with the parents. An older sibling helps reinforce rules and roles in the family by prompting and inhibiting certain patterns of behavior in the younger siblings. However, one sibling may test the waters by breaking a previously implicit rule to determine what rule flexibility is allowed in the family.

Children develop different personalities because of a need to establish distinct identities for themselves and be seen as unique in the family. It has not been possible to reproduce earlier research findings that birth order was associated with specific personality traits of individual children in a family (Craig & Baucum, 2002). Siblings may share some experiences, but they are often exposed to different environmental experiences that help shape their personalities (Craig & Baucum, 2002). First-born children do have some advantages, such as more favorable treatment in the family. They tend to have slightly higher IQs and greater achievement in school and in their careers (Craig & Baucum, 2002). Their intellectual development may be enhanced through experiences of teaching their younger siblings.

PARENTING

The family is an important component in the lives of all children, and it plays an essential role in fostering the development of infants, children, and youth. A significant concept in families is that of parenting. **Parenting** is a leadership role in the family in which children are guided to learn acceptable behaviors, beliefs, morals, and rituals of the family and to become socially responsible, contributing members of society. The manner in which children are parented, in combination with their individual personality traits and characteristics, influences their developmental outcomes.

Parents have responsibility for providing children stability through nurturance, safety, and structure in a family that undergoes frequent changes over time. The child needs to have physical and emotional space to grow and develop. Parents also provide their children with the values, beliefs, rituals, and behaviors learned and transmitted across family generations.

To be successful, parents should implement reasonable, consistent **limit setting** (established rules or guidelines for behavior) on children's autonomy while the children are still learning values and self-control. At the same time, parents need to foster their children's curiosity, initiative, and sense of competence. Parents use different styles to parent their children. Parental warmth and control are two major factors that are important in children's development. Parental warmth refers to the amount of affection and approval displayed. Parental control refers to how restrictive the parents are regarding rules. See Table 5–2 for the characteristics associated with parental warmth and control.

Diana Baumrind (1971), an important contemporary child developmentalist, proposed classifications of parenting styles that are still well accepted today. She identified three main types of parenting styles—(*authoritarian, authoritative*, and *permissive*)—and described the influences each style has on children. One additional parenting style, called *indifferent*, exists in some families. While families will generally tend to use one style, they may vary their style for certain situations. See Table 5–3 for characteristics or parenting styles defined by level of warmth and control, and the associated child outcomes.

Authoritarian Parents

Authoritarian parents tend to be punitive and adhere to rigid rules, or to be more dictatorial. Parents who use this style might say, "Because I'm your parent, that's why," "A rule is a rule," or "Just do what I say." While this style sets firm limits, those limits or rules are not negotiable or open to any discussion. Parents expect family beliefs and principles to be accepted without question. Children have no opportunity to participate in the family decision-making process. Children with authoritarian parents do not develop the skills to examine why a certain behavior is desirable or how their actions might influence others.

Authoritative Parents

Authoritative parents use firm control to set limits, but they establish an atmosphere with open discussion or are more democratic. Limits for behavior are clear, consistent, and reasonable, but the children are encouraged to talk about why certain behaviors occurred and how the situations might be handled differently another time. Parents set and stick to established routines, so children have clear expectations of appropriate behavior. Authoritative parents provide explanations about inappropriate behaviors at a child's level of understanding.

TABLE 5–2 Characteristics of Significant Parenting Attributes

PARENTING ATTRIBUTE	PARENTAL WARMTH	PARENTAL CONTROL
High level	■ Warm, nurturing ■ Expressing affection and smiling at children frequently ■ Limiting criticism, punishment ■ Expressing approval of child	■ Restrictive control of behavior ■ Surveying and enforcing compliance with rules ■ Encouraging children to fulfill their responsibilities ■ Sometimes limiting freedom of expression
Low level	■ Cool, hostile ■ Quick to criticize or punish ■ Ignoring children ■ Rarely expressing affection or approval ■ Sometimes rejecting children	■ Permissive, minimally controlling ■ Making fewer demands ■ Making fewer restrictions on behavior or expression of emotion ■ Permitting freedom in exploring environment

Source: Ball, J. W., & Bindler, R. C., (2008). *Pediatric nursing: Caring for children* (4th ed., p. 34). Upper Saddle River, NJ: Pearson Education.

Children are allowed to express their opinions and objections, and some flexibility is permitted when appropriate. However, parents make it clear that they are the ultimate authority for decisions. Children with authoritative parents develop a sense of social responsibility because they converse about their responsibilities and approaches.

Permissive Parents

Permissive parents show a great deal of warmth, but set few controls or restraints on the children's behavior. Parents are so intent on showing unconditional love that they fail to perform some important parenting functions. Children are allowed to

regulate their own behavior. Discipline is inconsistent, and parents may threaten punishment but not follow through. Both extremes result in excessive permissiveness, and the children do not learn socially acceptable limits of behavior. As the parents do not impose any controls on the children, the children end up controlling the parents.

Indifferent Parents

Indifferent parents do not display much interest in their children or in their roles as parents. They do not demonstrate affection or approval of the children, and they do not set limits or controls on the children. This may occur because they

TABLE 5–3 Parenting Styles by Level of Warmth and Control

PARENTING STYLE	WARMTH/CONTROL	BEHAVIOR OF PARENTS	CHILD OUTCOMES
Authoritarian	High control Low warmth	■ Highly controlling, issue commands and expect them to be obeyed ■ Little communication with children, avoid lengthy verbal discussions with children ■ Have inflexible rules ■ Permit little independence	■ Have no negotiation skills ■ Have no ability to direct and initiate own activities ■ Frustrated in efforts to achieve autonomy ■ May become fearful, withdrawn, and unassertive ■ Girls often passive and dependent during adolescence ■ Boys often rebellious and aggressive
Authoritative	Moderately high control High warmth	■ Set reasonable limits on behavior ■ Accept and encourage growing autonomy of children ■ Engage in open communication with children ■ Have flexible rules	■ More willingly accept restrictions ■ Tend to be more self-reliant, self-controlled, and socially competent ■ Have higher self-esteem ■ Perform better in school
Permissive	Low control High warmth	■ Have few or no restraints ■ Give unconditional love ■ Communication flows from child to parent ■ Provide much freedom and little guidance ■ Provide no limit setting	■ Often unable to cooperate and negotiate with others ■ May become rebellious, aggressive, or socially inept, self-indulgent, or impulsive ■ May have difficulty being accepted by peers or being accepted and effective in a work setting ■ May be creative, active, and outgoing
Indifferent	Low control Low warmth	■ Provide no limit setting ■ Lack affection for children ■ Focus on stress in own lives ■ May show hostility or neglect	■ Often have the worst outcomes such as destructive impulses and delinquent behavior

Source: Adapted from Craig, G. J., & Dunn, W. L. (2007). *Understanding human development* (9th ed., p. 230). Upper Saddle River, NJ: Prentice Hall.

CLIENT TEACHING **Guidelines for Promoting Acceptable Behavior in Children**

The nurse can assist parents in handling their child's misbehavior by helping them to:

- Set realistic expectations and directions for behavior based on the child's age and understanding; consistently enforce the expected directions and behaviors.
- Focus on promoting appropriate and desirable behaviors in the child.
- Model or suggest appropriate behavior.
- Review expected behavior for special situations, such as a family party, going to the movies, or other social event.
- Help the child distinguish between inside and outside voice and behaviors.
- Praise or reward the child using appropriate behaviors.
- Tell the child about his or her inappropriate behavior as soon as it begins, and offer guidelines for changing behavior or provide a distraction.
- When reprimanding the child, focus on the behavior rather than stating that the child is bad. Explain how the behavior is inappropriate,

how it makes you, as the parent, and any other person involved feel. Avoid ridicule or accusation that can take the form of shame or criticism, as these actions can affect the child's self-esteem if repeated often enough.

- Be alert for situations when the child could misbehave, such as when tired or overexcited. Use a distraction to control or calm the child.
- Help children gain self-control with friendly reminders (e.g., count to 3, as soon as the clothes are on the doll, as soon as you finish the game) regarding the timing for transition to the next event of the day, such as bedtime, putting the toys away, or washing hands before dinner.
- Discuss reasons and social rules for expected behaviors when the child is old enough to understand.

Source: Ball, J. W., & Bindler, R. C., (2008). *Pediatric nursing: Caring for children* (4th ed., p. 36). Upper Saddle River, NJ: Pearson Education.

do not care, or because their lives are so stressed that they have no time or energy left for the children (Craig & Baucum, 2002).

Assessing Parenting Styles

Nurses assess parenting styles by asking families how they handle situations that require limit setting. As previously described, an authoritative style is preferred because of its positive outcomes for child behavior and learning. The nurse in all settings is often in a position to discuss parenting styles and to offer suggestions for managing certain types of child behaviors that are frustrating to the family. Keep in mind that children are all different, and parents often must vary their parenting styles for different children in the family. For example, the child's temperament is often tied to her or his behavioral style. One child may need very clear limits, with discussion and reinforcement, while a sibling may immediately respond to the parents' limit setting without a need for discussion of the situation.

Discipline and Limit Setting

Discipline is a method for teaching children the rules for how to behave in society and what is expected in different circumstances. **Punishment** is the action taken to enforce the rules when the child misbehaves. Parenting styles play an important role in the type of discipline and punishment parents use with children. When clear limits are set and consistently maintained, as with authoritative parenting, punishment may be needed less often. Limit setting and firm control of those limits are important discipline methods that allow children to learn to what extent they can safely and independently operate within the environment. Firm limits also help children feel secure; they are reassured by consistency and the sense of protection the limits are perceived to provide. Punishment helps children learn that misbehavior has consequences, and may affect other individuals. This helps children develop a sense of responsibility for their behavior.

ALTERATIONS

The incidence of family violence has increased in recent years. Statistics are not accurate because many cases remain unreported. Family violence includes abuse between intimate partners, child abuse, and elder abuse, and it may include physical, mental, and verbal abuse as well as neglect. Nurses should be alert to the symptoms of family violence and take appropriate measures to report it and obtain resources for the family. More information about violence can be found in the Violence concept.

Family Assessment

The purpose of family assessment is to determine the level of family functioning, clarify family interaction patterns, identify family strengths and weaknesses, and describe the health status of the family and its individual members. Also important are family living patterns, including communication, childrearing, coping strategies, and health practices. Family assessment gives an overview of the family process and helps the nurse identify areas that need further investigation. Nurses carry out a detailed assessment in specific target areas as they become more acquainted with the family and begin to understand family needs and strengths more fully. The nurse's understanding of a family's structure helps provide insight into the family's support system and needs. In planning interventions, nurses need to focus not only on problems, but also on family strengths and resources as part of the nursing care plan (see Box 5–3).

To obtain an accurate and concise family assessment, the nurse needs to establish a trusting relationship with the parent(s) and the family. Data are best collected in a comfortable, private environment, free from interruptions.

Assessment begins with a complete health history. The nurse focuses first on the family unit and then on the individuals in that family. Taking a health history is one of the most effective ways to identify existing or potential health

Box 5–3 Family Assessment Guide

Family Structure
- Size and type of family
- Name, age, and gender of family members
- Family relationship of all people residing within the household

Family Roles and Functions
- Family members working outside the home; type of work and satisfaction with it
- Household roles and responsibilities and how tasks are distributed
- Ways childrearing responsibilities are shared
- Major decision maker and methods of decision making
- Family members' satisfaction with roles, the way tasks are divided, and the way decisions are made

Physical Health Status
- Current physical health status of each member
- Perceptions of own and other family members' health
- Preventive health practices (e.g., status of immunizations, oral hygiene practices, regularity of vision examinations)
- Routine health care; when and why primary care provider was last seen

Interaction Patterns
- Ways of expressing affection, love, sorrow, anger, and so on
- Most significant family member in person's life
- Openness of communication with all family members

Family Values
- Cultural and religious orientations; degree to which cultural and religious practices are followed
- Use of leisure time and whether leisure time is shared with total family unit
- Family's view of education, teachers, and the school system
- Health values: how much emphasis is put on exercise, diet, preventive health care

Coping Resources
- Degree of emotional support offered to one another
- Availability of support persons and affiliations outside the family (e.g., friends, church memberships, mentors)
- Sources of stress
- Methods of handling stressful situations and conflicting goals of family members
- Financial ability to meet current and future needs

Source: Berman, A., Snyder, S. J., Kozier, B., & Erb, G. (2008). *Kozier & Erb's fundamentals of nursing: Concepts, process, and practice* (8th ed., p. 433). Upper Saddle River, NJ: Pearson Education.

problems. Using a genogram will aid the nurse in visualizing how all family members are genetically related to each other and grasping how patterns of chronic conditions occur within the family unit. **Genograms** consist of visual representations of gender showing lines of birth descent through the generations (Figure 5–3 ■). The history is followed by physical assessment of family members. If further evaluation is indicated, a referral is made to the appropriate health care professional.

The nurse should also develop an ecomap for family members, individually and as a group, to document the family unit's energy expenditures within the community setting. **Ecomaps** visualize how the family unit interacts with the external community environment, including schools, religious commitments, occupational duties, and recreational pursuits (Figure 5–4 ■). When the focus is on health, the appraisal includes information on lifestyle behaviors and health beliefs. The nurse uses data from the health appraisal to formulate a health profile. The health profile provides the data necessary to determine wellness or establish a nursing diagnosis, and to plan appropriate nursing interventions to promote optimal health through lifestyle modification.

Health Beliefs

To promote health, the nurse must understand the health beliefs of individuals and families. Health beliefs may reflect a lack of information or misinformation about health or disease. They may also include folklore and practices from different cultures. Because of the many advances in medicine and health care during the last few decades, clients may have

outdated information about health, illness, treatment, and prevention. The nurse is frequently in a position to give information or correct misconceptions. This function is an important component of the nursing care plan.

Family Communication Patterns

Family communication is measured by focusing on the listening and speaking skills, self-disclosure, and tracking abilities of the family as a group. In high-functioning families each person does the following:
- Listens—is empathetic and attentive
- Speaks—speaks for oneself and does not speak for others
- Self-discloses—shares personal feelings about oneself and others in the family
- Tracks—stays on the topic at hand

Families who communicate well are better able to adapt and cope. Families who find communication difficult may experience lower levels of expressiveness, vague requests to one another, an inability to comprehend each other's messages, frequent interruption of one another, speaking for others, and high levels of verbalized hostility.

Another aspect of family communication is the family's strategy to resolve conflict. The ability to resolve differences is based on the family's capacity to talk about areas of disagreement and its mutual willingness to negotiate and reach acceptable solutions. Problem-solving skills are critical to smooth family functioning. Without these skills, families seem to use strategies such as confrontation or avoidance, which are ineffective in reducing stress and do not resolve conflict satisfactorily. Children who grow up in families that use appropriate

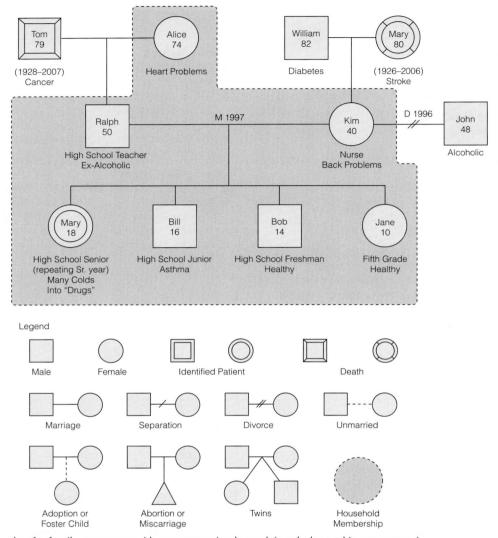

Figure 5–3 ■ Example of a family genogram with accompanying legend (symbols used in genograms).

problem-solving skills are more successful at avoiding and resolving conflicts both at home and in school.

The effectiveness of family communication determines the family's ability to function as a cooperative, growth-producing unit. Messages are constantly being communicated among family members, both verbally and nonverbally. The information transmitted influences how members work together, fulfill their assigned roles in the family, incorporate family values, and develop skills to function in society. Intrafamily communication plays a significant role in the development of self-esteem, which is necessary for the growth of personality.

Families that communicate effectively transmit messages clearly. Members are free to express their feelings without fear of jeopardizing their standing in the family. Family members support one another and have the ability to listen, empathize, and reach out to one another in times of crisis. When the needs of family members are met, they are more able to reach out to meet the needs of others in society.

When patterns of communication among family members are dysfunctional, messages are often communicated unclearly.

Verbal communication may be incongruent with nonverbal messages. Power struggles may be evidenced by hostility, anger, or silence. Members may be cautious in expressing their feelings because they cannot predict how others in the family will respond. When family communication is impaired, the growth of individual members is stunted. Members often turn to other systems to seek personal validation and gratification.

The nurse needs to observe intrafamily communication patterns closely. Nurses should pay special attention to who does the talking for the family, which members are silent, how disagreements are handled, and how well the members listen to one another and encourage the participation of others. Nonverbal communication is important because it gives valuable clues about what people are feeling.

Boundaries

Boundaries are the invisible lines that define the amount and kind of contact allowable among members of the family and between the family and outside systems. Boundaries determine the patterns of how, when, and to whom family members

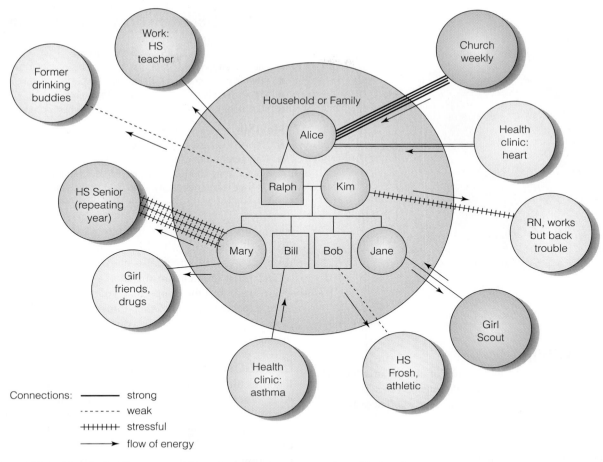

Figure 5–4 ■ Example of a family ecomap. Many more components may be added to the map.

relate. Boundaries define the divisions among the spousal, parental, and sibling subsystems.

- *Clear boundaries:* Firm yet flexible; family members are supported and nurtured but also allowed a certain degree of autonomy.
- *Rigid boundaries:* Family members are isolated from one another and there is little room for negotiation and individual development.
- *Diffuse boundaries:* Everyone is into everyone else's business; there is little distinction between family members and there is too much negotiation, resulting in a loss of autonomy.

In the modern Western nuclear family, competent families have clear hierarchical boundaries between generations in terms of power, authority, and responsibility. Competent adult leadership provides an emotional climate that considers everyone's needs and provides a sense of security. Members spend time apart, as well as time together. Mutual respect is also a boundary issue. Competent families respect and value the individual's opinions and feelings. The family system tolerates individual differences and honors different opinions.

Boundaries are a social construction and, as such, are culturally determined. What appears to be a boundary violation in one culture may be acceptable in another culture. For example,

how family members respect privacy in regard to toileting, bathing, changing clothes, and sleeping arrangements varies by culture. Multigenerational boundaries in terms of power and authority vary from culture to culture.

Family Cohesion

Family cohesion is defined as the emotional bonding between family members. There are four levels of cohesion (Figure 5–5 ■):

1. Disengaged (very low)
2. Separated (low to moderate)
3. Connected (moderate to high)
4. Enmeshed (very high)

In Western, developed societies, it is believed that the central ranges of cohesion (separated and connected) contribute to optimal family competency. The extremes (disengaged or enmeshed) are seen as less adaptive. Disengaged families seem almost like a group of strangers who happen to be living together. There is little loyalty or closeness in a disengaged family. Members of enmeshed families cannot develop a separate identity, and each person must yield autonomy to belong to the family. Uniqueness is experienced as distance, and individuality is viewed as alienation and disloyalty (Olson, 1996). See Box 5–4 for characteristics of family cohesion.

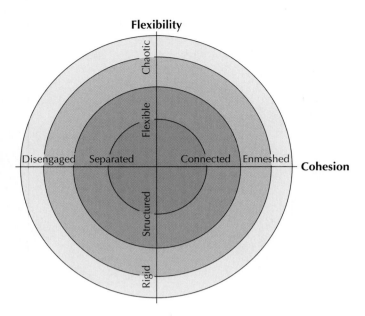

Figure 5–5 ■ Circumplex model.

Family Flexibility

Family flexibility includes the amount of change in a family's leadership, role relationships, and relationship rules, but it also refers to the family's ability to respond to stress. There are four levels of flexibility (see Figure 5–5):

1. Rigid (very low)
2. Structured (low to moderate)
3. Flexible (moderate to high)
4. Chaotic (very high)

As with the levels of family cohesion, it is believed that the central ranges (structured and flexible) are more conducive to family adaptation, with the extremes (rigid and chaotic) being less competent (Olson, 1996). See Box 5–5 for characteristics of family flexibility.

Rules determine appropriate roles and relationship patterns within the family. Rules express the family's values, forming a boundary around each family which screens outside information for compatibility with its value system. If the message is not congruent with the family's values, such

Box 5–5 **Characteristics of Family Flexibility**

Chaotic
- Lack of leadership
- Dramatic role shifts
- Erratic discipline
- Too much change

Structured
- Leadership sometimes shared
- Somewhat democratic discipline
- Roles stable
- Change when demanded

Flexible
- Shared leadership
- Democratic discipline
- Role-sharing change
- Change when necessary

Rigid
- Authoritarian leadership
- Strict discipline
- Roles seldom change
- Too little change

statements as, "That is not the way we do things in this family," or "I don't care what Marc is allowed to do; in this family, we . . ." will appear. To understand rules more clearly, reflect for a moment on the family in which you grew up. There were certain things that you just did, that you knew were expected of you. Other things were not permitted. To assess a few of the rules in your family of origin, complete the statements in Box 5–6.

Emotional Availability

Families that cope well encourage their members to express a wide variety of feelings. The emotional climate is one of intimacy and predictability. In other families, the emotional climate may be angry, cold, or distant and unpredictable. **Emotional availability** is another way to describe the quality of parent-child interactions. Areas for assessment include parental sensitivity, structuring, nonintrusiveness, and nonhostility. Parental sensitivity is assessed by how parents pick up on children's emotional signals and how appropriately parents express their own emotions. Parental structuring refers to the ability of parents to support learning and exploration without overwhelming the child's autonomy. Parental nonintrusiveness refers to the parents' availability to the child without being interfering, overprotective, or overwhelming. Nonhostility refers to ways of interacting with the child that are patient and pleasant. When angry, parents express their anger in an appropriately controlled manner (Biringen, 2000).

Box 5–4 **Characteristics of Family Cohesion**

Disengaged
- Little closeness
- Little loyalty
- High independence

Separated
- Low–moderate closeness
- Some loyalty
- Interdependent with more independence than dependence

Connected
- Moderate–high closeness
- High loyalty
- Interdependent with more dependence than independence

Enmeshed
- Very high closeness
- Very high loyalty
- High dependency

Box 5–6 **Assessing Rules in Your Family of Origin**

In my family, we were never allowed to . . .
In my family, we were always expected to . . .
In my family, girls were required to . . .
In my family, girls were allowed to . . .
In my family, girls were forbidden to . . .
In my family, boys were required to . . .
In my family, boys were allowed to . . .
In my family, boys were forbidden to . . .
In my family, household responsibilities were determined by . . .
In my family, we handled conflict by . . .
In my family, the most important thing in life for women is . . .
In my family, the most important thing in life for men is . . .

Family Competency

Competency is found in many family arrangements. More important than the form or type of family are the family's relational resources and adaptive abilities. The most distinctive trait of competent families is the ability to manage stress productively. Simply put, adaptive families evolve and shift with changing situations. This is often referred to as **resiliency**. Walsh (1998) describes family resiliency as the "process of coming to terms with all that has happened, reaching new emotional and relational equilibrium with changed circumstances, and becoming more resourceful in facing whatever lies ahead." Life crises and developmental transitions can stimulate family growth and transformation. Resilient families make it through crises such as disability and death with a renewed sense of confidence and purpose.

Family Coping Mechanisms

Family **coping** mechanisms are the behaviors families use to deal with stress or changes imposed from either within or without the family. Coping mechanisms can be viewed as an active method of problem solving developed to meet life's challenges. The coping mechanisms families and family members develop reflect their individual resourcefulness. Families may use coping patterns rather consistently over time or may change their coping strategies when new demands are made on the family. The success of a family largely depends on how well it copes with the stresses it experiences.

Nurses working with families realize the importance of assessing coping mechanisms as a way of determining how families relate to stress. Also important are the resources available to the family. Internal resources, such as knowledge, skills, effective communication patterns, and a sense of mutuality and purpose within the family, assist in the problem-solving process. In addition, external support systems promote coping and adaptation. These external systems may be extended family, friends, religious affiliations, health care professionals, or social service agencies. The development of social support systems is particularly valuable today because many families, due to stress, mobility, or poverty, are isolated from the resources that would traditionally have helped them cope with stress.

5.1 FAMILY RESPONSE TO HEALTH PROMOTION

KEY TERMS

Feedback, *142*
Input, *141*
Negative feedback, *142*
Output, *142*
Positive feedback, *142*
Structural-Functional theory, *142*
Subsystem, *141*
Suprasystem, *141*
System, *141*
Systems theory, *141*
Throughput, *142*

Basis for Selection of Exemplar

National Institute of Mental Health (NIMH)
ATI NCLEX®-RN test plan

LEARNING OUTCOMES

After learning about this exemplar, you will be able to do the following:

1. Describe the nurse's role in health promotion for the family.
2. Explain the definitions, functions, and developmental stages and tasks of the family.
3. Identify theoretical frameworks used in family health promotion.
4. Identify common risk factors regarding family health.
5. Assess family functioning using the family competency model.
6. Create caring plan of interventions using the nursing process for family health promotion.

OVERVIEW
Applying Theoretical Frameworks to Families

A variety of theoretical frameworks provide the nurse with a holistic overview of health promotion for families across the life span. The major theoretical frameworks nurses use in promoting the health of families are systems theory and structural-functional theory.

SYSTEMS THEORY   A **system** is a set of interacting identifiable parts or components. The basic concepts of general systems theory were proposed in the 1950s. One of its major proponents, Ludwig von Bertalanffy (1980), introduced **systems theory** as a universal theory that could be applied to many fields of study. Nurses are increasingly using systems theory to understand not only biologic systems but also systems in families, communities, and nursing and health care. General systems theory provides a way of examining interrelationships and deriving principles.

Systems may be complex and the systems components are often studied as **subsystems**. For family systems, the subsystems would be individuals. Looking back up the hierarchy, the systems above other systems are referred to as **suprasystems**—the family is the suprasystem of the individual. See Figure 5–6 ■ for a hierarchy of the human system.

A system depends on the quality and quantity of its input, throughput, output, and feedback. **Input** consists of information,

EVIDENCE-BASED PRACTICE **Are Adolescent Mothers Able to Promote a Healthy Life for Their Families?**

Much of the research on families headed by adolescent mothers has focused on the negative health aspects of these family units. Yet family and community theory suggest that no unit, family, or community will continue to exist with only negative factors. Black and Ford-Gilboe conducted a study with 41 adolescent mothers to test the families' resilience and ability to promote healthy lifestyles. The young mothers were asked to provide verbal responses to items on three questionnaires designed to gather information on the mothers' health-promoting lifestyle practices and demographic background. The results validated the theoretical relationships between increased family resilience and the teenage mother's ability to promote healthy lifestyles for herself and her children.

Implications

Nursing focuses on the complete individual by assessing for both positive and negative health behaviors and risks. In the past, families headed by young single mothers tended to be viewed only in negative terms. By conducting research to examine the positive strengths of these types of family units, nursing is helping to place these families in a more positive light.

Source: Black, C., & Ford-Gilboe, M. (2004). Adolescent mothers: Resilience, family health, work, and health promoting practices. *Journal of Advanced Nursing, 48,* 351–360. Reprinted with permission.

---

material, or energy that enters the system. After the input is absorbed by the system, it is processed into a form that is useful to the system. This transformation is called **throughput**. For example, food is input to the digestive system; it is digested (throughput) so that it can be used by the body. **Output** from a system is energy, matter, or information the system gives out as a result of its processes. Output from the digestive system includes caloric energy, nutrients, urine, and feces.

Feedback is the mechanism by which some of the output of a system is returned to the system as input. Feedback enables a system to regulate itself by redirecting the system's output back into the system as input, thus forming a feedback loop. This input influences the behavior of the system and its future output. **Negative feedback** inhibits change; **positive feedback** stimulates change.

The biologic system can be subdivided into the neurologic, musculoskeletal, respiratory, circulatory, gastrointestinal, and urinary subsystems, among others. Each subsystem can be subdivided in turn. For example, the urinary system consists of the kidneys, the ureters, and the bladder; the circulatory system consists of the heart and the blood vessels; the neurologic system consists of the brain, the spinal cord, and the nerves. The biologic system can also be subdivided into categories of needs or functional health patterns or activities of daily living, such as nutrition and hydration, sleep/rest, activity/exercise, elimination, and so on.

The family unit can also be viewed as a system. Its members are interdependent, working toward specific purposes and goals. Families, as open systems, are continually interacting with and influenced by other systems in the community. Boundaries regulate the input from other systems that interact with the family system; they also regulate output from the family system to the community or to society. Boundaries protect the family from the demands and influences of other systems. Families are likely to welcome input from without, encouraging individual members to adapt beliefs and practices to meet the changing demands of society, seek out health care information, and use community resources.

In understanding the complexity of family systems, consider how family members communicate, how they establish and maintain boundaries, how cohesive and flexible they are, and how emotionally available they are to others in the family. Understanding these interactions will provide a general idea of how well the family is able to adapt and function, both in everyday life and in the face of adversity.

STRUCTURAL-FUNCTIONAL THEORY The **structural-functional theory**, as the name implies, focuses on family structure and function. The structural component of the theory addresses the membership of the family and the relationships among family members. Intrafamily relationships are complex because of the numerous relationships that exist within the family structure—mother–daughter, brother–sister, spouse–partner, and so on. These relationships are constantly evolving as children mature and leave the family nest and as adults age and become more dependent on others to meet their daily needs.

The functional aspect of the theory examines the effects of intrafamily relationships on the family system, as well as their effects on other systems. Some of the main functions of the family include developing a sense of family purpose and affiliation,

National systems
State or provincial systems
Community systems
Family systems
Individual systems
Organ systems
Cellular systems
DNA chains

Figure 5–6 ■ A common system hierarchy.

adding and socializing new members, and providing and distributing care and services to members. A healthy family organizes its members and resources to meet family goals; it functions in harmony, working toward shared goals.

Nurses generally use a combination of theoretical frameworks in promoting the health of individuals and families. For example, the nurse may provide education for the mother of a toddler who is struggling to accomplish the developmental stage of autonomy described by Erikson (1963). Simultaneously, the nurse may guide the same family in its stressful transition period between developmental stages as their older school-age child becomes an adolescent.

Family Developmental Stages and Tasks

The family, like the individual, has developmental stages and tasks. Each stage brings change, requiring adaptation; each new stage also brings family-related risk factors for alterations in health. The nurse must consider the client's needs both at specific developmental stages and within a family with specific developmental tasks. Family developmental stages and developmental tasks are described next; related risk factors and health problems for each stage are listed in Table 5–4.

COUPLE Two people living together (with or without being married) are in a period of establishing themselves as a couple. The developmental tasks of the couple include adjusting to living together as a couple, establishing a mutually satisfying relationship, relating to kin, and deciding whether to have children (in those of child-bearing age).

FAMILY WITH INFANTS AND PRESCHOOLERS The family with infants or preschoolers must adjust to having and supporting the needs of more than two members, with at least one member who is incapable of supporting him- or herself. Other developmental tasks of the family at this stage are developing an attachment between parents and children, adjusting to the economic costs of having more members, coping with energy depletion and lack of privacy, and carrying out activities that enhance growth and development of the children.

FAMILY WITH SCHOOL-AGE CHILDREN The family with school-age children has the developmental tasks of adjusting to the expanded world of children in school and encouraging educational achievement. A further task is promoting joint decision making between children and parents.

FAMILY WITH ADOLESCENTS AND YOUNG ADULTS The developmental tasks of the family with adolescents and young adults focus on transition. While providing a supportive home base and maintaining open communications, parents must balance freedom with responsibility and release adult children as they seek independence.

FAMILY WITH MIDDLE ADULTS The family with middle adults (in which the parents are middle aged and children are no longer at home) has the developmental tasks of maintaining ties with older and younger generations and planning for retirement. If the family consists of just the middle-aged couple, they have the developmental task of reestablishing the relationship and (if necessary) acquiring the role of grandparents.

FAMILY WITH OLDER ADULTS The older adult family has the developmental tasks of adjusting to retirement, adjusting to aging, and coping with the loss of a spouse. If a spouse dies, further tasks include adjusting to living alone or closing the family home.

Risk Factors

RISK FOR HEALTH PROBLEMS Risk assessment helps the nurse identify individuals and groups at higher risk than the general population of developing specific health problems, such as stroke, diabetes, and lung cancer. The vulnerability of family units to health problems may be based on the maturity level of individual family members, heredity or genetic factors, sex or race, sociologic factors, and lifestyle practices.

MATURITY FACTORS Families with members at both ends of the age continuum are at risk of developing health problems. Families entering childbearing and child rearing phases experience many changes in roles, responsibilities, and expectations. The many, often conflicting, demands on the family cause stress and fatigue, either or both of which may impede growth of individual family members and the functioning of the group as a unit. Adolescent mothers, because of their developmental level and lack of knowledge about parenthood, are more likely to develop health problems, as are single-parent families, because of role overload experienced by the head of the household. Many elderly persons feel a lack of purpose and decreased self-esteem. These feelings can reduce their motivation to engage in health-promoting behaviors, such as exercise or community and family involvement.

HEREDITARY FACTORS Persons born into families with a history of certain diseases, such as diabetes or cardiovascular disease, are at greater risk of developing these conditions. A detailed family health history that includes genetically transmitted disorders is crucial to the identification of persons and families at risk. These data are used not only to monitor the health of individual family members, but also to recommend modifications in health practices that potentially reduce the risk, minimize the consequences, or postpone the development of genetically related conditions.

GENDER OR RACE FACTORS Some family units or family members may be at risk of developing a disease by reason of gender or race. Men, for example, are at greater risk of having cardiovascular disease at an earlier age than women, and women are at greater risk of developing osteoporosis, particularly after menopause. Although it is sometimes difficult to separate genetic factors from cultural factors, certain risk factors seem to be related to race. Sickle cell anemia, for example, is a hereditary disease limited to people of African descent, and Tay-Sachs is a neurodegenerative disease that occurs primarily in descendants of eastern European Jews.

SOCIOLOGIC FACTORS Poverty is a major problem that affects not only the family but also the community and society. Poverty is a real concern among the rising number of single-parent families. As the number of these families increases, poverty will affect a larger number of growing children.

TABLE 5–4 Family-Related Risk Factors for Alterations in Health

STAGE	RISK FACTORS	HEALTH PROBLEMS
Couple, or family with infants and preschoolers	■ Lack of knowledge about family planning, contraception, and sexual and marital roles ■ Inadequate prenatal care ■ Altered nutrition: inadequate nutrition, overweight, underweight ■ Smoking, alcohol/drug abuse ■ Lack of knowledge about child health and safety ■ Low socioeconomic status ■ First pregnancy before age 16 or after age 35 ■ Rubella, syphilis, gonorrhea, AIDS	■ Premature pregnancy ■ Low-birth-weight infant ■ Birth defects ■ Injury to infant or child ■ Accidents
Family with school-age children	■ Unsafe home environment ■ Working parents with inappropriate or inadequate resources for child care ■ Low socioeconomic status ■ Child abuse or neglect ■ Multiple, closely spaced children ■ Repeated infections, accidents, and hospitalizations ■ Unrecognized and unattended health problems ■ Poor or inappropriate nutrition ■ Toxic substances in the home	■ Behavior problems ■ Speech and vision problems ■ Learning disabilities ■ Communicable diseases ■ Physical abuse ■ Cancer ■ Developmental delay ■ Obesity, underweight
Family with adolescents and young adults	■ Family values of aggressiveness and competition ■ Lifestyle and behavior leading to chronic illness (substance abuse, inadequate diet) ■ Lack of problem-solving skills ■ Conflicts between parent and children	■ Violent death and injury ■ Alcohol/drug abuse ■ Unwanted pregnancy ■ Suicide ■ Sexually transmitted infections ■ Domestic abuse
Family with middle adults	■ High-cholesterol diet ■ Overweight ■ Hypertension ■ Smoking, alcohol abuse ■ Physical inactivity ■ Personality patterns related to stress ■ Exposure to environment: sunlight, radiation, asbestos, or water or air pollution ■ Depression ■ Age	■ Cardiovascular disease (coronary artery disease and cerebrovascular disease) ■ Cancer ■ Accidents ■ Suicide ■ Mental illness
Family with older adults	■ Depression ■ Drug interactions ■ Chronic illness ■ Death of spouse ■ Reduced income ■ Poor nutrition ■ Lack of exercise ■ Past environment and lifestyle	■ Impaired vision and hearing ■ Hypertension ■ Acute illness ■ Chronic illness ■ Infectious diseases (influenza, pneumonia) ■ Injuries from burns and falls ■ Depression ■ Alcohol abuse

Source: LeMone, P., & Burke, K. (2008). *Medical-surgical nursing: Critical thinking in client care* (4th ed., p. 32). Upper Saddle River, NJ: Pearson Education.

When ill, the poor are likely to put off seeking services until the illness reaches an advanced state and requires longer or more complex treatment. Although the health of the people of industrialized nations has improved significantly during the past century, this progress has not benefited all segments of society, particularly the poor.

LIFESTYLE FACTORS Many diseases are preventable, the effects of some diseases can be minimized, or the onset of disease can be delayed through lifestyle modifications. Certain cancers, cardiovascular disease, adult-onset diabetes, and tooth decay are among the lifestyle diseases. The incidence of lung cancer, for example, would be greatly reduced if people stopped smoking. Good nutrition, dental hygiene, and use of fluoride—in the water supply, in toothpaste, as a topical application, or as a supplement—have been shown to reduce dental decay or caries, one of America's most prevalent health problems.

Other important lifestyle considerations are exercise, stress management, and rest. Today, health professionals have the knowledge to prevent or minimize the effects of some of the main causes of disease, disability, and death. The challenge is to disseminate information about prevention and to motivate families to make lifestyle changes before the onset of illness.

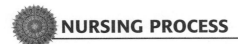

NURSING PROCESS

Assessment

Family Assessment Tools

Family assessment tools can be used to gather additional information about the family's functioning and can place particular focus on family stresses, coping strategies, and family strengths. Information about the way the family functions in nurturing its members, problem solving, and communicating may help identify strategies that are potentially more effective for managing the child's health care. These strategies, such as collaborating with the family in planning for health maintenance and health promotion strategies, enable the nurse to work more effectively with the family.

Family Ecomap

An ecomap illustrates the family's relationships and interactions with the social networks in the community, enabling the nurse and other health care providers to visualize the family's social network. By having family members participate in preparing the ecomap, it is possible to obtain information about how the family perceives or receives social support, as well as the strength of family relationships with significant other persons and organizations. The ecomap provides an opportunity to identify the community resources the family uses and to highlight any potential community resources that may help promote the family's health. See Figure 5–7 ■ for a sample ecomap.

Family APGAR

The Family APGAR is a quick five-item questionnaire that may be used as an initial screening tool for family assessment. The five family concepts measured are family adaptability, partnership, growth, affection, and resolve (Table 5–5). This five-item questionnaire can be administered quickly to family members over 10 years of age. Ask all family members to complete a separate copy of the questionnaire to gain a picture of the family's perspective on family functioning. Be concerned if the majority of responses fall in the "hardly ever" category or if responses vary a lot among family members. This may indicate a family that needs much more support to cope with the demands of daily life and provide insight into health maintenance and health promotion needs.

Home Observation for Measurement of the Environment (HOME)

The HOME Inventory is an assessment tool developed to measure the quality and quantity of stimulation and support available in the home environment (Caldwell & Bradley, 1984). Four age-specific scales are available (birth to 3 years, 3 to 6 years, 6 to 10 years, and 10 to 15 years). Examples of

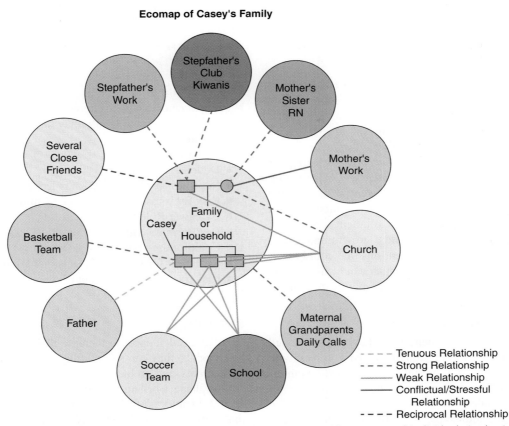

Ecomap of Casey's Family

- - - Tenuous Relationship
- - - Strong Relationship
—— Weak Relationship
——— Conflictual/Stressful Relationship
- - - - Reciprocal Relationship

Figure 5–7 ■ An ecomap illustrates the family's relationships and interactions with groups and individuals in the immediate external environment.

TABLE 5–5 The Family APGAR Questionnaire

Directions: The following questions have been designed to help us better understand you and your family. You should feel free to ask questions about any item in the questionnaire. The space for comments should be used when you wish to give additional information or if you wish to discuss how the question is applied to your family. Please try to answer all questions. Family is defined as the individual(s) with whom you usually live. If you live alone, your "family" consists of persons with whom you now have the strongest emotional ties.*

For each question, check only one box.

	ALMOST ALWAYS 2	SOME OF THE TIME 1	HARDLY EVER 0
I am satisfied that I can turn to my family for help when something is troubling me. Comments:_____			
I am satisfied with the way my family talks over things with me and shares problems with me. Comments:_____			
I am satisfied that my family accepts and supports my wishes to take on new activities or directions. Comments:_____			
I am satisfied with the way my family expresses affection and responds to my emotions, such as anger, sorrow, and love. Comments:_____			
I am satisfied with the way my family and I share time together. Comments:_____			

*Note: Depending on which member of the family is being interviewed, the interviewer may substitute for the word *family* either *spouse, significant other, parents,* or *children.*
Responses are scored 2, 1, 0 and totaled. The total score ranges from 0 to 10. The larger the score, the greater amount of satisfaction that family member has with family functioning.

Source: Adapted from: Smilkstein, G. (1978). The family APGAR: A proposal for a family function test and its use by physicians. *Journal of Family Practice,* (6), 1231–1239.

subscales within each age-specific scale are parental responsiveness, acceptance of child, the physical environment, learning materials, variety in experience, and parental involvement. Data are collected during an informal, low-stress interview and observation over 45–90 minutes in the home setting. The child and his or her primary caregiver must be present and awake during the interview. Observation of the parent–child interaction is an essential part of the assessment. The intent is to allow family members to act normally. Assessment of the home environment will help to identify factors that promote the child's growth and development. Examples of nursing interventions that could result from the HOME assessment are items that can be used in the home for toys and strategies for interacting with the child to promote learning.

Friedman Family Assessment Tool

The Friedman Family Assessment Tool (FFAM), developed by Marilyn Friedman, was designed to assist nurses with family assessment. This tool provides a method for examining the whole family in the context of the larger community where the family resides. The interview collects information about a family's relationships, functioning, strengths, and problems. The short form for this assessment tool is provided in Box 5–7.

Diagnosis

Nursing diagnoses will be chosen based on what type of health promotional needs the family may have and may include any of the following:

- Risk for Injury
- Deficient Knowledge
- Readiness for Enhanced Knowledge
- Risk for Impaired Parent/Infant/Child Attachment
- Caregiver Role Strain
- Readiness for Enhanced Communication
- Compromised Family Coping
- Readiness for Enhanced Decision Making
- Risk for Delayed Development
- Stress Overload

Planning

Families need support to increase their resources and coping behaviors so they can successfully manage the multiple stressors, strains, and problems of daily living.

The nurse working with a family to develop a care plan should identify potential resources in the community that match the child's and the family's needs for support. The nurse will collaborate with the family to discuss those resources and to select the ones that are acceptable to the family, to increase

Box 5–7 Friedman Family Assessment Tool

The following form is shortened for ease in assessing a family. If you are not sure what data should be covered in each of the assessment areas, please refer to the original reference, where more detailed questions/areas are presented.

Before using the following guidelines in completing family assessments, note that not all areas included will be germane for each of the families visited. The guidelines are comprehensive and allow depth when probing is necessary. Do not feel that every subarea needs to be covered when the broad area of inquiry poses no problems to the family or concern to the health worker. Second, by virtue of the interdependence of the family system, opportunities for repetition will arise. The assessor should try not to repeat data, but to refer the reader back to sections where this information has already been described.

Identifying Data
1. Family Name
2. Address and Phone
3. Family Composition: The Family Genogram
4. Type of Family Form
5. Cultural (Ethnic) Background
6. Religious Identification
7. Social Class Status
8. Social Class Mobility

Developmental Stage and History of Family
9. Family's Present Developmental Stage
10. Extent of Family Developmental Tasks Fulfillment
11. Nuclear Family History
12. History of Family of Origin of Both Parents

Environmental Data
13. Characteristics of Home
14. Characteristics of Neighborhood and Larger Community
15. Family's Geographical Mobility
16. Family's Associations and Transactions With Community

Family Structure
17. Communication Patterns
    - Extent of Functional and Dysfunctional Communication (types of recurring patterns)
    - Extent of Emotional (Affective) Messages and How Expressed
    - Characteristics of Communication Within Family Subsystems
    - Extent of Congruent and Incongruent Messages
    - Types of Dysfunctional Communication Processes Seen in Family
    - Areas of Closed Communication
    - Familial and Contextual Variables Affecting Communication
18. Power Structure
    - Power Outcomes
    - Decision-Making Process
    - Power Bases
    - Variables Affecting Family Power
    - Overall Family System and Subsystem Power (Family Power Continuum Placement)
19. Role Structure
    - Formal Role Structure
    - Informal Role Structure
    - Analysis of Role Models (optional)
    - Variables Affecting Role Structure
20. Family Values
    - Compare the family to American core values or family's reference group values and/or identify important family values and their importance (priority) in family
    - Congruence Between the Family's Values and the Family's Reference Group or Wider Community
    - Disparity in Value Systems
    - Presence of Value Conflicts in Family
    - Effect of the Above Values and Value Conflicts on Health
    - Status of Family

(continued)

Box 5–7 **Friedman Family Assessment Tool** (continued)

Family Functions

21. Affective Function
    - Mutual Nurturance, Closeness, and Identification
    - Separateness and Connectedness
    - Family's Need-Response Patterns
22. Socialization Function
    - Family Childrearing Practices
    - Adaptability of Childrearing Practices for Family Form and Family's Situation
    - Who Is (Are) Socializing Agent(s) for Child(ren)?
    - Value of Children in Family
    - Cultural Beliefs That Influence Family's Childrearing Patterns
    - Social Class Influence on Childrearing Patterns
    - Estimation About Whether Family Is at Risk for Childrearing Problems and if so, Indication of High-Risk Factors
    - Adequacy of Home Environment for Children's Needs to Play
23. Health Care Function
    - Family's Health Beliefs, Values, and Behavior
    - Family's Definitions of Health-Illness and Its Level of Knowledge
    - Family's Perceived Health Status and Illness Susceptibility
    - Family's Dietary Practices
    - Adequacy of Family Diet (recommended 3-day food history record)
    - Function of Mealtimes and Attitudes Toward Food and Mealtimes
    - Shopping (and its planning) Practices
    - Person(s) Responsible for Planning, Shopping, and Preparation of Meals
    - Sleep and Rest Habits
    - Physical Activity and Recreation Practices
    - Family's Therapeutic and Recreational Drug, Alcohol, and Tobacco Practices
    - Family's Role in Self-Care Practices
    - Medically Based Preventive Measures (physicals, eye and hearing tests, immunizations, dental care)
    - Complementary and Alternative Therapies
    - Family Health History (both general and specific diseases—environmentally and genetically related)
    - Health Care Services Received
    - Feelings and Perceptions Regarding Health Services
    - Emergency Health Services
    - Source of Payments for Health and Other Services
    - Logistics of Receiving Care

Family Stress, Coping, and Adaptation

24. Family Stressors, Strengths, and Perceptions
    - Stressors Family is Experiencing
    - Strengths That Counterbalance Stressors
    - Family's Definition of the Situation
25. Family Coping Strategies
    - How the Family Is Reacting to the Stressors
    - Extent of Family's Use of Internal Coping Strategies (past/present)
    - Extent of Family's Use of External Coping Strategies (past/present)
    - Dysfunctional Coping Strategies Used (past/present; extent of use)
26. Family Adaptation
    - Overall Family Adaptation
    - Estimation of Whether Family is in Crisis
27. Tracking Stressors, Coping, and Adaptation Over Time

Source: Friedman, M. M., Bowden, V. R., & Jones, E. G. (2003). *Family nursing: Research, theory, and practice* (5th ed., pp. 593–594). Upper Saddle River, NJ: Prentice Hall. Reprinted with permission.

the likelihood that the family will follow through with the plan. In some cases it may be necessary to collaborate with a multidisciplinary team, including social workers to help the family obtain assistance to overcome barriers such as transportation, financial, geographic, and any other that interfere with the child's health care. The nurse should make sure the family has a care coordinator, especially when a family member initially seems unable to assume the case management role. The nurse

NURSING CARE PLAN Family Response to Health Promotion

ASSESSMENT DATA	NURSING DIAGNOSIS	DESIRED OUTCOMES
Ms. Blankenship brings her 2-year-old son in for his routine immunizations. After receiving his immunizations, while waiting the required 20 minutes before leaving, Ms. Blankenship, a single mother, reveals that she has recently lost her job because her child became ill and she had to miss work. She says she has found a new job, but the salary is much lower than her previous job and she will not be able to afford day care for the child. She says she is considering taking the job anyway because she would be working nights and the child sleeps through the night, so she's considering leaving the child home alone and asking a next-door neighbor to keep an ear out for him in case he awakens.	Decisional conflict	Decision making as evidenced by ■ Identifying relevant information (090601)* ■ Identifying alternatives (090602) ■ Identifying potential consequences of each alternative (090604)

NURSING INTERVENTIONS	RATIONALE
Assess client's understanding of available choices.	*Talking with the mother in more detail about each of the choices she is considering helps the mother identify pros and cons of each choice.*
Provide information about risks associated with leaving child home alone.	*Helping the mother to understand risks of leaving a toddler home alone may aid her in making a more informed decision.*
Teach problem-solving and decision-making processes.	*These processes give the mother the tools to make better decisions.*
Provide referrals to social services to help meet financial needs.	*Social services may assist the mother in meeting financial obligations until alternative options can be explored.*
Provide decision-making support (5250).	

EVALUATION

Outcome is not met. Ms. Blankenship has an appointment to meet with social services and has decided not to make a decision until she has an opportunity to explore other options.

*The NOC # for desired outcomes and the NIC # for nursing interventions are shown in parentheses after the appropriate outcome or intervention. Outcomes, interventions, and activities selected are only a sample of those suggested by NOC and NIC and should be further individualized for each client.

---

may also assist the family in obtaining resources by such actions as role rehearsal, providing instructions and support when making an initial call, or connecting with another family support person who can help with resource linkage. The nurse will refer families with moderate or severe dysfunction to community resources for social support and counseling as appropriate.

Outcomes are determined based on the needs of the family and may include any of the following:

- Children will achieve developmental milestones in social, self-regulatory behavior or cognitive, language, or gross or fine motor skills.
- Family will display or describe actions to manage stressors that tax family resources.
- Family system will meet the needs of its members during developmental transitions.
- Family members will demonstrate actions to improve the overall health and social competence of family unit.

Implementation

Establishing a therapeutic relationship with the family is an important intervention in and of itself. This relationship should be characterized by empathy and trust, as well as the development of mutually identified goals for the family's needs. To help families develop resiliency, the nurse should focus on family competence and strengths, and acknowledge and validate their emotions. The nurse provides information in a clear, timely, and sensitive manner. Questions are asked to help direct the family's thinking rather than providing them with all of the answers. The nurse works with families by teaching them to identify solutions until they are able to problem solve independently. The family's ethnic and religious background need to be considered in developing intervention recommendations.

Evaluation

Evaluation will be based on the family's progress toward goals and outcomes mutually determined by the family and nurse. The following are indicators that outcomes are being met and progress is being achieved:

- Family members' behaviors collectively demonstrate cohesion, strength, and emotional bonding.
- The family system has the capacity to successfully adapt and function competently after adversity or crisis.

REVIEW Family Response to Health Promotion

RELATE: LINK THE CONCEPTS

Linking the concepts of Culture, Advocacy, and Development with the concept of Family:

1. What impact will culture have on the family?
2. Name activities that the nurse could become involved with in order to advocate for the family.
3. How can the nurse act to promote healthy development in family members?

REFLECT: CASE STUDY

The home health nurse has been visiting a 90-year-old woman and her younger sister who live alone in a large farmhouse. The women have been active in caring for each other and their residence. During one of the home visits, they confide that the farm is too much for them, but they admit that they do not want to tell their families because they are afraid that they will be put into a nursing home.

1. What community resources are available to assist the sisters to live independently?
2. How should the family be involved in the decision making?
3. What signs can alert the nurse that the sisters are unable to care for themselves?
4. Should the nurse contact the family without the sisters' knowledge? Why or why not?

5.2 FAMILY RESPONSE TO HEALTH ALTERATIONS

KEY TERMS

Family recovery, *152*
Family support, *153*
Friend support, *153*
Objective family burden, *151*
Professional support, *153*
Spiritual support, *153*
Stigma, *151*
Subjective family burden, *152*

Basis for Selection of Exemplar

Centers for Disease Control and Prevention (CDC)
The Joint Commission (JCAHO)
Institute for Healthcare Improvement (IHI)

LEARNING OUTCOMES

After reading about this exemplar, you will be able to do the following:

1. Create a nursing care plan utilizing the nursing process to support family functioning when facing health alterations in a family member.
2. List the categories of family strengths that help families develop and cope with stressors.
3. Identify a variety of family support services that might be available in a community.
4. Describe how family type may influence nursing care of the childbearing family.

OVERVIEW

Although some clients are totally alone in the world, most have one or more people who are significant in their lives. These significant others may be related or bonded to the client by birth, adoption, marriage, or friendship. Although not always meeting traditional definitions, people (or even pets) significant to the client are the client's family. The nurse includes the family as an integral component of care in all health care settings.

Illness of a family member is a crisis that affects the entire family system. The family is disrupted as members abandon their usual activities and focus their energy on restoring family equilibrium. Roles and responsibilities the ill person previously assumed are delegated to other family members, or those functions remain undone for the duration of the illness. The family experiences anxiety because members are concerned about the sick person and the resolution of the illness. This anxiety is compounded by additional responsibilities when there is less time or motivation to complete the normal tasks of daily living. See Box 5–8 for some factors that determine the impact of illness on the family unit.

The family's ability to deal with the stress of illness depends on the members' coping skills. Families with good communication skills are better able to discuss how they feel about the illness and how it affects family functioning. They can plan for the future and are flexible in adapting these plans as the situation changes. An established social support network provides strength, encouragement, and services to the family

Box 5–8 Factors Determining the Impact of Illness on the Family

- The nature of the illness, which can range from minor to life threatening
- The duration of the illness
- The residual effects of the illness, ranging from none to permanent disability
- The meaning of the illness to the family and its significance to family systems
- The financial impact of the illness, which is influenced by factors such as insurance and ability of the ill member to return to work
- The effect of the illness on future family functioning (for instance, previous patterns may be restored or new patterns may be established)

Source: Berman, A., Snyder, S. J., Kozier, B., & Erb, G. (2008). *Kozier & Erb's fundamentals of nursing: Concepts, process, and practice* (8th ed., p. 437). Upper Saddle River, NJ: Pearson Education

during the illness. During health crises, families must realize that turning to others for support is a sign of strength rather than weakness. Nurses can be part of the support system for families, or they can identify other sources of support in the community.

During a crisis, families are often drawn together by a common purpose. In this time of closeness, family members have the opportunity to reaffirm personal and family values and their commitment to one another. Indeed, illness may provide a unique opportunity for family growth.

The Nurse's Role With Families Experiencing Illness

Nurses committed to family-centered care involve both the ailing individual and the family in the nursing process. Through their interaction with families, nurses can give support and information, although the ailing individual needs to give permission regarding what information can be shared with family members. Nurses make sure that not only the individual but also each family member understands the disease, its management, and the effect of these two factors on family functioning.

The Family of the Client With a Chronic Illness

The client with a chronic illness may be hospitalized for diagnosis and treatment when he or she experiences acute exacerbations, but the care of the client is primarily and usually provided at home. Chronic illness in a family member is a major stressor that may cause changes in family structure and function, as well as in how family developmental tasks are performed.

Many different factors affect family responses to chronic illness; family responses in turn affect the client's response to and perception of the illness. Factors influencing response to chronic illness include personal, social, and economic resources; the nature and course of the disease; and demands of the illness as perceived by family members. Clients with chronic illness, and their families, may be at risk for depression. Nursing considerations for a client with a chronic illness include being alert to symptoms of depression, both in the client and in his or her close family members.

PATHOPHYSIOLOGY AND ETIOLOGY
Severe Mental Illness and the Family System

Family members of individuals with mental illness often share in the many losses that accompany the illness. Families are the major source of support and rehabilitation for their loved ones. Of clients discharged from acute care, 65% return to their families. At any given time, 40–50% of the 48 million Americans who are severely and persistently mentally ill live with their families on a regular basis. Even when clients do not live at home, the families are often the only source of support. In the United States, care for the mentally ill has become as much family based as community based. Caring for a mentally ill family member can result in overwhelming emotional and economic stress on the family system (Rose, Mallinson, & Gerson,

2006). In an ideal world, family members would be supportive and effective in dealing with an ill family member. The person with the mental disorder (client) would not act out (or threaten to act out). In reality, family relationships can be conflicted. When clients try to assert their autonomy, families worry about what will happen and become critical or try to control the situation. As families struggle with guilt and fear, clients feel rejected and abandoned. Clients may also experience shame over being mistrusted and monitored.

Family Burden

Families have important needs of their own in response to their loved one's mental illness. Severe and persistent mental illness often puts the family under catastrophic levels of stress. As families respond to the grief and trauma, they need empathy and support from health care professionals.

Family burden is the overall level of distress experienced as a result of the mental illness. The **objective family burden** is related to the actual, identifiable family problems associated with the person's mental illness. One burden the family must manage relates to *symptomatic behaviors*. The family's loved one's deficit behaviors—such as lack of motivation, difficulty in completing tasks, isolation from others, inability to manage money, poor grooming and personal care, and poor eating and sleeping behavior—can be of great concern to families. Intrusive or acting-out behaviors—such as lack of consideration for others, excessive arguing, conflicts with neighbors and friends, damaging material possessions, inappropriate sexual behavior, suicide attempts, substance abuse, and violent outbursts—are very disturbing to family members. These behaviors may be more episodic than the deficit behaviors but may have more severe immediate consequences. This family burden may lead to loss of independence and increased responsibility as families try to cope with day-to-day living. This burden includes disruption in household functioning, restriction of social activities, and financial hardship due to medical bills and the cost of their loved one's economic burden.

Another objective burden related to family problems is caregiving. Families may find that community services are not always available and not always satisfactory. Inadequate funding results in lack of treatment programs and lack of services for families themselves. Families also find themselves negotiating with the legal and criminal justice system. With few long-term psychiatric facilities available, many people who would have previously been cared for in state hospitals now find themselves in jails and prisons. Often, the "crimes" with which they are charged are misdemeanors resulting from their symptoms of mental illness, such as disorderly conduct, trespassing, and drunkenness.

A third objective burden that families must cope with is the burden of **stigma**, which is a collection of negative attitudes and beliefs that lead people to fear, reject, avoid, and discriminate against people with mental illness. In response to stigma, people with mental disorders internalize these attitudes and become ashamed of themselves and their illness. People with mental illness continue to be ostracized from mainstream society. Families may become isolated as they avoid others who misunderstand the illness. When a family member has cancer or heart disease, other people respond with kindness. When a family member has a mental disorder, the response is often avoidance because there is a perception of unpredictability and danger. Thus, stigma severely limits support from extended family and friends. As they and their loved one face multiple discriminations, families may feel isolated and shameful, may lose self-esteem, and may run the risk of self-stigmatization (Rose, Mallinson, & Gerson, 2006; Stengler-Wenzke, Trosbach, Dietrich, & Angermeyer, 2004).

The **subjective family burden** is defined as the psychological distress of the family members in relation to the objective burden. They often experience frustration, anxiety, depression, hopelessness, and helplessness. Families also experience intense feelings of grief and loss. They must mourn for the person they knew before the onset of the illness and the potential loss of hopes, dreams, and expectations. They live with a sense of chronic sorrow for those loved ones who experience periods of remission and relapse. There is also a sense of empathetic pain as they watch their family member become a victim of the illness. Living with and caring for a person with mental illness can have a tremendous impact on the family. Some families cope fairly well, whereas others are easily exhausted and give up (Jungbauer, Wittmund, Dietrich, & Angermeyer, 2003). See Box 5–9 for descriptions of the language of family pain.

Family Recovery

Family response to the mental illness of a family member can vary depending on what stage the family (or members of a family) is in. Family response, formally known as "**family recovery**" to mental illness within the family, has three pronounced stages. A nurse may adjust his or her approach adjust caring interventions for a family depending on the family's stage of recovery.

Box 5–9 The Language of Family Pain

Catastrophe: Watching as your loved one slips away. This is like a horror movie in which the hero/heroine (loved one) is utterly transformed by some unseen, monstrous force.

Torture: The agony of watching a loved one experience relentless pain and suffering without being able to make it stop. The absolute panic when he or she refuses your assistance, rejects your help, resists your protection at the time when it is most needed.

Anguish: The pain of having loved ones turn on those who are trying to help them, attack them angrily, or blame them for their difficulties.

Horror/fear: A dread that the ill person will do something terrible to his- or herself or others.

Nightmare: Rejection, labeling, and ostracism by the mental health system when we are trying to help.

Source: Reprinted with permission from Burland, J. (1999). *NAMI provided education program.* Arlington, VA: National Alliance for the Mentally Ill.

Stage 1 of family recovery involves discovery and denial. Family members are often the first to notice that another member is exhibiting unusual behavior. The family's initial response may range from minimizing (it's not so serious) to denial (it's just a phase). This response is a temporary, rather than maladaptive, reaction to avoid a painful reality. As the family members attempt to explain the changes to others, they may attribute the changes to something more socially acceptable than mental illness. For example, they might tell others that the person is suffering from exhaustion or an endocrine problem, or that stress at school or work is causing the difficulties. Others' prejudice and the family's avoidance of stigma can lead to family isolation and loss of relationships outside the immediate family system.

Stage 2 of family recovery involves recognition and acceptance. As it becomes more evident that a significant problem exists, families begin to search for reasons and solutions by gathering available information. Families start to develop their own image of the disease process and expectations of mental health professionals. Many families also hope for what was in the past and for what might be in the future. It is very sad to lose a close family member to mental illness. Many people do not believe that mental illness is a brain disease. If the disorder begins in childhood, it is easier to think that it is a result of bad parenting because good parenting should be able to fix it. That is like telling parents of a child with leukemia that if they were better parents they could stop those white cells from growing. When a person experiences a mental disorder, expectations and dreams may necessitate alteration. Some clients come through the experience of mental illness able to develop meaningful and productive lives. Others, who do not respond to current treatment strategies, may have to grieve the loss of their hopes and dreams (Tweedell, Forchuk, Jewell, & Steinnagel, 2004).

Stage 3 of family recovery involves coping and competence. This includes the day-to-day efforts necessary to cope with all the changes in the family. When people become persistently and severely mentally ill, they may have difficulty carrying out their family roles and responsibilities. In this case, other family members must assume those roles and come to terms with an altered family lifestyle. Family members develop cognitive, emotional, and behavioral coping strategies to live with their loved one who is experiencing a mental disorder. As they take stock of the challenges, constraints, and resources, they are better able to make the most of their options.

Coping strategies protect the affected family member and maintain the stability of family functioning. These strategies include expressing affection, suggesting alternatives, reducing conflict, seeking social support, and trying to make the best of the family members' experiences by focusing on the positive parts of the relationship with the ill family member.

Rose (1997) describes four family support sources:

- Professional support
- Friend support
- Family support
- Spiritual support

Professional support may come from any one or a number of professionals in the community who exhibit a nonblaming and respectful attitude toward families, and who provide information on how to respond to symptoms and help in locating community resources, such as housing or vocational training. **Friend support** comes from non-family members, such as close friends and coworkers. Friend support is most valued when the concern is genuine and stigma is minimized. **Family support** often comes in the form of tangible assistance, such as respite care for family members and physical presence in times of crisis. Many families find emotional strength from their religious faith. They find **spiritual support** as they search for meaning through relationships and feeling connected with others. Supportive relationships build and sustain courage, helping families make the best of their difficult lives.

When families learn to cope effectively, the intense focus on the ill family member lightens as other members, moving through the adjustment process, begin to focus on caring for themselves and reconnecting with others outside the family. The family adapts to its changed circumstances and continues to function successfully.

The final stage of family recovery is personal and political advocacy. This stage involves working with the mental health system to obtain treatment. Family members want to be seen as partners in treatment and do not want to be excluded from discussions and treatment recommendations. Ideally, professionals,

clients, and families all work together in joint problem solving. At times, the issue of client confidentiality is raised. Family members generally respect confidentiality but do need information about treatments, medications, resources, and ways to cope with certain behaviors.

Some families go on to educate the public about mental illness and lobby for improved public policy and legislation, often through the National Alliance on Mental Illness (NAMI), an organization composed of clients, families, and professionals. NAMI actively lobbies for improved legislation and improved health care benefits at local, state, and federal levels.

FAMILY-CENTERED CARE IN PEDIATRIC NURSING

Family-centered care is a philosophy of health care in which a mutually beneficial partnership develops between families, the nurse, and other health professionals as appropriate. In this way the priorities and needs of the family are addressed when the family seeks health care for the child. Each party respects the knowledge, skills, and experience that the other brings to the health care encounter (Table 5–6). This contrasts family-focused care, in which health professionals provide care from the position of an expert. In family-focused care, the expert health professional directs care, tells the family what to do, and intervenes for the child and family as a unit.

TABLE 5–6 Elements of Family-Centered Care and Recommendations for Nursing Practice

ELEMENTS	NURSING PRACTICE RECOMMENDATIONS
Family at the center: Incorporate into policy and practice the recognition that the family is the constant in a child's life, while the service systems and support personnel within those systems fluctuate, and that the illness or injury of a child affects all members of the family system.	■ Establish a therapeutic relationship with the family. ■ Perform a comprehensive family assessment in collaboration with the family, identifying both strengths and needs. ■ Use the family assessment when working with the family to plan, implement, and evaluate care, considering the impact of the child's illness or injury on the entire family, with special attention to the siblings. ■ Provide siblings with information about their sibling's illness/injury at an appropriate developmental level and answer questions honestly. ■ Promote sibling visitation in hospital settings and participation in home care activities. ■ Identify extended family members who should receive information and be included in the educational process.
Family-professional collaboration: Facilitate family professional collaboration at all levels of hospital, home, and community care for the following: ■ Care of an individual child ■ Program development, implementation, evaluation, and evolution ■ Policy formation	■ Develop provider–family relationships that are guided by goals and expectations of both the family and the provider. ■ Ensure that parents are integral and critical collaborators in the decision-making process about their child's care. Involve children and adolescents in the decision-making process as appropriate for their cognitive and emotional development. ■ Assure parents 24-hour access to their children and facilitate their participation in the child's care. ■ Provide parents with the option to stay with their child during procedures and tests, and provide ways for the parent to support the child during the procedure. ■ Provide comfort and hygiene facilities for families who spend long hours at the facility or travel great distances. ■ Promote the family's development of expertise in the special care of their child, fostering family independence and empowerment. ■ Incorporate parents and children into the quality assessment/improvement process. ■ Integrate family members into institutional and community advisory groups and in policy development.

TABLE 5–6 Elements of Family-Centered Care and Recommendations for Nursing Practice (continued)

ELEMENTS	NURSING PRACTICE RECOMMENDATIONS
Family-professional communication: Exchange complete and unbiased information between families and professionals in a supportive manner at all times.	■ Provide information about the child's problem, prognosis, and needs in a manner that respects the child and family as individuals and promotes two-way dialogue. ■ Encourage the family to share information about the child and the illness/injury so that care planning and decisions are made in the most informed and collaborative manner.
Cultural diversity of families: Incorporate into policy and practice the recognition and honoring of cultural diversity, strengths, and individuality within and across all families, including ethnic, racial, spiritual, social, economic, educational, and geographic diversity.	■ Practice family-centered care in a culturally competent manner with respect and sensitivity for the wide range of families with diverse values and beliefs. ■ Seek to understand the family's beliefs and practices related to race, culture, and ethnicity when developing relationships and collaborating in the child's health care. ■ Seek to understand and respect the family's religious/spiritual beliefs and practices and integrate these into the child's care, as the family desires. ■ Assist the family to address care issues related to socioeconomic status, insurance status, geography, and access to health care. ■ Integrate training programs on diversity, cultural understanding, and culturally competent care into staff development programs.
Coping differences and support: Recognize and respect different methods of coping. Implement comprehensive policies and programs that provide families with the developmental, educational, emotional, spiritual, environmental, and financial supports needed to meet their diverse needs.	■ Assess the strengths and weaknesses of the family's coping strategies and its resiliency factors and characteristics. Identify maladaptive coping mechanisms and assist the family to augment its coping efforts. ■ Assess and support the family's needs and desires for support and assist the family in accessing and accepting assistance from support networks as needed or desired.
Family-centered peer support: Encourage and facilitate family-to-family support and networking.	■ Educate parents about parent-to-parent and family support resources and assist them to access such resources in the institution and community. ■ Provide access to psychoeducational groups that might be useful to parents, siblings, or ill/injured children.
Specialized service and support systems: Ensure that hospital, home, and community service and support systems for children needing specialized health and developmental care and their families are flexible, accessible, and comprehensive in responding to diverse family-identified needs.	■ Provide collaborative, flexible, accessible, comprehensive, and coordinated services to children and their families. ■ Provide comprehensive case management/care coordination for children and families with ongoing care needs. ■ Along with families, take an active role in advocating for the needs of ill and injured children.
Holistic perspective of family-centered care: Appreciate families as families and children as children, recognizing that they possess a wider range of strengths, concerns, emotions, and aspirations beyond their need for specialized health and developmental services and support.	■ Encourage attention to the normal developmental needs and developmental tasks of the entire family unit and individual family members. ■ Encourage and facilitate the development of individual and family identities beyond a focus on illness or injury. ■ Facilitate "normalization" as valued and desired by the family.

Source: Reprinted with permission from Burland, J. (1999). NAMI provider education program. Arlington, VA: National Alliance for the Mentally Ill.

Promoting Family-Centered Care

Collaborating with families in providing health care is essential to promoting the best outcome when caring for children. Families have important knowledge to share about their child, their child's health condition, and how their child responds to various actions and events. They also need access to information that will make it possible for them to fully participate in planning and decision making.

PRACTICE ALERT

Some health care facilities are developing family resource centers to provide consumer information and support. In most cases, the resource center is a consumer-oriented health library with staffing, but peer support services may be coordinated through the center as well (Institute for Family Centered Care, 2004). Families can be supported in accessing useful information that helps them become informed decision makers about their child's care. Resources can often be provided in the preferred language and at appropriate reading level.

FOCUS ON DIVERSITY AND CULTURE
Family-Centered Care

When working to establish a family-centered relationship with families of various ethnic groups, consider the possibility that an extended family may need to be consulted. For example, Native Americans may consult tribal elders (considered part of the extended family) before agreeing to health care for their child. In some Hispanic cultures, major decisions for the child's health care include input from grandparents and other extended family members. It is important for the nurse to learn more about the strengths of the family network to better assist the family in planning the child's care at home (Ochieng, 2003).

Parents often need to assess their strengths in managing their ongoing family and caregiving responsibilities before planning how to add more caregiving responsibilities to their routine. Strategies that the nurse and parents collaboratively develop for the child's care must mesh with the family's cultural and ethnic illness-related behaviors, experiences, and beliefs (Sullivan-Bolyai, Sadler, Knafl et al., 2004). The child's opinions should also be integrated in the strategies for care. In almost all cases, the child leaves the health care setting and the family assumes responsibility for providing needed care in the home. The family caregivers must not feel alienated from a health care system they need for continuing assistance. See Box 5–10 for guidelines for effective collaboration.

Family involvement is also valuable in the development of policies and guidelines for family-centered care in all types of health care settings. A family's experiences while receiving care in the health care setting may reveal valuable insights, perspectives, and realities that could lead to improved quality of care and satisfaction with care. Feedback could be provided on such issues as how comfortable they felt in the setting; their understanding of information provided to them; and the attitudes they sensed from health professionals (Hanson & Randall, 1999). Parents who have been supported in developing leadership skills can be empowered to serve on advisory boards or councils representing the family and community perspectives. Guidelines for working with families as advisors and tools for assessing the family-centered policies in various health care settings are available from the Institute of Family-Centered Care.

Parents can also perform a valuable role in family-to-family support networks by serving as mentors to new families entering the health care system for a new chronic condition. In addition, parents may help raise awareness about specific health care issues, serve as advocates for public policy issues, and assist with fundraising activities.

PRACTICE ALERT

When providing care to children, recall that the family is central to all health care interventions with parents and child as the partners in care. It is important to consider how a health care setting's written policies, procedures, and literature for families refer to families and what attitudes these materials convey. Words like *policies, allowed,* and *not permitted* imply that hospital personnel have authority over families in matters concerning their children. Words like *guidelines, working together,* and *welcome* communicate an openness and appreciation for families in the care of their children.

Box 5–10 Guidelines for Effective Collaboration

Parents have a role in developing an effective collaborative relationship with nurses and other health professionals. Parents often become experts in their child's health condition, and learn to advocate for their child. They also must learn to communicate effectively with the health professionals caring for their child, and in the process develop a trusting relationship.

Tips for parents for improved communication follow (Allshouse & Goldberg, 2003):

- Keep a journal that includes your observations about your child's behavior, eating habits, illness, temperature, or anything else that might be helpful to the health care providers caring for your child.
- Keep a copy of your child's medical records, including test and procedure results.
- Write out questions and do not hesitate to ask for clarification if you don't understand an answer provided.
- Be realistic about what you can expect from your child's nurses and doctors. They cannot solve all your problems or answer all your questions. They also can become frustrated at times by a child's condition or lack of answers to questions. Try to let your health care providers know you appreciate their time and efforts on behalf of your child.

Communication tips for nurses include the following:

- Provide information and honestly discuss issues of concern to both the family and health care providers.
- Engage in creative problem solving and identify options for needed care that conform to the family's values and functioning.
- Demonstrate respect for the family's choices and methods for providing needed care.
- Continue to collaborate with the child and family and be willing to continue problem solving as new issues arise.

Source: Ball, J. W., & Bindler, R. C., (2008). *Pediatric nursing: Caring for children* (4th ed., p. 29). Upper Saddle River, NJ: Pearson Education.

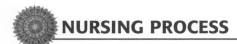

NURSING PROCESS

Assessment

The nurse assesses the family's readiness and ability to provide continued care and supervision at home when warranted. Support for the family is essential. The following information should be considered when performing any family assessment and developing a client's plan of care:

- Cohesiveness and communication patterns within the family
- Family interactions that support self-care
- Number of friends and relatives available
- Family values and beliefs about health and illness
- Cultural and spiritual beliefs
- Developmental level of the client and family

Family History

The family history is a review of the client's family to determine if any genetic or familial patterns of health or illness might shed light on the client's current health status. For example, if the client has a family history of type 1 diabetes, the nurse will question the client closely about signs of the disease. These signs include increased appetite, frequent urination, and weight loss. The family history begins with a review of the immediate family, parents, siblings, children, grandparents, aunts, uncles, and cousins. The nurse should encourage the client to recall as many generations as possible to develop a complete picture. If the client provides data about a genetic or familial disease, it is helpful to interview older members of the family for additional information. Adopted children, spouses, and other individuals living with the client may not be related by blood; however, their health history should be reviewed because the client's concern may have an environmental basis. For example, illnesses may be associated with secondhand smoke in the spouse or child of a smoker, or illness may be associated with exposure to toxins or fumes carried into the home on the clothing of a spouse or family member. The nurse documents information collected from the client and the family in a family genogram. The family genogram, also known as a pedigree or family tree, is the most effective method of recording the large amount of data gathered from a family's health history.

As nurses, we must focus our attention on the family, both as the context for the individual and as the unit of care. It is important to assess and involve families because they are in a position to be affected by and to influence the course of an individual's problems. The questions we ask influence how we view the family. For example, if we ask only about problems, we are likely to "find" problems in the family. On the other hand, if we also include questions about resourcefulness, we have an increased chance of discovering

family competency. Questions shape our experience of and our interactions with clients and families. The following questions are examples for assessing the resourcefulness of the family system:

- What do you hope for in the future?
- How will your life be different when your concerns are no longer problems?
- What strengths, resources, and knowledge do you have to deal with the problems?

Assessment includes gathering information on how partners, parents, and children in the family experience or react to the client's symptoms. Nurses must learn how others are affected by problems and how they have attempted to cope with problems. If we want to know the family, we must listen to its story. The family's story will tell us who the members are and what is meaningful to them. Telling their stories also allows families to make sense of any confusion.

Clients, families, and nurses collaborate to identify the family's strengths, resources, and social support and try to identify problems that might cause stress for any of the family members. Factors in assessing clients and their families include family communication, conflict resolution, boundaries, cohesion, flexibility, emotional availability, leadership patterns, and overall family functionality.

Diagnosis

Data gathered during a family assessment may lead to the following nursing diagnoses:

- Interrupted Family Processes, a change in family relationships
- Readiness for Enhanced Family Coping, effective management of adaptive tasks by family members involved with the client's health challenge, who now exhibits desire and readiness for enhanced health and growth in regard to self and in relation to the client
- Disabled Family Coping, behavior of significant person (family member or other primary person) that disables his or her capacities to effectively address tasks essential to either person's adaptation to the health challenge
- Impaired Parenting, inability of the primary caretaker to create, maintain, or regain an environment that promotes the optimum growth and development of the child
- Impaired Home Maintenance, inability to independently maintain a safe growth-promoting immediate environment
- Caregiver Role Strain, difficulty in performing family caregiver role

Examples of contributing factors for one selected diagnosis, desired outcomes to evaluate the achievement of client goals, and the effectiveness of nursing interventions are listed in Table 5–7.

Planning

Being sensitive to cultural differences is important in assessment and planning care. Knowing who makes most of the decisions in the family, especially in health care, helps the

TABLE 5–7 Identifying Nursing Diagnoses, Outcomes, and Interventions: Clients With Disruption in Family Health

DATA CLUSTER: Mr. and Mrs. G's 6-year-old son has just been diagnosed with acute leukemia. they also have a 9-year-old daughter and a 4-year-old son

NURSING DIAGNOSIS/ DEFINITION	SAMPLE DESIRED OUTCOMES*: DEFINITION	NOC INDICATORS	SELECTED INTERVENTIONS	SAMPLE NIC ACTIVITIES
Interrupted family processes: Change in family relationships	Family coping [2600]: Family actions to manage stressors that tax family resources	Often demonstrated: ■ Involves family members in decision making ■ Uses stress reduction strategies ■ Arranges for respite care	Family integrity promotion [7100]: Promotion of family cohesion and unity Normalization promotion [7200]: Assisting parents and other family members of children with chronic illness or disabilities in providing normal life experiences for their children and families	■ Determine family understanding of illness. ■ Tell family members it is safe and acceptable to use typical expressions of affection. ■ Refer for family therapy as indicated. ■ Deemphasize uniqueness of child's condition. ■ Involve siblings in care and activities of child as appropriate.
	Psychosocial adjustment: Life change [1305]: Adaptive psychosocial response of an individual to a significant life change	Sometimes demonstrated: ■ Sets realistic goals ■ Reports of feeling empowered	Family process maintenance [7130]: Minimization of family process disruption effects	■ Determine typical family processes. ■ Discuss strategies for normalizing family life with family members.

*The NOC# for desired outcomes and the NIC# for nursing interventions are listed in brackets after the appropriate outcome or intervention. Outcomes, indicators, interventions, and activities in this table are only a sample of those suggested by NOC and NIC and should be further individualized for each client.

nurse know to whom to direct questions in order to obtain information and also whom to instruct. The extended family unit is found in many cultures, and different health beliefs and health practices may exist within the family. Older members of the family may continue their traditional practices, whereas younger members may have had more exposure to modern practices. Building a trusting relationship with these families by talking with them about their beliefs and practices is the first step toward planning more effective care.

Nursing needs to focus on assisting the family to plan realistic goals/outcomes and strategies that enhance family functioning, such as improving communication skills, identifying and utilizing support systems, and developing and rehearsing parenting skills. Anticipatory guidance may assist well-functioning families in preparing for predictable developmental transitions that occur in the life of families.

In helping families reintegrate the ill person into the home, nurses use data gathered during family assessment to identify family resources and deficits. By formulating mutually acceptable goals for reintegration, nurses help families cope with the realities of the illness and the changes it may have brought about. Such changes may include new roles and functions of family members or the need to provide continued medical care to the ill or recovering person. Working together, nurses and families can create environments that restore or reorganize family functioning during illness and throughout the recovery process.

Implementation

Nursing interventions are based on the medical diagnoses, nursing diagnoses, and selected goals or outcomes (see Table 5–7).

After carefully planned instruction and practice, families are given an opportunity to demonstrate their ability to provide care under the supportive guidance of the nurse. When the care indicated is beyond the capability of the family, nurses work with families to identify available resources that are socially and financially acceptable.

It is important to remember that standardized teaching plans may not be effective for clients with chronic illness and their families. Rather, these clients and their families should be given the freedom to choose appropriate literature, self-help or support groups, and interactions with others who have the same illness.

Evaluation

In evaluating the success of the family care plan, the nurse assesses for the presence of the indicators identified for the chosen outcomes. If the indicators are present, it is likely that the outcome has been achieved. If the indicators or outcomes are partially or not met, all aspects of the family situation must be reexamined: Have the intervention activities been carried out? Are the indicators and outcomes appropriate? Is the nursing diagnosis proper? Has the medical condition or diagnosis changed?

Recognition of individual and family strengths helps to maintain wellness and also directs behavior in crisis situations. If a plan of care has to be modified to be more effective, these strengths should be identified and utilized.

REVIEW Family Response to Health Alterations

RELATE: LINK THE CONCEPTS

Mrs. Ann Bell, an 82-year-old widow, was diagnosed with Alzheimer's disease several years ago. She lives with her daughter and son-in-law and their two children, aged 16 and 10 years. Mrs. Bell has begun wandering, especially at night, and has started small fires when she attempts to cook and forgets about the pot on the stove. Mrs. Bell's daughter, Laura, accompanies her mother to her physician's appointment today and relates that the stress of caring for her mother, in addition to her other obligations to her family, is becoming increasingly difficult.

Linking the concepts of Advocacy, Cognition, Development, and Ethics with the concept of Family:

1. How can the nurse advocate for this daughter?
2. How can the nurse help the client to improve cognition?
3. What questions would the nurse ask to determine how the presence of their sick grandmother may be impacting the development of the children in the family?
4. What ethical obligations does this daughter have toward the care of her mother?

REFLECT: CASE STUDY

Casey, a 16-year-old, is recuperating from injuries sustained in a motor vehicle crash in which he was the passenger. He was not wearing a seatbelt and experienced a brain injury after striking the windshield. His cognitive and motor functions are impaired. After a 7-day acute care hospital stay, he was moved to an inpatient rehabilitation hospital, where he has been for the past 5 days. He is much more responsive to stimuli and to family members 12 days after his injury. Physical therapy is provided twice a day to promote range of motion and muscle tone and to prevent contractures. Plans are being made to discharge him home with outpatient rehabilitation care within the next 5 days. A case manager will be assigned to coordinate his health care services.

Casey lives with his mother, two half-brothers (10 and 6 years old), and stepfather. Both his mother and stepfather are employed full time and are trying to determine how to manage care for Casey once he returns home. Casey's father has not been actively involved in his life since the divorce 12 years ago. Casey's grandparents reside in the same town and may provide the family some support.

1. What family supports will Casey need as he continues his rehabilitation for the brain injury?
2. What family assessment information is needed to effectively plan nursing care for this adolescent and his family?
3. Does this family have strengths and coping strategies that will help them adapt to Casey's disability?

Casey's family is coping with his initial survival of a serious brain injury, and facing a long rehabilitation process. The family is just now recognizing that life as they have known it is changing. Casey is totally dependent for care, including bathing, toileting, feeding, and mobilizing. While he is expected to regain self-care abilities, the impact of the injury on his cognitive ability and future functioning is unknown.

Casey's extended family has provided support for the family during the past 12 days, but the level of support in the future weeks will decrease because of other family obligations. Casey's mother has already initiated a leave of absence from work so she can care for him when he returns home; however, this will mean the family has reduced income during that time period. Casey's younger brothers have been able to visit him, and they are very anxious because Casey cannot talk with them. They have been trying to avoid bothering their mother and father during this time, but they are wondering when life will be more normal and they can again participate in their usual afterschool activities.

1. What information about the family strengths, needs, and resilience can be identified from the chapter opening scenario, the ecomap on page 000, and the previous information?
2. What additional information would be helpful to know about family strengths and needs prior to developing a nursing care plan?
3. Based on your assessment of the family and challenges facing them, list at least one nursing diagnosis (additional to those listed on page 000) that addresses issues important in planning nursing care for Casey and his family.
4. Describe the use of family-centered care principles in planning Casey's nursing care in collaboration with the family.
5. What potential parenting issues could this family anticipate for Casey and his brothers?

REFERENCES

Alan Guttmacher Institute. (2004). *U.S. teenage pregnancy statistics: Overall trends, trends by race and ethnicity and state-by-state information.* New York: Author.

Allshouse, C., & Goldberg, P. F. (2003). *Working with doctors: A parent's guide to navigating the health system.* Minneapolis, MN: Pacer Center.

American Academy of Pediatrics. (2004). Fathers and pediatricians: Enhancing men's roles in the care and development of their children. *Pediatrics, 113*(5), 1406–1411.

American Academy of Pediatrics Committee on Early Childhood, Adoption, and Dependent Care. (2000). Developmental issues for young children in foster care. *Pediatrics, 106*(5), 1145–1150.

American Academy of Pediatrics Committee on Early Childhood, Adoption, and Dependent Care. (2002). Health care of young children in foster care. *Pediatrics, 109*(3), 536–541.

American Academy of Pediatrics Committee on Hospital Care and the Institute of Family Centered Care. (2003). Family-centered care and the pediatrician's role. *Pediatrics, 112*(3), 691–696.

American Academy of Pediatrics Committee on Psychosocial Aspects of Child and Family Health. (2002). Coparent or second parent adoption by same-sex parents. *Pediatrics, 111*(6), 1541–1571.

American Academy of Pediatrics Task Force on the Family. (2003). Family pediatrics: Report on the Task Force on the Family. *Pediatrics, 111*(6), 1541–1571.

American Nurses Association. (1998). *Culturally competent assessment for family violence.* Washington, DC: American Nurses Association.

American Psychological Association. (2004). *Sexual orientation, parents, and children: APA Policy Statement.* Retrieved May 6, 2006, from http://www.apa.org/pi/lgbc/policy/parents.html

Baumrind, D. (1971). Current patterns of parental authority. *Developmental Psychology, 4,* 1–103.

Biringen, Z. (2000). Emotional availability: Conceptualization and research findings. *American Journal of Orthopsychiatry, 70*(1), 104–114.

Black, C., & Ford-Gilboe, M. (2004). Adolescent mothers: Resilience, family health work and health-promoting practices. *Journal of Advanced Nursing, 48,* 351–360.

Byrd, M., & Garwick, A. (2004). A feminist critique of research on interracial family identity: Implications for family health. *Journal of Family Nursing, 10,* 302–320.

Caldwell, B. M., & Bradley, R. H. (1984). *The home observation for measurement of the environment.* Little Rock: University of Arkansas.

Craig, G. J., & Baucum, D. (2002). *Human development* (9th ed.). Upper Saddle River, NJ: Prentice Hall.

Denham, S. A. (2005). Family structure, function, and process. In S. M. H. Hanson, V. Gedaly-Duff, & J. R. Kaakinen, *Family health care nursing* (3rd ed., pp. 119–156). Philadelphia: F. A. Davis.

Doane, G. H., & Varcoe, C. (2004). *Family nursing as relational inquiry.* Philadelphia: Lippincott Williams & Wilkins.

Dochterman, J., & Bulechek, G. B. (Eds.). (2004). *Nursing interventions classification (NIC)* (4th ed.). St. Louis, MO: Mosby.

Duvall, E.M. (1977). *Marriage and family development* (5th ed.). New York: Harper & Row.

Erikson, E. (1963). *Childhood and society* (2nd ed.). New York: W.W. Norton.

Family and Medical Leave, Public Law 103-3, February 5, 1999. 5 U.S.C. 6381–6387; 5 CFR part 630, subpart L. Retrieved July 9, 2004, from http://www.opm.gov/pca/leave/HTMS/fmlafac2.asp

Fields, J. (2003). *America's families and living arrangements: 2003.* Current Population Reports, P20–553. Washington, DC: U.S. Bureau of the Census.

Friedman, M. M., Bowden, V. R., & Jones, E. G. (2003). *Family nursing: Research, theory and practice* (5th ed.). Upper Saddle River, NJ: Prentice Hall.

Hanson, J. L., & Randall, V. F. (1999). Evaluating and improving the practice of family-centered care. *Pediatric Nursing, 25*(4), 445–449.

Institute for Family Centered Care. (2004). Patient and family resource centers. Retrieved May 7, 2009, from http://www.familycenteredcare.org/advance/topics/pafam-resource.html

Jungbauer, J., Wittmund, B., Dietrich, S., & Angermeyer, M. C. (2003). Subjective burden over 12 months in parents of patients with schizophrenia. *Archives of Psychiatric Nursing, 17*(3), 126–134

Lewandowski, L. A., & Tesler, M. D. (Eds.). (2003). *Family-centered care: Putting it into action. The SPN/ANA guide to family-centered care.* Washington, DC: American Nurses Association.

Locsin, R. C. (2003). Culture perspectives. The integration of family health, culture, and nursing: Prescriptions and practices. *Holistic Nursing Practice, 17*(1), 8–10.

Lugaila, T., & Overturf, J. (2004). *Children and the households they live in: 2000. CENSR-14.* Washington, DC: U.S. Bureau of the Census.

McGuinness, T. M., Noonan, P., & Dyer, J. G. (2005). Family history as a tool for psychiatric nurses. *Archives of Psychiatric Nursing, 19*(3), 116–124.

Meyers, T. A., Eichhorn, D. J., & Guzzetta, C. E. (1998). Do family members want to be present during CPR? A retrospective study. *Journal of Emergency Nursing, 24*(5), 400–405.

Moorhead, S., Johnson, M., & Maas, M. (Eds.). (2004). *Nursing outcomes classification (NOC)* (3rd ed.). St. Louis, MO: Mosby.

Munro, H., & D'Errico, C. (2000). Parental involvement in perioperative anesthetic management. *Journal of PeriAnesthesia Nursing, 15*(6), 397–400.

NANDA International. (2007). *NANDA nursing diagnoses: Definitions and classification 2007–2008.* Philadelphia: NANDA.

Ochieng, B. M. N. (2003). Minority ethnic families and family-centered care. *Journal of Child Health Care, 7*(2), 123–132.

Olson, D. H. (1996). Clinical assessment and treatment interventions using the family circumplex model. In F. W. Kaslow (Ed.), *Handbook of relational diagnosis and dysfunctional family patterns* (pp. 59–77). New York: John Wiley & Sons.

Peterson, K. S. (2003, September 18). Unmarried with children: For better or worse? *USA Today*, pp. 1A, 8A.

Powers, K. S., & Rubenstein, J. S. (1999). Family presence during invasive procedures in pediatric intensive care unit: A prospective study. *Archives of Pediatric and Adolescent Medicine, 153,* 955–958.

Rigazio-DiGilio, S. A. (2005). *Community genograms: Using individual, family, and cultural narratives with clients.* New York: Teacher's College Press.

Rose, L. E. (1997). Caring for caregivers: Perceptions of social support. *Journal of Psychosocial Nursing, 35* (2), 17–24.

Rose, L. E., Mallinson, R. K., & Gerson, L. D. (2006). Mastery, burden and areas of concern among family caregivers of mentally ill persons. *Archives of Psychiatric Nursing, 20*(1), 41–51.

Sacchetti, A., Paston, C., & Carraccio, C. (2005). Family members do not disrupt care when present during invasive procedures. *Academic Emergency Medicine, 12*(5), 477–479.

Sgarbossa, D., & Ford-Gilboe, M. (2004). Mother's friendship quality, parental support, quality of life, and family health work in families led by adolescent mothers with preschool children. *Journal of Family Nursing, 10,* 232–261.

Stengler-Wenzke, K., Trosbach, J., Dietrich, S., & Angermeyer, M. C. (2004). Experience of stigmatization of relatives of patients with obsessive compulsive disorder. *Archives of Psychiatric Nursing, 18*(3),88–96.

Sullivan-Bolyai, S., Sadler, L., Knafl, K. A., & Gillis, C. L. (2004). Great expectations: A position description for parents as caregivers: Part II. *Pediatric Nursing, 30*(1), 52–56.

Tweedell, D., Forchuk, C., Jewell, J., & Steinnagel, L. (2004). Families' experience during recovery of nonrecovery from psychosis. *Archives of Psychiatric Nursing, 18*(1), 17–25.

U.S. Census Bureau. (2002). Living arrangements of children under 18 years of age: 1960 to present. Retrieved May 6, 2009, from http://www.census.gov/population/socdemo/hh-fam/cps2002/tabC3-all.pdf

U.S. Census Bureau. (2004). *"Stay-at-home" parents top 5 million.* Washington, DC: Author. Retrieved May 6, 2009, from http://www.census.gov/Press-Release/www/releases/archives/families_households/003118.html

U.S. Census Bureau (2006). *Definition: Household and family.* Retrieved May 6, 2009, from http://www.census.gov/population/www/cps/cpsdef.html

U.S. Conference of Mayors. (2004). *A status report on hunger and homelessness in America's cities: 2004.* Retrieved May 5, 2006, from http://www.usmayors.org/uscm/us_mayor_newspaper/documents/01_10_05/hunger_survey.asp

U.S. Department of Health and Human Services. (2001). Indicators of welfare reform. Annual Report to Congress 2001. Table Birth 4. Washington, DC: Author.

Urban Institute. (2003). *Gay and lesbian families in the Census: Couples with children.* Washington, DC: Author. Retrieved January 28, 2004, from http://www.urban.org

von Bertalanffy, L. (1980). *General system theory* (revised from original 1969). New York: George Braziller.

Wilkerson, S. A., & Loveland-Cherry, C. J. (2004). Johnson's behavioral system model. In J. J. Fitzpatrick & A. L. Whall (Eds.), *Conceptual models of nursing: Analysis and application* (4th ed., pp. 83–103). Upper Saddle River, NJ: Prentice Hall Health.

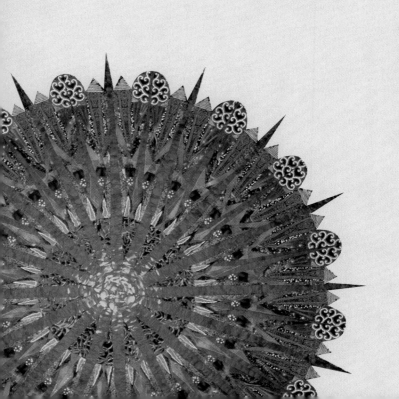

Fluids and Electrolytes

6

Concept at-a-Glance

Concept Learning Outcomes

After reading about this concept, you will be able to do the following:

1. Discuss the function, distribution, movement, regulation and importance of fluids and electrolytes in the body.
2. Identify factors affecting normal body fluids and electrolytes and recognize normal fluid and electrolyte balance in individuals.
3. Collect assessment data related to the client's fluid and electrolyte balances.
4. Describe normal fluid and electrolyte status for children at various ages.
5. Identify regulatory mechanisms for fluid and electrolyte balance.
6. Describe conditions for which intravenous fluid therapy may be indicated.
7. Explain how changes in the osmolality or tonicity of a fluid can cause water to move to a different compartment.
8. Explain the pharmacotherapy of fluid and electrolyte imbalance.
9. Compare the use of colloids and crystalloids in intravenous therapy.

Concept Key Terms

About Fluids and Electrolytes

The body is largely composed of fluid in many forms. Blood, serum, saline, albumin, urine, bile, hormones, cerebrospinal fluid—these are just a few of the fluids required for homeostasis, the delicate balance of fluids and electrolytes that promotes the body's functions.

Within each of these fluids are **electrolytes**, charged ions capable of conducting electricity, in various concentrations and combinations. Learning what fluids contain specific electrolytes can help you identify causes of electrolyte imbalances in clients. This will allow you to specifically design care to restore homeostasis.

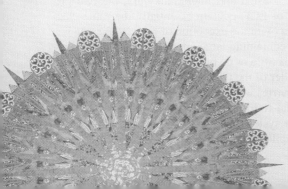

Homeostasis depends on multiple physiologic processes. Fluid and electrolyte balance is critical to maintaining good health. Fluid and electrolyte imbalance can result in a variety of conditions, such as dehydration and renal failure, and can also impact both chronic and acute illnesses. In turn, almost every illness has the potential to threaten this crucial balance. Even in daily living, excessive temperatures or vigorous activity can disturb the balance if adequate intake of water and salt is not maintained. Therapeutic measures can also disturb the body's homeostasis unless water and electrolytes are replaced. ●

NORMAL PRESENTATION

The proportion of the human body composed of fluid is surprisingly large. Approximately 60% of the average healthy adult's weight is water, the primary body fluid. In good health, this volume remains relatively constant and the person's weight varies by less than 0.2 kg (0.5 lb) in 24 hours, regardless of the amount of fluid ingested.

Water is vital to health and normal cellular function, serving as

- a medium for metabolic reactions within cells;
- transporter for nutrients, waste products, and other substances;
- a lubricant;
- an insulator and shock absorber;
- one means of regulating and maintaining body temperature.

Age, sex, and body fat affect total body water. Infants have the highest proportion of water, accounting for 70–80% of their body weight. The proportion of body water decreases with aging. In people older than 60 years of age, water represents only about 50% of the total body weight. Women also have a lower percentage of body water than men. Women and older adults have reduced body water due to lower muscle mass and a greater percentage of fat tissue. Fat tissue is essentially free of water, whereas lean tissue contains a significant amount of water. Water makes up a greater percentage of a lean person's body weight than that of an obese person.

Distribution and Composition of Body Fluids

The body's fluid is divided into two major compartments, intracellular and extracellular.

Both of these contain oxygen from the lungs, dissolved nutrients from the gastrointestinal tract, excretory products of metabolism such as carbon dioxide, and charged particles called **ions**. The composition of fluids varies from one body compartment to another.

Many salts dissociate in water; that is, they break up into electrically charged ions. The salt sodium chloride breaks up into one ion of sodium (Na^+) and one ion of chloride (Cl^-). These charged particles are called electrolytes because they are capable of conducting electricity. The number of ions that carry a positive charge, called **cations**, and ions that carry a negative charge, called **anions**, should be equal. Examples of cations are sodium (Na^+), potassium (K^+), calcium (Ca^{2+}), and magnesium (Mg^{2+}). Examples of

anions are chloride (Cl^-), bicarbonate HCO_3^-, phosphate HPO_4^{2-}, and sulfate SO_4^{2-}.

Electrolytes generally are measured in milliequivalents per liter of water (mEq/L) or milligrams per 100 mL (mg/100 mL). The term **milliequivalent** refers to the chemical combining power of the ion, or the capacity of cations to combine with anions to form molecules. This combining activity is measured in relation to the combining activity of the hydrogen ion (H^+). Thus, 1 mEq of any anion equals 1 mEq of any cation. Clinically, the milliequivalent system is most often used. However, nurses need to be aware that different systems of measurement may be found when interpreting laboratory results. For example, calcium levels frequently are reported in milligrams per deciliter (1 dL = 100 mL) instead of milliequivalents per liter. It also is important to remember that laboratory tests are usually performed using blood plasma, an extracellular fluid. Although these results may reflect what is happening in the ECF, it generally is not possible to directly measure electrolyte concentrations within the cell.

INTRACELLULAR FLUID Intracellular fluid (ICF) is found within the cells of the body. It constitutes approximately two-thirds of the total body fluid in adults.

Intracellular fluid is vital to normal cell functioning. It contains **solutes** (substances that dissolve in liquid) such as oxygen, electrolytes, and glucose, and provides a medium in which metabolic processes of the cell take place.

The composition of intracellular fluid differs significantly from that of extracellular fluid (ECF). Potassium and magnesium are the primary cations present in ICF, and phosphate and sulfate the major anions. As in ECF, other electrolytes are present within the cell, but in much smaller concentrations (Figure 6–1 ■).

EXTRACELLULAR FLUID Extracellular fluid (ECF) is found outside the cells and accounts for about one-third of total body fluid. It is subdivided into compartments. The two main compartments of ECF are intravascular and interstitial. **Intravascular fluid**, or plasma, accounts for approximately 20% of the ECF and is found within the vascular system. **Interstitial fluid**, accounting for approximately 75% of the ECF, surrounds the cells. The other compartments of ECF are the lymph and transcellular fluids. Examples of **transcellular fluid** are cerebrospinal, pericardial, pancreatic, pleural, intraocular, biliary, peritoneal, and synovial fluids.

In extracellular fluid, the principal electrolytes are sodium, chloride, and bicarbonate. Other electrolytes such as potassium, calcium, and magnesium are also present but in much smaller quantities. Plasma and interstitial fluid, the two primary components of ECF, contain essentially the same electrolytes and solutes, with the exception of protein. Plasma is a protein-rich fluid, containing large amounts of albumin; interstitial fluid contains little or no protein. Although extracellular fluid is in the smaller of the two compartments, it is the transport system that carries nutrients to and waste products from the cells. Interstitial fluid transports wastes from the cells by way of the lymph system as well as directly into the blood plasma through capillaries.

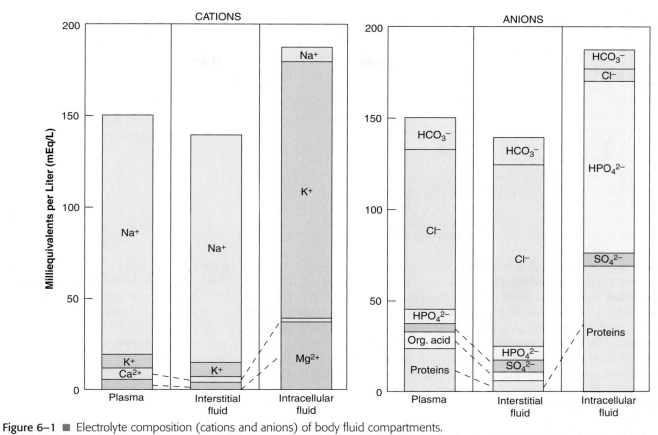

Figure 6–1 ■ Electrolyte composition (cations and anions) of body fluid compartments.

Maintaining a balance of fluid volumes and electrolyte compositions in the fluid compartments of the body is essential to health. Normal and unusual fluid and electrolyte losses must be replaced if homeostasis is to be maintained (Box 6–1).

Other body fluids such as gastric and intestinal secretions also contain electrolytes. Excessive loss of these fluids from the body (for example, with severe vomiting or diarrhea or when gastric suction removes the gastric secretions) is of particular concern, as fluid and electrolyte imbalances can result. Table 6–1 shows electrolyte concentrations in body fluid compartments.

Movement of Body Fluids

The body fluid compartments are separated from one another by cell membranes and the capillary membrane. While these membranes are completely permeable to water, they are considered to be selectively permeable to solutes as substances move across them with varying degrees of ease. Small particles such as ions, oxygen, and carbon dioxide move easily across these membranes, but larger molecules such as glucose and proteins have more difficulty moving between fluid compartments. The methods by which electrolytes and other solutes move are osmosis, diffusion, filtration, and active transport.

OSMOSIS **Osmosis** is the movement of water across cell membranes, from the less concentrated solution to the more concentrated solution (Figure 6–2 ■). In other words, water moves toward the higher concentration of solute in an attempt to equalize the concentrations.

Solutes may be **crystalloids** (salts that dissolve readily into true solutions) or **colloids** (substances such as large protein molecules that do not readily dissolve into true solutions). A

Box 6–1 **Linking Concepts**

Fluid and electrolyte imbalance is critical to maintaining homeostasis. Just two examples of the important role that fluids and electrolytes play are given here.

Fluids, Electrolytes, and Cognition

Imbalance of fluids and electrolytes can severely affect cognition. Moderate to severe dehydration can result in confusion in the healthiest adult. Fluid and electrolyte imbalance can also be a factor in delirium, and best practice dictates that fluid and electrolyte levels be assessed through diagnostic testing when a patient presents with symptoms of delirium.

Fluids, Electrolytes, and Perfusion

Clients with imbalance in fluid and electrolytes, particularly fluid and sodium, may increase intravascular fluid content resulting in stress on the cardiovascular system. Clients with perfusion disorders are frequently placed on medications that can cause a fluid and/or electrolyte imbalance.

TABLE 6–1 Electrolyte Concentrations in Body Fluid Compartments

COMPONENTS	EXTRACELLULAR FLUID (ECF)		INTRACELLULAR FLUID (ICF)
	VASCULAR	INTERSTITIAL	
Na+	High	High	Low
K+	Low	Low	High
Ca++	Low	Low	Low (higher than ECF)
Mg++	Low	Low	High
Pi	Low	Low	High
Cl-	High	High	Low
Proteins	High	Low	High

Source: Ball, J.W., & Bindler, R.C.(2008). *Pediatric Nursing: Caring for Children* (4th ed.) Upper Saddle River, NJ: Pearson, Inc.

solvent is the component of a solution that can dissolve a solute. An example of the solute/solvent relationship is sugar added to coffee: Sugar is the solute and coffee is the solvent.

In the body, water is the solvent; the solutes include electrolytes, oxygen and carbon dioxide, glucose, urea, amino acids, and proteins. Osmosis occurs when the concentration of solutes is higher on one side of a selectively permeable membrane, such as the capillary membrane, than on the other side. For example, a marathon runner loses a significant amount of water through perspiration, increasing the concentration of solutes in the plasma because of water loss. This higher solute concentration draws water from the interstitial space and cells into the vascular compartment to equalize the concentration of solutes in all fluid compartments. Osmosis is an important mechanism for maintaining homeostasis and fluid balance.

The concentration of solutes in body fluids is usually expressed as the **osmolality**. Osmolality is determined by the total solute concentration within a fluid compartment and is measured as parts of solute per kilogram of water.

Osmolality is reported as milliosmols per kilogram (mOsm/kg). Sodium is by far the greatest determinant of osmolality, with glucose and urea also contributing. Potassium,

glucose, and urea are the primary contributors to the osmolality of intracellular fluid. The term **tonicity** may be used to refer to the osmolality of a solution. Solutions may be termed isotonic, hypertonic, or hypotonic. An **isotonic** solution has the same osmolality as body fluids. Normal **saline**, 0.9% sodium chloride, is an isotonic solution. **Hypertonic** solutions have a higher osmolality than body fluids; 3% sodium chloride is a hypertonic solution. **Hypotonic** solutions such as one-half normal saline (0.45% sodium chloride), by contrast, have a lower osmolality than body fluids.

Osmotic pressure is the power of a solution to draw water across a semipermeable membrane. When two solutions of different solute concentrations are separated by a semipermeable membrane, the solution of higher solute concentration exerts a higher osmotic pressure, drawing water across the membrane to equalize the concentrations of the solutions. For example, infusing a hypertonic intravenous solution such as 3% sodium chloride will draw fluid out of red blood cells (RBCs), causing them to shrink. On the other hand, a hypotonic solution administered intravenously will cause the RBCs to swell as water is drawn into the cells by their higher osmotic pressure. In the body, plasma proteins exert an osmotic draw called **colloid osmotic pressure** or **oncotic pressure**, pulling water from the interstitial space into the vascular compartment. This is an important mechanism in maintaining vascular volume.

DIFFUSION **Diffusion** is the continual intermingling of molecules in liquids, gases, or solids brought about by the random movement of the molecules. For example, two gases become mixed by the constant motion of their molecules. The process of diffusion occurs even when two substances are separated by a thin membrane. In the body, diffusion of water, electrolytes, and other substances occurs through the "split pores" of capillary membranes.

The rate of diffusion of substances varies according to (a) the size of the molecules, (b) the concentration of the solution, and (c) the temperature of the solution. Larger molecules move less quickly than smaller ones because they require more energy to move about. With diffusion, the molecules move from a solution of higher concentration to a

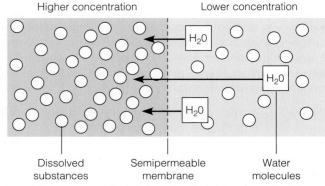

Higher concentration   Lower concentration

Dissolved substances   Semipermeable membrane   Water molecules

Figure 6–2 ■ Osmosis: Water molecules move from the less concentrated area to the more concentrated area in an attempt to equalize the concentration of solutions on two sides of a membrane.

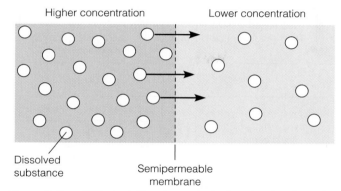

Higher concentration   Lower concentration

Dissolved substance

Semipermeable membrane

Figure 6–3 ■ Diffusion: The movement of molecules through a semipermeable membrane from an area of higher concentration to an area of lower concentration.

solution of lower concentration (Figure 6–3 ■). Increases in temperature increase the rate of motion of molecules and therefore the rate of diffusion.

FILTRATION **Filtration** is a process whereby fluid and solutes move together across a membrane from one compartment to another. The movement is from an area of higher pressure to one of lower pressure. An example of filtration is the movement of fluid and nutrients from the capillaries of the arterioles to the interstitial fluid around the cells. The pressure in the compartment that results in the movement of the fluid and substances dissolved in fluid out of the compartment is called filtration pressure. **Hydrostatic pressure** is the pressure a fluid exerts within a closed system on the walls of its container. The hydrostatic pressure of blood is the force blood exerts against the vascular walls (e.g., the artery walls). The principle involved in hydrostatic pressure is that fluids move from the area of greater pressure to the area of lesser pressure. Using the example of the blood vessels, the plasma proteins in the blood exert a colloid osmotic or oncotic pressure (see the earlier section on Osmosis) that opposes the hydrostatic pressure and holds the fluid in the vascular compartment to maintain the vascular volume. When the hydrostatic pressure is greater than the osmotic pressure, the fluid filters out of the blood vessels. The filtration pressure

in this example is the difference between the hydrostatic pressure and the osmotic pressure (Figure 6–4 ■).

ACTIVE TRANSPORT Substances can move across cell membranes from a less concentrated solution to a more concentrated one by **active transport** (Figure 6–5 ■). This process differs from diffusion and osmosis in that metabolic energy is expended. In active transport, a substance combines with a carrier on the outside surface of the cell membrane, and together they move to the inside surface of the cell membrane. Once inside, they separate, and the substance is released to the inside of the cell. Each substance requires a specific carrier; active transport requires enzymes; and energy is expended.

Active transport is particularly important in maintaining the differences in sodium and potassium ion concentrations of ECF and ICF. Under normal conditions, sodium concentrations are higher in the extracellular fluid, and potassium concentrations are higher inside the cells. To maintain these proportions, the active transport mechanism (the sodium-potassium pump) is activated, moving sodium from the cells and potassium into the cells.

Regulating Body Fluids

In a healthy person, the volumes and chemical composition of the fluid compartments stay within narrow, safe limits. Normally, fluid intake and fluid loss are balanced. Illness can upset this balance so that the body has too little or too much fluid. Fluid imbalance can result in a number of illnesses and conditions. The most common example is probably **dehydration**, a condition that occurs when a body does not take in as much water as it loses or lacks sufficient reserves to maintain proper function.

FLUID INTAKE During periods of moderate activity at moderate temperature, the average adult drinks about 1,500 mL per day but needs 2,500 mL per day, an additional 1,000 mL. This added volume is acquired from foods and the oxidation of these foods during metabolic processes. Interestingly, the water content of food is relatively large, contributing about 750 mL per day. The water content of fresh vegetables is approximately 90%, of fresh fruits about 85%, and of lean meats around 60%.

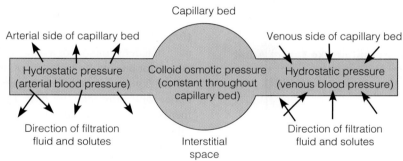

Capillary bed

Arterial side of capillary bed

Venous side of capillary bed

Hydrostatic pressure (arterial blood pressure)

Colloid osmotic pressure (constant throughout capillary bed)

Hydrostatic pressure (venous blood pressure)

Direction of filtration fluid and solutes

Interstitial space

Direction of filtration fluid and solutes

Figure 6–4 ■ Schematic of filtration pressure changes within a capillary bed. On the arterial side, arterial blood pressure exceeds colloid osmotic pressure, so that water and dissolved substances move out of the capillary into the interstitial space. On the venous side, venous blood pressure is less than colloid osmotic pressure, so that water and dissolved substances move into the capillary.

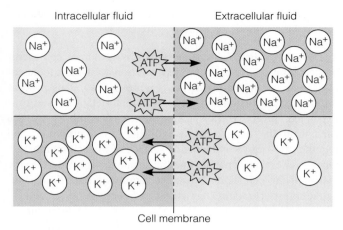

Figure 6–5 ■ An example of active transport. Energy (ATP) is used to move sodium molecules and potassium molecules and across a semipermeable membrane against sodium's and potassium's concentration gradients (i.e., from areas of lesser concentration to areas of greater concentration).

Water as a byproduct of food metabolism accounts for most of the remaining fluid volume required. This quantity is approximately 200 mL per day for the average adult (Table 6–2).

The thirst mechanism is the primary regulator of fluid intake. The thirst center is located in the hypothalamus of the brain. A number of stimuli trigger this center, including the osmotic pressure of body fluids, vascular volume, and angiotensin (a hormone released in response to decreased blood flow to the kidneys). For example, a long-distance runner loses significant amounts of water through perspiration and rapid breathing during a race, increasing the concentration of solutes and the osmotic pressure of body fluids. This increased osmotic pressure stimulates the thirst center, causing the runner to experience the sensation of thirst and the desire to drink to replace lost fluids.

Thirst is normally relieved immediately after drinking a small amount of fluid, even before it is absorbed from the gastrointestinal tract. However, this relief is only temporary, and the thirst returns in about 15 minutes. The thirst is again temporarily relieved after the ingested fluid distends the upper gastrointestinal tract. These mechanisms protect the individual

TABLE 6–2 Average Daily Fluid Intake for an Adult

SOURCE	AMOUNT (ML)
Oral fluids	1,200–1,500
Water in foods	1,000
Water as by-product of food metabolism	200
Total	2,400–2,700

Source: Berman, A., Snyder, S.J., Kozier, B., & Erb, G. (2008). *Kozier & Erb's Fundamentals of Nursing: Concepts, Process, and Practice* (8th ed.). Upper Saddle River, NJ: Pearson, Inc.

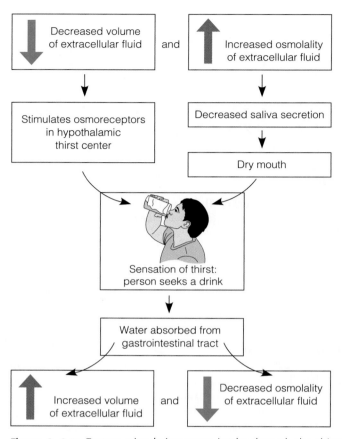

Figure 6–6 ■ Factors stimulating water intake through the thirst mechanism.

from drinking too much, because it takes from 30 minutes to 1 hour for the fluid to be absorbed and distributed throughout the body. See Figure 6–6 ■.

FLUID OUTPUT Fluid losses from the body counterbalance the adult's 2,500-mL average daily intake of fluid, as shown in Table 6–3. There are four routes of fluid output:

1. Urine
2. Insensible loss through the skin as perspiration and through the lungs as water vapor in the expired air
3. Noticeable loss through the skin
4. Loss through the intestines in feces

Urine Urine formed by the kidneys and excreted from the urinary bladder is the major avenue of fluid output. Normal urine output for an adult is 1,400–1,500 mL per 24 hours, or at least 0.5 mL/kg per hour. In healthy people, urine output may vary noticeably from day to day. Urine volume automatically increases as fluid intake increases. If fluid loss through perspiration is large, however, urine volume decreases to maintain fluid balance in the body.

Insensible Losses **Insensible fluid loss** occurs through the skin and lungs. It is called insensible because it is usually not noticeable and cannot be measured. Insensible fluid loss

TABLE 6–3 Average Daily Fluid Output for an Adult

ROUTE	AMOUNT (ML)
Urine	1,400–1,500
Insensible losses	
Lungs	350–400
Skin	350–400
Sweat	100
Feces	100–200
Total	2,300–2,600

Source: Berman, A., Snyder, S.J., Kozier, B., & Erb, G. (2008). *Kozier & Erb's Fundamentals of Nursing: Concepts, Process, and Practice* (8th ed.). Upper Saddle River, NJ: Pearson, Inc.

through the skin occurs in two ways. Water is lost through diffusion and perspiration (which is noticeable but not measurable). Water losses through diffusion are not noticeable but normally account for 300–400 mL per day. This loss can be significantly increased if the protective layer of the skin is lost due to burns or large abrasions. Perspiration varies depending on factors such as environmental temperature and metabolic activity. Fever and exercise increase metabolic activity and heat production, thereby increasing fluid losses through the skin.

Another type of insensible loss is the water in exhaled air. In an adult, this is normally 300–400 mL per day. When respiratory rate accelerates due to changes such as exercise or an elevated body temperature, this loss can increase.

Feces The chyme that passes from the small intestine into the large intestine contains water and electrolytes. The volume of chyme entering the large intestine in an adult is normally about 1,500 mL per day. Of this amount, all but about 100 mL is reabsorbed in the proximal half of the large intestine.

Certain fluid losses are required to maintain normal body function. These are known as **obligatory losses**. An adult must excrete approximately 500 mL of fluid through the kidneys each day to eliminate metabolic waste products from the body. Losses of water through respirations, through the skin, and in feces are also obligatory losses, necessary for temperature regulation and elimination of waste products. The total of all these losses is approximately 1,300 mL per day.

MAINTAINING HOMEOSTASIS The volume and composition of body fluids are regulated through several homeostatic mechanisms. The body's systems work together to contribute to this regulation. As the kidneys regulate and filter waste, they return electrolytes such as potassium and sodium back to the blood for use. The cardiovascular and respiratory systems ensure the body has adequate oxygen to function and use fluids and electrolytes appropriately. The immune system destroys foreign particles and pathogens that can undermine homeostasis. Hormones such as antidiuretic hormone (ADH; also known as arginine vasopressin or AVP), the renin-angiotensin-aldosterone system, and atrial natriuretic factor

are involved, as are mechanisms to monitor and maintain vascular volume.

Illness or injury to any one system can negatively impact homeostasis. Some illnesses and diseases, such as cancers, impact homeostasis directly by their very presence in the body. They also impact homeostasis indirectly by the nature of the treatments required to rid the body of the illness itself. Chemotherapy, which can wreak havoc on fluid and electrolyte balance, is a prime example of such a treatment.

Kidneys The kidneys are the primary regulator of body fluids and electrolyte balance. They regulate the volume and osmolality of extracellular fluids by regulating water and electrolyte excretion. The kidneys adjust the reabsorption of water from plasma filtrate and ultimately the amount excreted as urine. Although 135–180 L of plasma per day is normally filtered in an adult, only about 1.5 L of urine is excreted. Electrolyte balance is maintained by selective retention and excretion by the kidneys. The kidneys also play a significant role in acid-base regulation, excreting hydrogen ion (H^+) and retaining bicarbonate.

Antidiuretic Hormone Antidiuretic hormone, which regulates water excretion from the kidney, is synthesized in the anterior portion of the hypothalamus and acts on the collecting ducts of the nephrons. When serum osmolality rises, ADH is produced, causing the collecting ducts to become more permeable to water. This increased permeability allows more water to be reabsorbed into the blood. As more water is reabsorbed, urine output falls and serum osmolality decreases because the water dilutes body fluids. Conversely, if serum osmolality decreases, ADH is suppressed, the collecting ducts become less permeable to water, and urine output increases. Excess water is excreted, and serum osmolality returns to normal. Other factors also affect the production and release of ADH, including blood volume, temperature, pain, stress, and some drugs such as opiates, barbiturates, and nicotine. (See Figure 6–7 ■.)

Renin-Angiotensin-Aldosterone System Specialized receptors in the juxtaglomerular cells of the kidney nephrons respond to changes in renal perfusion. This initiates the renin-angiotensin-aldosterone system. If blood flow or pressure to the kidney decreases, renin is released. Renin causes the conversion of angiotensinogen to angiotensin I, which is then converted to angiotensin II by angiotensin-converting enzyme. Angiotensin II acts directly on the nephrons to promote sodium and water retention. In addition, it stimulates the release of aldosterone from the adrenal cortex. Aldosterone also promotes sodium retention in the distal nephron. The net effect of the renin-angiotensin-aldosterone system is to restore blood volume (and renal perfusion) through sodium and water retention.

Atrial Natriuretic Factor Atrial natriuretic factor (ANF) is a peptide-hormone released from cells in the atrium of the heart in response to excess blood volume and stretching of the atrial walls. Acting on the nephrons, ANF promotes sodium wasting and acts as a potent diuretic, thus reducing vascular volume. ANF also inhibits thirst, reducing fluid intake.

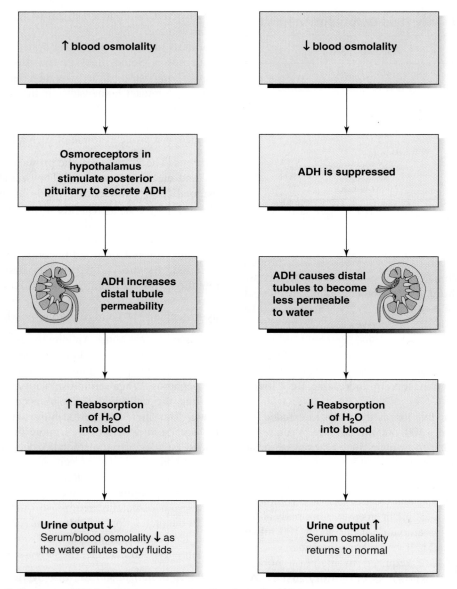

Figure 6–7 ■ Antidiuretic hormone (ADH) regulates water excretion from the kidneys.

Regulating Electrolytes

Electrolytes are present in all body fluids and fluid compartments. Just as maintaining the fluid balance is vital to normal body function, so is maintaining electrolyte balance. Although the concentration of specific electrolytes differs between fluid compartments, a balance of cations (positively charged ions) and anions (negatively charged ions) always exists. Electrolytes are important for the following:

■ Maintaining fluid balance
■ Contributing to acid–base regulation
■ Facilitating enzyme reactions
■ Transmitting neuromuscular reactions

Most electrolytes enter the body through dietary intake and are excreted in the urine. The body does not store some electrolytes, such as sodium and chloride, which must be consumed daily to maintain normal levels. Potassium and calcium,

on the other hand, are stored in the cells and bone, respectively. When serum levels drop, ions can shift out of the storage "pool" into the blood to maintain adequate serum levels for normal functioning. The regulatory mechanisms and functions of the major electrolytes are summarized in Table 6–4.

SODIUM (NA⁺) Sodium is the most abundant cation in extracellular fluid and a major contributor to serum osmolality. Normal serum sodium levels are 135–145 mEq/L. Sodium functions largely in controlling and regulating water balance. When sodium is reabsorbed from the kidney tubules, chloride and water are reabsorbed with it, thus maintaining ECF volume. Sodium is found in many foods including bacon, ham, processed and canned foods and processed cheeses, and table salt.

POTASSIUM (K⁺) Potassium is the major cation in intracellular fluids, with only a small amount found in plasma and interstitial fluid. ICF levels of potassium are usually 125–140 mEq/L,

TABLE 6–4 Regulation and Functions of Electrolytes

ELECTROLYTE	REGULATION	FUNCTION
Sodium (Na^+)	■ Renal reabsorption or excretion ■ Aldosterone increases Na^+ reabsorption in collecting duct of nephrons	■ Regulating ECF volume and distribution ■ Maintaining blood volume ■ Transmitting nerve impulses and contracting muscles
Potassium (K^+)	■ Renal excretion and conservation ■ Aldosterone increases K^+ excretion ■ Movement into and out of cells ■ Insulin helps move K^+ into cells; tissue damage and acidosis shift K^+ out of cells into ECF	■ Maintaining ICF osmolality ■ Transmitting nerve and other electrical impulses ■ Regulating cardiac impulse transmission and muscle contraction ■ Skeletal and smooth muscle function ■ Regulating acid–base balance
Calcium (Ca^{2+})	■ Redistribution between bones and ECF ■ Parathyroid hormone and calcitriol increase serum Ca^{2+} levels; calcitonin decreases serum levels	■ Forming bones and teeth ■ Transmitting nerve impulses ■ Regulating muscle contractions ■ Maintaining cardiac pacemaker (automaticity) ■ Blood clotting ■ Activating enzymes such as pancreatic lipase and phospholipase
Magnesium (Mg^{2+})	■ Conservation and excretion by kidneys ■ Intestinal absorption increased by vitamin D and parathyroid hormone	■ Intracellular metabolism ■ Operating sodium-potassium pump ■ Relaxing muscle contractions ■ Transmitting nerve impulses ■ Regulating cardiac function
Chloride (Cl^-)	■ Excreted and reabsorbed along with sodium in the kidneys ■ Aldosterone increases chloride reabsorption with sodium	■ HCl production ■ Regulating ECF balance and vascular volume ■ Regulating acid–base balance ■ Buffer in oxygen–carbon dioxide exchange in RBCs
Phosphate (PO_4^-)	■ Excretion and reabsorption by the kidneys ■ Parathyroid hormone decreases serum levels by increasing renal excretion ■ Reciprocal relationship with calcium: increasing serum calcium levels decrease phosphate levels; decreasing serum calcium increases phosphate	■ Forming bones and teeth ■ Metabolizing carbohydrate, protein, and fat ■ Cellular metabolism; producing ATP and DNA ■ Muscle, nerve, and RBC function ■ Regulating acid–base balance ■ Regulating calcium levels
Bicarbonate (HCO_3^-)	■ Excretion and reabsorption by the kidneys ■ Regeneration by kidneys	■ Major body buffer involved in acid–base regulation

Source: Berman, A., Snyder, S.J., Kozier, B., & Erb, G. (2008). *Kozier & Erb's Fundamentals of Nursing: Concepts, Process, and Practice* (8th ed.). Upper Saddle River, NJ: Pearson, Inc.

whereas normal serum potassium levels are 3.5–5.0 mEq/L. The ratio of intracellular to extracellular potassium must be maintained for neuromuscular response to stimuli. Potassium is a vital electrolyte for skeletal, cardiac, and smooth muscle activity. It is involved in maintaining acid–base balance as well, and it contributes to intracellular enzyme reactions. Potassium must be ingested daily because the body does not conserve it. Many fruits and vegetables, meat, fish, and other foods contain potassium.

CALCIUM (CA²⁺) The vast majority, 99%, of calcium in the body is in the skeletal system, with a relatively small amount in extracellular fluid. Although this calcium outside the bones and teeth amounts to only about 1% of the total calcium in the body, it is vital in regulating muscle contraction and relaxation, neuromuscular function, and cardiac function. ECF calcium is regulated by a complex interaction of parathyroid hormone, calcitonin, and calcitriol, a metabolite of vitamin D. When calcium levels in the ECF fall, parathyroid hormone and calcitriol cause calcium to be released from bones into ECF and increase the absorption of calcium in the intestines, thus raising serum calcium levels. Conversely, calcitonin stimulates the deposition of calcium in bone, reducing the concentration of calcium ions in the blood.

With aging, the intestines absorb calcium less effectively and more calcium is excreted via the kidneys. Calcium shifts out of the bone to replace these ECF losses, increasing the risk of osteoporosis and fractures of the wrists, vertebrae, and hips. Lack of weight-bearing exercise (which helps keep calcium in the bones) and vitamin D deficiency (usually due to inadequate exposure to sunlight) contribute to this risk.

Milk and milk products are the richest sources of calcium, with other foods such as dark green leafy vegetables and canned salmon containing smaller amounts. Many clients benefit from calcium supplements.

Serum calcium levels are often reported in two ways, based on how it circulates in the plasma. Approximately 50% of serum calcium circulates in a free, ionized, or unbound form. The other 50% circulates in the plasma bound to either plasma proteins or other nonprotein ions. The normal total serum calcium levels, which range from 8.5–10.5 mg/dL, represent both bound and unbound calcium. The normal ionized serum calcium, which ranges from 4.0–5.0 mg/dL, represents calcium circulating in the plasma in free, or unbound, form (Hayes, 2004b).

MAGNESIUM (MG²⁺) Magnesium is primarily found in the skeleton and intracellular fluid. It is the second most abundant intracellular cation, with normal serum levels of

1.5–2.5 mEq/L. It is important for intracellular metabolism, particularly in the production and use of adenosine triphosphate (ATP). Magnesium also is necessary for protein and DNA synthesis within the cells. Only about 1% of the body's magnesium is in ECF; here it is involved in regulating neuromuscular and cardiac function. Maintaining and ensuring adequate magnesium levels are an important part of care of clients with cardiac disorders. Cereal grains, nuts, dried fruit, legumes, and green leafy vegetables are good sources of magnesium in the diet, as are dairy products, meat, and fish.

CHLORIDE (CL⁻) Chloride is the major anion of ECF, and normal serum levels are 95–108 mEq/L. Chloride functions with sodium to regulate serum osmolality and blood volume. The concentration of chloride in ECF is regulated secondarily to sodium; when sodium is reabsorbed in the kidney, chloride usually follows. Chloride is a major component of gastric juice, as hydrochloric acid (HCl) and is involved in regulating acid–base balance. It also acts as a buffer in the exchange of oxygen and carbon dioxide in RBCs. Chloride is found in the same foods as sodium.

PHOSPHATE PO₄⁻ Phosphate is the major anion of intracellular fluids. It also is found in ECF, bone, skeletal muscle, and nerve tissue. Normal adult serum levels of phospate range from 2.5 to 4.5 mg/dL. Children have much higher phosphate levels than adults, with that of a newborn nearly twice that of an adult. Higher levels of growth hormone and a faster rate of skeletal growth probably account for this difference. Phosphate is involved in many chemical actions of the cell; it is essential for functioning of muscles, nerves, and red blood cells. It is also involved in the metabolism of protein, fat, and carbohydrate. Phosphate is absorbed from the intestine and is found in many foods such as meat, fish, poultry, milk products, and legumes.

BICARBONATE HCO₃⁻ Bicarbonate is present in both intracellular and extracellular fluids. Its primary function is regulating acid–base balance as an essential component of the carbonic acid–bicarbonate buffering system. Extracellular bicarbonate levels are regulated by the kidneys: Bicarbonate is excreted when too much is present; if more is needed, the kidneys both regenerate and reabsorb bicarbonate ions. Unlike other electrolytes that must be consumed in the diet, bicarbonate is produced through metabolic processes in adequate amounts to meet the body's needs.

Factors Affecting Body Fluid and Electrolyte Balance

The ability of the body to adjust fluid and electrolyte balance is influenced by age, gender and body size, environmental temperature, and lifestyle.

AGE *Pediatric Differences* Infants and young children differ physiologically from adults in ways that make them vulnerable to fluid and electrolyte imbalances. Infants lose more fluid through the kidneys because immature kidneys are less able to conserve water than adult kidneys. In addition, infants' respirations are more rapid and their **body surface area** (BSA; relationship between height and weight measured in square meters) is proportionately greater than that of adults, increasing insensible fluid losses. This greater percentage of body surface area also puts them at greater risk when burned.

The percentage of body weight that is composed of water also varies with age (Figure 6–8 ■). The percentage is highest at birth (and higher in premature than in full-term infants) and decreases with age (see As Children Grow, Figure 6–9 ■). Neonates and young infants have a proportionately larger extracellular fluid volume than older children and adults because their brain and skin (both rich in interstitial fluid) constitute a greater proportion of their body weight. Because much of our extracellular fluid is exchanged each day, infants have a high daily fluid requirement with little fluid volume reserve, making them vulnerable to dehydration. As an infant grows, the proportion of water inside the cells increases, the extracellular amount decreases in comparison, and the risk of fluid imbalance begins to decrease.

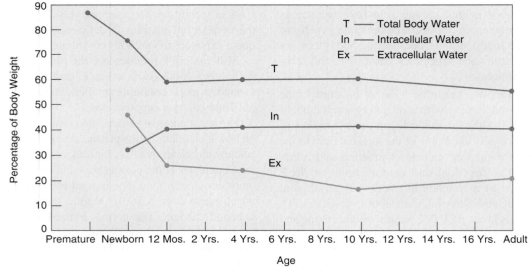

Figure 6–8 ■ The major body fluid compartments at various ages. *Extracellular fluid* is composed mainly of vascular fluid (fluid in blood vessels) and interstitial fluid (fluid between the cells and outside the blood and lymphatic vessels.) *Intracellular fluid* is that within cells.

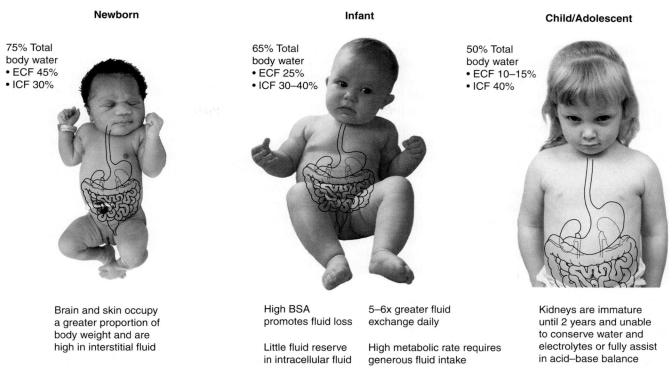

Newborn	Infant	Child/Adolescent
75% Total body water • ECF 45% • ICF 30%	65% Total body water • ECF 25% • ICF 30–40%	50% Total body water • ECF 10–15% • ICF 40%

Brain and skin occupy a greater proportion of body weight and are high in interstitial fluid

High BSA promotes fluid loss

Little fluid reserve in intracellular fluid

5–6x greater fluid exchange daily

High metabolic rate requires generous fluid intake

Kidneys are immature until 2 years and unable to conserve water and electrolytes or fully assist in acid–base balance

Figure 6–9 ■ The newborn and infant have a high percentage of body weight comprised of water, especially extracellular fluid, which is lost from the body easily. Note the small stomach size which limits ability to rehydrate quickly.

Infants and children under 2 years of age lose a greater proportion of fluid each day than do older children and adults and are thus more dependent on adequate intake. Respiratory illnesses, stomach viruses resulting in vomiting or diarrhea, and burns can all result in fluid or electrolyte imbalance in an infant or young child, increasing the risk for serious complications. A nurse working with parents of a young child presenting with these conditions should take time to explain the importance of monitoring the child's hydration until the child returns to health.

In addition, respiratory and metabolic rates are high during early childhood. These factors lead to greater water loss from the lungs and greater water demand to fuel the body's metabolic processes (Figure 6–10 ■). Because of these factors, the exercising child dehydrates easily and must consume more fluid during physical activity, particularly during hot weather (Committee on Sports Medicine and Fitness, 2000).

When fluid status is compromised, a number of body mechanisms activate to help restore balance. Several of these mechanisms occur in the kidneys. The kidneys conserve water and needed electrolytes while excreting waste products and drug metabolites. In children under 2 years of age, however, the glomeruli, tubules, and nephrons of the kidneys are immature. They are therefore unable to conserve or excrete water and solutes effectively. Because more water is generally excreted, the infant and young child can become dehydrated or develop electrolyte imbalances quickly. Children under 2 years of age also have difficulty regulating electrolytes such as sodium and calcium. Renal response to high solute loads is slower and less developed, with function improving gradually during the first year of life.

Older Adults In elderly people, the normal aging process may affect fluid balance. The thirst response often is blunted. Antidiuretic hormone levels remain normal or may even be elevated, but the nephrons become less able to conserve water in response to ADH. Increased levels of ANF seen in older adults may also contribute to this impaired ability to conserve water. These normal changes of aging increase the risk of dehydration. When combined with the increased likelihood of heart diseases, impaired renal function, and multiple drug regimens, the older adult's risk for fluid and electrolyte imbalance is significant. Nurses should take the opportunity to remind

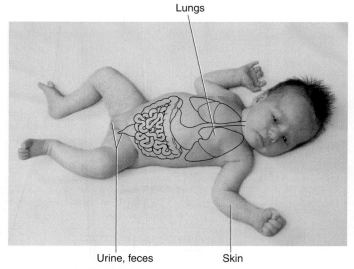

Figure 6–10 ■ Normal routes of fluid excretion from infants and children.

older adults and caregivers of the importance of adequate hydration at each interaction within the health care system.

GENDER AND BODY SIZE Total body water is also affected by gender and body size. Because fat cells contain little or no water, and lean tissue has a high water content, people with a higher percentage of body fat have less body fluid. Women have proportionately more body fat and less body water than men. Water accounts for approximately 60% of an adult man's weight, but only 52% for an adult woman. In an obese individual, this percentage may be even less, with water being responsible for only 30–40% of the person's weight.

ENVIRONMENTAL TEMPERATURE People with an illness and those participating in strenuous activity are at risk for fluid and electrolyte imbalances when the environmental temperature is high. Fluid losses through sweating are increased in hot environments as the body attempts to dissipate heat. These losses are even greater in people who have not been acclimatized to the environment.

Both salt and water are lost through sweating. When only water is replaced, salt depletion is a risk. The person with salt depletion may experience fatigue, weakness, headache, and gastrointestinal symptoms such as loss of appetite and nausea. The risk of adverse effects is even greater if lost water is not replaced. Body temperature rises, and the person becomes at risk for heat exhaustion or heatstroke. Heatstroke may occur in older adults or ill people during prolonged periods of heat; it can also affect athletes and laborers when their heat production exceeds the body's ability to dissipate heat. Consuming adequate amounts of cool liquids, particularly during strenuous activity, reduces the risk of adverse effects from heat. Balanced electrolyte solutions and carbohydrate–electrolyte solutions such as sports drinks are recommended because they replace both water and electrolytes lost through sweat.

LIFESTYLE Other factors such as diet, exercise, and stress affect fluid and electrolyte balance. The intake of fluids and electrolytes is affected by the diet. Regular weight-bearing physical exercise such as walking, running, or bicycling has a beneficial effect on calcium balance. Stress can increase cellular metabolism, blood glucose concentration, and catecholamine levels. In addition, stress can increase production of ADH, which in turn decreases urine production.

Other lifestyle factors can also affect fluid, electrolyte, and acid–base balance. Heavy alcohol consumption affects electrolyte balance, increasing the risk of low calcium, magnesium, and phosphate levels.

ALTERATIONS

Many health conditions cause changes in body fluids that must be regulated and managed. Sometimes management of fluid status in the home or in a short-term ambulatory facility can prevent

---

ALTERATIONS AND TREATMENTS Fluids and Electrolytes

Alterations	Description	Treatment
Fluid volume deficit–dehydration	Fluids are lost secondary to diarrhea, vomiting, inability to take in fluids, excessive perspiration, or increased basal metabolic rate due to fever, hyperthyroidism, or medications.	Administer fluids via either the oral or intravenous route and treat the underlying cause.
Fluid volume excess	Too much fluid in the body may be caused by excessive fluid intake (intravenous fluid administration, water intoxication) or inadequate fluid excretion (e.g., kidney failure, poor perfusion to the kidneys secondary to congestive heart failure, low cardiac output, hypertension).	Administer diuretics to increase fluid excretion, reduce fluid intake, and elevate head of bed if dyspnea results from pulmonary edema.
Elevated electrolyte level	Any electrolyte level may be elevated. Hyponatremia and hypokalemia are the most common and significant extracellular findings.	Limit intake of the elevated electrolyte. Administration of glucose and insulin will lower serum potassium levels by driving potassium from the extracellular space into the intracellular space. Diuretics will increase potassium and sodium loss but will also remove fluid.
Low electrolyte level	Any electrolyte level can decrease, but hypokalemia (low potassium) is the most common result of diuretics unless a potassium sparing diuretic is administered.	Administer electrolyte supplement, monitor serum electrolyte levels, monitor for symptoms associated with electrolyte imbalance. For example, low potassium levels can cause cardiac arrhythmias, and client should be placed on cardiorespiratory monitor.
Chronic renal failure	Damage to the kidney over time causes progressive decline in kidney function; may be caused by diabetes mellitus, hypertension, or cardiac disease.	Initially may be treated with diuretics, progresses to need for dialysis and/or kidney transplant.
Acute renal failure	Rapidly progressive loss of kidney function is characterized by oliguria and fluid and electrolyte imbalances. Can be the result of disturbed blood supply to the kidneys, toxins, or kidney trauma; may be reversible or permanent.	Administer dialysis, monitor fluid and electrolyte balance, transplant kidney, treat the underlying cause.

more serious illness or hospitalization. Examples of conditions that commonly require fluid, electrolyte, or acid–base balance include gastroenteritis, burns, kidney disorders, oral fluid restriction for surgery, anorexia or bulimia, and dehydration and electrolyte imbalances that can result from athletics in hot weather.

PHYSICAL ASSESSMENT

Evaluating clients for fluid and electrolyte status is an important nursing care function. Components of the assessment include (a) the nursing history, (b) physical assessment of the client, (c) clinical measurements, and (d) review of laboratory test results.

Nursing History

The nursing history is particularly important for identifying clients who are at risk for fluid and electrolyte imbalances. The current and past medical history reveals conditions such as chronic cardiac disease or diabetes mellitus that can disrupt normal balances. Medications prescribed to treat acute or chronic conditions (e.g., diuretic therapy for hypertension) also may put the client at risk for altered homeostasis. Functional, developmental, and socioeconomic factors must also be considered in assessing the client's risk. Older people and very young children, clients who must depend on others to meet their needs for food and fluid intake, and people who cannot afford or do not have the means to cook food for a balanced diet (e.g., homeless people) are at greater risk for fluid and electrolyte imbalances.

When obtaining the nursing history, the nurse needs not only to recognize risk factors but also to obtain data about the client's food and fluid intake, fluid output, and the presence of signs or symptoms suggesting altered fluid and electrolyte balance. The Assessment Interview provides examples of questions to elicit information regarding fluid and electrolyte balance.

Physical Assessment

Physical assessment to evaluate a client's fluid and electrolyte status focuses on the skin, the oral cavity and mucous membranes, the eyes, the cardiovascular and respiratory systems, and neurologic and muscular status. Often, the agency will use a standardized form or computer software to help the nurse make sure that certain elements of physical assessment are conducted consistently between visits and from one patient to the next. In addition to these important tools, the nurse should also make note of anything unusual in the client's physical appearance. For example, **edema**, which is swelling caused by excess fluid trapped in bodily tissue, may be readily observed in a client's extremities and recorded during the physical assessment. Data from the physical assessment are used to expand and verify information obtained in the nursing history.

Clinical Measurements

Three simple clinical measurements that the nurse can initiate without a primary care provider's order are daily weights, vital signs, and fluid intake and output.

DAILY WEIGHTS Daily weight measurements provide a relatively accurate assessment of a client's fluid status. Significant changes in weight over a short time (e.g., more than 5 lbs in a week or less) indicate acute fluid changes.

Each kilogram (2.2 lbs) of weight gained or lost is equivalent to 1 L of fluid gained or lost. Such fluid gains or losses indicate changes in total body fluid volume rather than in any specific compartment. Rapid losses or gains of 5–8% of total body weight indicate moderate to severe fluid volume deficits or excesses. Regular assessment of weight is particularly important for clients in the community and extended care facilities who are at risk for fluid imbalance. For these clients, measuring intake and output may be impractical because of lifestyle or problems with incontinence. Regular weight measurement, taken daily, every other day, or weekly, provides valuable information about the client's fluid volume status.

VITAL SIGNS Changes in the vital signs may indicate, or in some cases precede, fluid, electrolyte, and acid–base imbalances. For example, elevated body temperature may be a result of dehydration or a cause of increased body fluid losses.

Tachycardia is an early sign of hypovolemia. Pulse volume will decrease in fluid volume deficit and increase in fluid volume excess. Irregular pulse rates may occur with electrolyte imbalances.

Blood pressure, a sensitive measure to detect blood volume changes, may fall significantly with fluid volume deficit (FVD) and hypovolemia or increase with fluid volume excess (FVE). Postural, or orthostatic, hypotension may also occur with FVD and hypovolemia.

FLUID INTAKE AND OUTPUT The measurement and recording of all fluid intake and output (I & O) during a 24-hour period provides important data about the client's fluid and electrolyte balance.

Most agencies have a form for recording I & O, usually a bedside record on which the nurse lists all items measured and the quantities per shift. Some agencies have another form for recording the specifics of intravenous fluids, such as the type of solution, additives, time started, amounts absorbed, and amounts remaining per shift.

It is important to inform clients, family members, and all caregivers that accurate measurements of the client's fluid intake and output are required. Explain why and emphasize the need to use a bedpan, urinal, commode, or in-toilet collection device (unless a urinary drainage system is in place). Instruct the client not to put toilet tissue into the container with urine. Clients who wish to be involved in recording fluid intake measurements need to be taught how to compute the values and which foods are considered fluids.

To measure fluid intake, the nurse records each fluid item taken (if the client has not already done so) on the I & O form, specifying the time and type of fluid. All of the following fluids need to be recorded:

- Oral fluids
- Ice chips
- Foods that are or tend to become liquid at room temperature
- Tube feedings
- Parenteral fluids
- Intravenous medications
- Catheter or tube irrigants

Fluid and Electrolyte Assessments

System	Assessment Focus	Technique	Possible Abnormal Findings
Skin	Color, temperature, moisture	Inspection, palpation	Flushed, warm, very dry Moist or diaphoretic Cool and pale
	Turgor	Gently pinch up a fold of skin over sternum or inner aspect of thigh for adults, on the abdomen or medial thigh for children	Poor turgor: Skin remains tented for several seconds instead of immediately returning to normal position
	Edema	Inspect for visible swelling around eyes, in fingers, and in lower extremities	Skin around eyes is puffy, lids appear swollen; rings are tight; shoes leave impressions on feet
		Compress the skin over the dorsum of the foot, around the ankles, over the tibia, in the sacral area	Depression remains (pitting)
Mucous membranes	Color, moisture	Inspection	Mucous membranes dry, dull in appearance; tongue dry and cracked
Eyes	Firmness	Gently palpate eyeball with lid closed	Eyeball feels soft to palpation
Fontanels (infant)	Firmness, level	Inspect and gently palpate anterior fontanel	Fontanel bulging, firm Fontanel sunken, soft
Cardiovascular system	Heart rate	Auscultation, cardiac monitor	Tachycardia, bradycardia; irregular; dysrhythmias
	Peripheral pulses	Palpation	Weak and thready; bounding
	Blood pressure	Auscultation of Korotkoff's sounds	Hypotension
		BP assessment lying and standing	Postural hypotension
	Capillary refill	Palpation	Slowed capillary refill
	Venous filling	Inspection of jugular veins and hand veins	Jugular venous distention; flat jugular veins, poor venous refill
Respiratory system	Respiratory rate and pattern	Inspection	Increased or decreased rate and depth of respirations
	Lung sounds	Auscultation	Crackles or moist rales
Neurologic	Level of consciousness (LOC)	Observation, stimulation	Decreased LOC, lethargy, stupor, or coma
	Orientation, cognition	Questioning	Disoriented, confused; difficulty concentrating
	Motor function	Strength testing	Weakness, decreased motor strength
	Reflexes	Deep-tendon reflex (DTR) testing	Hyperactive or depressed DTRs
	Abnormal reflexes	*Chvostek's sign:* Tap over facial nerve about 2 cm anterior to tragus of ear	Facial muscle twitching including eyelids and lips on side of stimulus
		Trousseau's sign: Inflate a blood pressure cuff on the upper arm to 20 mmHg greater than the systolic pressure, leave in place for 2–5 minutes	Carpal spasm: contraction of hand and fingers on affected side

Assessment Interview Fluid and Electrolyte Balance

CURRENT AND PAST MEDICAL HISTORY

- Are you currently seeing a health care provider for treatment of any chronic diseases such as kidney disease, heart disease, high blood pressure, diabetes insipidus, or thyroid or parathyroid disorders?
- Have you recently experienced any acute conditions such as gastroenteritis, severe trauma, head injury, or surgery? If so, describe them.

MEDICATIONS AND TREATMENTS

- Are you currently taking any medications on a regular basis such as diuretics, steroids, potassium supplements, calcium supplements, hormones, salt substitutes, or antacids?
- Have you recently undergone any treatments such as dialysis, parenteral nutrition, or tube feedings or been on a ventilator? If so, when and why?

FOOD AND FLUID INTAKE

- How much and what type of fluids do you drink each day?
- Describe your diet for a typical day. (The nurse should pay particular attention to the client's intake of protein, whole grains, fruits, vegetables, and foods high in sodium content.)
- Have you made any recent changes in your food or fluid intake, for example, as a result of following a weight-loss program?
- Are you on any type of restricted diet?
- Has your food or fluid intake recently been affected by changes in appetite, nausea, or other factors such as pain or difficulty breathing?

FLUID OUTPUT

- Have you noticed any recent changes in the frequency or amount of urine output?
- Have you recently experienced any problems with vomiting, diarrhea, or constipation? If so, when and for how long?
- Have you noticed any other unusual fluid losses such as excessive sweating?

FLUID AND ELECTROLYTE IMBALANCES

- Have you gained or lost weight in recent weeks?
- Have you recently experienced any symptoms such as excessive thirst, dry skin or mucous membranes, dark or concentrated urine, or low urine output?
- Do you have problems with swelling of your hands, feet, or ankles? Do you ever have difficulty breathing, especially when lying down or at night? How many pillows do you use to sleep?
- Have you recently experienced any of the following symptoms: difficulty concentrating or confusion; dizziness or feeling faint; muscle weakness, twitching, cramping, or spasm; excessive fatigue; abnormal sensations such as numbness, tingling, burning, or prickling; abdominal cramping or distention; heart palpitations?

Source: Berman, A., Snyder, S. J., Kozier, B., & Erb, G. (2008). *Kozier & Erb's fundamentals of nursing: Concepts, process, and practice* (8th ed., p. 1445). Upper Saddle River, NJ: Pearson Education.

To measure fluid output, measure the following fluids (remember to observe appropriate infection control precautions):
- Urinary output
- Vomitus and liquid feces (The amount and type of fluid and the time of output need to be specified.)
- Tube drainage, such as gastric or intestinal drainage
- Wound drainage and draining fistulas

Fluid intake and output measurements are totaled at intervals pursuant to agency protocol or physician instruction, and the totals are recorded in the client's permanent record.

To determine whether the fluid output is proportional to fluid intake or whether there are any changes in the client's fluid status, the nurse (a) compares the total 24-hour fluid output measurement with the total fluid intake measurement, and (b) compares both to previous measurements. Urinary output is normally equivalent to the amount of fluids ingested; the usual range is 1,500–2,000 mL in 24 hours, or 40–80 mL in 1 hour (0.5 mL/kg per hour). Clients whose output substantially exceeds intake are at risk for **fluid volume deficit**. By contrast, clients whose intake substantially exceeds output are at risk for **fluid volume excess**. In assessing the client's fluid balance, it is important to consider additional factors that may affect intake and output. The client who is extremely diaphoretic or who has rapid, deep respirations has fluid losses that cannot be measured but must be considered in evaluating fluid status.

When there is a significant discrepancy between intake and output or when fluid intake or output is inadequate (for example, a urine output of less than 500 mL in 24 hours or less than 0.5 mL/kg per hour in an adult), this information should be reported to the charge nurse or primary care provider.

DIAGNOSTIC TESTS

Many laboratory studies may be conducted to determine the client's fluid and electrolyte status. Some of the more common tests are discussed here.

Serum Electrolytes

Serum electrolyte levels are often routinely ordered for any client admitted to the hospital as a screening test for electrolyte imbalances. The most commonly ordered serum tests are for sodium, potassium, chloride, magnesium, and bicarbonate ions. Normal values of commonly measured electrolytes are shown in Box 6–2. Some primary care providers use a diagram format (Figure 6–11 ■) for keeping track of the client's electrolytes when documenting in their progress notes.

Complete Blood Count (CBC)

The complete blood count, another basic screening test, includes information about the hematocrit (Hct). The **hematocrit** measures the volume (percentage) of whole blood that is composed of RBCs. Because the hematocrit is a measure of the volume of cells in relation to plasma, it is affected by changes in plasma volume. Thus, the hematocrit increases with severe dehydration and decreases with severe overhydration. Normal hematocrit values are 40–54% (men) and 37–47% (women).

Box 6–2 Normal Electrolyte Values for Adults*

Venous Blood

Sodium	135–145 mEq/L
Potassium	3.5–5.0 mEq/L
Chloride	95–108 mEq/L
Calcium (total)	4.5–5.5 mEq/L or 8.5–10.5 mg/dL
(ionized)	56% of total calcium (2.5 mEq/L or 4.0–5.0 mg/dL)
Magnesium	1.5–2.5 mEq/L or 1.6–2.5 mg/dL
Phosphate (phosphorus)	1.8–2.6 mEq/L or 2.5 – 4.5 mg/dL
Serum osmolality	280–300 mOsm/kg water

*Note: Normal laboratory values vary from agency to agency.

Osmolality

Serum osmolality is a measure of the solute concentration of the blood. The particles included are sodium ions, glucose, and urea (blood urea nitrogen, or BUN). Serum osmolality can be estimated by doubling the serum sodium, because sodium and its associated chloride ions are the major determinants of serum osmolality. Serum osmolality values are used primarily to evaluate fluid balance. Normal values are 280–300 mOsm/kg. An increase in serum osmolality indicates a fluid volume deficit; a decrease reflects a fluid volume excess.

Urine osmolality is a measure of the solute concentration of urine. The particles included are nitrogenous wastes, such as creatinine, urea, and uric acid. Normal values are 500–800 mOsm/kg. An increased urine osmolality indicates a fluid volume deficit; a decreased urine osmolality reflects a fluid volume excess.

Urine Specific Gravity

Specific gravity is an indicator of urine concentration that can be performed quickly and easily by nursing personnel. Normal specific gravity ranges from 1.005–1.030 (usually 1.010–1.025). When the concentration of solutes in the urine is high, the specific gravity rises; in very dilute urine with few solutes, it is abnormally low.

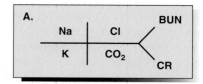

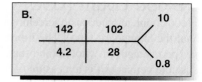

Figure 6–11 ■ *A*, Format for a diagram of serum electrolyte results. *B*, Example that may be seen in a primary care provider's documentation notes.

Urine Sodium and Chloride Excretion

These are indicators of renal perfusion that can provide useful information about a client's fluid status. With hypovolemia, aldosterone is secreted. This will cause reabsorption of sodium and chloride, which results in decreased levels of sodium and chloride, less than 20 mEq/L each (Elgart, 2004).

CARING INTERVENTIONS

Alterations in fluid and electrolytes may occur as a primary event or as a secondary response to a preexisting disease state or a sudden traumatic event. When alterations of fluid and electrolytes exceed the narrow limits consistent with health, the body needs to adjust quickly. The severity of fluid and electrolyte imbalance determines whether treatment will consist of oral replacements or the initiation of intravenous therapy. Intravenous fluids may be ordered for the client with a fluid volume deficit if replacement oral fluids cannot be taken in sufficient quantity. Electrolyte supplements may be used to replace electrolyte deficits. Diuretics may be ordered to reduce fluid volume excess.

Consult your skills manual for step-by-step descriptions of the following caring interventions related to fluids and electrolytes:

- Initiating intravenous therapy
- Intravenous management
- Monitoring fluid balance
- Medication administration
- Blood transfusions

PHARMACOLOGIC THERAPIES

Pharmacological therapies are aimed at replacing what has been lost or deleting what may be excessive in order to restore a normal balance to the body's fluid and electrolytes. Fluids are replaced in an attempt to put back what is lost so blood loss is replaced with blood transfusions, albumins, or other large-molecule protein solutions (colloid). Fluids lost secondary to excessive diuresis, perspiration, inadequate intake, or insensible water loss are replaced using crystalloids.

Electrolyte correction is highly dependent on the specific electrolyte and whether the body is in deficit or in excess. For example, elevated potassium levels (sometimes referred to as **hyperkalemia**) are ultimately corrected by dialysis, but treatments such as administration of glucose and insulin can help to drive potassium back into the cell where elevated levels will create less risk. A deficit in potassium is known as **hypokalemia**, and is frequently a side-effect of diuretics. Sodium excess, often seen in clients with reduced production of antidiuretic hormone (ADH), may be corrected by administration of ADH. Sodium excess may be referred to as **hypernatremia**, whereas a deficit in sodium is known as **hyponatremia**. Sodium deficiency may be treated with oral supplementation or, if the deficiency is severe or life threatening, intravenous supplementation may be administered.

MEDICATIONS

Drug Groups	Mechanism of Action	Common Drugs	Nursing Considerations
Electrolyte supplements	Restore electrolyte balance by replacing.	Sodium chloride–sodium supplement Potassium chloride–potassium supplement	■ Monitor serum electrolyte levels, intake and output, vital signs.
Colloids	Proteins, starches, or other large molecules remain in the blood for a long time and act as a volume expander.	Serum albumin, dextran 40	■ Carefully monitor client's condition, laboratory values, and renal function.
Crystalloids	Intravenous solutions that contain electrolytes and other agents that mimic the body's extracellular fluid are used to replace depleted fluid and promote urine output.	5% dextrose and water, normal saline solution, lactated ringer's, 5% dextrose and 1/2 normal saline	■ Monitor client's fluid and electrolyte status.
Diuretics	Promote urine output.	Furosemide, hydrochlorothiazide, aldactone	■ Monitor intake and output, daily weight, serum electrolytes, and hydration status.

REFERENCES

Adams, M.P., Holland, Jr., L.N., & Bostwick, P.M. (2008). *Pharmacology for nurses: A pathophysiologic approach* (2nd ed.). Upper Saddle River, NJ: Pearson, Inc.

Allen, K. (2005). Four-step method of interpreting arterial blood gas analysis. *Nursing Times, 101*(1), 42–45.

American Medical Association, American Nurses Association–American Nurses Foundations, Centers for Disease Control and Prevention, Center for Food Safety and Applied Nutrition, Food and Drug Administration, Food Safety and Inspection Service, U.S. Department of Agriculture. (2004). Diagnosis and management of foodborne illnesses: A primer for physicians and other health care professionals. *Morbidity and Mortality Weekly Report, 53* (RR-4), 1–33.

Anderson, N. R. (2005). When to use a midline catheter. *Nursing, 35*(4), 28.

Andrews, M. M., & Boyle, J. S. (2003). *Transcultural concepts in nursing Care* (4th ed.). Philadelphia: Lippincott Williams & Wilkins.

Astle, S. M. (2005). Restoring electrolyte balance. *RN, 68*(5), 34–39.

Ball, J.W., & Bindler, R.C.(2008). *Pediatric nursing: Caring for children* (4th ed.) Upper Saddle River, NJ: Pearson, Inc.

Bennett, J. A., Thomas, V., & Riegel, B. (2004). Unrecognized chronic dehydration in older adults. Examining prevalence rate and risk factors. *Journal of Gerontological Nursing, 30*(1), 22–28.

Berman, A., Snyder, S.J., Kozier, B., & Erb, G. (2008). *Kozier & Erb's fundamentals of nursing: Concepts, process, and practice* (8th ed.). Upper Saddle River, NJ: Pearson, Inc.

Bunce, M. (2003). Troubleshooting central lines. *RN, 66*(12), 28–33.

Burger, C. M. (2004a). Hyperkalemia: When serum K+ is not okay. *American Journal of Nursing, 104*(10), 66–70.

Burger, C. M. (2004b). Hypokalemia: Averting crisis with early recognition and intervention. *American Journal of Nursing, 104*(11), 61–65.

Centers for Disease Control and Prevention. (2002). Guidelines for the prevention of intravascular catheter-related infections. *Morbidity and Mortality Weekly Report, 51*(10), 1–29.

Committee on Sports Medicine and Fitness. (2000). Climatic heat stress and the exercising child and adolescent. *Pediatrics, 106,* 158–159.

Corbett, J. V. (2004). *Laboratory tests and diagnostic procedures with nursing diagnoses* (6th ed.). Upper Saddle River, NJ: Pearson Prentice Hall.

Deglin, J. H., & Vallerand, A. H. (2004). *Davis's Drug Guide for Nurses* (9th ed.). Philadelphia: F. A. Davis.

Dochterman, J. M., & Bulechek, G. M. (Eds.). (2004). *Nursing Interventions Classification (NIC)* (4th ed.). St. Louis, MO: Mosby.

Dulak, S. B. (2005). Technology today: Smart IV pumps. *RN, 68*(12), 38–43.

Elgart, H. N. (2004). Assessment of fluids and electrolytes. *AACN Clinical Issues, 15*(4), 607–621.

Food and Drug Administration (FDA). (2004). Bar code label requirements for human drug products and biological products. *Federal Register, 69*(38), 9119–9171.

Hadaway, L. C. (2003). Infusing without infecting. *Nursing, 33*(10), 58–64.

Hadaway, L. C. (2004). Preventing and managing peripheral extravasation. *Nursing, 34*(5), 66–67.

Hadaway, L. C. (2005). Reopen the pipeline for I.V. therapy. *Nursing, 35*(8), 54–61.

Hadaway, L. C. (2006). Keeping central line infection at bay. *Nursing, 36*(4), 58–63.

Hayes, D. D. (2004a). Balancing act: What happens when sodium and water are off-kilter? *Nursing Made Incredibly Easy, 2*(1), 52–57.

Hayes, D. D. (2004b). Calcium in the balance. *Nursing Made Incredibly Easy, 2*(2), 46–53.

Hayes, D. D. (2004c). Magnesium's balancing act. *Nursing Made Incredibly Easy, 2*(4), 44–50.

Hayes, D. D. (2004d). Phosphorus: Here, there, everywhere. *Nursing Made Incredibly Easy, 2*(6), 36–41.

Hogan, M. A., & Wane, D. (2003). *Fluids, electrolytes, & acid-base balance: Reviews & rationales*. Upper Saddle River, NJ: Prentice Hall.

Just the Facts: Fluids & Electrolytes. (2005). Philadelphia: Lippincott Williams & Wilkins.

Lynes, D. (2003). Respiratory care skills: An introduction to blood gas analysis. *Nursing Times, 99*(11), 54–55.

Marders, J. (2005). Sounding the alarm for I.V. infiltration. *Nursing, 35*(4), 19–20.

Masoorli, S., & Angeles, T. (2002). Getting a line on central vascular access devices. *Nursing, 32*(4), 36–43.

Moorhead, S., Johnson, M., & Maas, M. (Eds.). (2004). *Nursing outcomes classification (NOC)* (3rd ed.). St. Louis, MO: Mosby.

Moureau, N. L. (2003). Is your skin-prep technique up-to-date? *Nursing, 33*(11), 17.

Moureau, N. L. (2004). Tips for inserting an I.V. in an older patient. *Nursing, 34*(7), 18.

NANDA International. (2007). *NANDA Nursing Diagnoses: Definitions and classification 2007–2008*. Philadelphia: Author.

Newberry, N. (Ed.). (2003). *Sheehy's emergency nursing* (5th ed.). St. Louis, MO: Mosby.

Phillips, L. D. (2005). *Manual of I.V. therapeutics* (4th ed.). Philadelphia: F. A. Davis.

Pruitt, W. C., & Jacobs, M. (2004). Interpreting arterial blood gases: Easy as ABC. *Nursing, 34*(8), 50–53.

Quillen, T. F. (2005). Myths & facts: About hypercalcemia. *Nursing, 35*(7), 74.

Rosenthal, K. (2004a). Avoiding bad blood: Key steps to safe transfusions. *Nursing Made Incredibly Easy, 2*(5), 20–29.

Rosenthal, K. (2004b). It's not magic! The tricks to cannulating difficult veins. *Nursing Made Incredibly Easy, 2*(2), 4–7.

Rosenthal, K. (2004c). The line—for central venous access—forms here. *Nursing Made Incredibly Easy, 2*(5), 4–7.

Rosenthal, K. (2004d). What you should know about needleless I.V. systems. *Nursing, 34*(9), 76.

Rosenthal, K. (2005a). Documenting peripheral I.V. therapy. *Nursing, 35*(7), 28.

Rosenthal, K. (2005c). Tailor your I.V. insertion techniques for special populations. *Nursing, 35*(5), 37–41.

Rosenthal, K. (2005b). Ports: The gateway to central lines. *Nursing Made Incredibly Easy, 3*(1), 53–56.

Simpson, H. (2004). Interpretation of arterial blood gases: A clinical guide for nurses. *British Journal of Nursing, 13*(9), 522–528.

Spandorfer, P. R., Alessandrini, E. A., Joffe, M. D., Localio, R., & Shaw, K. N. (2005). Oral versus intravenous rehydration of moderately dehydrated children: A randomized, controlled trial. *Pediatrics, 115*(2), 295–301.

Sweeney, J. (2005a). What causes sudden hypokalemia? *Nursing, 35*(4), 12.

Sweeney, J. (2005b). What causes hyponatremia? *Nursing, 35*(6), 18.

Trimble, T. (2003). Peripheral I.V. starts: Securing and removing the catheter. *Nursing, 33*(9), 26.

Wilburn, S. Q. (2004). Needlestick and sharps injury prevention. *Online Journal of Issues in Nursing, 9*(3), manuscript 4. Retrieved July 15, 2006, from http://www.nursingworld.org/ojin/topic25/tpc25_4.htm

Yucha, C. (2004). Renal regulation of acid–base balance. *Nephrology Nursing Journal, 31*(2), 201–208.

Health, Wellness, and Illness

7

Concept at-a-Glance

Concept Learning Outcomes

After reading about this concept, you will be able to do the following:

1. Define health, illness, wellness, and disease.
2. Explain the health-illness continuum and the concept of high-level wellness.
3. Define health promotion.
4. Describe the nurse's role in health promotion.
5. Identify characteristics of health, disease, and illness.
6. Differentiate illness from disease and acute illness from chronic illness.
7. Develop and evaluate plans for health promotion across the life span.

Concept Key Terms

Acute illness, *182*
Autonomy, *183*
Chronic illness, *182*
Disease, *182*
Exacerbation, *182*
Health, *180*
Health promotion, *183*
Illness, *182*
Illness behavior, *182*

Lifestyle, *189*
Modeling, *192*
Positive reinforcement, *192*
Remission, *182*
Risk factors, *189*
Well-being, *181*
Wellness, *181*
Wellness diagnoses, *191*

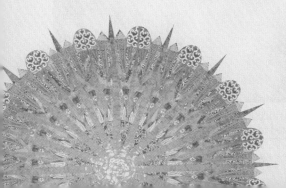

About Health, Wellness, and Illness

Nurses' understanding of health and wellness largely determines the scope and nature of nursing practice. Clients' health beliefs also influence health practices. Some people think of health and wellness (or well-being) as the same thing or, at the very least, as accompanying one another. However, health may not always accompany well-being: A person who has a terminal illness may have a sense of well-being; conversely, another person may lack a sense of well-being, yet be in a state of good health.

For many years the concept of disease was the yardstick by which health was measured. In the late 19th Century, the "how" of disease (pathogenesis) was the major concern of health professionals. The 20th Century focused on finding cures for diseases. Currently, health care providers are increasing their emphasis on promoting health and wellness in individuals, families, and communities. ●

CONCEPTS OF HEALTH, WELLNESS, AND WELL-BEING

Health, wellness, and well-being have many definitions and interpretations. The nurse should be familiar with the most common aspects of these concepts and consider how they may be individualized with specific clients.

Health

Traditionally **health** has been defined in terms of the presence or absence of disease. Nightingale defined health as a state of being well and using every power the individual possesses to the fullest extent (Nightingale, 1860/1969). The World Health Organization (WHO) takes a more holistic view of health. Its constitution defines health as "a state of complete physical, mental, and social well-being, and not merely the absence of disease or infirmity" (WHO, 1948). This definition serves the following purposes:

- It reflects concern for the individual as a total person functioning physically, psychologically, and socially. Mental processes determine people's relationships with their physical and social surroundings, their attitudes about life, and their interaction with others.
- It places health in the context of environment. People's lives, and therefore their health, are affected by everything they interact with—not only environmental influences, such as climate and the availability of food, shelter, clean air, and water to drink, but also other people, including family, lovers, employers, coworkers, friends, and associates.

In 1980, the American Nurses Association (ANA) defined health in its social policy statement as "a dynamic state of being in which the developmental and behavioral potential of an individual is realized to the fullest extent possible" (ANA, 1980, p. 5). In this definition, health is more than a state or the absence of disease; it includes striving toward optimal functioning. In 2004, the ANA also stated that health was "An experience that is often expressed in terms of wellness and illness, and may occur in the presence or absence of disease or injury" (2004, p. 48).

PERSONAL DEFINITIONS OF HEALTH Health is a highly individual perception. Consider the following examples of individuals who would probably say they are healthy, even though they have physical impairments that some people would consider illnesses:

- A 15-year-old boy with diabetes takes injectable insulin each morning. He plays on the school soccer team and is editor of the high school newspaper.

- A 32-year-old man is paralyzed from the waist down and needs a wheelchair for mobility. He is taking accounting at a nearby college and uses a specially designed automobile for transportation.
- A 72-year-old woman takes antihypertensive medications to treat high blood pressure. She bowls once a week, is a member of the neighborhood golf club, makes handicrafts for a local charity, and travels 2 months each year.

Many people define and describe health as being free from symptoms of disease and pain as much as possible, being able to be active and to do what they want or must, and being in good spirits most of the time. These characteristics indicate that health is not something that a person achieves suddenly at a specific time. It is an ongoing process, a way of life through which a person develops and encourages every aspect of the body, mind, and feelings to interrelate harmoniously as much as possible (Figure 7–1 ■).

Many factors affect individual definitions of health—the individual's previous experiences, expectations of self, age, and sociocultural influences. Nurses should be aware of their own personal definitions of health and appreciate that other people have their individual definitions as well. How a person

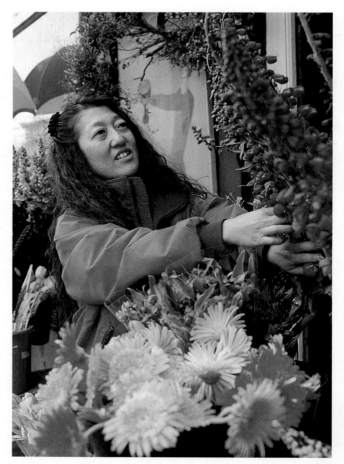

Figure 7–1 ■ Satisfaction with work enhances a sense of well-being and contributes to wellness.

defines health influences his or her behavior related to health and illness. By understanding clients' perceptions of health and illness, nurses can provide more meaningful assistance to help them regain or attain a state of health. For aid in developing a personal definition of health see Box 7–1.

Wellness and Well-Being

Wellness is a state of well-being. Basic aspects of wellness include self-responsibility; an ultimate goal; a dynamic, growing process; daily decision making in the areas of nutrition, stress management, physical fitness, preventive health care, and emotional health; and, most important, the whole being of the individual.

Anspaugh, Hamrick, and Rosato (2006) propose seven components of wellness (Figure 7–2 ■). To realize optimal health and wellness, people must deal with the factors within each component:

1. *Physical:* The ability to carry out daily tasks, achieve fitness (e.g., pulmonary, cardiovascular, gastrointestinal), maintain adequate nutrition and proper body fat levels, avoid abusing drugs and alcohol or using tobacco products, and generally practice positive lifestyle habits.
2. *Social:* The ability to interact successfully with people and within the environment of which each person is a part, to develop and maintain intimacy with significant others, and to develop respect and tolerance for those with different opinions and beliefs.
3. *Emotional:* The ability to manage stress and to express emotions appropriately. Emotional wellness involves the ability to recognize, accept, and express feelings and to accept one's limitations.
4. *Intellectual:* The ability to learn and use information effectively for personal, family, and career development.

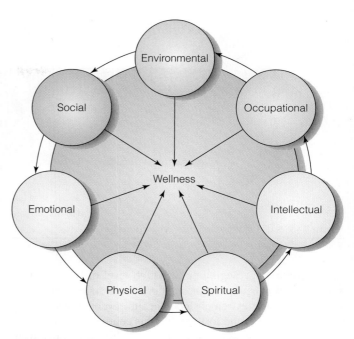

Figure 7–2 ■ The seven components of wellness.

Source: Reproduced with permission from Anspaugh, D. J., Hamrick, M. H., & Rosato, F. D. (2006). *Wellness: Concepts and applications* (6th ed., p. 4). New York: McGraw-Hill.

Intellectual wellness involves striving for continued growth and learning to deal with new challenges effectively.

5. *Spiritual:* The belief in some force (nature, science, religion, or a higher power) that serves to unite human beings and provide meaning and purpose to life. It includes a person's own morals, values, and ethics.
6. *Occupational:* The ability to achieve a balance between work and leisure time. A person's beliefs about education, employment, and home influence personal satisfaction and relationships with others.
7. *Environmental:* The ability to promote health measures that improve the standard of living and quality of life in the community. This includes influences such as food, water, and air.

The seven components overlap to some extent, and factors in one component often directly affect factors in another. For example, a person who learns to control daily stress levels from a physiologic perspective is also helping to maintain the emotional stamina needed to cope with a crisis. Wellness involves working on all aspects of the model.

Well-being is a component of health. Hood and Leddy (2003) describe well-being as "a subjective perception of vitality and feeling well …[that] can be described objectively, experienced, and measured … and can be plotted on a continuum" (p. 264).

HEALTH-ILLNESS CONTINUA

Health-illness continua (grids or graduated scales) can be used to measure a person's perceived level of wellness. Health and illness or disease can be viewed as the opposite ends of a

---

Box 7–1 Developing a Personal Definition of Health

Answering the following questions can help nurses develop a personal definition of health:

■ Is a person more than a biophysiologic system?
■ Is health more than the absence of disease symptoms?
■ Is health the ability of an individual to perform work?
■ Is health the ability of an individual to adapt to the environment?
■ Is health a condition of a person's actualization?
■ Is health a state or a process?
■ Is health the effective functioning of self-care activities?
■ Is health static or changing?
■ Are health and wellness the same?
■ Are disease and illness different?
■ Are there levels of health?
■ Are wellness, health, and illness separate entities or points along a continuum?
■ Is health socially determined?
■ How do you rate your health and why?

Source: Berman, A., Snyder, S. J., Kozier, B., & Erb, G. (2008). *Kozier & Erb's fundamentals of nursing: Concepts, process, and practice* (8th ed., p. 296). Upper Saddle River, NJ: Pearson Education.

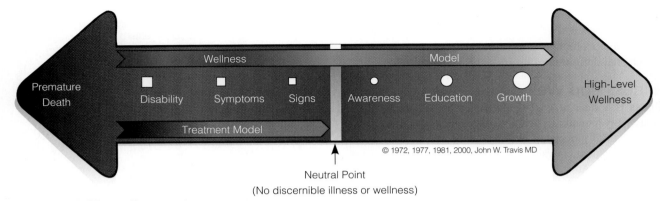

Figure 7–3 ■ An illness-wellness continuum.

Source: Reprinted with permission from Travis, J. W., & Ryan, R. S. (1988). *Wellness workbook.*, Berkeley, CA: Ten Speed Press.

health continuum. Beginning at a high level of health, a person's condition can move through good health, normal health, poor health, and extremely poor health, eventually to death. People move back and forth within this continuum day by day. There is no distinct boundary across which people move from health to illness or from illness back to health. How people perceive themselves and how others see them in terms of health and illness will also affect their placement on the continuum. The ranges in which people can be thought of as healthy or ill are considerable (Figure 7–3 ■).

ILLNESS AND DISEASE

Illness is a highly personal state in which the person's physical, emotional, intellectual, social, developmental, or spiritual functioning is thought to be diminished. It is not synonymous with disease and may or may not be related to disease. An individual could have a disease, for example, a growth in the stomach, and not feel ill. Similarly a person can feel ill, that is, feel uncomfortable, and yet have no discernible disease.

Disease can be described as an alteration in body functions that results in a reduction of capacities or a shortening of the normal life span. Disease occurs when microorganisms produce a detectable alteration in normal tissue function that results in a reduction of capacities or a shortening of the normal life span. Primitive people thought "forces" or spirits caused disease. Later, this belief was replaced by the single-causation theory. Traditionally, the goal of intervention by primary care providers was to eliminate or ameliorate disease processes. Today, multiple factors are considered to interact in causing disease and determining an individual's response to treatment.

Illness and disease can be classified in many ways. The terms acute and chronic are commonly used. **Acute illness** is typically characterized by severe symptoms of relatively short duration. The symptoms often appear abruptly and subside quickly and, depending upon the cause, may or may not require intervention by health care professionals. Some acute illnesses are serious (for example, appendicitis may require surgical intervention), but many acute illnesses, such as colds, subside without medical intervention or with only the help of over-the-counter medications. Following an acute illness, most people return to their normal level of wellness.

A **chronic illness** is one that lasts for an extended period, usually 6 months or longer, and often for the duration of person's life. Chronic illnesses usually have a slow onset and often have periods of **remission**, when the symptoms disappear, and **exacerbation**, when the symptoms reappear. Some chronic diseases with intermittent or recurring symptoms may be termed persistent. For example, a client with severe asthma that is normally well-controlled may be diagnosed with severe persistent asthma.

Examples of chronic illnesses include arthritis, heart and lung diseases, and diabetes mellitus. Nurses are involved in caring for chronically ill individuals of all ages in all types of settings—homes, nursing homes, hospitals, clinics, and other institutions. Care needs to be focused on promoting the highest possible level of independence, sense of control, and wellness. Clients often need to modify their activities of daily living, social relationships, and perception of self and body image. In addition, many must learn how to live with increasing physical limitations and discomfort. Client teaching regarding compliance with medications and treatment plans, even when the client is feeling well, is an essential nursing intervention for individuals with chronic illnesses.

Illness Behaviors

When people become ill, they behave in certain ways that sociologists refer to as illness behavior. **Illness behavior**, a coping mechanism, involves ways that individuals describe, monitor, and interpret their symptoms, take remedial actions, and use the health care system. How people behave when they are ill is highly individualized and is affected by many variables such as age, sex, occupation, socioeconomic status, religion, ethnic origin, psychologic stability, personality, education, and modes of coping.

Effects of Illness on the Client and Family

Illness brings about changes in both the involved individual and the family. The changes vary depending upon the nature, severity, and duration of the illness; attitudes associated with the illness by the client and others; the financial costs associated with the illness; the lifestyle changes incurred; adjustments to usual roles; and so on.

Ill clients may experience behavioral and emotional changes, changes in self-concept and body image, and lifestyle changes. Behavioral and emotional changes associated with short-term illness are generally mild and short lived. The individual, for example, may become irritable and lack the energy or desire to interact with family members or friends in the usual fashion. More acute responses are likely with severe, life-threatening, chronic, or disabling illness. Anxiety, fear, anger, withdrawal, denial, a sense of hopelessness, and feelings of powerlessness are all common responses to severe or disabling illness. For example, a client experiencing a heart attack fears for his or her life and the financial burden it may place on the client's family. Another client informed about a diagnosis of cancer or AIDS or crippling neurologic disease may, over time, experience episodes of denial, anger, fear, and hopelessness. For a client with a life-long chronic illness, these feelings can recur each time the client experiences an acute attack of the illness. Repeated acute attacks, the financial expense that they incur, and the emotional strain that they put on the client and family can cause both the client and family a great deal of stress.

Certain illnesses can also change the client's body image or physical appearance, especially if there is severe scarring or loss of a limb or special sense organ. The client's self-esteem and self-concept may also be affected. Many factors play a part in low self-esteem and a disturbance in self-concept and include: loss of body parts and function, pain, disfigurement, dependence on others, unemployment, financial problems, inability to participate in social functions, strained relationships with others, and spiritual distress. Nurses need to help clients express their thoughts and feelings, and to provide care that helps the client effectively cope with change.

Ill individuals are vulnerable to loss of **autonomy**—the state of being independent and self-directed without outside control. Family interactions may change so that clients are no longer involved in making family decisions or even in making decisions about their own health care. Nurses need to support clients' right to self-determination and autonomy as much as possible by providing them with sufficient information to participate in decision-making processes and to maintain a feeling of being in control.

Illness often necessitates a change in lifestyle. In addition to participating in treatments and taking medications, the ill person may need to change diet, activity and exercise, and rest and sleep patterns.

Nurses can help clients adjust their lifestyles in the following ways:

■ Providing explanations about necessary adjustments
■ Making arrangements wherever possible to accommodate the client's lifestyle
■ Encouraging other health professionals to become aware of the person's lifestyle practices and to support healthy aspects of that lifestyle
■ Reinforcing desirable changes in practices with a goal of making them a permanent part of the client's lifestyle

HEALTH PROMOTION

The vision of **health promotion** was initially expressed in 1979 with the Surgeon General's report *Healthy People,* which emphasized health promotion and disease prevention. *Healthy People 2000* followed in 1990, providing a framework for national health promotion, health protection, and preventive service strategy. The current *Healthy People 2010: Understanding and Improving Health* (U.S. Department of Health and Human Services [USDHHS], 2000) presents a comprehensive 10-year strategy for promoting health and preventing illness, disability, and premature death. The two major goals of *Healthy People 2010* reflect the nation's changing demographics:

1. "Increase quality and years of healthy life" indicates the aging or "graying" of the population.
2. "Eliminate health disparities" reflects the diversity of the population.

To support these goals, *Healthy People 2010* is organized into 28 focus areas to improve health (Box 7–2). *Healthy People 2010* also establishes a set of leading health indicators that reflect the major public health concerns in the United States at the beginning of the 21st Century (Box 7–3). Each indicator relates to a number of the health objectives. It is

---

Box 7–2 The 28 Focus Areas in *Healthy People 2010*

1. Access to quality health services
2. Arthritis, osteoporosis, and chronic back conditions
3. Cancer
4. Chronic kidney disease
5. Diabetes
6. Disability and secondary conditions
7. Educational and community-based programs
8. Environmental health
9. Family planning
10. Food safety
11. Health communication
12. Heart disease and stroke
13. HIV
14. Immunization and infectious diseases
15. Injury and violence prevention
16. Maternal, infant, and child health
17. Medical product safety
18. Mental health and mental disorders
19. Nutrition and overweight
20. Occupational safety and health
21. Oral health
22. Physical activity and fitness
23. Public health infrastructure
24. Respiratory diseases
25. Sexually transmitted diseases
26. Substance abuse
27. Tobacco use
28. Vision and hearing

Source: U.S. Department of Health and Human Services. (2007). Retrieved July 6, 2009, from http://www.cdc.gov/nchs/about/otheract/hpdata2010/2010fa28.htm.

Box 7–3 The Leading Health Indicators in *Healthy People 2010*

- Physical activity
  - Regular physical activity throughout life is important for maintaining a healthy body, enhancing psychological well-being, and preventing premature death (p. 26).
- Overweight and obesity
  - Overweight and obesity are major contributors to many preventable causes of death. On average, higher body weights are associated with higher death rates. The number of overweight children, adolescents, and adults has risen over the past four decades (p. 28).
- Tobacco use
  - Cigarette smoking is the single most preventable cause of disease and death in the United States (p. 30).
- Substance abuse
  - Alcohol and illicit drug use are associated with many of this country's most serious problems, including violence, injury, and HIV infection (p. 32).
- Responsible sexual behavior
  - Unintended pregnancies and sexually transmitted diseases (STDs), including infection with the human immunodeficiency virus that causes AIDS, can result from unprotected sexual behaviors (p. 34).
- Mental health
  - Approximately 20% of the U.S. population is affected by mental illness during a given year; no one is immune. Of all mental illnesses, depression is the most common disorder.

Major depression is the leading cause of disability and is the cause of more than two thirds of suicides each year (p. 36).
- Injury and violence
  - More than 400 Americans die each day from injuries due primarily to motor vehicle crashes, firearms, poisonings, suffocation, falls, fires, and drowning (p. 38).
- Environmental quality
  - An estimated 25% of preventable illnesses worldwide can be attributed to poor environmental quality. Two indicators of air quality are ozone (outdoor) and environmental tobacco smoke (indoor) (p. 40).
- Immunization
  - Vaccines are among the greatest public health achievements of the 20th century. Immunizations can prevent disability and death from infectious diseases for individuals and can help control the spread of infections within communities (p. 42).
- Access to health care
  - Strong predictors of access to quality health care include having health insurance, a higher income level, and a regular primary care provider or other source of ongoing health care. Use of clinical preventive services, such as early prenatal care, can serve as indicators of access to quality health care services (p. 44).

Source: U.S. Department of Health and Human Services. (2007). Retrieved July 6, 2009, from http://www.cdc.gov/nchs/about/otheract/hpdata2010/2010indicators.htm.

---

expected that these indicators will help develop action plans to improve the health of both individuals and communities.

The foundation for *Healthy People 2010* is the belief that individual health is closely linked to community health and the reverse. For example, community health is affected by the beliefs, attitudes, and behaviors of the individuals who live in the community. Thus, the vision for *Healthy People 2010* is "Healthy People in Healthy Communities" (USDHHS, 2000, p. 3). As a result, partnerships are important to improving individual and community health. Businesses, local government, and civic, professional, and religious organizations can all participate. Examples include sponsoring a health fair, establishing fitness programs, beginning community recycling, and printing immunization schedules.

Health Promotion, Health Protection, and Disease Prevention

Considerable differences appear in the literature regarding the use of the terms *health promotion, primary prevention, health protection,* and *illness/disease prevention.* Edelman and Mandle (2006) state that "prevention, in a narrow sense, means avoiding the development of disease in the future, and, in the broader sense, consists of all interventions to limit progression of a disease" (p. 13). Pender, Murdaugh, and Parsons (2006) consider health promotion to be different from disease prevention or health protection. They define *health promotion* as "behavior motivated by the desire to increase well-being and actualize human health potential," and *disease prevention* or *health protection* as "behavior motivated by a desire to actively

avoid illness, detect it early, or maintain functioning within the constraints of illness" (p. 7). The individual's underlying motivation for the behavior is the major difference. Box 7–4 provides an overview of the differences between health promotion and health protection.

The difficulty in separating the terms *health promotion* and *disease prevention/health protection* lies in the fact that an activity may be carried out for numerous reasons. For example, a 40-year-old male may begin a program of walking 3 miles each day. If the goal of his program was to "decrease the risk of cardiovascular disease," then the activity would be considered disease prevention or health protection. By contrast, if the motivation for his walking regimen were to "increase his overall health and feeling of well-being," then the activity would be considered a health promotion behavior. It is

Box 7–4 Differences Between Health Promotion and Health Protection

HEALTH PROMOTION	HEALTH PROTECTION
Not disease oriented	Illness or injury specific
Motivated by personal, positive "approach" to wellness	Motivated by "avoidance" of illness
Seeks to expand positive potential for health	Seeks to thwart the occurrence of insults to health and well-being

Source: Pender, N. J., Murdaugh, C. L., & Parsons, M. A. (2006). *Health promotion in nursing practice* (5th ed., p. 8). Upper Saddle River, NJ: Prentice Hall. Reprinted with permission.

most helpful to think of health promotion and health protection as being complementary processes because both affect quality of health.

Health promotion can be offered to all clients regardless of their health and illness status or age. For example, weight-control measures can benefit both overweight clients without disease and clients with cardiac or joint disease. See Developmental Considerations feature for examples.

The Nurse's Role in Health Promotion

Health promotion is an important component of nursing practice. It is a way of thinking that revolves around a philosophy of wholeness, wellness, and well-being. In the past two decades, the public has become increasingly aware of and interested in health promotion. Many people are aware of the relationship between lifestyle and illness and have begun developing health-promoting habits, such as getting adequate exercise, rest, and relaxation; maintaining good nutrition; and controlling the use of tobacco, alcohol, and other drugs.

Individuals and communities that seek to increase their responsibility for personal health and self-care require health education. The trend toward health promotion has created new opportunities for nurses to strengthen the profession's influence on health promotion. Nurses also have more opportunity to disseminate information that promotes an educated public and to assist individuals and communities to change long-standing health behaviors. Today, nurses serve in a wide variety of organizations and committees.

A variety of programs can be used to promote health, including (a) information dissemination, (b) health risk appraisal and wellness assessment, (c) lifestyle and behavior change, and (d) environmental control programs.

Information dissemination is the most basic type of health promotion program. This method makes use of a variety of media to offer information to the public about the risk of particular lifestyle choices and personal behavior, as well as the benefits of changing that behavior and improving the quality of life. Billboards, posters, brochures, newspaper features, books, and health fairs all offer opportunities for disseminating health promotion information. Alcohol and drug abuse, driving under the influence of alcohol, hypertension, and the need for immunizations are some of the topics frequently discussed. Information dissemination is a useful strategy for raising the level of knowledge and awareness of individuals and groups about health habits.

When planning information dissemination, it is important to consider factors such as culture and age group. Knowing the best place and method for distributing information will increase the effectiveness. For example, churches often provide older Black individuals with social support while serving as a spiritual home. The church is often the appropriate place to hold health fairs or even small group discussions on various health topics. It offers a stepping-stone for providing information and suggesting resources for special needs—all done in a comfortable, nonthreatening environment.

It is just as critical to know where people get misinformation. Sending multiple mailings has become a marketing ploy for advertising "miracle" vitamins, herbs, and food supplements. These are heavily directed toward older adults, who may choose this route to purchase items if they have transportation problems.

DEVELOPMENTAL CONSIDERATIONS **Health Promotion Topics Across the Life Span**

INFANTS
- Infant-parent attachment/bonding
- Breast-feeding
- Sleep patterns
- Playful activity to stimulate development
- Immunizations
- Safety promotion and injury control

CHILDREN
- Nutrition
- Dental checkups
- Rest and exercise
- Immunizations
- Safety promotion and injury control

ADOLESCENTS
- Communicating with the teen
- Hormonal changes
- Nutrition
- Exercise and rest
- Peer group influences
- Self-concept and body image
- Sexuality
- Safety promotion and accident prevention

OLDER ADULTS
- Adequate sleep
- Appropriate use of alcohol
- Dental/oral health
- Drug management
- Exercise
- Foot health
- Health screening recommendations
- Hearing aid use
- Immunizations
- Medication instruction
- Mental health
- Nutrition
- Physical fitness
- Preventive health services
- Safety precautions
- Smoking cessation
- Weight control

Source: Berman, A., Snyder, S. J., Kozier, B., & Erb, G. (2008). *Kozier & Erb's fundamentals of nursing: Concepts, process, and practice* (8th ed., p. 278). Upper Saddle River, NJ: Pearson Education.

Health risk appraisal and wellness assessment programs are used to teach individuals about the risk factors inherent in their lives and to motivate them to reduce specific risks and develop positive health habits. Wellness assessment programs are focused on more positive methods of enhancement, in contrast to the risk factor approach used in the health appraisal. A variety of tools are available to facilitate these assessments; some are computer based and can therefore be offered to educational institutions and industries at a reasonable cost.

Lifestyle and behavior change programs require the participation of the individual and are geared toward enhancing the quality of life and extending the life span. Individuals generally consider lifestyle changes after they have been informed of the need to change their health behavior and have become aware of the potential benefits of the process. Many programs are available to the public, on both a group and individual basis and may include topics such as stress management, nutrition awareness, weight control, smoking cessation, and exercise.

Environmental control programs have been developed in response to the continuing increase of contaminants of human origin being introduced into our environment. The amount of contaminants that are already present in the air, food, and water will affect the health of our descendants for several generations. The most common concerns of community groups are toxic and nuclear wastes, nuclear power plants, air and water pollution, and herbicide and pesticide use.

Health promotion activities, such as the variety of programs previously discussed, involve collaborative relationships with both clients and primary care providers. The role of the nurse is to work *with* people, not *for* them—that is, to act as a facilitator of the process of assessing, evaluating, and understanding health. The nurse may act as advocate, consultant, teacher, or coordinator of services. For examples of the nurse's role in health promotion, see Box 7–5.

In these roles, the nurse may work with individuals of all age groups and diverse family units or concentrate on a specific population, such as new parents, school-age children, or older adults. In any case, the nursing process is a basic tool for the nurse in a health promotion role. Although the process is the same, the nurse emphasizes teaching the client (either an individual or a family unit) self-care responsibility. Adult clients decide the goals, determine the health promotion plans, and take responsibility for the success of the plans.

As increasingly knowledgeable health care consumers, clients expect and deserve quality care. Whether assisting an individual, family, or an entire community, quality nursing care seeks to emphasize illness prevention and health promotion. Nurses recognize that a client's state of health and wellness encompasses many dimensions, including social, spiritual, cultural, sexual, environmental, physical, and psychological. Each client encounter affords the nurse an opportunity to influence and encourage both traditional and innovative health-seeking behaviors.

Assessing and planning health care of the individual client are enhanced when the nurse understands the concepts of individuality, holism, homeostasis, and human needs. The beliefs and values of each person and the support he or she receives come in large part from the family and are reinforced by the community. The reverse is also true—the health of a community is affected by the beliefs, attitudes, and behaviors of the individuals in the community.

VARIABLES INFLUENCING HEALTH

Many variables influence a person's health status, beliefs, and behaviors or practices. These factors may or may not be under conscious control. People can usually control their health behaviors and can choose healthy or unhealthy activities (external variables). In contrast, people have little or no choice over their genetic makeup, age, sex, culture, and sometimes their geographic environments (internal variables).

Internal variables include biologic, psychologic, and cognitive dimensions. They are often described as nonmodifiable variables because, for the most part, they cannot be changed. However, when internal variables are linked to health problems, the nurse must be even more diligent about working with the client to influence external variables (such as exercise and diet) that may assist in health promotion and illness prevention. Regular health exams and appropriate screening for early detection of health problems become even more important. See Table 7–1 for health screening guidelines across the life span.

Biologic Dimension

Genetic makeup, gender, age, and developmental level all significantly influence a person's health. Genetic makeup influences biologic characteristics, innate temperament, activity level, and intellectual potential. It can impact susceptibility to specific disease, such as diabetes and breast cancer. In some cases, genetic predisposition for health or illness is enhanced when parents are from the same ethnic genetic pool. For example, people of African heritage have a higher incidence of sickle-cell anemia and hypertension than the general population but may be less susceptible to malaria.

Box 7–5 **The Nurse's Role in Health Promotion**

- Model healthy lifestyle behaviors and attitudes.
- Facilitate client involvement in the assessment, implementation, and evaluation of health goals.
- Teach clients self-care strategies to enhance fitness, improve nutrition, manage stress, and enhance relationships.
- Assist individuals, families, and communities to increase their levels of health.
- Educate clients to be effective health care consumers.
- Assist clients, families, and communities to develop and choose health-promoting options.
- Guide clients' development in effective problem solving and decision making.
- Reinforce clients' personal and family health-promoting behaviors.
- Advocate in the community for changes that promote a healthy environment.

Source: Berman, A., Snyder, S. J., Kozier, B., & Erb, G. (2008). *Kozier & Erb's fundamentals of nursing: Concepts, process, and practice* (8th ed., p. 283). Upper Saddle River, NJ: Pearson Education.

TABLE 7–1 Health Screenings and Immunization Guidelines Across the Life Span

AGE GROUP	RECOMMENDED SCREENINGS AND HEALTH PROMOTION
Newborn and infant	■ Screening of newborns for hearing loss; follow-up at 3 months and early intervention by 6 months if appropriate ■ Health examinations at 2 weeks and 2, 4, 6, and 12 months ■ Immunizations: diphtheria, tetanus, acellular pertussis (DTaP), inactivated poliovirus vaccine (IPV), pneumococcal, measles-mumps-rubella (MMR), *Haemophilus influenzae* type B (HIB), hepatitis B (HepB), varicella and influenza vaccines as recommended ■ Fluoride supplements if there is inadequate water fluoridation (less than 0.7 ppm) ■ Screening for tuberculosis ■ Screening for phenylketonuria (PKU) and other metabolic conditions ■ Denver II or other developmental screening
Toddler	■ Health examinations at 15 and 18 months and then as recommended by the primary care provider ■ Dental visit starting at age 3 or earlier ■ Immunizations: continuing DTaP, IPV series, pneumococcal, MMR, *Haemophilus influenzae* type B, hepatitis B, hepatitis A, and influenza vaccines as recommended ■ Screenings for tuberculosis and lead poisoning ■ Fluoride supplements if there is inadequate water fluoridation (less than 0.7 ppm)
Preschool	■ Health examinations every 1–2 years ■ Immunizations: continuing DTaP, IPV series, MMR, hepatitis, pneumococcal, influenza, and other immunizations as recommended ■ Screenings for tuberculosis ■ Vision and hearing screening ■ Regular dental screenings and fluoride treatment
School-age	■ Annual physical examination or as recommended ■ Immunizations as recommended (e.g., MMR, meningococcal, tetanus-diphtheria, adult preparation [Td]) ■ Screening for tuberculosis ■ Periodic vision, speech, and hearing screenings ■ Regular dental screenings and fluoride treatment
Adolescent	■ Health examination as recommended by the primary care provider ■ Immunizations as recommended, such as adult tetanus-diphtheria vaccine, MMR, pneumococcal, and hepatitis B vaccine ■ Screening for tuberculosis ■ Periodic vision and hearing screenings ■ Regular dental assessments
Young adults	■ Routine physical examination (every 1–3 years for females; every 5 years for males) ■ Immunizations as recommended, such as tetanus-diphtheria boosters every 10 years, meningococcal vaccine if not given in early adolescence (Bilukha & Rosenstein, 2005), and hepatitis B vaccine ■ Regular dental assessments (every 6 months) ■ Periodic vision and hearing screenings ■ Professional breast examination every 1–3 years ■ Papanicolaou smear annually within 3 years of onset of sexual activity ■ Testicular examination every year ■ Screening for cardiovascular disease (e.g., cholesterol test every 5 years if results are normal; blood pressure to detect hypertension; baseline electrocardiogram at age 35) ■ Tuberculosis skin test every 2 years ■ Smoking: history and counseling, if needed

(continued)

TABLE 7–1 **Health Screenings and Immunization Guidelines Across the Life Span** (continued)

AGE GROUP	RECOMMENDED SCREENINGS AND HEALTH PROMOTION
Middle-aged adults	■ Physical examination (every 3–5 years until age 40, then annually)
	■ Immunizations as recommended, such as a tetanus booster every 10 years, and current recommendations for influenza vaccine
	■ Regular dental assessments (e.g., every 6 months)
	■ Tonometry for signs of glaucoma and other eye diseases every 2–3 years or annually if indicated
	■ Breast examination annually by primary care provider
	■ Testicular examination annually by primary care provider
	■ Screenings for cardiovascular disease (e.g., blood pressure measurement; electrocardiogram and cholesterol test as directed by the primary care provider)
	■ Screenings for colorectal, breast, cervical, uterine, and prostate cancer
	■ Screening for tuberculosis every 2 years
	■ Smoking: history and counseling, if needed
Older adults	■ Total cholesterol and high-density lipid protein measurement every 3–5 years until age 75
	■ Aspirin, 81 mg, daily, if in high-risk group
	■ Diabetes mellitus screen every 3 years, if in high-risk group
	■ Smoking cessation
	■ Screening mammogram every 1–2 years (women)
	■ Clinical breast exam annually (women)
	■ Pap smear annually if there is a history of abnormal smears or previous hysterectomy for malignancy (U.S. Preventive Services Task Force, 2003)
	■ Older women who have regular, normal Pap smears or hysterectomy for nonmalignant causes do NOT need Pap smears beyond the age of 65 (U.S. Preventive Services Task Force, 2003)
	■ Annual digital rectal exam
	■ Annual prostate-specific antigen (PSA)
	■ Annual fecal occult blood test (FOBT)
	■ Sigmoidoscopy every 5 years; colonoscopy every 10 years
	■ Visual acuity screen annually
	■ Hearing screen annually
	■ Depression screen periodically
	■ Family violence screen periodically
	■ Height and weight measurements annually
	■ Sexually transmitted disease testing, if in high-risk group
	■ Annual flu vaccine if over 65 or in high-risk group
	■ Pneumococcal vaccine at 65 and every 10 years thereafter
	■ Td vaccine every 10 years

Gender influences the distribution of disease. Certain acquired and genetic diseases are more common in one sex than in the other. Disorders more common among women include osteoporosis and autoimmune diseases such as rheumatoid arthritis. Those more common among men are stomach ulcers, abdominal hernias, and respiratory diseases.

Age is also a significant factor in the distribution of disease. For example, arteriosclerotic heart disease is common in middle-aged men but occurs infrequently in younger people; communicable diseases such as whooping cough and measles are common in children but rare in older adults, who have acquired immunity to them.

Developmental level has a major impact on health status. Consider these examples:

■ Because infants lack physiologic and psychologic maturity, their defenses against disease are lower during the first years of life.

■ Toddlers who are learning to walk are more prone to falls and injury.

■ Adolescents who need to conform to peers are more prone to risk-taking behavior and subsequent injury.

■ Declining physical and sensory-perceptual abilities limit the ability of older adults to respond to environmental hazards and stressors.

Psychologic Dimension

Psychologic (emotional) factors influencing health include mind-body interactions and self-concept.

Mind-body interactions can affect health status positively or negatively. Emotional responses to stress affect body function. For example, a student who is extremely anxious before a test may experience urinary frequency or diarrhea. A person worried about the outcome of surgery or about the behavior of a teenager may chain smoke. Prolonged emotional distress may increase susceptibility to organic disease or precipitate it. Emotional distress may influence the immune system through central nervous system and endocrine alterations. Alterations in the immune system are related to the incidence of infections, cancer, and autoimmune diseases.

Increasing attention is being given to the mind's ability to direct the body's functioning. Relaxation, meditation, and biofeedback techniques are gaining wider recognition among individuals and health care professionals. For example, women often use relaxation techniques to decrease pain during childbirth. Other people may learn biofeedback skills to reduce hypertension.

Emotional reactions also occur in response to body conditions. For example, a person diagnosed with a terminal illness may experience fear and depression. *Self-concept* is how a person feels about self (self-esteem) and perceives the physical self (body image) and his or her needs, roles, and abilities. Self-concept affects how people view and handle situations. Such attitudes can affect health practices, responses to stress and illness, and when treatment is sought. An example is the anorexic woman who deprives herself of needed nutrients because she believes she is too fat even though she is well below an acceptable weight level. Self-perceptions are also associated with a person's definition of health. For example, a 75-year-old man who can no longer move large objects as he was accustomed to doing may need to examine and redefine his concept of health in view of his age and abilities.

Cognitive Dimension

Cognitive or intellectual factors influencing health include lifestyle choices and spiritual and religious beliefs. Some clients are better at problem solving and come equipped with better coping skills than others. Nurses must be aware of cognitive and intellectual factors that support or hinder a client's compliance with treatment.

Lifestyle refers to a person's general way of living, including living conditions and individual patterns of behavior that are influenced by sociocultural factors and personal characteristics. In brief, lifestyle is often considered as behavior and activities over which people have control. Lifestyle choices may have positive or negative effects on health. Practices that have potentially negative effects on health are often referred to as **risk factors**. For example, overeating, getting insufficient exercise, and being overweight are closely related to the incidence of heart disease, arteriosclerosis, diabetes, and hypertension. Excessive use of tobacco is clearly implicated in lung cancer, emphysema, and cardiovascular diseases. See Box 7–6 for examples of healthy lifestyle choices.

Box 7–6 Examples of Healthy Lifestyle Choices

- Regular exercise
- Weight control
- Avoidance of saturated fats
- Alcohol and tobacco avoidance
- Seat belt use
- Bike helmet use
- Immunization updates
- Regular dental checkups
- Regular health maintenance visits for screening examinations or tests

Source: Berman, A., Snyder, S. J., Kozier, B., & Erb, G. (2008). *Kozier & Erb's fundamentals of nursing: Concepts, process, and practice* (8th ed., p. 301). Upper Saddle River, NJ: Pearson Education.

Spiritual and religious beliefs can significantly affect health behavior. For example, Jehovah's Witnesses oppose blood transfusions; some fundamentalists believe that a serious illness is a punishment from God; some religious groups are strict vegetarians; and religious Jews perform circumcision on the eighth day of a male baby's life. The influence of spirituality and religion is discussed further in the Spirituality concept.

 ## NURSING PROCESS

Health Promotion

A thorough assessment of the individual's health status is basic to health promotion. As nurses move toward greater autonomy in client care, expanded assessment skills are essential to providing the meaningful data needed for health planning.

Assessment

Components of this assessment are the health history and physical examination, physical fitness assessment, lifestyle assessment, spiritual assessment, social support systems review, health risk assessment, health beliefs review, and life-stress review.

HEALTH HISTORY AND PHYSICAL EXAMINATION The health history and physical examination provide a means for detecting any existing problems. The age of the individual must be considered when collecting data. For example, an environmental safety assessment and immunization history must be appropriate to the person's age. A nutritional assessment is another important part of the health history. The nurse must consider both age and body build of the client when gathering information on dietary patterns.

PHYSICAL FITNESS ASSESSMENT During an evaluation of physical fitness, the nurse assesses several components of the body's physical functioning: muscle endurance, flexibility, body composition, and cardiorespiratory endurance. See exemplar 7.2 Physical Fitness and Exercise.

LIFESTYLE ASSESSMENT Lifestyle assessment focuses on the personal lifestyle and habits of the client as they affect health. Categories of lifestyle generally assessed include physical activity, nutritional practices, stress management, and such habits as smoking, alcohol consumption, and drug use. Other

DEVELOPMENTAL CONSIDERATIONS Factors Affecting Health Promotion and Illness Prevention in Children and Older Adults

CHILDREN

Childhood obesity is becoming a serious health problem. Data collected by the Centers for Disease Control and Prevention (CDC) show that nearly 16% of American children are overweight, up from 6.5% in 1980 (National Center for Health Statistics, 2004). Obesity and overweight in children contribute to long-term health problems such as heart disease and diabetes mellitus.

Although specific causes of obesity and appropriate strategies to reduce weight will vary from child to child, healthy eating habits and adequate exercise patterns form the basis for healthy growth and prevention of obesity in children. It is the responsibility of parents and caregivers to provide children with healthy food choices and an environment that makes eating a pleasure. It is the responsibility of children to decide how much and what foods to eat. Adults must be role models for their children, eating well and exercising regularly themselves.

OLDER ADULTS

In older adults, health promotion and illness prevention are important, but often the focus is on learning to adapt to and live with increasing changes and limitations. Maximizing strengths continues to

be of prime importance in maintaining optimal function and quality of life. Factors that may indicate a need for additional information or resources include the following:

- An increase in physical limitations
- Presence of one or more chronic illnesses
- Change in cognitive status
- Difficulty in accessing health care services due to transportation problems
- Poor support system
- Need for environmental modifications for safety and to maintain independence
- Attitude of hopelessness and depression, which decreases the motivation to use resources or learn new information

Source: Berman, A., Snyder, S. J., Kozier, B., & Erb, G. (2008). *Kozier & Erb's fundamentals of nursing: Concepts, process, and practice* (8th ed., p. 285). Upper Saddle River, NJ: Pearson Education.

---

categories may be included. Several tools are available to assess lifestyle. The goals of lifestyle assessment tools are to provide the following:

- An opportunity for clients to assess the impact of their present lifestyle on their health
- A basis for decisions related to desired behavior and lifestyle change
- Special consideration may need to be given to the lifestyles of children and older adults (see the Developmental Considerations feature box).

SPIRITUAL HEALTH ASSESSMENT Spiritual health is the ability to develop one's inner nature to its fullest potential, including the ability to discover and articulate one's basic purpose in life; learn how to experience love, joy, peace, and fulfillment; and learn how to help ourselves and others achieve their fullest potential (Pender et al., 2006, p. 108). Spiritual beliefs can affect a person's interpretation of events in his or her life and, therefore, an assessment of spiritual well-being is a part of evaluating the person's overall health. (See the Spirituality concept for more information.)

SOCIAL SUPPORT SYSTEMS REVIEW Understanding the social context in which a person lives and works is important in health promotion. Individuals and groups, through

interpersonal relationships, can provide comfort, assistance, encouragement, and information. Social support fosters successful coping and promotes satisfying and effective living.

Social support systems contribute to health by creating an environment that encourages healthy behaviors, promotes self-esteem and wellness, and provides feedback to ensure that the person's actions will lead to desirable outcomes. Examples of social support systems include family, peer support groups (including Internet-based support groups), community-organized religious support systems (e.g., churches), and self-help groups (e.g., Mended Hearts, Weight Watchers). The Focus on Diversity and Culture box addresses aspects of social support within the context of culture.

LIFE STRESS REVIEW There is abundant literature about the impact of stress on mental and physical well-being. A variety of stress-related instruments can be found in the literature.

Validating Assessment Data

Following the collection of assessment data, the nurse and client together need to review, validate, and summarize the information. During this process, the nurse verbally reviews the current practices and attitudes of the client. This allows

---

FOCUS ON DIVERSITY AND CULTURE Cultural Aspects of Social Support

It is important to understand how various subgroups of American society may define social support.

- In the Black community, the family and church traditionally are major providers of social support.
- Hispanic-Latin Americans and Asian Americans view the family as a major social support system.

- Asian Americans respect older adults and use shame and harmony in giving and receiving support.
- Native Americans live in social networks that foster mutual assistance and support.

Source: Pender, N. J., Murdaugh, C. L., & Parsons, M. A. (2006). *Health promotion in nursing practice* (5th ed., pp. 239–240). Upper Saddle River, NJ: Prentice Hall. Reprinted with permission.

validation of the information by the client and may increase awareness of the need to change behavior. The nurse and client need to consider the following:

- Any existing health problems
- The client's perceived degree of control over health status
- Key health beliefs
- Level of physical fitness and nutritional status
- Illnesses for which the client is at risk
- Current positive health practices
- Spirituality
- Sources of life stress and ability to handle stress
- Social support systems
- Information needed to enhance health care practices

Diagnoses

Nursing diagnoses accepted by the North American Nursing Diagnosis Association (NANDA) have generally focused on impaired or imbalanced health patterns or problems. The NANDA **wellness diagnoses** definition, however, states "Describes human responses to levels of wellness in an individual, family, or community that have a readiness for enhancement" (2005, p. 277).

Wellness diagnoses can be applied at all levels of prevention but are particularly useful for healthy clients who require teaching for health promotion, disease prevention, and personal growth. When the nurse and client conclude that the client has positive function in a certain pattern area, such as adequate nutrition or effective coping, the nurse can use this information to help the client reach a higher level of functioning.

A wellness diagnosis is preceded by the modifier "readiness for enhanced." The following examples are included in the NANDA taxonomy:

- Readiness for Enhanced Spiritual Well-being
- Readiness for Enhanced Coping
- Readiness for Enhanced Nutrition
- Readiness for Enhanced Knowledge (Specify)
- Readiness for Enhanced Parenting
- Readiness for Enhanced Self-Concept
- Readiness for Enhanced Immunization Status
- Readiness for Enhanced Self-Care

Wellness diagnoses provide a clear focus for planning interventions without indicating that a problem exists.

Planning

Health promotion plans need to be developed according to the needs, desires, and priorities of the client. The client decides on health promotion goals, the activities or interventions to achieve those goals, the frequency and duration of the activities, and the method of evaluation. During the planning process, the nurse acts as a resource person rather than as an advisor or counselor. The nurse provides information when asked, emphasizes the importance of small steps to behavioral change, and reviews the client's goals and plans to make sure they are realistic, measurable, and acceptable to the client.

STEPS IN PLANNING   Pender et al. (2006, pp. 127–141) outline several steps in the process of developing a joint health promotion-prevention plan. These steps actively involve both the nurse and the client:

1. *Review and summarize data from assessment.* The nurse shares with the client a summary of the data collected from the various assessments (e.g., physical health and fitness, nutrition, sources of stress, spirituality, health practices).
2. *Reinforce strengths and competencies of the client.* The nurse and the client come to consensus about areas in which the client is doing well and areas that need further development.
3. *Identify health goals and related behavior-change options.* The client selects two or three top priority personal health goals, prioritizes them, and reviews behavior-change options.
4. *Identify behavioral or health outcomes.* For each of the selected goals or areas in step 1, the nurse and client determine what specific behavioral changes are needed to bring about the desired outcome. For example, to reduce the risk of cardiovascular disease, the client may need to stop smoking, lose weight, and increase activity level.
5. *Develop a behavior-change plan.* A constructive program of change is based on client "ownership" of those behavior changes selected for implementation within everyday life (Pender et al., 2006, p. 134). Nurses may need to assist clients in examining value-behavior inconsistencies and in selecting behavioral options that are most appealing and that clients are most willing to try. The client's priorities will reflect personal values, activity preferences, and expectations for success.
6. *Reiterate benefits of change.* The positive benefits will probably need to be reiterated by both the nurse and the client even though the client is committed to the change. The nurse should encourage the client to keep the health-related and non-health-related benefits before the client as central motivating factors.
7. *Address environmental and interpersonal facilitators and barriers to change.* Environmental and interpersonal factors that support positive change should be used to reinforce the client's efforts to change lifestyle. All people experience barriers, some of which can be anticipated and planned for, thereby making the change more likely to occur.
8. *Determine a time frame for implementation.* A time frame allows the client to develop the appropriate knowledge and skills before a new behavior is implemented. The time frame may be several weeks or months. Scheduling short-term goals and rewards can offer encouragement to achieve long-term objectives. Clients require help to be realistic and to deal with one behavior at a time.
9. *Formalize commitment to behavior-change plan.* Commitments to changing behaviors have usually been verbal. Increasingly, a formal, written behavioral contract is being used to motivate the client to follow

through with selected actions. Motivation to follow through is provided by a **positive reinforcement** or reward stated in the contract. Contracting is based on the belief that all people have the potential for growth and the right of self-determination, that is, to be able to make decisions independently without outside interference or compulsion, even though their choices may differ from the norm.

EXPLORING AVAILABLE RESOURCES Another essential aspect of planning is identifying support resources available to the client. These may be community resources such as a fitness program at a local gymnasium, or educational programs about important topics such as stress management, breast self-examination, nutrition, smoking cessation, and health lectures.

Implementation

Implementation is the "doing" part of behavior change. Self-responsibility is emphasized for implementing the plan. Depending on the client's needs, the nursing interventions may include supporting, counseling, facilitating, teaching, consulting, enhancing the behavior change, and modeling.

A major nursing role is to support the client. A vital component of lifestyle change is ongoing support that focuses on the desired behavior change and is provided in a nonjudgmental manner. Support can be offered by the nurse on an individual basis or in a group setting. The nurse can also facilitate the development of support networks for the client, including family members and friends.

INDIVIDUAL COUNSELING SESSIONS Counseling sessions may be routinely scheduled as part of the plan, or may be provided if the client encounters difficulty in carrying out interventions or meets insurmountable barriers to change. In a counseling relationship, the nurse and client share ideas. In this sharing relationship, the nurse acts as a facilitator, promoting the client's decision-making in regard to the health promotion plan.

TELEPHONE OR INTERNET COUNSELING Regular telephone sessions or Internet interaction may be provided to the client to help in answering questions, reviewing goals and strategies, and reinforcing progress. The client may find that scheduling a weekly interaction is helpful or may wish to initiate a call if a problem occurs. The nurse asks the client, "Is your plan working?" If the plan is not working, the nurse asks, "What would you like to do?" The client may wish to continue or may wish to change the plan to a more realistic one. Telephone or Internet support is efficient for the busy client who may not have the time for regular, in-person sessions.

GROUP SUPPORT Group sessions provide an opportunity for participants to learn from the experiences of others in changing behavior. Group contact gives individuals a renewed commitment to their goals. Groups can be scheduled at a variety of time intervals to best suit the group.

FACILITATING SOCIAL SUPPORT Social networks, such as family and friends, can facilitate or impede the efforts directed toward health promotion and prevention. The nurse's role is to assist the client to assess, modify, and develop the social support necessary to achieve the desired change. To provide the necessary support, families must communicate effectively, be aware of and support each other's needs and goals, and provide help and assistance to one another to achieve those goals. The client may wish the nurse to meet with the family or significant others to help enlist their understanding and support.

PROVIDING HEALTH EDUCATION Health education programs on a variety of topics discussed earlier can be provided to groups, individuals, or communities. Group programs need to be planned carefully before they are implemented. The decision to establish a health promotion program must be based upon the health needs of the people; also, specific health promotion goals must be set. After the program is implemented, outcomes must be evaluated.

ENHANCING BEHAVIOR CHANGE Whether people will make and maintain changes to improve health or prevent disease depends upon many interrelated factors. To help clients succeed in implementing behavior changes, the nurse needs to understand the stages of change and choose effective interventions that focus on helping the individual progress through the stages of change. Figure 7–4 ■ and the Client Teaching feature provide suggested strategies to assist clients depending upon their stage of change. As Saarmann, Daugherty, and Riegel (2000) point out, the nursing goal is not necessarily to change behavior but to advance the client to the next stage of change (p. 285).

MODELING In **modeling**, the client acquires ideas for behavior and coping strategies that can be used with specific problems by observing a model or role model. The client is not expected to mimic the sequence of actions or behavior patterns of the model, but can adapt them to fit with or modify the client's own behaviors. The nurse and client should mutually select models with whom the client can identify, since the cultural and ethnic backgrounds and age of the nurse and client often differ. Models should be people the client respects. Nurses should also serve as models of wellness. To model effectively, nurses need to adopt a personal philosophy and lifestyle that demonstrate good health habits.

Evaluation

Evaluation takes place on an ongoing basis as short-term goals are attained and after long-term goals have been completed. Goals are written during the planning phase, and a date is determined for attaining the specific results or behaviors that are desired to promote health or prevent illness. During evaluation, the client may decide to continue with the plan, reorder priorities, change strategies, or revise the health protection–promotion contract. Evaluation of the plan is a collaborative effort between the nurse and the client.

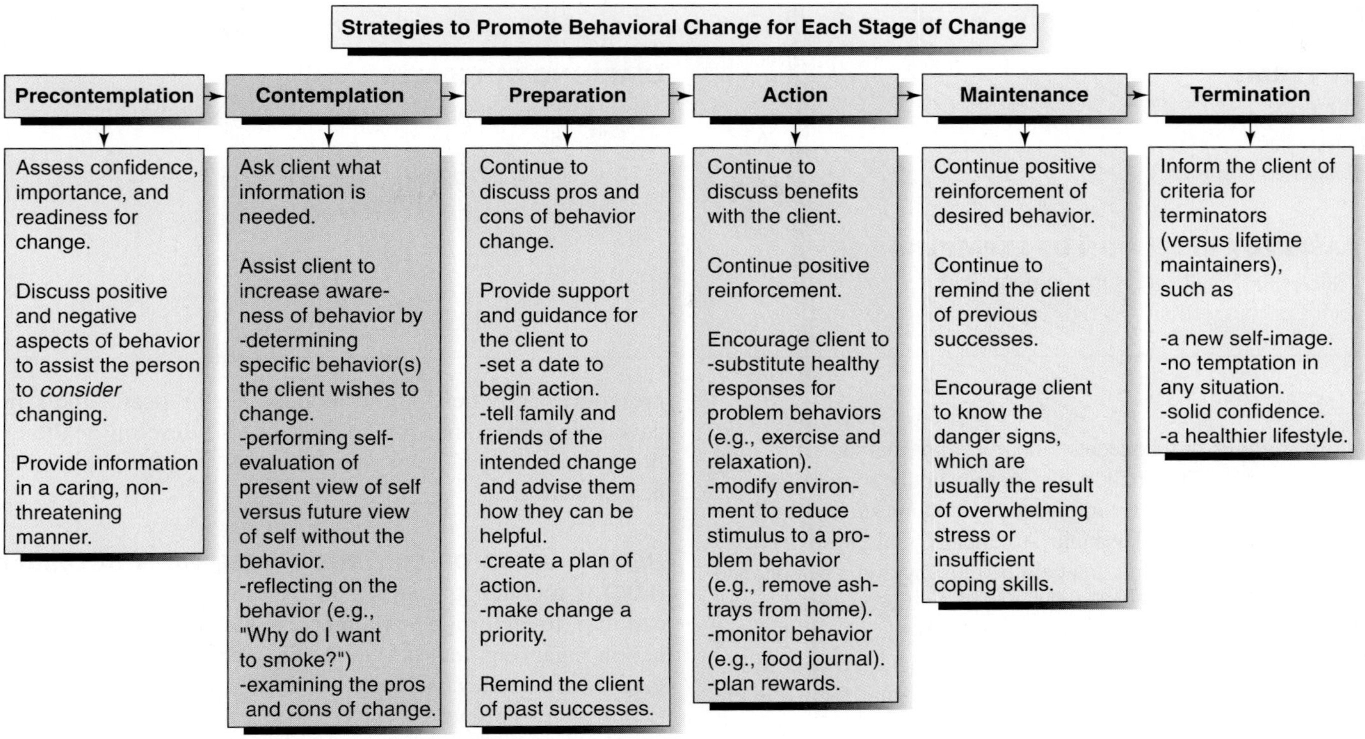

Strategies to Promote Behavioral Change for Each Stage of Change

Precontemplation	Contemplation	Preparation	Action	Maintenance	Termination
Assess confidence, importance, and readiness for change. Discuss positive and negative aspects of behavior to assist the person to *consider* changing. Provide information in a caring, non-threatening manner.	Ask client what information is needed. Assist client to increase awareness of behavior by -determining specific behavior(s) the client wishes to change. -performing self-evaluation of present view of self versus future view of self without the behavior. -reflecting on the behavior (e.g., "Why do I want to smoke?") -examining the pros and cons of change.	Continue to discuss pros and cons of behavior change. Provide support and guidance for the client to -set a date to begin action. -tell family and friends of the intended change and advise them how they can be helpful. -create a plan of action. -make change a priority. Remind the client of past successes.	Continue to discuss benefits with the client. Continue positive reinforcement. Encourage client to -substitute healthy responses for problem behaviors (e.g., exercise and relaxation). -modify environment to reduce stimulus to a problem behavior (e.g., remove ashtrays from home). -monitor behavior (e.g., food journal). -plan rewards.	Continue positive reinforcement of desired behavior. Continue to remind the client of previous successes. Encourage client to know the danger signs, which are usually the result of overwhelming stress or insufficient coping skills.	Inform the client of criteria for terminators (versus lifetime maintainers), such as -a new self-image. -no temptation in any situation. -solid confidence. -a healthier lifestyle.

Figure 7–4 ■ Strategies to promote behavioral change for each stage of change.

CLIENT TEACHING **Enhancing Behavior Change**

ESTABLISH RAPPORT

■ Provide privacy and a perception of a collaborative, equal-power relationship.

■ If time allows, ask the client to describe a "typical" day. Usually the problematic behavior is described; however, even if it is not, the listening will strengthen rapport and the personal information may be helpful in understanding the client's current situation.

SET AGENDA

■ Allow the client to identify concerns. If there are multiple concerns (e.g., smoking, exercise, diet, stress), it is best to focus on one specific behavior at a time. Ask the client which behavior he or she feels most ready to *think* about changing.

ASSESS IMPORTANCE, CONFIDENCE, AND READINESS

■ A client's readiness to change is often influenced by his or her perception of importance and confidence.

■ Importance refers to the personal value of change. Questions that elicit this information can include the following: "How do you feel at the moment about [state the change]?" "How important is it to you to [state the change]?" "On a scale of 1–10, with 1 being not important and 10 very important, what number would you give yourself?"

■ Confidence relates to mastering the skills needed to achieve the behavior and the situations in which behavior change will be challenging to the client. A potential question to use to assess confidence is "If you decided right now to change, how confident would you feel about succeeding?"

EXCHANGE INFORMATION AND REDUCE RESISTANCE

■ These two tasks are performed throughout the various stages of behavior change.

■ Ask clients if they would like information; if so, ask what specific information they need.

■ Present information in a neutral tone of voice, and avoid using the word "you" too much. Referring to other people (versus "you") and what happens to them makes the information less threatening to the client.

■ After presenting the information, ask for the client's interpretation of the information.

■ There are three *traps* that increase resistance. The traps and strategies to avoid them include the following:

a. *Trap:* Taking control away. *Instead:* Emphasize personal choice and control.

b. *Trap:* Misjudging importance, confidence, or readiness. Often this results in talking about action before the client is ready. *Instead:* It is important to reexamine the client's feelings about importance and confidence as they influence readiness to make a specific change.

c. *Trap:* Meeting force with force (attacking or defending through argument). *Instead:* Sit back and use reflective listening. Try to understand how the client is feeling. The resistance usually subsides and the discussion can move in a different direction.

Source: Rollnick, S., Mason, P., & Butler, C. (1999). *Health behavior change: A guide for practitioners.* Philadelphia: Elsevier. Reprinted with permission.

7.1 HEALTH BELIEFS

KEY TERMS

Adherence, *194*
Health beliefs, *194*
Locus of control (LOC), *194*

BASIS FOR SELECTION OF EXEMPLAR

Institute for Healthcare Improvement (IHI)
Joint Commission (JCAHO)

LEARNING OUTCOMES

After reading about this exemplar, you will be able to do the following:

1. Describe health belief.
2. Identify factors that modify health beliefs.

OVERVIEW

Health beliefs are concepts about health that an individual believes are true. Such beliefs may or may not be founded on fact.

Some health beliefs are influenced by culture, such as the "hot-cold" belief of some Hispanic Americans. This system views health as a balance of hot and cold qualities within a person, and foods are classified as hot or cold as well. In this context, hot and cold do not denote temperature or spiciness but innate qualities of the food. Citrus fruits and some fowl are considered cold foods, and meats and bread are hot foods. A Hispanic family might believe that a fever is caused by an excess of hot foods, so the person with a fever would be given cold foods as a remedy.

Another example of a culturally related health belief is the belief that health and illness are closely associated with the amount and quality of blood in the body. For example, some southerners say that "high blood," meaning too much blood in the body, causes headaches and dizziness. For additional information about cultural views of health and illness, see the Culture concept.

Health Beliefs Review

Clients' health beliefs must be clarified, particularly those that determine how clients perceive control of their own health status. Several instruments are available that assess a person's health-belief measures. Assessment of clients' health beliefs provides the nurse with an indication of how much the clients believe they can influence or control health through personal behaviors.

Several cultures have a strong belief in fate, that is, "Whatever will be, will be." When people hold this belief, they do not think they can do anything to change the course of their disease. An example is a client with diabetes who must make many lifestyle changes in diet and exercise and closely control glucose levels to prevent complications. If the diabetic client believes he or she has no control over the outcome, it is difficult to teach the client to make the necessary changes. These health beliefs can provide a better indication of the client's readiness and motivation to engage in healthy behaviors.

Health Belief Models

Several theories or models of health beliefs and behaviors have been developed to help determine whether an individual is likely to participate in disease prevention and health promotion activities. These models can be useful tools in developing programs for helping people develop healthier lifestyles and a more positive attitude toward preventive health measures.

HEALTH LOCUS OF CONTROL MODEL Locus of control (LOC) is a concept from social learning theory that nurses can use to determine whether clients are likely to take action regarding health, that is, whether clients believe that their health status is under their own or others' control. People who believe they have a major influence on their own health status—that health is largely self-determined—are called *internals*. People who exercise internal control are more likely than others to take the initiative in their own health care, be more knowledgeable about their health, and adhere to prescribed health care regimens such as taking medication, making and keeping appointments with primary care providers, maintaining diets, and giving up smoking. By contrast, people who believe their health is largely controlled by outside forces (e.g., chance or powerful others) are referred to as *externals*.

Research has shown that locus of control plays an important role in clients' choices about health behaviors. In some cases, externals demonstrate better **adherence** (compliance) to medical regimens, while in others, internals have increased adherence. For example, Leong, Molassiotis, and Marsh (2004) found externals adhered better to weight loss regimens whereas internals adhered better to exercise programs.

Locus of control is a measurable concept that can be used to predict which people are most likely to change their behavior. Many measurement instruments are available to assess LOC. One widely used example is the Multidimensional Health Locus of Control (MHLC) Scale (Wallston, Wallston, & DeVellis, 1978), most recently expanded to Form C (Wallston, Stein, & Smith, 1994). Nurses can use LOC results to plan internal reinforcement training if necessary to improve client efforts toward better health.

Nurses play a major role in helping clients implement healthy behaviors. They help clients monitor health, supply anticipatory guidance, and impart knowledge about health. Nurses can also reduce barriers to action (e.g., by minimizing inconvenience or discomfort) and support positive actions.

REVIEW   Health Beliefs

RELATE: LINK THE CONCEPTS

Linking the concepts of Development and Culture with the concept of Health, Wellness, and Illness:

1. Explain how developmental stages from childhood through older adult would affect locus of control.
2. Compare the health beliefs of the various cultures within your community. What challenges would they present in providing health care?

REFLECT: CASE STUDY

A home care nurse visits a 79-year-old woman client recently diagnosed with diabetes mellitus. The client takes her oral medication for diabetes only sporadically, and she is not following her new diet. The client says, "I don't really think I have diabetes. I feel fine, except that I'm always thirsty."

1. How would you deal with this belief?

7.2 PHYSICAL FITNESS AND EXERCISE

KEY TERMS

Activity-exercise pattern, *195*
Activity tolerance, *196*
Aerobic exercise, *196*
Anaerobic exercise, *196*
Exercise, *196*
Functional strength, *196*
Hypertrophy, *196*
Isokinetic exercise, *196*
Isometric exercise, *196*
Isotonic exercise, *196*
Physical activity, *196*

BASIS FOR SELECTION OF EXEMPLAR

Healthy People 2010

LEARNING OUTCOMES

After reading about this exemplar, you will be able to do the following:

1. Differentiate isotonic, isometric, isokinetic, aerobic, and anaerobic exercise.
2. Describe the effects of exercise on body systems.
3. Assess activity-exercise pattern and activity tolerance.
4. Develop nursing diagnoses and outcomes related to activity and exercise.

OVERVIEW

Physical fitness is to the human body what fine-tuning is to an engine. It enables the body to perform to its potential. Fitness can be described as a condition that helps individuals look, feel, and do their best. More specifically, physical fitness is the ability to perform daily tasks vigorously and alertly, with energy left over for enjoying leisure-time activities and meeting emergency demands. It is the ability to endure, to bear up, to withstand stress, to carry on in circumstances where an unfit person could not continue, and it is a major basis for good health and well-being (President's Council on Physical Fitness and Sports, 2003).

Physical fitness involves the performance of the body's heart, lungs, and muscles. Fitness, to some degree, influences qualities such as mental alertness and emotional stability, because what humans do with their bodies also affects what they can do with their minds. To maintain fitness, one must meet the needs for exercise, nutrition, rest, and relaxation, and follow practices to promote and preserve health.

Many *Healthy People 2010* objectives pertain to exercise and activity. Following are some of these objectives:

- Increase the proportion of people who engage in moderate physical activity for at least 30 minutes a day
- Increase the proportion of adults and children who perform physical activities that enhance and maintain muscle strength, endurance, and flexibility

- Increase the proportion of work sites offering employer-sponsored physical activity and fitness programs
- Reduce activity limitation due to chronic back conditions
- Reduce the number of overweight people (Edelman & Mandle, 2006)

A strong, well-developed body of research evidence supports the role of exercise in improving the health status of individuals with cardiovascular disease, pulmonary dysfunction, disabilities of aging, and depression. Integrating well-researched exercise protocols with conventional nursing and medical approaches will result in optimal treatment of these common disorders. Evidence shows that exercise can prevent and even reverse many of the chronic diseases experienced by aging adults. A growing body of research supports the preventive and therapeutic effects of exercise for individuals with diabetes, cancer, arthritis, chronic fatigue syndrome, fibromyalgia, menopause, urinary incontinence, Parkinson's, Alzheimer's, and HIV/AIDS (Freeman, 2004; Micozzi, 2006).

An **activity-exercise pattern** refers to a person's routine of exercise, activity, leisure, and recreation. It includes (a) activities of daily living (ADLs) that require energy expenditure, such as hygiene, dressing, cooking, shopping, eating, working, and home maintenance; and (b) the type, quality, and quantity of exercise, including sports.

People often define their health and physical fitness by their activity because mental well-being and the effectiveness of body functioning depend largely on their mobility status. For example, when a person is upright, the lungs expand more easily, intestinal activity (peristalsis) is more effective, and the kidneys are able to empty completely. In addition, motion is essential for proper functioning of bones and muscles.

PHYSICAL ACTIVITY AND EXERCISE

The U.S. Department of Health and Human Services defines physical activity and exercise as follows (Edelman & Mandle, 2006):

- **Physical activity** is bodily movement produced by skeletal muscle contraction that increases energy expenditure.
- **Exercise** is a type of physical activity defined as a planned, structured, and repetitive bodily movement performed to improve or maintain one or more components of physical fitness.

People participate in exercise programs to decrease risk factors for cardiovascular disease and to increase their health and well-being. **Activity tolerance** is the type and amount of exercise or daily living activities an individual is able to perform without experiencing adverse effects. **Functional strength** is another goal of exercise, and it is defined as the body's ability to perform work.

Types of Exercise

Exercise involves the active contraction and relaxation of muscles. Exercises can be classified according to the type of muscle contraction (isotonic, isometric, or isokinetic) and the source of energy (aerobic or anaerobic).

Isotonic exercises, which are dynamic exercises, are those in which the muscle shortens to produce muscle contraction and active movement. Most physical conditioning exercises—running, walking, swimming, cycling, and other such activities—are isotonic, as are ADLs and active ROM (range of motion) exercises (those initiated by the client). Examples of isotonic bed exercises are pushing or pulling against a stationary object, using a trapeze to lift the body off the bed, lifting the buttocks off the bed by pushing with the hands against the mattress, and pushing the body to a sitting position.

Isotonic exercises increase muscle tone, mass, and strength and maintain joint flexibility and circulation. During isotonic exercise, both heart rate and cardiac output quicken to increase blood flow to all parts of the body.

Isometric exercises, which are static or setting exercises, are those in which muscles contract without moving the joint (muscle length does not change). These exercises involve exerting pressure against a solid object and are useful for strengthening abdominal, gluteal, and quadriceps muscles used in ambulation; for maintaining strength in immobilized muscles in casts or traction; and for endurance training. These are often called "quad sets." Isometric exercises produce a mild increase in heart rate and cardiac output, but no appreciable increase in blood flow to other parts of the body.

Isokinetic exercises, which are resistive exercises, involve muscle contraction or tension against resistance; thus, they can be either isotonic or isometric. During isokinetic exercises, the person moves (isotonic) or tenses (isometric) against resistance. Special machines or devices provide the resistance to the movement. These exercises are used in physical conditioning and are often done to build up certain muscle groups; for example, the pectorals (chest muscles) may be increased in size and strength by lifting weights. An increase in blood pressure and blood flow to muscles occurs with resistance training (Burke & Laramie, 2004).

Aerobic exercise is an activity during which the amount of oxygen taken into the body is greater than that used to perform the activity. Aerobic exercises use large muscle groups that move repetitively. Aerobic exercises improve cardiovascular conditioning and physical fitness. Aerobic exercise brings more oxygen into the body than is used to perform the activity.

1. *Target Heart Rate:* The goal is to work up to and sustain a target heart rate during exercise; the target rate is based on the person's age. To determine target heart rate, first calculate the person's maximum heart rate by subtracting his or her current age in years from 220. Then obtain the target heart rate by taking 60–85% of the maximum. Because heart rates vary among individuals, the Talk Test is one of several tests that is being used to replace this measure.
2. *Talk Test:* This test is easier to implement and keeps most people at 60% of maximum heart rate or higher. The test is simple: When exercising, the person should experience labored breathing, yet still be able to carry on a conversation.

Anaerobic exercise involves activity in which the muscles cannot draw out enough oxygen from the bloodstream, and anaerobic pathways are used to provide additional energy for a short time. This type of exercise, such as weight lifting and sprinting, is used in endurance training for athletes.

Benefits of Exercise

In general, regular exercise is essential for maintaining mental and physical health. Table 7–2 summarizes the benefits of exercise on body systems.

MUSCULOSKELETAL SYSTEM The size, shape, tone, and strength of muscles (including the heart muscle) are maintained with mild exercise and increased with strenuous exercise. With strenuous exercise, muscles **hypertrophy** (enlarge), and the efficiency of muscular contraction increases. Hypertrophy is commonly seen in the arm muscles of a tennis player, the leg muscles of a skater, and the arm and hand muscles of a carpenter.

Joints lack a discrete blood supply. It is through activity that joints receive nourishment. Exercise increases joint flexibility, stability, and range of motion. A growing number of randomized, controlled clinical trials have shown that exercise interventions significantly reduce weakness, frailty, depression, and the risk and incidence of falling in older adults (Burke & Laramie, 2004).

Bone density and strength is maintained through weight bearing. The stress of weight-bearing and high-impact movement maintains a balance between osteoblasts (bone-building cells) and osteoclasts (bone-resorption and breakdown cells). Weight-bearing activity is particularly important for individuals at risk for osteoporosis. Examples of weight-bearing activity

TABLE 7–2 Benefits of Exercise by Body System

BODY SYSTEM	BENEFITS
Musculoskeletal	■ Increases joint flexibility, stability, and range of motion ■ Maintains bone density and strength ■ Reduces weakness, frailty, and depression ■ Decreases risk and incidence of falling in older adults
Cardiovascular	■ Increases strength of heart muscle contraction and blood supply to heart and muscles ■ Mediates harmful effects of stress ■ Lowers resting heart rate ■ Raises HDL level ■ Lowers blood pressure ■ Improves circulation
Respiratory	■ Increases tidal volume ■ Increases vital capacity ■ Improves gas exchange ■ Increases oxygen to the brain ■ Improves stamina and immune function
Gastrointestinal	■ Facilitates peristalsis ■ Relieves constipation ■ May improve symptoms of conditions such as IBS
Metabolic/Endocrine	■ Elevates metabolic rate ■ Stabilizes blood sugar
Urinary	■ Promotes efficient blood flow and waste excretion
Psychoneurologic	■ Elevates mood ■ Relieves stress and anxiety ■ Relieves depressive symptoms

are walking, dancing, and weight lifting. Non-weight-bearing exercises offer great benefit for individuals with a variety of health considerations. Examples of non-weight-bearing exercise are swimming and bicycling.

CARDIOVASCULAR SYSTEM The American Heart Association's most recent guidelines for primary prevention of stroke and cardiovascular disease place great emphasis on physical activity (Freeman, 2004). Adequate moderate-intensity exercise (40–60% of maximum capacity such as walking a mile in 15–20 minutes) increases the heart rate, the strength of heart muscle contraction, and the blood supply to the heart and muscles through increased cardiac output. In two studies with male participants, levels of "good" (high-density lipoprotein [HDL]) cholesterol were increased through regular endurance (walking/jogging) exercise. Exercise also promotes heart health by mediating the harmful effects of stress. The types of exercise that provide cardiac benefit vary. They include aerobic exercise such as walking and cycling (Freeman, 2004). Recent research supports the benefits of yoga practice on cardiovascular health. Statistically significant effects include lowered systolic and diastolic blood pressure, improved oxygen uptake, improved heart rate variability, improved circulation, and self-reported stress reduction (Fontaine, 2005; Freeman, 2004; McCaffrey, Ruknui, Hatthakit, & Kasetsomboon, 2005).

RESPIRATORY SYSTEM Ventilation (air circulating into and out of the lungs) and oxygen intake increase during exercise, thereby improving gas exchange. More toxins are eliminated with deeper breathing, and problem solving and emotional stability are enhanced by increased oxygen to the brain. Adequate exercise also prevents pooling of secretions in the bronchi and bronchioles, decreasing breathing effort and risk of infection (Freeman, 2004). Attention to exercising muscles of respiration (by deep breathing) throughout activity as well as during rest enhances oxygenation (improving stamina) and circulation of lymph (improving immune function). A strong body of evidence supports the use of lower extremity exercise forms (e.g., walking, treadmill, stationary bike, stair climbing) for treating individuals with chronic obstructive pulmonary disease (COPD) (Freeman, 2004). Research reports citing the benefits of yogic breathing and postures for persons with asthma are increasing in the literature (Fontaine, 2005; Freeman, 2004; Micozzi, 2006).

GASTROINTESTINAL SYSTEM Exercise improves the appetite and increases gastrointestinal tract tone, facilitating peristalsis. Activities such as rowing, swimming, walking, and sit-ups work the abdominal muscles and can help relieve constipation (Fontaine, 2005). Abdominal compressive exercise, such as with twisting and forward bending yoga postures, has been shown to improve symptoms of irritable bowel syndrome (Fontaine, 2005; Micozzi, 2006).

METABOLIC/ENDOCRINE SYSTEM Exercise elevates the metabolic rate, thus increasing the production of body heat, waste products, and calorie use. During strenuous exercise, the metabolic rate can increase to as much as 20 times the normal rate. This elevation lasts after exercise is completed. Exercise increases the use of triglycerides and fatty acids, resulting in a reduced level of serum triglycerides and cholesterol. Weight loss and exercise stabilize blood sugar and make cells more responsive to insulin. The Diabetes Prevention Program, a large 3-year study, showed that even a modest 5% decrease in body weight (about 10 pounds in most participants) achieved through exercise and dietary modification reduced the risk of diabetes by a striking 58%. In those over 60 years of age, the reduction was 71% (Freeman, 2004).

URINARY SYSTEM As adequate exercise promotes efficient blood flow, the body excretes wastes more effectively. In addition, adequate exercise usually prevents stasis (stagnation) of urine in the bladder.

IMMUNE SYSTEM As respiratory and musculoskeletal effort increase with exercise and as gravity is enlisted with postural changes, lymph fluid is more efficiently pumped from tissues into lymph capillaries and vessels throughout the body. Circulation through lymph nodes, where destruction of pathogens and removal of foreign antigens can occur, is also improved. Research in older adults has shown benefits of moderate exercise on natural killer cell function, circulating T-cell function, and cytokine production, potentially increasing resistance to viral infections and preventing formation of malignant cells (Freeman, 2004).

While moderate exercise seems to enhance immunity, strenuous exercise may reduce immune function, leaving a window of opportunity for infection during the recovery phase. Adequate rest is important after vigorous training to allow the body to recover (Edelman & Mandle, 2006).

PSYCHONEUROLOGIC SYSTEM Mental or affective disorders such as depression or chronic stress may affect a person's desire to move. The depressed person may lack enthusiasm for taking part in any activity and may even lack energy for usual hygiene practices. Lack of visible energy is seen in a slumped posture with head bowed. Chronic stress can deplete the body's energy reserves to the point that the resulting fatigue discourages the desire to exercise, even though exercise can energize the person and facilitate coping. By contrast, individuals with eating disorders may exercise excessively in an effort to prevent weight gain.

A strong and growing body of evidence supports the role of exercise in elevating mood and relieving stress and anxiety across the life span. Solid data examining relationships between both aerobic and nonaerobic styles of exercise support the use of this modality to relieve symptoms of depression. The mechanism of action is thought to be a result of one or more of the following: Exercise increases levels of metabolites for neurotransmitters such as norepinephrine and serotonin; exercise releases endogenous opioids, thus increasing levels of endorphins; exercise increases levels of oxygen to the brain and other body systems, inducing euphoria; and through muscular exertion (especially with movement modalities such as yoga and t'ai chi) the body releases stored stress associated with accumulated emotional demands. Regular exercise also improves quality of sleep for most individuals (Freeman, 2004).

COGNITIVE FUNCTION Current research supports the positive effects of exercise on cognitive functioning, in particular decision-making and problem-solving processes, planning, and paying attention. Physical exertion induces cells in the brain to strengthen and build neuronal connections. Research evidence demonstrates that athletic older adults have denser brains than their inactive counterparts (Freeman, 2004). Brain Gym (educational kinesiology) is a series of easy, mostly cross-lateral movements that enhance right- and left-brain integration, thus improving mood, learning, problem solving, and performance in persons of all ages. These contralateral movements have been shown to help individuals with attention deficit disorder (ADD), attention deficit/hyperactivity disorder (ADHD), learning disorders, and mood disorders. Recent research indicates that physical exercise also provides positive effects in individuals with Parkinson's and Alzheimer's diseases.

SPIRITUAL HEALTH Jackson (2003) found that a program of Pilates and yoga-style exercise significantly enhanced students' experiences of mind-body-spirit connection and relationship with God. The emphasis on breathing in both Pilates and yoga is thought to soothe the nervous and cardiorespiratory systems, promoting relaxation and preparedness for contemplative experience. Recitation of a word or phrase (mantra) and rosary prayer were both found to powerfully enhance and synchronize cardiovascular rhythms because of the resulting decrease in respiratory rate. Slow breathing enhances heart rate variability and baroreflex sensitivity, both beneficial for those with heart disease (Micozzi, 2006). (See the Spirituality concept.)

REVIEW Physical Fitness and Exercise

RELATE: LINK THE CONCEPTS

Linking the concept of Metabolism with the concept of Health, Wellness, and Illness:

1. Identify the benefits of physical activity for a client with (1) type 2 diabetes, and (2) osteoporosis.

REFLECT: CASE STUDY

Mary Martin is a 75-year-old female who was recently widowed. She has limited income because her husband's pension terminated when he died, so she has moved in with her son, his wife, and their three teenage children. Mary has cataracts and glaucoma, for which she sees an ophthalmologist on a regular basis, but otherwise she is in good health. Mary recently learned she has low bone density.

1. What kind of physical activity and exercise is appropriate for Mary?
2. What are the benefits of these activities on body systems?

7.3 ORAL HEALTH

KEY TERMS

Cheilosis, *202*

Dental caries, *200*

Gingiva, *200*

Gingivitis, *202*

Periodontal disease, *200*

Plaque, *200*

Pyorrhea, *202*

Tartar, *200*

Xerostomia, *204*

BASIS FOR SELECTION OF EXEMPLAR

Healthy People 2010

LEARNING OUTCOMES

After reading about this concept, you will be able to do the following:

1. Identify factors influencing oral health.
2. Identify normal and abnormal assessment findings across the life span.
3. Describe the significance of oral hygiene across the life span.
4. Develop nursing diagnoses and outcomes related to oral health.

OVERVIEW

The mouth, also called the oral or buccal cavity, is lined with mucous membranes and is enclosed by the lips, cheeks, palate, and tongue (Figure 7–5 ■).

The lips and cheeks are skeletal muscle covered externally by skin. Their function is to keep food in the mouth during chewing. The palate consists of two regions: the hard palate and the soft palate. The hard palate covers bone in the roof of the mouth and provides a hard surface against which the tongue forces food. The soft palate, extending from the hard palate and ending at the back of the mouth as a fold called the uvula, is primarily muscle. When food is swallowed, the soft palate rises as a reflex to close off the oropharynx.

The tongue, composed of skeletal muscle and connective tissue, is located in the floor of the mouth. It contains mucous and serous glands, taste buds, and papillae. The tongue mixes food with saliva during chewing, forms the food into a mass (called a *bolus*), and initiates swallowing. Some papillae provide surface roughness to facilitate licking and moving food; other papillae house the taste buds.

Saliva moistens food so it can be made into a bolus, dissolves food chemicals so they can be tasted, and provides enzymes (such as amylase) that begin the chemical breakdown of starches. Saliva is produced by salivary glands, most of which lie superior or inferior to the mouth and drain into it. The salivary glands include the parotid, the submaxillary, and the sublingual glands.

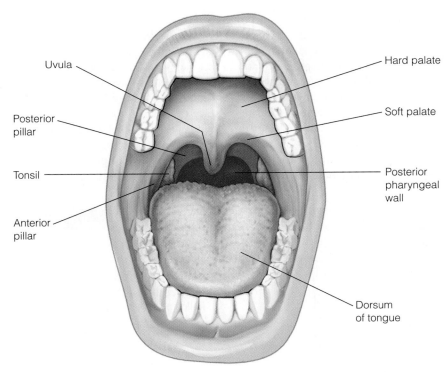

Figure 7–5 ■ Oral cavity.

The teeth chew (masticate) and grind food to break it down into smaller parts. As the food is masticated, it is mixed with saliva.

Each tooth has three parts: the crown, the root, and the pulp cavity. The crown is the exposed part of the tooth, which is outside the gum. It is covered with a hard substance called enamel. The ivory-colored internal part of the crown below the enamel is the dentin. The root of a tooth is embedded in the jaw and covered by a bony tissue called cementum. The pulp cavity in the center of the tooth contains the blood vessels and nerves.

DEVELOPMENTAL VARIATIONS

Teeth usually appear 5–8 months after birth. Baby-bottle syndrome may result in decay of all of the upper teeth and the lower posterior teeth (Pillitteri, 2003, p. 824). This syndrome occurs when an infant is put to bed with a bottle of sugar water, formula, milk, or fruit juice. The carbohydrates in the solutions cause demineralization of the tooth enamel, which leads to tooth decay.

By the time children are 2 years old, they usually have all 20 of their deciduous (temporary) teeth. At about age 6 or 7, children start losing their deciduous teeth, and these are gradually replaced by the 33 permanent teeth. By age 25, most people have all of their permanent teeth (Figure 7–6 ■).

The incidence of periodontal disease increases during pregnancy because the rise in female hormones affects gingival tissue and increases its reaction to bacterial plaque. Many pregnant women experience more bleeding from the gingival sulcus during brushing and increased redness and swelling of the **gingiva** (the gum).

Teeth turn yellowish as a part of the aging process. Teeth are normally off-white. With age, the enamel thins and the yellow-gray color of the inner portion of the teeth begins to show. In addition, coffee drinking and cigarette smoking can stain the teeth. Commercial teeth whitening products and whitening treatments offered at dental offices are available to consumers who desire whiter teeth for cosmetic reasons.

Lack of fluoridated water and preventive dentistry during their developmental years caused tooth and gum problems in older adults (Edelman & Mandle, 2006, p. 582). As a result, some older adults may have few permanent teeth left, and some have dentures. Loss of teeth occurs mainly because of

periodontal disease (gum disease) rather than **dental caries** (cavities); however, caries are also common in middle-aged adults.

Some receding of the gums and a brownish pigmentation of the gums occur with age. Because saliva production decreases with age, dryness of the oral mucosa is a common finding in older people.

 # NURSING PROCESS

Assessment

Assessment of the client's mouth and hygiene practices includes (a) a nursing health history, (b) physical assessment of the mouth, and (c) identification of clients at risk for developing oral problems.

Health History

During the nursing health history, the nurse obtains data about the client's oral hygiene practices, including dental visits, self-care abilities, and past or current mouth problems. Data about the client's oral hygiene help the nurse determine learning needs and incorporate the client's needs and preferences in the plan of care. Assessment of the client's self-care abilities determines the amount and type of nursing assistance to provide. Clients whose hand coordination is impaired, whose cognitive function is impaired, whose illness alters energy levels and motivation, or whose therapy imposes restrictions on activities will need assistance from the nurse. Information about past or current problems alerts the nurse to specific interventions required or referrals that may be necessary. Questions to elicit this information are shown in the accompanying Assessment Interview.

Physical Assessment

Dental caries (cavities) and periodontal disease are the two problems that most frequently affect the teeth. Both problems are commonly associated with plaque and tartar deposits. **Plaque** is an invisible soft film that adheres to the enamel surface of teeth; it consists of bacteria, molecules of saliva, and remnants of epithelial cells and leukocytes. When plaque is unchecked, tartar (dental calculus) is formed. **Tartar** is a visible, hard deposit of plaque and dead bacteria that forms at the gum lines. Tartar buildup can alter the fibers that attach the

---

Assessment Interview   Oral Hygiene

ORAL HYGIENE PRACTICES
- What are your usual mouth care and/or denture care practices?
- What oral hygiene products do you routinely use (e.g., mouthwash, type of toothpaste, dental floss, denture cleaner)?
- When was your last dental examination, and how often do you see your dentist?

SELF-CARE ABILITY
- Do you have any problems managing your mouth care?

PAST OR CURRENT MOUTH PROBLEMS
- Have you had or do you have any problems such as bleeding, swollen or reddened gums, ulcerations, lumps, or tooth pain?

Source: Berman, A., Snyder, S. J., Kozier, B., & Erb, G. (2008). *Kozier & Erb's fundamentals of nursing: Concepts, process, and practice* (8th ed., p. 765). Upper Saddle River, NJ: Pearson Education.

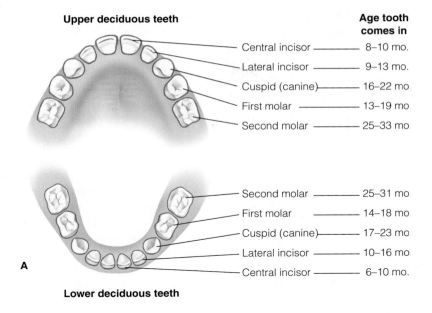

Upper deciduous teeth

	Age tooth comes in
Central incisor	8–10 mo.
Lateral incisor	9–13 mo.
Cuspid (canine)	16–22 mo
First molar	13–19 mo
Second molar	25–33 mo

	Age tooth comes in
Second molar	25–31 mo
First molar	14–18 mo
Cuspid (canine)	17–23 mo
Lateral incisor	10–16 mo
Central incisor	6–10 mo.

A

Lower deciduous teeth

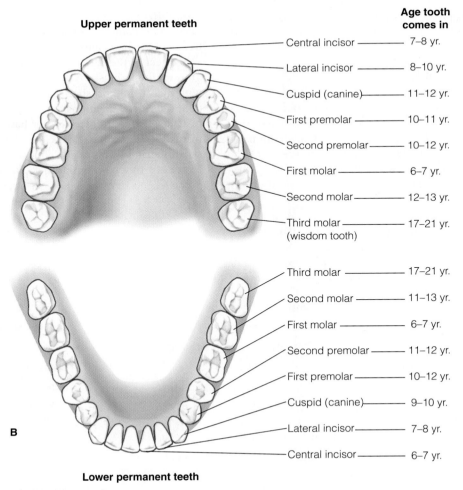

Upper permanent teeth

	Age tooth comes in
Central incisor	7–8 yr.
Lateral incisor	8–10 yr.
Cuspid (canine)	11–12 yr.
First premolar	10–11 yr.
Second premolar	10–12 yr.
First molar	6–7 yr.
Second molar	12–13 yr.
Third molar (wisdom tooth)	17–21 yr.

	Age tooth comes in
Third molar	17–21 yr.
Second molar	11–13 yr.
First molar	6–7 yr.
Second premolar	11–12 yr.
First premolar	10–12 yr.
Cuspid (canine)	9–10 yr.
Lateral incisor	7–8 yr.
Central incisor	6–7 yr.

B

Lower permanent teeth

Figure 7–6 ■ Deciduous and permanent teeth.

teeth to the gum and eventually disrupt bone tissue. Periodontal disease is characterized by **gingivitis** (red, swollen gingiva), bleeding, receding gum lines, and the formation of pockets between the teeth and gums. In **pyorrhea** (advanced periodontal disease), the teeth are loose and pus is evident when the gums are pressed. Table 7–3 lists additional problems of the mouth.

PRACTICE ALERT

Always wear gloves when assessing the oral cavity.
To perform an oral health assessment complete the following:

- Inspect and palpate the lips. Lips should be of normal color for race without lesions.
- Inspect and palpate the tongue. Tongue should be pink, smooth, and have good turgor.
- Inspect and palpate the buccal mucosa. Mucosa should be moist, without lesions and of appropriate color.
- Inspect and palpate the teeth. Teeth should be in a state of good hygiene without caries.
- Inspect and palpate the gums. Gums should be of even color without swelling.
- Inspect the throat and tonsils. Tonsils (if present) should be of appropriate color and size.
- Note the client's breath. Breath should not have unusual or foul odors.

Identifying Clients at Risk

Certain clients are prone to oral problems because of lack of knowledge or the inability to maintain oral hygiene. Among these are seriously ill, confused, comatose, depressed, illiterate, and dehydrated clients. In addition, clients with nasogastric tubes and clients receiving oxygen are likely to develop dry oral mucous membranes, especially if they breathe through their mouths. Clients who have had oral or jaw surgery must maintain meticulous oral hygiene care to prevent the development of infections.

PRACTICE ALERT

Clients in long-term care settings are at high risk for oral health problems. The nurse must assess the client's oral health and teach the importance of and methods to promote oral hygiene.

Healthy appearing individuals, too, may be at risk. High-risk variables such as inadequate nutrition, lack of money and/or insurance for dental care, excessive intake of refined sugars, and family history of periodontal disease also need to be identified. Some older people may also be at risk, for example, those who choose salty and enamel-eroding sugary foods because of a decline in their number of taste buds. Decreased saliva production in older adults, which produces a dry mouth and thinning of the oral mucosa, is another factor.

A dry mouth can be aggravated by poor fluid intake, heavy smoking, alcohol use, high salt intake, anxiety, and many medications. Medications that can cause dryness of the mouth include diuretics; laxatives, if used excessively; and tranquilizers, such as chlorpromazine (Thorazine) and diazepam (Valium). Some chemotherapeutic agents used to treat cancer also cause oral dryness and lesions. A common side effect of the anticonvulsant drug phenytoin (Dilantin) is gingival hyperplasia. Optimal oral hygiene (e.g., brushing with a soft toothbrush and flossing) is necessary for clients taking these medications.

Clients who are receiving or have received radiation treatments to the head and neck may have permanent damage to salivary glands. This results in a very dry mouth and can often be treated by providing a thick liquid called artificial saliva. Some clients prefer to just sip on liquids to moisten their

---

TABLE 7–3 Common Problems of the Mouth

PROBLEM	DESCRIPTION	NURSING IMPLICATIONS
Halitosis	Bad breath	Teach or provide regular oral hygiene.
Glossitis	Inflammation of the tongue	Teach or provide regular oral hygiene.
Gingivitis	Inflammation of the gums	Teach or provide regular oral hygiene.
Periodontal disease	Gums appear spongy and bleeding	Teach or provide regular oral hygiene.
Reddened or excoriated mucosa		Check for ill-fitting dentures.
Excessive dryness of the buccal mucosa		Increase fluid intake as health permits.
Cheilosis	Cracking of lips	Lubricate lips, use antimicrobial ointment to prevent infection.
Dental caries	Darkened areas on teeth, may be painful	Advise client to see a dentist.
Sordes	Accumulation of foul matter (food, microorganisms, and epithelial elements) on the teeth and lips	Teach or provide regular cleaning.
Stomatitis	Inflammation of the oral mucosa	Teach or provide regular cleaning.
Parotitis	Inflammation of the parotid salivary glands	Teach or provide regular oral hygiene.

Source: Berman, A., Snyder, S. J., Kozier, B., & Erb, G. (2008). *Kozier & Erb's fundamentals of nursing: Concepts, process, and practice* (8th ed., p. 765). Upper Saddle River, NJ: Pearson Education.

mouth. Radiation can also cause damage to teeth and jaw structure, with actual damage occurring years after the radiation.

Diagnosis

Three nursing diagnoses are related to problems with oral hygiene and the oral cavity:

- Self-Care Deficit
- Impaired Oral Mucous Membrane
- Deficient Knowledge

Note that the North American Nursing Diagnosis Association (NANDA, 2007) includes oral hygiene in the diagnostic label Self-Care Deficit: Bathing/Hygiene. In this book, the diagnosis Self-Care Deficit: Oral Hygiene will be used for clients unable to perform oral care independently. This includes the inability to brush or floss teeth or clean dentures.

The nursing diagnosis Impaired Oral Mucous Membrane refers to the state in which an individual experiences disruptions in the tissue layers of the oral cavity. Manifestations include a coated tongue, dry mouth, halitosis, gingivitis, oral pain, discomfort, erythema, oral lesions or ulcers, and dry mouth. These may be the result of ineffective oral hygiene, physical injury or drying effect (e.g., mouth breathing, oxygen therapy, dehydration), mechanical trauma (e.g., oral surgery, braces, or ill-fitting dentures), chemical trauma (e.g., side effects of medications), or radiation therapy.

Planning

In planning care, the nurse and, if appropriate, the client and/or family set outcomes for each nursing diagnosis. The nurse then performs nursing interventions and activities to achieve the client outcomes.

During the planning phase, the nurse also identifies interventions that will help the client achieve these goals. Specific, detailed nursing activities taken by the nurse may include the following:

- Monitor for dryness of the oral mucosa.
- Monitor for signs and symptoms of glossitis (inflammation of the tongue) and stomatitis (inflammation of the mouth).
- Assist dependent clients with oral care.
- Provide special oral hygiene for clients who are debilitated, are unconscious, or have lesions of the mucous membranes or other oral tissues.
- Teach clients about good oral hygiene practices and other measures to prevent tooth decay.
- Reinforce the oral hygiene regimen as part of health promotion and discharge teaching.

Implementation

Good oral hygiene includes daily stimulation of the gums, mechanical brushing and flossing of the teeth, and flushing of the mouth. The nurse is often in a position to help people maintain oral hygiene by helping or teaching them to clean the teeth and oral cavity, by inspecting whether clients (especially children) have done so, or by actually providing mouth care to clients who are ill or incapacitated. The nurse can also be instrumental in identifying problems that require the intervention of a dentist or oral surgeon and arranging a referral.

Promoting Oral Health Throughout the Life Span

A major role of the nurse in promoting oral health is teaching clients about specific oral hygienic measures.

INFANTS AND TODDLERS Most dentists recommend that dental hygiene begin when the first tooth erupts and be practiced after each feeding. Cleaning can be accomplished by using a wet washcloth or small gauze moistened with water.

Dental caries occur frequently during the toddler period, often as a result of the excessive intake of sweets or a prolonged use of the bottle during naps and at bedtime. The nurse should give parents the following instructions to promote and maintain dental health:

- Beginning at about 18 months of age, brush the child's teeth with a soft toothbrush. Use only a toothbrush moistened with water at first and introduce toothpaste later. Use a toothpaste that contains fluoride.
- Give a fluoride supplement daily or as recommended by the primary care provider or dentist, unless the drinking water is fluoridated.
- Schedule an initial dental visit for the child at about 2 or 3 years of age, as soon as all 20 primary teeth have erupted.
- Some dentists recommend an inspection type of visit when the child is about 18 months old to provide an early, pleasant introduction to the dental examination.
- Seek professional dental attention for any problems such as discoloring of the teeth, chipping, or signs of infection such as redness and swelling.

PRESCHOOLERS AND SCHOOL-AGE CHILDREN Because deciduous teeth guide the entrance of permanent teeth, dental care is essential to keep these teeth in good repair and to establish good dental habits early. Abnormally placed or lost deciduous teeth can cause misalignment of permanent teeth. Fluoride remains important at this stage to prevent dental caries. Preschoolers need to be taught to brush their teeth after eating and to limit their intake of refined sugars. Parental supervision may be needed to ensure the completion of these self-care activities. Regular dental checkups are required during these years when permanent teeth appear.

PRACTICE ALERT

Many parents are unaware of the importance of dental health in very young children. They may see their child's teeth as "baby teeth," and think they can put off dental visits until the child begins to lose his or her primary teeth. Nurses working with parents of very young children may need to provide teaching opportunities to help parents learn that care of primary teeth is essential to healthy permanent teeth.

ADOLESCENTS AND ADULTS Proper diet and tooth and mouth care should be evaluated and reinforced for adolescents and adults. Specific measures to prevent tooth decay and periodontal disease are listed in Client Teaching.

OLDER ADULTS Over 50% of older adults have their own teeth (Gooch, Eke, & Malvitz, 2004), and they are at risk for dental cavities and periodontal disease. Older adults who

CLIENT TEACHING   Measures to Prevent Tooth Decay

- Brush the teeth thoroughly after meals and at bedtime. Assist children or inspect their mouths to be sure the teeth are clean. If the teeth cannot be brushed after meals, vigorous rinsing of the mouth with water is recommended.
- Floss the teeth daily.
- Ensure an adequate intake of nutrients, particularly calcium, phosphorus, vitamins A, C, and D, and fluoride.
- Avoid sweet foods and drinks between meals. Take them in moderation at meals.
- Eat coarse, fibrous foods (cleansing foods), such as fresh fruits and raw vegetables.
- Have topical fluoride applications as prescribed by the dentist.
- Have a checkup by a dentist every 6 months.

Source: Berman, A., Snyder, S. J., Kozier, B., & Erb, G. (2008). *Kozier & Erb's fundamentals of nursing: Concepts, process, and practice* (8th ed., p. 768). Upper Saddle River, NJ: Pearson Education.

have self-care deficits are at an increased risk because they cannot maintain their oral hygiene practices and/or may not be able to visit the dentist on a routine basis. Furthermore, those who suffer the worst oral health and hygiene include older adults residing in nursing homes (Coleman, 2002, 2004). Coleman (2004) reported that poor oral hygiene among the frail and among dependent nursing home residents can place them at risk for serious illness such as pneumonia (p. 3). Nurses have an important role in promoting optimal geriatric oral health care.

Brushing and Flossing the Teeth Thorough brushing of the teeth is important in preventing tooth decay. The mechanical action of brushing removes food particles that can harbor and incubate bacteria. It also stimulates circulation in the gums, thus maintaining their healthy firmness. One of the techniques recommended for brushing teeth is called the sulcular technique, which removes plaque and cleans under the gingival margins. Fluoride toothpaste is often recommended because of its antibacterial protection.

Caring for Artificial Dentures Some people have artificial teeth in the form of a plate—a complete set of teeth for one jaw. A person may have a lower plate or an upper plate or both. When only a few artificial teeth are needed, the individual may have a bridge rather than a plate. A bridge may be fixed or removable. Artificial teeth are fitted to the individual and usually will not fit another person. People who wear dentures or other types of oral prostheses should be encouraged to use them. Ill-fitting dentures or other oral prostheses can cause discomfort and chewing difficulties. They may also contribute to oral problems as well as poor nutrition and enjoyment of food. Those who do not wear their prostheses are prone to shrinkage of the gums, which results in further tooth loss.

Like natural teeth, artificial dentures collect microorganisms and food. They need to be cleaned regularly, at least once a day. They can be removed from the mouth, scrubbed with a toothbrush, rinsed, and reinserted. Some people use a dentifrice for cleaning teeth, and others use commercial cleaning compounds for plates.

Assisting Clients With Oral Care When providing mouth care for partially or totally dependent clients, the nurse should wear gloves to guard against infections. Other required equipment includes a curved basin that fits snugly under the client's chin (e.g., a kidney basin) to receive the rinse water, and a towel to protect the client and the bedclothes.

Foam swabs are often used in health care agencies to clean the mouths of dependent clients. These swabs are convenient and effective in removing excess debris from the teeth and mouth but should be used infrequently and for short periods (i.e., less than 3 days) because they do not remove plaque that is at the base of the teeth.

Most people prefer privacy when they take their artificial teeth out to clean them. Many do not like to be seen without their teeth; one of the first requests of many postoperative clients is "May I have my teeth in, please?"

Clients With Special Oral Hygiene Needs For the client who is debilitated or unconscious or who has excessive dryness, sores, or irritations of the mouth, it may be necessary to clean the oral mucosa and tongue in addition to the teeth. Agency practices differ in regard to special mouth care and the frequency with which it is provided. Depending on the health of the client's mouth, special care may be needed every 2–8 hours; see Developmental Considerations for Oral Hygiene in Older Adults.

Mouth care for unconscious or debilitated people is important because their mouths tend to become dry, predisposing them to tooth decay and infections. Saliva has antiviral, antibacterial, and antifungal effects (Walton, Miller, & Tordecilla, 2001, p. 40). Dry mouth—also called **xerostomia**—occurs

DEVELOPMENTAL CONSIDERATIONS   Oral Hygiene in Older Adults

- Oral care is often difficult for certain older adults to perform due to problems with dexterity or cognitive problems with dementia.
- Some long-term health care facilities have dentists who come on a regular basis to see clients with special needs.
- Dryness of the oral mucosa is a common finding in older adults. Because this can lead to tooth decay, advise clients to discuss it with their dentist or primary care provider.

- Decay of the tooth root is common among older adults. When the gums recede, the tooth root is more vulnerable to decay.
- Promoting good oral hygiene can have a positive effect on the older adults' ability to eat.

Source: Berman, A., Snyder, S. J., Kozier, B., & Erb, G. (2008). *Kozier & Erb's fundamentals of nursing: Concepts, process, and practice* (8th ed., p. 296). Upper Saddle River, NJ: Pearson Education.

when the supply of saliva is reduced (American Dental Association, n.d.). This condition can be caused by certain medications (e.g., antihistamines, antidepressants, antihypertensives), oxygen therapy, tachypnea, and NPO status, where the client cannot take fluids by mouth (Anonymous, 2003).

For clients with special oral hygiene needs, the nurse needs to focus on removing plaque and microorganisms as well as client comfort. If possible, a soft-bristled toothbrush should be used, as it provides the best means of removing plaque. A sodium bicarbonate toothpaste will help dissolve mucus and reduce the saliva's acidity, which helps decrease bacteria (Nainar & Mohummed, 2004). If the client cannot tolerate the use of a toothbrush, the nurse can use an oral swab or a gauze soaked with saline to swab the teeth and tongue. A foam swab can be used to provide oral hygiene for dependent clients. The swab, however, is not effective for plaque removal (Munro, Grap, & Kleinpell, 2004). Lemon-glycerin swabs are not recommended as they irritate and dry the oral mucosa and can decalcify teeth. Mouthwashes containing alcohol can irritate the oral mucosa as well as cause dryness. The Food and Drug Administration approves hydrogen peroxide as a mouth rinse (Anonymous, 2003, p. 12). It provides a cleaning action as well

as an antimicrobial effect. Diluting the hydrogen peroxide with saline or a nonalcohol–based mouthwash will help decrease the potential for the client to experience a burning sensation. Mineral oil is contraindicated as a moisturizer for the lips or inside the mouth because aspiration of it can initiate an infection (lipid pneumonia). A water-soluble moisturizer, absorbed by the skin and tissue, provides important hydration. Saliva substitutes can also help moisturize the oral cavity.

Evaluation

Using data collected during care (e.g., status of oral mucosa, lips, tongue, and teeth), the nurse judges whether desired outcomes have been achieved.

If outcomes are not achieved, the nurse and client need to explore the reasons before modifying the care plan. Following are examples of questions to consider:

- Did the nurse overestimate the client's functional abilities?
- Is the client's hand coordination or cognitive function impaired?
- Did the client's condition change?
- Has there been a change in the client's energy level and/or motivation?

REVIEW **Oral Health**

RELATE: LINK THE CONCEPTS

Linking the concept of Development with the concept of Health, Wellness, and Illness:

1. What are the dental concerns of age groups across the life span?

READY: GO TO COMPANION SKILLS MANUAL

1. Providing oral care
2. Brushing and flossing the teeth
3. Providing special oral care for the unconscious or debilitated client

REFLECT: CASE STUDY

Tyler Martin is a 2-year-old boy. Since he was 4 weeks old, Tyler has been going to various babysitters while his parents worked. He and his father have recently moved in with Tyler's grandparents. Tyler loves living at

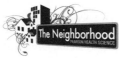

his grandfather's home because of all the attention he gets. Tyler also no longer has to go to day care.

Tyler has generally been in good health; he is of normal weight and has a good appetite. Tyler still loves his bottle, and each night he is given a bottle of milk or juice to help him go to sleep. If he doesn't receive a bottle to sleep with, he screams until someone gives in and brings him one.

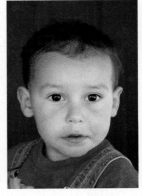

1. Are there any concerns that require intervention and teaching in this scenario?
2. What teaching would you provide to Tyler and his family?

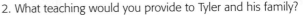

7.4 NUTRITION SCREENING

KEY TERMS

Diet recall, *208*
Malnutrition, *206*
Nutritional health, *206*
Overnutrition, *206*
Protein-calorie malnutrition, *206*
Undernutrition, *206*

BASIS FOR SELECTION OF EXEMPLAR

Healthy People 2010

LEARNING OUTCOMES

After reading about this exemplar, you will be able to do the following:

1. Define nutritional health.

2. Outline risk factors that affect nutritional health status.
3. Identify physical and laboratory parameters utilized in a nutrition assessment.
4. Identify components of a diet history and techniques for gathering diet history data.
5. Describe existing validated nutritional assessment tools.
6. Identify specific nutritional assessment techniques and tools appropriate for unique stages in the life span.
7. Discuss strategies for integrating a complete nutritional assessment into the nursing care process.

OVERVIEW

Nutritional health is a crucial component of overall health across the life span. The nutritional health of a pregnant female will influence pregnancy outcome. Nutritional health in growing children plays a central role in growth and development. In adults and older adults, nutritional health can be associated with prevention or development of chronic disease in conditions involving both undernutrition and overnutrition. **Undernutrition**, also called **malnutrition**, is defined as health effects of insufficient nutrient intake or stores. **Overnutrition** results from excesses in nutrient intake or stores and can manifest itself in conditions such as obesity, hypertension, hypercholesterolemia, or toxic levels of stored vitamins or minerals.

The determination of an individual's nutritional status is based on a thorough nutritional assessment. The assessment portion of the nursing care process incorporates the gathering and interpretation of data often used as part of a nutritional assessment. These data then create the foundation for later development of appropriate nursing and nutritional interventions aimed at preserving or improving nutritional health.

Nutritional health can be defined as the physical result of the balance between nutrient intake and nutritional requirements. For example, an individual who consumes excess saturated fat may be at risk for elevated blood cholesterol and cardiovascular disease. This person may therefore be considered to have poor nutritional health due to overnutrition. A pregnant female who consumes less than the required amounts of folic acid may place her unborn child at risk for certain birth defects, such as neural tube defects, and could be considered in poor nutritional health due to undernutrition. A client who consumes adequate nutrition to meet individual needs and avoids habitual excesses and insufficiencies would be considered in good nutritional health.

Many factors can influence nutritional health. When gathering data for a nutritional assessment, it is important to know common risk factors for poor nutritional status. Overnutrition in the form of excess dietary intake of fat, especially saturated fat, has been associated with an increased risk of atherosclerosis. Overweight and obesity are linked to increased risk of hypertension, cardiovascular disease, type 2 diabetes, some cancers, degenerative joint disease, and other conditions. Additionally, excess body weight has been shown to increase the risk of all-cause mortality in adults 30–74 years of age. In the United States, 63% of males and 55% of females 20–74 years of age are considered overweight or obese, a statistic that has increased by 25% over the past 30 years. The prevalence of obesity and overweight has doubled in children and adolescents in the last 30 years to 13 and 14%, respectively. Excess alcohol intake is associated with chronic liver disease and cirrhosis, the 12th leading cause of death in the United States, according to the National Center for Health Statistics at the Centers for the CDC.

Undernutrition is less common than overnutrition in the United States, but it can have devastating physical health consequences when **protein-calorie malnutrition** or other nutrient deficiencies develop. Undernutrition can lead to growth faltering, compromised immune status, poor wound healing, muscle loss, physical and functional decline, and lack of proper development. Generally, individuals at risk for undernutrition include those who have a chronic illness or who are poor, elderly, hospitalized, restrictive eaters (from chronic dieting or disordered eating), or alcoholics. An individual can have both overnutrition and undernutrition, such as an overweight child who consumes no fruit or vegetables. Box 7–7 outlines additional risk factors for overnutrition and undernutrition to consider when conducting a nutrition assessment.

Healthy People 2010's objectives for targeting overweight, obesity, and issues of undernutrition are important reminders to the clinician of the central role nutrition plays in overall health across the life span. The increasing prevalence of overweight and obesity in the United States and the statistics on nutritional health

---

Box 7–7 Risk Factors for Poor Nutritional Health

UNDERNUTRITION
- Chronic disease, acute illness, or injury
- Multiple medications
- Food insecurity—lack of free access to adequate and safe food
- Restrictive eating due to chronic dieting, disordered eating, faddism, or food beliefs
- Alcohol abuse
- Depression, bereavement, loneliness, social isolation
- Poor dental health
- Decreased knowledge or skills about food preparation and recommendations
- Extreme age—premature infants or adults over 80 years of age

OVERNUTRITION
- Excess intake of fat, sugar, calories, or nutrients
- Alcohol abuse
- Sedentary lifestyle
- Decreased knowledge or skills about food preparation and recommendations

Source: D'Amico, D., & Barbarito, C. (2007). *Health & physical assessment in nursing* (p. 137). Upper Saddle River, NJ: Pearson Education.

Box 7–8 Cultural and Socioeconomic Influences on Nutritional Health

OVERWEIGHT AND OBESITY

- More than than 60% of adults 20–74 years of age are overweight; 27% are classified as obese.
- Up to 15% of children 6–19 years of age are overweight.
- Prevalence of obesity has increased in the three major racial and ethnic groups.
- Prevalence of overweight is highest among Mexican American males.
- Prevalence of obesity is highest among Mexican American females.
- Hypertension, a comorbid condition of overweight and obesity, affects 23% of adults in the United States.
- Prevalence of hypertension is highest among Black persons.
- Adults of low socioeconomic status have twice the rate of overweight or obesity than those of medium and high socioeconomic status.

UNDERNUTRITION

- Undernutrition can contribute to growth retardation. By definition, 5% of children would be expected to be at the 5th percentile for height. However, up to 15% of Black children have growth retardation in the first year of life, and 11% of Asian and Pacific Islander children have growth retardation during the second year.
- Up to 60% of older adults in dependent care or hospitals are malnourished.

- Adequate folic acid and iron status are important for healthy outcomes during pregnancy. Pregnant Mexican American females are more likely than those of other ethnic groups to have iron deficiency and low folic acid levels. Females of lower economic status and those with less education are also more likely to have inadequate folic acid or iron status.
- Black women and adolescents under age 15 years are more likely to have insufficient gestational weight gain and deliver low-birth-weight babies than women of other populations.

POVERTY AND FOOD INSECURITY

- Poverty is a major risk factor for food insecurity and malnutrition. Public programs such as Women, Infants and Children (WIC) and the Supplemental Nutrition Assistance Program (formerly the Food Stamp program) assist families in poverty with accessing healthy food for their children.
- Among Americans, the prevalence of poverty was 12.5% in 2007.
- Children under age 18 experience a 17.6% poverty rate, although this rate is higher in some states.
- Prevalence of poverty is highest among Black (24.5%) and Hispanic populations (21.5%).

Sources: Healthy People 2010. 19. Nutrition and Overweight. Retrieved June 24, 2005, at www.healthypeople.gov/Document/HTML/VOLUME2/ 19Nutrition.htm; and *Income, Poverty, and Health Insurance Coverage in the United States: 2007.* Retrieved May 31, 2009 at www.census.gov/prod/ 2008pubs/p60-235.pdf.

disparities illustrate the importance of nutritional screening and assessment as the first step toward reaching these important goals. Box 7–8 outlines the cultural and socioeconomic influences that may affect nutritional health. And the Focus on Culture and Diversity lists cultural influences on diet.

Laboratory Data

Laboratory tests provide objective data for the nutritional assessment, but because many factors can influence these tests, no single test specifically predicts nutritional risk or measures the presence or degree of a nutritional problem. The

FOCUS ON DIVERSITY AND CULTURE Cultural Diet Influences

- Cultural and religious beliefs and traditions can affect food choices, beliefs, and practices in many ways from the number of meals eaten in a day to food choices, preparation methods, and overall food beliefs.
- Diversity exists within cultural and religious groups. It is important to avoid applying general knowledge about cultural and religious food practices to all people within a group; instead explore individual interpretation and influences.
- Assess common dietary staples as well as foods believed to be associated with health or symbolic benefits. Some food is thought to promote health or cure conditions, such as making a "hot" condition "colder." Other beliefs may be related to life span issues, such as the proper diet during pregnancy for easy delivery.
- Many religious groups have dietary laws that are observed differently by subgroups within the population. Consumption of kosher meats, fasting, and avoidance of certain foods such as pork, crustaceans, birds of prey, beef, or other animal products are examples.

- Ask about food practices and particular meals for special occasions and holidays. Some religious groups fast during parts of some holy days.
- Discuss food preparation methods. A variety of cultures make similar dishes but prepare them differently—for example, using different fats such as bacon drippings, lard, oils, or ghee clarified butter.
- Ask about medicinal herb use as this varies among cultures and is often an important aspect of health beliefs.
- Explore to what extent any acculturation has taken place and which traditional practices changed once the client was living in a new dominant culture. Ask whether new foods have been added to traditional foods, newer versions have been substituted for traditional foods, and any traditional foods have been omitted. In some cases, traditional diets are healthier than the diet in the new culture, and encouragement to maintain healthy traditions may be helpful.

Source: D'Amico, D., & Barbarito, C. (2007). *Health & physical assessment in nursing* (p. 137). Upper Saddle River, NJ: Pearson Education.

tests most commonly used are serum proteins, urinary urea nitrogen and creatinine, and total lymphocyte count.

Food Guide Pyramid

Dietary Guidelines for Americans is published jointly every 5 years by the Department of Health and Human Services (HHS) and the Department of Agriculture (USDA). The most recent guidelines, released in January 2005, provide a new comprehensive Food Guide Pyramid and an interactive Web site that may be used for individual food guide planning and diet analysis. The nurse can compare the **diet recall** or nutrition history data to the distribution of food groups recommended and make a general assessment of diet adequacy. The benefit of the new pyramid is that it is flexible and molds to the individual. Instead of requiring special food pyramids for various age or culture groups, the new Web site (www.usda.gov) has the richness of choice to meet all needs.

The Minimum Data Set

The Minimum Data Set (MDS) is a component of the Residential Assessment Instrument mandated for all clients in Medicare-certified health care facilities. The MDS nutritional components are to be included in admission assessments for all residents as well as in quarterly and annual updates. Any changes in client status that involve a nutritional component of the MDS require a complete reassessment of nutritional status.

Mini Nutritional Assessment and Subjective Global Assessment

The Mini Nutritional Assessment (MNA) and Subjective Global Assessment (SGA) have both been validated for use in the nutritional assessment of older adults. The SGA has also been used in assessing other populations since its development over 20 years ago. The MNA is a newer tool with extensive data validating its use with older adults. The MNA can be included as a routine component of a physical examination or as a quick bedside tool.

NURSING PROCESS

Diagnosis

NANDA (2007) includes the following diagnostic labels for nutritional problems:
- Imbalanced Nutrition: More Than Body Requirements
- Imbalanced Nutrition: Less Than Body Requirements
- Readiness for Enhanced Nutrition
- Risk for Imbalanced Nutrition: More Than Body Requirements

Many other NANDA nursing diagnoses may apply to certain individuals, because nutritional problems often affect other areas of human functioning. In this case, the nutritional diagnostic label may be used as the etiology of other diagnoses. Examples include the following:
- Activity intolerance related to inadequate intake of iron-rich foods resulting in iron-deficiency anemia
- Constipation related to inadequate fluid intake and fiber intake
- Low self-esteem related to obesity
- Risk for infection related to immunosuppression secondary to insufficient protein intake

Planning

Major goals for clients with or at risk for nutritional problems include the following:
- Maintain or restore optimal nutritional status.
- Promote healthy nutritional practices.
- Prevent complications associated with malnutrition.
- Decrease weight.
- Regain specified weight.

Specific nursing activities associated with each of these interventions can be selected to meet the individual needs of the client.

Implementation

Nursing interventions to promote optimal nutrition for hospitalized clients are often provided in collaboration with the primary care provider who writes the diet orders and the dietitian who informs clients about special diets. The nurse reinforces this instruction and, in addition, creates an atmosphere that encourages eating, provides assistance with eating, monitors the client's appetite and food intake, administers enteral and parenteral feedings, and consults with the primary care provider and dietitian about nutritional problems that arise.

In the community setting, the nurse's role is largely educational. For example, nurses promote optimal nutrition at health fairs, in schools, at prenatal classes, and with well or ill clients and support people in their homes. In the home setting, nurses also initiate nutritional screens, refer clients at risk to appropriate resources, instruct clients about enteral and parenteral feedings, and offer nutrition counseling as needed. Nutrition counseling involves more than simply providing information. The nurse must help clients integrate diet changes into their lifestyle and provide strategies to motivate them to change their eating habits.

Evaluation

The goals established in the planning phase are evaluated according to specific desired outcomes, also established in that phase. If the outcomes are not achieved, the nurse should explore the reasons. The nurse might consider the following questions:
- Were the outcomes unrealistic for this person?
- Were the client's food and religious preferences considered?
- Is anything interfering with digestion or absorption of nutrients (e.g., diarrhea)?
- Was the family included in the teaching plan? Are family members supportive?
- Is the client experiencing symptoms that cause loss of appetite (e.g., pain, nausea, fatigue)?

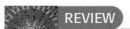 REVIEW **Nutrition Screening**

RELATE: LINK THE CONCEPTS

Linking the concept of Culture with the concept of Health, Wellness, and Illness:

1. Describe how you would provide nutrition teaching to a recent immigrant whose religious practices and comforting food choices available from his country of origin have caused him to be malnourished.

READY: GO TO COMPANION SKILLS MANUAL

1. Measuring body mass index
2. Assessing height and weight

REFLECT: CASE STUDY

Madison, a 17-month-old, is brought to the Pediatric Clinic by her mother, who is worried because it seems Madison is eating less. Madison is always moving and doing something. The mother asks you what are some good snack foods to give Madison. Her mother says Madison wants milk and juice when she is "on the move."

1. Madison seems to eat less to her mother. What phenomenon is occuring?
2. What are the elements of a healthy diet for a toddler? What are examples of healthy snacks?
3. How much milk and juice should Madison be drinking?
4. Describe a typical daily dietary intake for Madison.

7.5 NORMAL SLEEP/REST PATTERNS

KEY TERMS

Biological rhythms, *210*
Nocturnal emissions, *212*
NREM (non-rapid-eye-movement) sleep, *210*
REM (rapid-eye-movement) sleep, *210*
Sleep, *209*
Sleep architecture, *210*
Somnology, *209*

BASIS FOR SELECTION OF EXEMPLAR

Institute of Medicine (IOM)

LEARNING OUTCOMES

After reading this exemplar, you will be able to do the following:

1. Explain the functions and the physiology of sleep.
2. Identify the characteristics of the sleep states.
3. Describe variations in sleep patterns throughout the life span.
4. Describe interventions that promote normal sleep.

OVERVIEW

Sleep is a basic human need; it is a universal biological process common to all people. Humans spend about one third of their lives asleep. We require sleep for many reasons: to cope with daily stresses, to prevent fatigue, to conserve energy, to restore the mind and body, and to enjoy life more fully. Sleep enhances daytime functioning. It is vital for not only optimal psychological functioning but also physiological functioning, as the rate of healing of damaged tissue is greatest during sleep (Robinson, Weitzel, & Henderson, 2005, p. 263).

Sleep is an important factor in a person's quality of life, yet a 2006 report from the Institute of Medicine (IOM) states that sleep disorders and sleep deprivation is an unmet public health problem. It is estimated that 50 million to 70 million Americans suffer from a chronic disorder of sleep and wakefulness that hinders daily functioning and adversely affects health (IOM, 2006, p. 24). Numerous *Sleep in America* polls by the National Sleep Foundation reflect that Americans, from infants to older adults, need more sleep. Furthermore, many members of the general public and health professionals are unaware of the consequences of chronic sleep loss (e.g., increased risk of hypertension, diabetes, obesity, depression, heart attack, and stroke).

Almost 20% of all serious car crash injuries are associated with driver sleepiness (IOM, 2006, p. 25).

As a result of these studies, the IOM report made a number of recommendations, including to (a) increase financial investments in interdisciplinary **somnology** (the study of sleep) and sleep medicine research training; (b) increase public awareness by establishing a multimedia public education campaign; (c) increase education and training of health care professionals in somnology and sleep medicine; (d) develop new technologies for the diagnosis and treatment of sleep disorders; and (e) monitor the American population's sleep patterns and the prevalence and health outcomes associated with sleep disorders (IOM, 2006).

PHYSIOLOGY OF SLEEP

Historically, sleep was considered a state of unconsciousness. More recently, **sleep** has come to be considered an altered state of consciousness in which the individual's perception of and reaction to the environment are decreased. Sleep is characterized by minimal physical activity, variable levels of consciousness, changes in the body's physiologic processes, and decreased responsiveness to external stimuli. Some environmental stimuli, such as a smoke detector alarm, will usually awaken a sleeper, whereas many other noises will not. It appears that individuals respond to meaningful stimuli while sleeping and selectively disregard nonmeaningful stimuli. For example, a mother may respond to her baby's crying but not to the crying of another baby.

The cyclic nature of sleep is thought to be controlled by centers located in the lower part of the brain. Neurons within the reticular formation, located in the brainstem, integrate sensory information from the peripheral nervous system and relay the information to the cerebral cortex. The upper part of the reticular formation consists of a network of ascending nerve fibers called the reticular activating system (RAS), which is involved with the sleep-wake cycle. An intact cerebral cortex and reticular formation are necessary for the regulation of sleep and waking states.

Neurotransmitters, located within neurons in the brain, affect the sleep-wake cycles. For example, serotonin is thought to lessen the response to sensory stimulation and gamma-aminobutyric acid (GABA) to shut off the activity in the neurons of the RAS. Another key factor to sleep is exposure to darkness. Darkness and preparing for sleep cause a decrease in RAS stimulation. During this time, the pineal gland in the brain begins actively to secrete the natural hormone melatonin, and the person feels less alert. During sleep, the growth hormone is secreted and cortisol is inhibited.

With the beginning of daylight, melatonin is at its lowest level in the body and the stimulating hormone cortisol is at its highest. Wakefulness is also associated with high levels of acetylcholine, dopamine, and noradrenaline. Acetylcholine is released in the reticular formation, dopamine in the midbrain, and noradrenaline in the pons. These neurotransmitters are localized within the reticular formation and influence cerebral cortical arousal.

Circadian Rhythms

Biological rhythms exist in plants, animals, and humans. In humans, these are controlled from within the body and synchronized with environmental factors, such as light and darkness. The most familiar biological rhythm is the circadian rhythm. The term *circadian* is from the Latin *circa dies,* meaning "about a day." Although sleep and waking cycles are the best known of the circadian rhythms, body temperature, blood pressure, and many other physiologic functions also follow a circadian pattern.

Sleep is a complex biological rhythm. When a person's biological clock coincides with the sleep-wake cycles, the person is said to be in circadian synchronization; that is, the person is awake when the body temperature is highest, and asleep when the body temperature is lowest. Circadian regularity begins to develop by the sixth week of life, and by 3–6 months most infants have a regular sleep-wake cycle.

Types of Sleep

Sleep architecture refers to the basic organization of normal sleep. There are two types of sleep: **NREM (non-rapid-eye-movement) sleep** and **REM (rapid-eye-movement) sleep**. During sleep, NREM and REM sleep alternate in

cycles. Irregular cycling and/or absent sleep stages are associated with sleep disorders (IOM, 2006, p. 42).

NREM SLEEP NREM sleep occurs when activity in the RAS is inhibited. About 75–80% of sleep during a night is NREM sleep. NREM sleep is divided into four stages, each associated with distinct brain activity and physiology. Stage I is the stage of very light sleep and lasts only a few minutes. During this stage, the person feels drowsy and relaxed, the eyes roll from side to side, and the heart and respiratory rates drop slightly. The sleeper can be readily awakened and may deny that he or she was sleeping.

Stage II is the stage of light sleep during which body processes continue to slow down. The eyes are generally still, the heart and respiratory rates decrease slightly, and body temperature falls. Stage II constitutes 44–55% of total sleep (IOM, 2006, p. 44). An individual requires more intense stimuli in stage II than in stage I to awaken.

Stages III and IV are the deepest stages of sleep, differing only in the percentage of delta waves recorded during a 30-second period. During *deep sleep* or *delta sleep,* the sleeper's heart and respiratory rates drop 20–30% below those exhibited during waking hours. The sleeper is difficult to arouse. The person is not disturbed by sensory stimuli, the skeletal muscles are very relaxed, reflexes are diminished, and snoring is most likely to occur. Even swallowing and saliva production are reduced during delta sleep (Orr, 2000). These stages are essential for restoring energy and releasing important growth hormones (Box 7–9).

PRACTICE ALERT

In a sleep-deprived client, the loss of NREM sleep causes immunosuppression, slows tissue repair, lowers pain tolerance, triggers profound fatigue, and increases susceptibility to infection (Lower, Bonsack, & Guion, 2003, p. 40D).

REM SLEEP REM sleep usually recurs about every 90 minutes and lasts 5–30 minutes. Most dreams take place during REM sleep but usually will not be remembered unless the person arouses briefly at the end of the REM period.

Box 7–9 **Physiologic Changes During NREM Sleep**

- Arterial blood pressure falls.
- Pulse rate decreases.
- Peripheral blood vessels dilate.
- Cardiac output decreases.
- Skeletal muscles relax.
- Basal metabolic rate decreases 10–30%.
- Growth hormone levels peak.
- Intracranial pressure decreases.

Source: Berman, A., Snyder, S. J., Kozier, B., & Erb, G. (2008). *Kozier & Erb's fundamentals of nursing: Concepts, process, and practice* (8th ed., p. 1165). Upper Saddle River, NJ: Pearson Education.

During REM sleep, the brain is highly active, and brain metabolism may increase as much as 20%. For example, during REM sleep, levels of acetylcholine and dopamine increase, with the highest levels of acetylcholine release occurring during REM sleep. Since both of these neurotransmitters are associated with cortical activation, it makes sense that their levels would be high during dreaming sleep. This type of sleep is also called paradoxical sleep because electroencephalogram (EEG) activity resembles that of wakefulness. Distinctive eye movements occur, voluntary muscle tone is dramatically decreased, and deep tendon reflexes are absent. In this phase, the sleeper may be difficult to arouse or may wake spontaneously, gastric secretions increase, and heart and respiratory rates often are irregular. It is thought that the regions of the brain used in learning, thinking, and organizing information are stimulated during REM sleep.

PRACTICE ALERT

In a sleep-deprived client, the loss of REM sleep causes psychologic disturbances such as apathy, depression, irritability, confusion, disorientation, hallucinations, impaired memory, and paranoia (Lower, Bonsack, & Guion, 2003, p. 40D).

Sleep Cycles

During a sleep cycle, people typically pass through NREM and REM sleep, with the complete cycle usually lasting about 90–110 minutes in adults. In the first sleep cycle, a sleeper usually passes through all of the first three NREM stages in a total of about 20–30 minutes. Then, stage IV may last about 30 minutes. After stage IV NREM, the sleeper passes back through stages III and II over about 20 minutes. Thereafter, the first REM stage occurs, lasting about 10 minutes, completing the first sleep cycle. It is not unusual for the first REM period to be very brief or even skipped entirely. The healthy adult sleeper usually experiences four to six cycles of sleep during 7–8 hours (Figure 7–7 ■). The sleeper who is awakened during any stage must begin anew at stage I NREM sleep and proceed through all the stages to REM sleep.

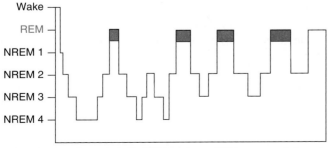

Figure 7–7 ■ Time spent in REM and non-REM stages of sleep in an adult.

The duration of NREM stages and REM sleep varies throughout the sleep period. During the early part of the night, the deep sleep periods are longer. As the night progresses, the sleeper spends less time in stages III and IV of NREM sleep. REM sleep increases and dreams tend to lengthen. Before sleep ends, periods of near wakefulness occur, and stages I and II NREM sleep and REM sleep predominate.

FUNCTIONS OF SLEEP

The effects of sleep on the body are not completely understood. Sleep exerts physiologic effects on both the nervous system and other body structures. Sleep in some way restores normal levels of activity and normal balance among parts of the nervous system. Sleep is also necessary for protein synthesis, which allows repair processes to occur.

The role of sleep in psychological well-being is best noticed by the deterioration in mental functioning related to sleep loss. Persons with inadequate amounts of sleep tend to become emotionally irritable, have poor concentration, and experience difficulty making decisions.

NORMAL SLEEP PATTERNS AND REQUIREMENTS

Although it used to be believed that maintaining a regular sleep-wake rhythm is more important than the number of hours actually slept, recent research has shown that sleep deprivation is associated with significant cognitive and health problems. Although reestablishing the sleep-wake rhythm (e.g., after the disruption of surgery) is an important aspect of nursing, it is not appropriate to curtail or decrease daytime napping in hospitalized clients.

Newborns

Newborns sleep 16–18 hours a day, on an irregular schedule with periods of 1–3 hours spent awake. Unlike older children and adults, newborns enter REM sleep (called active sleep during the newborn period) immediately. Rapid eye movements are observable through closed lids, and the body movements and irregular respirations may be observed. NREM sleep (also called quiet sleep during the newborn period) is characterized by regular respirations, closed eyes, and the absence of body and eye movements. Newborns spend nearly 50% of their time in each of these states, and the sleep cycle is about 50 minutes.

It is best to put newborns to bed when they are sleepy but not asleep. Newborns can be encouraged to sleep less during the day by exposing them to light and by playing more with them during the day hours. As evening approaches, the environment can be less bright and quieter, with less activity (National Sleep Foundation, n.d.d). It is important to teach new parents and caregivers of newborns to put the baby "back to sleep," to make sure the newborn who is lying down while sleeping is sleeping on the back, as babies who sleep on their stomachs are at greater risk for sudden infant death syndrome.

Infants

At first, infants awaken every 3 or 4 hours, eat, and then go back to sleep. Periods of wakefulness gradually increase during the first months. By 6 months, most infants sleep through the night (from midnight to 5 a.m.) and begin to establish a pattern of daytime naps. At the end of the first year, an infant usually takes two naps per day and should get about 14–15 hours of sleep in 24 hours.

About half of the infant's sleep time is spent in light sleep. During light sleep, the infant exhibits a great deal of activity, such as movement, gurgles, and coughing. Parents need to make sure that infants are truly awake before picking them up for feeding and changing. Putting infants to bed when they are drowsy but not asleep helps them to become "self-soothers." This means that they fall asleep independently, and if they do awake at night, they can put themselves back to sleep. Infants who become used to parental assistance at bedtime may become "signalers" and cry for their parents to help them return to sleep at night (National Sleep Foundation, n.d.a).

Toddlers

Between 12 and 14 hours of sleep are recommended for children 1–3 years of age. Most still need an afternoon nap, but the need for midmorning naps gradually decreases. The toddler may exhibit a great deal of resistance to going to bed and may awaken during the night. Nighttime fears and nightmares are also common. A security object such as a blanket or stuffed animal may help. Parents need assurance that if the child has had adequate attention from them during the day, maintaining a daily sleep schedule and consistent bedtime routine will promote good sleep habits for the entire family.

Preschoolers

The preschool child (3–5 years of age) requires 11–13 hours of sleep per night, particularly if the child is in preschool. Sleep needs fluctuate in relation to activity and growth spurts. Many children of this age dislike bedtime and resist by requesting another story, game, or television program. The 4–5-year-old may become restless and irritable if sleep requirements are not met.

Parents can help children who resist bedtime by maintaining a regular and consistent sleep schedule. It also helps to have a relaxing bedtime routine that ends in the child's room. Preschool children wake up frequently at night, and they may be afraid of the dark or experience night terrors or nightmares. Often limiting or eliminating TV will reduce the number of nightmares.

School-Age Children

The school-age child (5–12 years of age) needs 10–11 hours of sleep, but most receive less because of increasing demands (e.g., homework, sports, social activities). They may also be spending more time at the computer and watching TV. Some may be drinking caffeinated beverages. All of these activities can lead to difficulty falling asleep and fewer hours of sleep. Nurses can teach parents and school-age children about healthy sleep habits. A regular and consistent sleep schedule and bedtime routine need to be continued.

Adolescents

Adolescents (12–18 years of age) require 9–10 hours of sleep each night; however, few actually get that much sleep (IOM, 2006, p. 56). The National Sleep Foundation's 2006 *Sleep in America* poll found that teens are sleepy at times and places where they should be fully awake—at school, at home, and on the road. This can result in lower grades, negative moods (e.g., unhappy, sad, tense), and increased potential for car accidents. Interestingly, while more than half of the adolescents knew they were not getting enough sleep, 90% of the parents believed their adolescent was getting enough sleep. Nurses can teach parents to recognize signs and symptoms that indicate their teen is not getting enough sleep.

As children reach adolescence, their circadian rhythms tend to shift. Research in the 1990s found that later sleep and wake patterns among adolescents are biologically determined; the natural tendency for teenagers is to stay up late at night and wake up later in the morning (National Sleep Foundation, n.d.a). Many schools, however, start at 7 a.m., which is in conflict with adolescents' sleep patterns and needs and contribute to their sleep deprivation. As a result, some members of Congress have introduced resolutions to encourage schools and school districts to reconsider the early school start times.

During adolescence, boys begin to experience **nocturnal emissions** (orgasm and emission of semen during sleep), known as "wet dreams," several times each month. Boys need to be informed about this normal development to prevent embarrassment and fear.

Adults

Most healthy adults need 7–9 hours of sleep a night (National Sleep Foundation, n.d.b). However, there is individual variation as some adults may be able to function well (e.g., without sleepiness or drowsiness) with 6 hours of sleep and others may need 10 hours to function optimally. Signs that may indicate a person is not getting enough sleep include falling asleep or becoming drowsy during a task that is not fatiguing (e.g., listening to a boring or monotonous presentation), not being able to concentrate or remember information, and being unreasonably irritable with others.

The National Sleep Foundation (n.d.b) reports that certain adults are particularly vulnerable to getting insufficient sleep: students, shift workers, travelers, and persons suffering from acute stress, depression, or chronic pain. Adults working long hours or multiple jobs may find their sleep less refreshing. Also, the sleep habits of children have an impact on the adults caring for them. Parents and caregivers whose children get the least amount of sleep are twice as likely to say they sleep less than 6 hours a night (National Sleep Foundation, n.d.b). Parents of infants lose the most sleep— nearly an hour on a typical night. Women may experience more disrupted sleep during pregnancy, menses, and the perimenopausal period.

Nurses need to teach adults the importance of obtaining sufficient sleep and tips on how to promote sleep that result in the client waking up feeling restored or refreshed.

Older Adults

A hallmark change with age is a tendency toward earlier bedtime and wake times. Older adults (65–75 years) usually awaken 1.3 hours earlier and go to bed approximately 1 hour earlier than younger adults (ages 20–30). Older adults may show an increase in disturbed sleep that can create a negative impact on their quality of life, mood, and alertness. Although sleeping becomes more difficult, the need to sleep does not decrease with age (IOM, 2006, pp. 57–59).

The National Sleep Foundation's 2003 *Sleep in America* poll was the first poll to look at the sleep habits of Americans between the ages of 55 and 84. It found that older adults are sleeping 7–9 hours on both weeknights and weekends. Of interest, however, was the striking relationship between the older adult's health and quality of life and the person's sleep quantity and quality. The poll found that the better the health of older adults, the more likely they are to sleep well. And, conversely, the more diagnosed medical conditions, the more likely they were to report sleep problems (National Sleep Foundation, n.d.c). Older adults who have several medical conditions and complain of having sleeping problems should discuss this with their primary care provider: They may have a major sleep disorder that is complicating treatment of the other conditions. It is important for the nurse to teach about the connection between sleep, health, and aging.

Some older adult clients with dementia may experience *sundown syndrome*. Although not a sleep disorder directly, it refers to a pattern of symptoms (e.g., agitation, anxiety, aggression, and sometimes delusions) that occur in the late afternoon (thus the name). These symptoms can last throughout the night, further disrupting sleep (Arnold, 2004).

FACTORS AFFECTING SLEEP

Both the quality and the quantity of sleep are affected by a number of factors. *Sleep quality* is a subjective characteristic and is often determined by whether or not a person wakes up feeling energetic. *Quantity of sleep* is the total time the individual sleeps.

Following an irregular morning and nighttime schedule can affect sleep. Moderate exercise in the morning or early afternoon usually is conducive to sleep, but exercise late in the day can delay sleep. The person's ability to relax before retiring is an important factor affecting the ability to fall asleep. It is best, therefore, to avoid doing homework or office work before or after getting into bed.

Night shift workers frequently obtain less sleep than other workers and have difficulty falling asleep after getting off work. Wearing dark wraparound sunglasses during the drive home and light-blocking shades can minimize the alerting effects of exposure to daylight, thus making it easier to fall asleep when body temperature is rising.

Emotional Stress

Most sleep experts consider stress to be the number one cause of short-term sleeping difficulties (National Sleep Foundation, n.d.b). A person preoccupied with personal problems (e.g., school- or job-related pressures, financial difficulties, family or marriage problems) may be unable to relax sufficiently to get to sleep. Anxiety increases the norepinephrine blood levels through stimulation of the sympathetic nervous system. This chemical change results in less deep sleep and REM sleep and more stage changes and awakenings.

Stimulants and Alcohol

Caffeine-containing beverages act as stimulants of the central nervous system. Drinking beverages containing caffeine in the afternoon or evening may interfere with sleep. People who drink an excessive amount of alcohol often find their sleep disturbed. Although it may hasten the onset of sleep, alcohol disrupts REM sleep. While making up for lost REM sleep after some of the effects of the alcohol have worn off, people often experience nightmares. The alcohol-tolerant person may be unable to sleep well and become irritable as a result.

Diet

Weight gain has been associated with reduced total sleep time as well as broken sleep and earlier awakening. Weight loss, on the other hand, seems to be associated with an increase in total sleep time and less broken sleep. Dietary L-tryptophan—found, for example, in cheese and milk—may induce sleep, a fact that might explain why warm milk helps some people get to sleep.

Smoking

Nicotine has a stimulating effect on the body, and smokers often have more difficulty falling asleep than nonsmokers do. Smokers are usually easily aroused and often describe themselves as light sleepers. Refraining from smoking after the evening meal usually helps the person sleeps better; moreover, many former smokers report that their sleeping patterns improved once they stopped smoking.

Motivation

Motivation can increase alertness in some situations (e.g., a tired person can probably stay alert while attending an interesting concert or surfing the Web late at night). Motivation alone, however, is usually not sufficient to overcome the normal circadian drive to sleep during the night. Nor is motivation sufficient to overcome sleepiness due to insufficient sleep. Boredom alone is not sufficient to cause sleepiness, but when insufficient sleep combines with boredom, sleep is likely to occur.

Medications

Some medications affect the quality of sleep. Most hypnotics can interfere with deep sleep and suppress REM sleep. Beta-blockers have been known to cause insomnia and nightmares. Narcotics, such as meperidine hydrochloride (Demerol) and morphine, are known to suppress REM sleep and to cause frequent awakenings and drowsiness. Tranquilizers interfere with REM sleep. Although antidepressants suppress REM sleep, this effect is considered a therapeutic action. In fact, selectively depriving a depressed client of REM sleep will result in an immediate but transient improvement in mood. Clients accustomed to taking hypnotic medications and antidepressants may experience a REM rebound (increased REM sleep) when these medications are discontinued. Warning clients to expect a period of more intense dreams when these medications are discontinued may reduce their anxiety about this symptom.

REVIEW Normal Sleep/Rest Patterns

RELATE: LINK THE CONCEPTS

Linking the concept of Cognition with the concept of Health, Wellness, and Illness:

1. What is the effect of inadequate sleep on thought process?

REFLECT: CASE STUDY

Ms. Smith, a 70-year-old woman, reports that she is having difficulty falling asleep at night. This has been occurring more frequently over the past year. She says, "I am so tired in the mornings, I can hardly get out of bed."

1. Which assessment tools might be used to determine her problem?
2. Identify life span issues that might be influencing her condition.
3. What will Ms. Smith report if the interventions are successful?

7.6 CONSUMER EDUCATION

KEY TERMS

Health literacy, *216*
Teaching, *215*

BASIS FOR SELECTION OF EXEMPLAR

Healthy People 2010

LEARNING OUTCOMES

After reading this exemplar, you will be able to do the following:

1. Explain the importance of the teaching role of the nurse in consumer education.
2. Explain the implications of using the Internet as a source of health information.
3. Identify methods to evaluate learning.
4. Demonstrate effective documentation of teaching–learning activities.

OVERVIEW

Teaching client education is a major aspect of nursing practice and an important independent nursing function. In 1992, the American Hospital Association passed *A Patient's Bill of Rights*, mandating client education as a right of all clients. State nurse practice acts include client teaching as a function of nursing, thereby making teaching a legal and professional responsibility. In addition, the Joint Commission on Accreditation of Healthcare Organizations (JCAHO) recently expanded its standards of client education by nurses to include "evidence that patients and their significant others understand what they have been taught. This requirement means that providers must consider the literacy level, educational background, language skills, and culture of every client during the education process" (Bastable, 2003, p. 5).

Client education is multifaceted, involving promoting, protecting, and maintaining health. It involves teaching about reducing health risk factors, increasing a person's level of wellness, and taking specific protective health measures. Box 7–10 lists specific areas of health teaching.

Box 7–10 **Areas for Client Education**

PROMOTION OF HEALTH

- Increasing a person's level of wellness
- Growth and development topics
- Fertility control
- Hygiene
- Nutrition
- Exercise
- Stress management
- Lifestyle modification
- Resources within the community

PREVENTION OF ILLNESS/INJURY

- Health screening (e.g., blood glucose levels, blood pressure, blood cholesterol, Pap test, mammograms, vision, hearing, routine physical examinations)
- Reducing health risk factors (e.g., lowering cholesterol level)
- Specific protective health measures (e.g., immunizations, use of condoms, use of sunscreen, use of medication, umbilical cord care)
- First aid
- Safety (e.g., using seat belts, helmets, walkers)

RESTORATION OF HEALTH

- Information about tests, diagnosis, treatment, and medications
- Self-care skills or skills needed to care for family member
- Resources within health care setting and community

ADAPTING TO ALTERED HEALTH AND FUNCTION

- Adaptations in lifestyle
- Problem-solving skills
- Adaptation to changing health status
- Strategies to deal with current problems (e.g., home IV skills, medications, diet, activity limits, prostheses)
- Strategies to deal with future problems (e.g., fear of pain with terminal cancer, future surgeries, or treatments)
- Information about treatments and likely outcomes
- Referrals to other health care facilities or services
- Facilitation of strong self-image
- Grief and bereavement counseling

Source: Berman, A., Snyder, S. J., Kozier, B., & Erb, G. (2008). *Kozier & Erb's fundamentals of nursing: Concepts, process, and practice* (8th ed., p. 487). Upper Saddle River, NJ: Pearson Education.

TEACHING

Teaching is a system of activities intended to produce learning. The teaching-learning process involves dynamic interaction between teacher and learner. Each participant in the process communicates information, emotions, perceptions, and attitudes to the other. The teaching process and the nursing process are much alike.

Nurses teach a variety of learners in various settings. They teach clients and their families or significant others in the hospital, primary care clinics, urgent care, managed care, the home, and assisted living and long-term care facilities. Nurses teach large and small groups of learners in community health education programs.

Nurses also teach professional colleagues and other health care personnel in academic institutions such as vocational schools, colleges, and universities, and in health care facilities such as hospitals or nursing homes.

Teaching Clients and Their Families

Nurses may teach individual clients in one-to-one teaching episodes. For example, the nurse may teach about wound care while changing a client's dressing or may teach about diet, exercise, and other lifestyle behaviors that minimize the risk of a heart attack for a client who has a cardiac problem. The nurse may also be involved in teaching family members or other support people who are caring for the client. Nurses working in obstetric and pediatric areas teach parents and sometimes grandparents how to care for children.

The Internet has become a source of information for many clients. See Box 7–11 for more information on how Americans are using the Internet for health care information.

Teaching in the Community

Nurses are often involved in community health education programs. Such teaching activities may be voluntary, as part of the nurse's involvement in an organization such as the Red Cross

---

Box 7–11 **The Internet and Health Information**

The Internet has become a part of the lives of many Americans, allowing them to communicate and obtain information quickly. Internet technology has dramatically changed the activities of business, including health care. The term *e-health* is defined as "the application of Internet and other related technologies in the healthcare industry to improve the access, efficiency, effectiveness, and quality of clinical and business processes utilized by healthcare organizations, practitioners, patients, and consumers in an effort to improve the health status of patients" (Healthcare Information and Management Systems Society E-Health Special Interest Group, 2003, p. 4). E-health includes many aspects such as online appointment access, billing review, e-mail access between the client and health care provider, online health information, and online support groups.

ONLINE HEALTH INFORMATION
The Pew Internet & American Life Project (2006) reports that 73% of American adults use the Internet. Using the Internet to locate health information is common. Health care online usage is growing twice as fast as any other online type of usage (Curran & Curran, 2005, p. 496). Eight out of 10 American Internet users have searched for information on at least one major health topic online. Certain groups of users are more likely to search the Internet for health information: women, adults younger than 65, college graduates, people with online experience, and those with broadband (high-speed) access (Pew Internet & American Life Project, 2005a, p. 1).

ACCESS
The Pew Internet & American Life Project (2005b, p. 7) reported on three groups of adults in the United States: those who do not use the Internet, those with a modest connection, and those highly engaged with the Internet. Each group has its distinct characteristics.

Twenty-two percent of American adults have never used the Internet. They tend to have a high school or less education or to be over the age of 65. Forty percent of adults have a loose connection to the Internet. That is, they have access (usually dial-up) but do not use the Internet regularly. They are younger and more educated than the previous group. Thirty-three percent of American adults are

highly engaged by using the Internet daily. They tend to have college educations and are under age 50; however, there are "pockets" of older adults who are also highly engaged in Internet use.

OLDER ADULTS AND USE OF THE INTERNET
The Kaiser Family Foundation (2005, pp. 3–10) conducted a survey research study that provided the first close look at how older adults use the Internet for health information. Following are key findings of the report:
- Only 4 in 10 adults age 65 and over have used a computer.
- Seventy percent of "Baby Boomers" (age 50–64) use the Internet. Thus, the number of older adults using the Internet will increase over the next decade.
- There is a "digital divide" among older adults. Those whose annual income is under $20,000, those who have a high school degree or less, those who are older (e.g., 75 and above), and older women are less likely to use the Internet.
- One in five older adults (65 and over) use the Internet for health information. These elders are more likely to use TV and books for their health information.
- Many older adults do not trust the Internet as a source for health information except for the 50–64 age group, who trust the Internet "a lot."
- Seeking information on prescription drugs is the top reason for using the Internet for health information.
- Of those older adults who have used the Internet for health information, about half say it helped them and the other half say it wasn't helpful.
- Most older adults do not check the source of health information they find online.

IMPLICATIONS
The Internet is an important source of health information for many adult clients in the United States. Therefore, nurses need to know and be able to integrate this technology into the teaching plans for those clients who use the Internet. On the other hand, nurses also need to apply effective teaching strategies for those clients who do not use the Internet.

or Planned Parenthood, or they may be compensated as part of the nurse's work role, such as school nurses. Community teaching activities may be aimed at large groups of people who have an interest in some aspect of health, such as nutrition classes, cardiopulmonary resuscitation (CPR) or cardiac risk factor reduction classes, and bicycle or swimming safety programs. Community education programs can also be designed for small groups or individual learners, such as childbirth or family planning classes.

Health Literacy

A 1993 National Adult Literacy Study reported that the average reading ability of many American adults is at the fifth-grade level (Edmunds, 2005). A report from the Institutes of Medicine (IOM, 2004) titled *Health Literacy: A Prescription to End Confusion* states that nearly half of all American adults—90 million people—have difficulty understanding and acting on health information (p. 1). Moreover, studies that assessed a variety of health-related materials found that the reading level exceeded the twelfth-grade level.

Health literacy is the ability to read, understand, and act on health information, and includes such tasks as comprehending prescription labels, interpreting appointment slips, completing health insurance forms, and following instructions for diagnostic tests (Redman, 2004, pp. 30–31). Limited health literacy skills are often greater among certain groups: older adults, people with limited education, poor people, minority populations, and people with limited English proficiency.

Low health literacy skills are associated with poor health outcomes and higher health care costs (IOM, 2004). For example, a client may not be able to read a prescription to know how many pills to take, and may take the wrong number of pills (e.g., "once" reads as "eleven" in Spanish). Clients with low literacy skills have less information about health promotion and/or management of a disease process for themselves and their families because they are unable to read the educational materials. As a result, they have higher rates of hospitalization than people with adequate health literacy.

It is a challenge for the nurse to teach clients with low or no reading and writing skills. However, such teaching is vital because clients with low literacy skills need learning opportunities to improve their health practices.

PRACTICE ALERT

The majority of people at the lowest reading levels will report that they "read well." Often clients will not admit to having difficulty reading because of the embarrassment it brings them. A nurse who suspects a client has difficulty reading may ask the client tactful questions, such as "Would you like me to go over it with you?"

CLIENT TEACHING **Developing Written Teaching Aids**

- Keep language level at or below the fifth-grade level.
- Use active, not passive, voice.
- Use easy, common words of one or two syllables (e.g., *use* instead of *utilize*, or *give* instead of *administer*).
- Use the second person (*you*) rather than the third person (*the client*).
- Use a large type size (14–16 point).
- Write short sentences.
- Avoid using all capital letters.
- Place priority information first and repeat more than once.
- Use bold for emphasis.
- Use simple pictures, drawings, or cartoons, if appropriate.
- Leave plenty of white space.
- Obtain feedback from nurses and clients.

Source: Berman, A., Snyder, S. J., Kozier, B., & Erb, G. (2008). *Kozier & Erb's fundamentals of nursing: Concepts, process, and practice* (8th ed., p. 497). Upper Saddle River, NJ: Pearson Education.

It is difficult, however, to assess a client's literacy skills because the shame and stigma associated with limited health literacy skills are major barriers. Clients may be too embarrassed to admit they cannot read. The following client behaviors may cause a nurse to suspect a literacy problem:

- Pattern of noncompliance
- Insisting that they already know the information
- Having a friend or family member read the document for them
- Pattern of excuses for not reading the instructions (e.g., glasses broken, stating will read later or when they get home)

CLIENT TEACHING **Teaching Clients With Low Literacy Levels**

- Use multiple teaching methods: Show pictures. Read important information. Lead a small group discussion. Role play. Demonstrate a skill. Provide hands-on practice.
- Emphasize key points in simple terms and provide examples.
- Limit the amount of information in a single teaching session. Instead of one long session with a great deal of information, it is better to have more frequent sessions with a major point at each session.
- Associate new information with something the client already knows and/or associates with his or her job or lifestyle.
- Reinforce information through repetition.
- Involve the client in the teaching.
- Obtain feedback: Ask the client specific questions about the information presented or ask the client to repeat it in his or her own words.
- Avoid handouts with many pages and classroom lecture format with a large group.

Source: Berman, A., Snyder, S. J., Kozier, B., & Erb, G. (2008). *Kozier & Erb's fundamentals of nursing: Concepts, process, and practice* (8th ed., p. 497). Upper Saddle River, NJ: Pearson Education.

Box 7–12 Can Animated Cartoons Increase Knowledge of Educational Information?

Printed client information may not be helpful because of low English-language literacy levels. The researchers in this study compared the gain of knowledge about polio vaccination from information presented in two formats: printed pamphlet and videotape of animated cartoons. Both formats contained the same information. The participants were parents/caretakers of pediatric clinic clients. Ninety-six participants were in the treatment group who watched the videotape in the clinic waiting room in the midst of intense client traffic. The comparison group consisted of 96 participants who were given a written pamphlet to read. Both groups completed a pretest that included demographics and five questions related to understanding polio vaccine. After the two groups completed either reading the pamphlet or viewing the videotape, the participants completed a posttest, which included the same five pretest questions and three additional questions.

There was no statistical difference between the two groups regarding demographic information or pretreatment knowledge. There was a significant statistical difference between the two groups in posttest knowledge. Both groups scored higher on the post-test compared to the pretest. However, 30% of the participants in the videotape group answered all of the posttest questions correctly while none of the participants in the pamphlet group responded correctly to all the questions.

IMPLICATIONS

This study showed that animated cartoons can improve client knowledge independent of the level of literacy. The production cost of the videotape used in this study was $6,000 with a production time of 6 weeks. Printed material is less costly and can be developed more quickly. However, if the client does not or cannot read the material, what is the ultimate cost to the client and the health care system?

Source: Health Education Research. New York: Oxford University Press. Copyright 2004 by Oxford University Press Journals. Reproduced with permission of Oxford University Press Journals in the format Textbook via Copyright Clearance Center.

There are many formulas for assessing reading level of written material. Most word processing programs have a feature that will calculate the readability. Nurses involved in developing written health teaching materials should write for lower reading levels (see Client Teaching). The goal is to have the education materials at a fifth- or sixth-grade level (Aldridge, 2004). People with good reading skills are not offended by simple reading material and prefer easy-to-read information. Even the simplest written directions, however, won't be helpful for the client with low or no reading skills. See the following Client Teaching box for suggestions on how to teach clients with low literacy levels; see also Box 7–12.

REVIEW   Consumer Education

RELATE: LINK THE CONCEPTS

Linking the concepts of Development and Culture with the concept of Health, Wellness, and Illness:

1. Select a developmental theorist, and identify the factors to consider when planning a literacy program for school-age children through older adulthood.
2. How would you teach non-English-speaking clients about using the Internet as a source of health information?

REFLECT: CASE STUDY

Marge Loder is a 48-year-old client with diabetes. Her husband of 20 years recently died in a car crash; 2 days later, Marge was admitted with diabetic ketoacidosis. After she was stabilized, Marge told the nurse that she does not know how to read and her husband managed all of her care.

1. What are Marge's immediate needs?
2. How will you implement teaching?

REFERENCES

Aldridge, M. D. (2004). Writing and designing readable patient education materials. *Nephrology Nursing Journal, 31*(4), 373–377.

American Dental Association. (n.d.). *Cleaning your teeth and gums (oral hygiene).* Retrieved June 13, 2006, from http://www.ada.org/public/ topics/cleaning_faq.asp

American Dental Association. (n.d.). *Oral changes with age.* Retrieved June 13, 2006, from http://www.ada.org/public/ topics/oral_ changes_faq.asp

American Nurses Association. (1980). *Nursing: A social policy statement.* Kansas City, MO: Author.

American Nurses Association. (2004). *Nursing: Scope and standards of practice.* Washington, DC: Author.

Anonymous. (2003). Oral care update. *Nursing Management, 34*(5), S1–S16.

Anspaugh, D. J., Hamrick, M. H., & Rosato, F. D. (2006). *Wellness: Concepts and applications* (6th ed., p. 4). New York: McGraw-Hill.

Arnold, E. (2004). Sorting out the 3 D's: Delirium, dementia, and depression. *Nursing, 34*(6), 36–42.

Bastable, S. (2003). *Nurse as educator: Principles of teaching and learning for nursing practice* (2nd ed.). Boston: Jones & Bartlett.

Bilukha, O. O., & Rosenstein, N. (2005). Prevention and control of meningococcal disease. Recommendations of the Advisory Committee on Immunization Practices (ACIP). *Morbidity and Mortality Weekly Report, 54* (RR-7), 1–21.

Burke, M., & Laramie, J. (2004). *Primary care of the older adult: A multidisciplinary approach* (2nd ed.). Philadelphia: Mosby/Elsevier.

Coleman, P. R. (2002). Improving oral health care for the frail elderly: A review of widespread problems and best practices. *Geriatric Nursing, 23,* 189–199.

Coleman, P. R. (2004). Promoting oral health in elder care: Challenges and opportunities. *Journal of Gerontological Nursing, 30*(4), 3.

Curran, M. A., & Curran, K. E. (2005). The e-health revolution: Competitive options for nurse practitioners as local providers. *Journal of the American Academy of Nurse Practitioners, 17*(12), 495–498.

Edelman, C., & Mandle, C. (2006). *Health promotion throughout the life span* (6th ed.). St. Louis, MO: Mosby.

Edmunds, M. (2005). Health literacy a barrier to patient education. *Nurse Practitioner, 30*(3), 54.

Fontaine, K. L. (2005). *Complementary & alternative therapies for nursing practice* (2nd ed.). Upper Saddle River, NJ: Prentice Hall. *This practical guide covers the principles, techniques, research, and health promotion methods and healing practices of specific illnesses and symptoms. It discusses over 40 alternative therapies.*

Freeman, L. (2004). *Mosby's complementary & alternative medicine: A research-based approach* (2nd ed.). Philadelphia: Mosby/Elsevier.

Gooch, B. F., Eke, P. I., & Malvitz, D. M. (2004). Public health and aging: Retention of natural teeth among older adults—United States, 2002. *Journal of the American Medical Association, 291*(3), 292.

Healthcare Information and Management Systems Society E-Health Special Interest Group (SIG). (2003). *HIMSS e-health SIG white paper.* Retrieved June 9, 2006, from http://www. himss.org/content/files/ehealth_whitepaper.pdf

Hood, L., & Leddy, S. K. (2003). *Leddy & Pepper's conceptual bases of professional nursing* (5th ed.). Philadelphia: Lippincott Williams & Wilkins.

Institute of Medicine. (2004). *Health literacy: A prescription to end confusion.* Washington, DC: National Academies Press.

Institute of Medicine (IOM). (2006). *Sleep disorders and sleep deprivation: An unmet public health problem.* Washington, DC: Institute of Medicine.

Jackson, C. (2003). Movement, breathing and Christian meditation: Catalysts for spiritual growth. *International Journal of Healing and Caring On-Line, 3*(2), 1–24.

Kaiser Family Foundation. (2005). *E-health and the elderly: How seniors use the Internet for health information. Key findings from a national survey of older Americans.* Menlo Park, CA: Kaiser Family Foundation.

Leiner, M., Handal, G., & Williams, D. (2004). Patient communication: A multidisciplinary approach using animated cartoons. *Health Education Research, 19*(5), 591–595.

Leong, J., Molassiotis, A., & Marsh, H. (2004). Adherence to health recommendations after a cardiac rehabilitation programme in post-myocardial infarction patients: The role of health beliefs, locus of control and psychological status. *Clinical Effectiveness in Nursing, 8*(1), 26–38.

Lower, J., Bonsack, C., & Guion, J. (2003). Peace and quiet. *Nursing Management, 34*(4), 40A–40D. *The authors reviewed factors that make it difficult for clients to rest in hospitals and steps that are needed to help provide a healing environment (e.g., uninterrupted sleep, massage, music). They describe their vision, implementation, and outcomes of providing quiet time between 2 and 4 p.m. for clients in two ICUs.*

McCaffrey, R., Ruknui, P., Hatthakit, U., & Kasetsomboon, P. (2005). The effects of yoga on hypertensive persons in Thailand. *Holistic Nursing Practice, 19*(4), 173–180.

McCaffrey, Ruknui, Hatthakit, & Kasetsomboon (2005).

Micozzi, M. (2006). *Fundamentals of complementary and alternative medicine* (3rd ed.). Philadelphia: Mosby/Elsevier.

Munro, C. L., Grap, M. J., & Kleinpell, R. (2004). Oral health and care in the intensive care unit: State of the science. *American Journal of Critical Care, 13*(1), 25–34.

Nainar, S. M., & Mohummed, S. (2004). Role of infant feeding practices on the dental health of children. *Clinical Pediatrics, 43*(2), 129–133.

NANDA International. (2005). *NANDA nursing diagnoses: Definitions and classification 2005–2006.* Philadelphia: Author.

National Center for Health Statistics. (2004). *Health, United States, 2004. With chartbook on trends in the health of Americans.* Hyattsville, MD: National Center for Health Statistics.

National Sleep Foundation. (n.d.a). *A look at the school start times debate.* Retrieved June 29, 2006, from http://www .sleepfoundation.org/hottopics/index.php?secid=18&id=206

National Sleep Foundation. (n.d.b). *ABCs of ZZZZ—When you can't sleep.* Retrieved June 29, 2006, from http://www .sleepfoundation.org/sleeplibrary/index.php?secid=id=53

National Sleep Foundation. (n.d.c). *Aging gracefully and sleeping well.* Retrieved June 29, 2006, from http://www .sleepfoundation.org/hottopics/index.php?secid=12&id=225

National Sleep Foundation. (n.d.d). *Children's sleep habits.* Retrieved June 29, 2006, from http://www.sleepfoundation. org/hottopics/index.php?secid=11&id=39

National Sleep Foundation. (n.d.e). *Parents of teens: Recognize the signs and symptoms of sleep deprivation and sleep problems.* Retrieved July 2, 2006, from http://www .sleepfoundation.org/_content/hottopics/teensigns.pdf

National Sleep Foundation. (2006). National *Sleep Foundation 2006 Sleep in America poll highlights and key findings.* Retrieved July 4, 2006, from http://www.sleepfoundation .org/_content/hottopics/Highlights_facts_06.pdf

Nightingale, F. (1860; 1969). *Notes on nursing: What it is, and what it is not.* New York: Dover Books.

North American Nursing Diagnosis Association (NANDA). (2005). *Nursing diagnoses: Definitions & classification 2005–2006.* Philadelphia: NANDA.

North American Nursing Diagnosis Association (NANDA). (2007). *Nursing diagnoses: Definitions & classification 2007–2008.* Philadelphia: NANDA.

Orr, W. C. (2000). Editorial: Sleep and functional bowel disorders: Can bad bowels cause bad dreams? *American Journal of Gastroenterology, 95,* 1118–1121.

Pender, N. J., Murdaugh, C. L., & Parsons, M. J. (2006). *Health promotion in nursing practice* (5th ed.). Upper Saddle River, NJ: Prentice Hall.

Pew Internet & American Life Project. (2005a). *Health information online.* Retrieved June 9, 2006, from http://www.pewinternet.org/PPF/r/165/report_display.asp

Pew Internet & American Life Project. (2005b). *Digital sections.* Retrieved June 9, 2006, from http://www.pewinternet.org/ PPF/r/165/report_display.asp

Pew Internet & American Life Project. (2006). *Demographics of Internet users.* Retrieved June 9, 2006, from http://www .pewinternet. org/trends.asp

Pillitteri, A. (2003). *Maternal and child health nursing: Care of the childbearing and childrearing family* (2nd ed.). Philadelphia: Lippincott Williams & Wilkins.

President's Council on Physical Fitness and Sports. (2003). Washington, DC: U. S. Department of Health and Human Services.

President's Council on Physical Fitness and Sports. (2003). *Fitness Fundamentals: Guidelines for Personal Exercise Programs.* Washington DC.

Redman, B. K. (2004). *Advances in patient education.* New York: Springer.

Robinson, S. B., Weitzel, T., & Henderson, L. (2005). The sh-h-h-h project. Nonpharmacological interventions. *Holistic Nursing Practice, 19*(6), 263–266.

Rollnick, S., Mason, P., & Butler, C. (1999). *Health behavior change. A guide for practitioners.* Edinburgh: Churchill Livingstone.

Saarmann, L., Daugherty, J., & Riegel, B. (2000). Patient teaching to promote behavioral change. *Nursing Outlook, 48*(6), 281–287.

Travis, J. W., & Ryan, R. S. (1988). *Wellness workbook.* Berkeley, CA: Ten Speed Press.

U. S. Department of Health and Human Services. (2000). *Healthy people 2010: Understanding and improved health* (2nd ed.). Washington, DC: U. S. Government Printing Office.

U.S. Preventive Services Task Force. *Screening for Cervical Cancer. Recommendations and Rationale.* AHRQ Publication No. 03-515A. January 2003. Agency for Healthcare Research and Quality, Rockville, MD. Retrieved June 30, 2006, from, http://www.ahrq.gov/clinic/ 3rduspstf/cervcan/cervcanrr.htm

Wallston, K. A., Stein, M. J., & Smith, C. A. (1994). Form C of the MHLC scales: A condition-specific measure of locus of control. *Journal of Personality Assessment, 63,* 534–553.

Wallston, K. A., Wallston, B. S., & DeVellis, R. (1978, Spring). Development of the Multidimensional Locus of Control (MHLC) scales. *Health Education Monographs, 6,* 160–170.

Walton, J. C., Miller, J., & Tordecilla, L. (2001). Elder oral assessment and care. *Medsurg Nursing, 10*(1), 37–44.

World Health Organization. (1948). *Preamble to the constitution of the World Health Organization as adopted by the International Health Conference.* New York, June 19–22, 1946; signed on July 22, 1946, by the representatives of 61 states (Official Records of the World Health Organization, no. 2, p. 100) and entered into force on April 7, 1948.

Infection

8

Concept at-a-Glance

Concept Learning Outcomes

After reading about this concept, you will be able to do the following:

1. Summarize the structure and physiologic processes of the immune system related to infection prevention.
2. List factors that increase the risk for infection.
3. Identify commonly occurring alterations in the immune system that increase the risk for or occurrence of infection and their related treatments.
4. Explain common physical assessment procedures used to evaluate for the presence of infection in clients across the life span.
5. Outline diagnostic and laboratory tests and expected findings to determine whether an individual has an infection.
6. Explain the management of immune health and prevention of infection.
7. Demonstrate the nursing process in providing culturally competent care across the life span for individuals with infection.
8. Identify pharmacologic interventions used in caring for individuals with infection.

Concept Key Terms

Acute infections, *221*
Airborne precautions, *229*
Antibody, *227*
Antiseptics, *227*
Asepsis, *221*
Bacteremia, *221*
Bacteria, *221*
Bactericidal agent, *227*
Bacteriostatic agent, *227*
Bloodborne pathogens, *228*
Body substance isolation (BSI), *228*
Carrier, *222*
Chronic infections, *221*
Clean, *221*
Colonization, *221*
Communicable disease, *220*
Compromised host, *223*
Contact precautions, *229*
Cultures, *254*
Dirty, *221*
Disease, *220*
Disease surveillance, *241*
Disinfectants, *227*
Droplet nuclei, *223*
Droplet precautions, *229*
Endogenous, *237*
Endotoxins, *236*

Exogenous, *237*
Exotoxins, *236*
Fungi, *221*
Iatrogenic infections, *237*
Infection, *220*
Infectious disease, *220*
Isolation, *228*
Local infection, *221*
Medical asepsis, *221*
Nosocomial infections, *237*
Occupational exposure, *235*
Opportunistic pathogen, *221*
Parasites, *221*
Pathogenicity, *220*
Pathogens, *220*
Reservoirs, *222*
Sepsis, *221*
Septicemia, *221*
Specific defenses, *223*
Sterile field, *232*
Sterile technique, *221*
Sterilization, *228*
Surgical asepsis, *221*
Systemic infection, *221*
Universal precautions, *228*
Virulence, *220*
Viruses, *221*

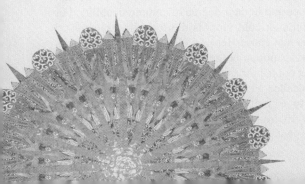

About Infection

Infection is the invasion of body tissue by microorganisms with the potential to cause illness or disease. The human body is continually threatened by foreign substances, infectious agents, and abnormal cells. Recent years have seen the emergence of resistant microorganisms, such as methicillin-resistant *Staphylococcus aureus,* and altered strains of familiar diseases, such as multiple-drug-resistant tuberculosis. New diseases have also emerged, including Lyme disease, *Clostridium difficile,* and HIV. ●

The immune system is the body's major defense mechanism against infectious organisms and abnormal or damaged cells. Any illness or injury can result in an infection if it is left untreated or if the body's immune system is compromised in some way. More than any other group of health care providers, nurses think about infection prevention all the time: They know that if they move from client room to client room with contaminated hands or equipment, they risk infecting everyone they touch. It does not matter how effective the other care delivered might be if the nurse is not protecting the client against infection. As a result, nurses are directly involved in providing a biologically safe environment. Infection control is a central tenant to delivering quality nursing care. This concept explains the steps to take to prevent the spread of infection, how infection is shared, and the impact an infection can have on the human body.

Microorganisms exist everywhere: in water, in soil, and on body surfaces such as the skin, intestinal tract, and other areas open to the outside (e.g., mouth, upper respiratory tract, vagina, and lower urinary tract). Most microorganisms are harmless, and some are even beneficial because they perform essential functions in the body. Some microorganisms found in the intestines (e.g., enterobacteria) produce substances called bacteriocins, which are lethal to related strains of bacteria. Others produce substances that repress the growth of other microorganisms. Some microorganisms are normal resident flora (the collective vegetation in a given area) in one part of the body, yet produce infection in another. For example, *Escherichia coli* is a normal inhabitant of the large intestine, but a common cause of infection of the urinary tract. Table 8–1 provides a list of common resident microorganisms by body area.

Recall that an infection is an invasion of body tissue by microorganisms. If the microorganisms produce no clinical evidence of disease, the infection is *asymptomatic* or *subclinical*. **Disease** occurs when the microorganisms produce a detectable alteration in normal tissue function. A **communicable disease** is an illness that is directly transmitted from one person or animal to another by contact with body fluids, or indirectly transmitted by contact with contaminated objects or vectors (e.g., ticks, mosquitoes, other insects). An **infectious disease** is any communicable disease that is caused by microorganisms that are commonly transmitted from one person to another or from an animal to a person. Infectious and communicable diseases are a major cause of disease and death in infants and children in the United States. Some subclinical infections can cause considerable damage. For example, cytomegalovirus (CMV) infection in a pregnant woman can lead to significant disease in the unborn child.

TABLE 8–1 Examples of Common Resident Microorganisms

BODY AREA	RESIDENT MICROORGANISMS
Skin	*Staphylococcus epidermidis*
	Propionibacterium acnes
	Staphylococcus aureus
	Corynebacterium xerosis
	Pityrosporum oxale (yeast)
Nasal passages	*Staphylococcus aureus*
	Staphylococcus epidermidis
Oropharynx	*Streptococcus pneumoniae*
Mouth	*Streptococcus mutans*
	Lactobacillus
	Bacteroides
	Actinomyces
Intestine	*Bacteroides*
	Fusobacterium
	Eubacterium
	Lactobacillus
	Streptococcus
	Enterobacteriaceae
	Shigella
	Escherichia coli
Urethral orifice	*Staphylococcus epidermidis*
Urethra (lower)	*Proteus*
Vagina	*Lactobacillus*
	Bacteroides
	Clostridium
	Candida albicans

Source: Berman, A., Snyder, S. J., Kozier, B., Erb, G. (2008). *Kozier & Erb's fundamentals of nursing: Concepts, process, and practice* (8th ed.). Upper Saddle River, NJ: Pearson Education.

NORMAL PRESENTATION

Microorganisms vary in **virulence** (i.e., their ability to produce disease). Microorganisms also vary in the severity of the diseases they produce and in their degree of communicability. For example, the common cold virus is more readily transmitted than the bacillus that causes leprosy (*Mycobacterium leprae*). If the infectious agent can be transmitted to an individual by direct or indirect contact or as an airborne infection, the resulting condition is called a communicable disease.

Pathogenicity is the ability to produce disease; thus a **pathogen** is a microorganism that causes disease. Many microorganisms that are normally harmless can cause disease under certain circumstances. A "true" pathogen causes disease or infection in a healthy individual, whereas an **opportunistic pathogen** causes disease only in susceptible individuals.

Infectious diseases are a major cause of death worldwide. The spread of microorganisms is controlled and people are protected from communicable diseases and infections on the international, national, state, community, and individual levels. The World Health Organization (WHO) is the major regulatory agency at the international level. In the United States, the Centers for Disease Control and Prevention (CDC) is the principal public health agency concerned with disease prevention and control at the national level. State and county or city health departments track epidemics and illnesses as reports are made throughout those areas.

Asepsis is the absence of disease-causing microorganisms. Aseptic technique is used to decrease the possibility of transferring microorganisms from one place to another. There are two basic types of asepsis: medical and surgical. **Medical asepsis** includes all practices intended to confine a specific microorganism to a specific area, thus limiting the number, growth, and transmission of microorganisms. In medical asepsis, objects are referred to as **clean**, which means that almost all microorganisms are absent, or **dirty** (soiled, contaminated), which means that microorganisms are likely to be present, some of which may be capable of causing infection.

Surgical asepsis, or **sterile technique**, refers to those practices that keep an area or object free of all microorganisms; it includes practices that destroy all microorganisms and spores (microscopic dormant structures formed by some pathogens that are very hardy and often survive common cleaning techniques). Surgical asepsis is used for all procedures involving sterile areas of the body. **Sepsis** refers to the whole body inflammatory process, resulting in acute illness; however, the term is often used generally to refer to the state of infection.

Types of Microorganisms Causing Infections

Four major categories of microorganisms cause infection in humans: bacteria, viruses, fungi, and parasites. **Bacteria** are by far the most common infection-causing microorganisms. Several hundred species can cause disease in humans and can live and be transported through air, water, food, soil, body tissues and fluids, and inanimate objects. Most of the microorganisms listed in Table 8–1 are bacteria. **Viruses** consist primarily of nucleic acid and therefore must enter living cells in order to reproduce. Common virus families include the rhinovirus (causes the common cold), hepatitis, herpes, and HIV. **Fungi** include yeasts and molds. *Candida albicans* is a yeast considered to be normal flora in the human vagina. **Parasites** live on other organisms. They include protozoa, such as the one that causes malaria, helminths (worms), and arthropods (mites, fleas, ticks).

Types of Infections

Colonization is the process by which strains of microorganisms become resident flora. In this state, the microorganisms may grow and multiply, but they do not cause disease.

Infection occurs when newly introduced or resident microorganisms succeed in invading a part of the body where the host's defense mechanisms are ineffective, and the pathogen causes tissue damage. The infection becomes a disease when the signs and symptoms of the infection are unique, can be differentiated from other conditions, and alter bodily function or processes.

Infections can be local or systemic. A **local infection** is limited to the specific part of the body where the microorganisms remain. If the microorganisms spread and damage different parts of the body, it is a **systemic infection**. When a culture of the person's blood reveals microorganisms, the condition is called **bacteremia**. When bacteremia results in systemic infection, it is referred to as **septicemia**. Unfortunately, these infections have become more common in recent times.

Infections are also classified as acute or chronic. **Acute infections** generally appear suddenly and last a short time. A **chronic infection** may develop slowly, over a very long period, and often persist for months and sometimes years.

It is important to note that a person does not need to have an identified infection in order to transmit potentially infective microorganisms to another person. Even microorganisms that are normal for one person can infect another person.

Chain of Infection

The chain of infection consists of six links (Figure 8–1 ■): the etiologic agent, or microorganism; the place where the organism naturally resides (reservoir); a portal of exit from the

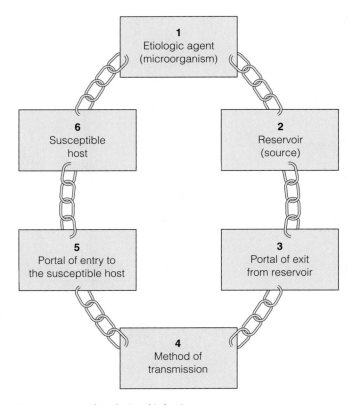

Figure 8–1 ■ The chain of infection.

reservoir; a method (mode) of transmission; a portal of entry into a susceptible host; and a susceptible host.

ETIOLOGIC AGENT   The extent to which any microorganism is capable of producing an infectious process depends on the number of microorganisms present, the virulence and potency of the microorganisms (pathogenicity), the ability of the microorganisms to enter the body, the susceptibility of the host, and the ability of the microorganisms to live in the host's body.

Some microorganisms, such as the smallpox virus, have the ability to infect almost all susceptible people after exposure. By contrast, microorganisms such as the tuberculosis bacillus infect a relatively small number of the population who are susceptible and exposed. Those at risk are usually people who are poorly nourished or living in crowded conditions, or those whose immune systems are less competent (such as older adults and individuals with HIV or cancer).

RESERVOIR   There are many **reservoirs**, or sources of microorganisms. Common sources are other humans, the client's own microorganisms, plants, animals, and the general environment. People are the most common source of infection for others and for themselves. For example, a person with an influenza virus frequently spreads it to others. A **carrier** is a human or animal reservoir of a specific infectious agent that usually does not manifest any clinical signs of disease. For example, the *Anopheles* mosquito reservoir carries the malaria parasite but is unaffected by it. The carrier state may also exist in individuals with a clinically recognizable disease, such as a dog with rabies. Under either circumstance, the carrier state may be of short duration (temporary or transient carrier) or long duration (chronic carrier). Food, water, and feces also can be reservoirs.

PORTAL OF EXIT FROM RESERVOIR   Before an infection can establish itself in a host, the microorganisms must leave the reservoir. Common human reservoirs and their associated portals of exit are summarized in Table 8–2.

METHOD OF TRANSMISSION   After a microorganism leaves its source or reservoir, it requires a means of transmission to reach another person or host through a receptive portal of entry. There are three modes of transmission:

1. *Direct transmission.* Direct transmission involves the immediate and direct transfer of microorganisms from person to person through touching, biting, kissing, or sexual

TABLE 8–2   Human Body Area Reservoirs, Common Infectious Microorganisms, and Portals of Exit

BODY AREA RESERVOIR	COMMON INFECTIOUS MICROORGANISMS	PORTALS OF EXIT
Respiratory tract	Parainfluenza virus	Nose or mouth through sneezing, coughing, breathing, or talking
	Mycobacterium tuberculosis	
	Staphylococcus aureus	
Gastrointestinal tract	Hepatitis A virus	Mouth: saliva, vomitus; anus: feces; ostomies
	Salmonella species	
	Clostridium difficile	Anus: feces, colostomies
Urinary tract	*Escherichia coli, enterococci*	Urethral meatus and urinary diversion
	Pseudomonas aeruginosa	
Reproductive tract	*Neisseria gonorrhoeae*	Vagina: vaginal discharge; urinary meatus: semen, urine
	Treponema pallidum	
	Herpes simplex virus type 2	
	Hepatitis B virus (HBV)	
Blood	Hepatitis B virus	Open wound, needle puncture site, any disruption of intact skin or mucous membrane surfaces
	HIV	
	Staphylococcus aureus	
	Staphylococcus epidermidis	
Tissue	*Staphylococcus aureus*	Drainage from cut or wound
	Escherichia coli	
	Proteus species	
	Streptococcus beta-hemolytic A or B	

Source: Berman, A., Snyder, S. J., Kozier, B., Erb, G. (2008). *Kozier & Erb's fundamentals of nursing: Concepts, process, and practice* (8th ed.). Upper Saddle River, NJ: Pearson Education.

intercourse. Droplet spread is also a form of direct transmission, but it can occur only if the source and the host are within 3 feet of each other. Sneezing, coughing, spitting, singing, or talking can project droplet spray into the conjunctiva or onto the mucous membranes of the eye, nose, or mouth of another person.

2. *Indirect transmission.* Indirect transmission can be either vehicle-borne or vector-borne.

    a. *Vehicle-borne transmission.* A *vehicle* is any substance that serves as an intermediate means to transport and introduce an infectious agent into a susceptible host through a suitable portal of entry. Fomites (inanimate materials or objects), such as handkerchiefs, toys, soiled clothes, cooking or eating utensils, and surgical instruments or dressings, can act as vehicles. Water, food, blood, serum, and plasma are also vehicles. For example, food can become contaminated by a food handler who carries the hepatitis A virus, and the food is then ingested by a susceptible host.

    b. *Vector-borne transmission.* A *vector* is an animal or flying or crawling insect that serves as an intermediate means of transporting the infectious agent. Transmission can occur by injecting salivary fluid during biting or by depositing feces or other materials on the skin through the bite wound or a traumatized skin area.

3. *Airborne transmission.* Airborne transmission can involve droplets or dust. **Droplet nuclei**, the residue of evaporated droplets emitted by an infected host, such as an individual with tuberculosis, can remain in the air for long periods of time. Dust particles containing the infectious agent (e.g., *Clostridium difficile,* commonly referred to as *C. difficile,* spores from the soil) can also become airborne. The material is transmitted by air currents to a suitable portal of entry on another person, usually the respiratory tract.

PORTAL OF ENTRY TO THE SUSCEPTIBLE HOST Before a person can become infected, microorganisms must enter the body. The skin is a barrier to infectious agents; however, any break in the skin can readily serve as a portal of entry. Often, microorganisms enter the body of a host by the same route they used to leave the source. For example, an airborne infection escapes its host or carrier via sneezing or coughing and is transmitted to a new host, who inhales the microorganism through his or her nose or mouth. The mouth, throat, nose, ears, eyes, and genitalia are open to outside exposure, and thus are the most frequent portals of entry for microorganisms. Cuts and tears in the skin also provide portals through which microorganisms can enter and cause disease.

SUSCEPTIBLE HOST A susceptible host is any person who is at risk for infection. Infants and young children are often susceptible hosts. Their immune systems have not fully matured, and they have not yet developed antibodies to many agents. Therefore, they cannot defend themselves against infectious and communicable diseases as well as older children and adults. A **compromised host** is a person at increased risk, that is, an individual who for one or more reasons is more likely than others to acquire an infection. Impairment of the body's natural defenses and a number of other factors can also affect susceptibility to infection. Examples include age (the very young or the very old); individuals who receive immune suppression treatment for cancer or chronic illness, or following a successful organ transplant; and immune deficiency conditions.

Table 8–3 outlines nursing interventions that break the chain of infection, including their rationales.

Body Defenses Against Infection

Individuals normally have defenses that protect the body from infection. Nonspecific defenses include anatomic and physiological barriers and the inflammatory response. **Specific defenses** involve the immune system when an antigen induces a state of sensitivity and antibodies respond to contain or destroy the antigen.

Intact skin and mucous membranes are the body's first line of defense against microorganisms. Unless the skin and mucosa become cracked and broken, they act as an effective barrier against bacteria. Fungi can live on the skin, but they cannot penetrate it. The dryness of the skin also is a deterrent to bacteria. Bacteria are most plentiful in moist areas of the body, such as the perineum and axillae. Resident bacteria of the skin also prevent other bacteria from multiplying. They use up the available nourishment, and the end products of their metabolism inhibit other bacterial growth. Normal secretions make the skin slightly acidic, which also inhibits bacterial growth.

The nasal passages have a defensive function. As entering air follows the tortuous route of the passage, it comes in contact with moist mucous membranes and cilia. These structures trap microorganisms, dust, and foreign materials. The lungs have alveolar macrophages (large phagocytes). Phagocytes are cells that ingest microorganisms, other cells, and foreign particles.

Each body orifice also has protective mechanisms. The oral cavity regularly sheds mucosal epithelium to rid the mouth of colonizers. The flow of saliva and its partially buffering action help prevent infections. Saliva contains microbial inhibitors, such as lactoferrin, lysozyme, and secretory immunoglobulin A (IgA).

The eye is protected from infection by tears, which continually wash microorganisms away and contain inhibiting lysozyme. The gastrointestinal tract also has defenses against infection. The high acidity of the stomach normally prevents microbial growth. The resident flora of the large intestine help prevent the establishment of disease-producing microorganisms. Peristalsis also tends to move microbes out of the body.

The vagina also has natural defenses against infection. When a girl reaches puberty, lactobacilli ferment sugars in the vaginal secretions, creating a vaginal pH of 3.5–4.5. This low pH inhibits the growth of many disease-producing microorganisms. The entrance to the urethra normally harbors many microorganisms, including *Staphylococcus epidermidis coagulase* (from the skin) and *Escherichia coli* (from feces). It is believed that the urine flow has a flushing and bacteriostatic action that keeps the bacteria from ascending the urethra. An intact mucosal surface also acts as a barrier.

TABLE 8–3 Nursing Interventions That Break the Chain of Infection

LINK IN CHAIN OF INFECTION	INTERVENTIONS	RATIONALES
Etiologic agent (microorganism)	Ensure that articles are correctly cleaned and disinfected or sterilized before use.	Correct cleaning, disinfecting, and sterilizing reduce or eliminate microorganisms.
	Educate clients and support persons about appropriate methods to clean, disinfect, and sterilize articles.	Knowledge of ways to reduce or eliminate microorganisms reduces the numbers of microorganisms present and the likelihood of transmission.
Reservoir (source)	Change dressings and bandages when they are soiled or wet.	Moist dressings are ideal environments for microorganisms to grow and multiply.
	Assist clients to carry out appropriate skin and oral hygiene.	Hygienic measures reduce the numbers of resident and transient microorganisms and the likelihood of infection.
	Dispose of damp, soiled linens appropriately.	Damp, soiled linens harbor more microorganisms than dry linens.
	Dispose of feces and urine in appropriate receptacles.	Urine and feces in particular contain many microorganisms.
	Ensure that all fluid containers, such as bedside water jugs and suction and drainage bottles, are covered or capped.	Prolonged exposure increases the risk of contamination and promotes microbial growth.
	Empty suction and drainage bottles at the end of each shift, before they become full, or according to agency policy.	Drainage harbors microorganisms that, if left for long periods, proliferate and can be transmitted to others.
Portal of exit from the reservoir	Avoid talking, coughing, or sneezing over open wounds and sterile fields, and cover the mouth and nose when coughing and sneezing.	These measures limit the number of microorganisms that escape from the respiratory tract.
Method of transmission	Cleanse hands between client contacts, after touching body substances, and before performing invasive procedures or touching open wounds.	Hand cleansing is an important means of controlling and preventing the transmission of microorganisms.
	Instruct clients and support persons to cleanse hands before handling food or eating, after eliminating, and after touching infectious material.	Hand cleansing helps prevent the transfer of microorganisms from one person to another.
	Wear gloves when handling secretions and excretions.	Gloves and gowns prevent soiling of the hands and clothing.
	Wear gowns if there is danger of soiling clothing with body substances.	
	Place discarded soiled materials in moisture-proof refuse bags.	Moisture-proof bags prevent the spread of microorganisms to others.
	Hold used bedpans steadily to prevent spillage, and dispose of urine and feces in appropriate receptacles.	Feces in particular contain many microorganisms.
	Initiate and implement aseptic precautions for all clients.	All clients can harbor potentially infectious microorganisms that can be transmitted to others.
	Wear masks and eye protection when in close contact with clients who have infections transmitted by droplets from the respiratory tract.	Masks and eyewear reduce the spread of droplet-transmitted microorganisms.
	Wear masks and eye protection when sprays of body fluid are possible (e.g., during irrigation procedures).	Masks and eye protection provide protection from microorganisms in clients' body substances.
Portal of entry to the susceptible host	Use sterile technique for invasive procedures (e.g., injections, catheterizations).	Invasive procedures penetrate the body's natural protective barriers to microorganisms.

TABLE 8–3 **Nursing Interventions That Break the Chain of Infection** (continued)

LINK IN CHAIN OF INFECTION	INTERVENTIONS	RATIONALES
	Use sterile technique when exposing open wounds and handling dressings.	Open wounds are vulnerable to microbial infection.
	Place used disposable needles and syringes in puncture-resistant containers for disposal.	Injuries from needles contaminated by blood or body fluids from an infected client or carrier are a primary cause of HBV and HIV transmission to health care workers.
	Provide all clients with their own personal care items.	People have less resistance to another person's microorganisms than to their own.
Susceptible host	Maintain the integrity of the client's skin and mucous membranes.	Intact skin and mucous membranes protect against invasion by microorganisms.
	Ensure that the client receives a balanced diet.	A balanced diet supplies proteins and vitamins necessary to build and maintain body tissues.
	Educate the public about the importance of immunizations.	Immunizations protect people against virulent infectious diseases.

Source: Berman, A., Snyder, S. J., Kozier, B., Erb, G. (2008). *Kozier & Erb's fundamentals of nursing: Concepts, process, and practice* (8th ed.). Upper Saddle River, NJ: Pearson Education.

Factors Increasing Susceptibility to Infection

Whether or not a microorganism causes an infection depends on a number of factors that have been identified above. One of the most important factors is host susceptibility, which is affected by age, heredity, level of stress, nutritional status, current medical therapy, and preexisting disease processes.

Age influences the risk of infection. Newborns and older adults have reduced defenses against infection. Infections are a major cause of death in newborns, who have immature immune systems and are protected only for the first 2 or 3 months by immunoglobulins passively received from the mother. Between 1 and 3 months of age, infants begin to synthesize their own immunoglobulins. Immunizations against diphtheria, tetanus, and pertussis are usually started at 2 months, when the infant's immune system can respond (see Table 8–3).

With advancing age, the immune responses again become weak. Although there is still much to learn about aging, it is known that immunity to infection decreases with advancing age. Because of the prevalence of influenza and its potential for causing death, the CDC recommends annual immunization against influenza for older adults and persons with chronic cardiac, respiratory, metabolic, and renal disease. Pneumococcal vaccine is recommended for older adults who were last vaccinated more than 5 years previously.

Special considerations related to infection in children and older adults are further described in the following Developmental Considerations feature.

Heredity also influences the development of infection in that some people have a genetic susceptibility to certain infections. For example, some individuals are deficient in serum immunoglobulins, which play a significant role in the internal defense mechanism of the body.

The nature, number, and duration of physical and emotional stressors can influence susceptibility to infection. Stressors elevate blood cortisone, and the prolonged elevation of blood cortisone decreases anti-inflammatory responses, depletes energy stores, leads to a state of exhaustion, and decreases resistance to infection. For example, a person recovering from a major operation or injury is more likely to develop an infection than a healthy person.

Resistance to infection also depends on adequate nutritional status. Because antibodies are proteins, inadequate nutrition can impair the body's ability to synthesize them, especially when protein reserves are depleted (e.g., as a result of injury, surgery, or debilitating diseases such as cancer).

Some medical therapies may predispose a person to infection. For example, radiation treatments for cancer destroy not only cancerous cells but also some normal cells, thereby rendering the client more vulnerable to infection. Some diagnostic procedures may also predispose the client to infection, especially when the skin is broken or sterile body cavities are penetrated during the procedure.

Certain medications also increase susceptibility to infection. Antineoplastic (anticancer) medications can depress bone marrow function, resulting in the inadequate production of white blood cells necessary to combat infections. Anti-inflammatory medications, such as adrenal corticosteroids, inhibit the inflammatory response, which is an essential defense against infection. Even some antibiotics used to treat infections can have adverse effects. Antibiotics can kill resident flora, allowing for the proliferation of strains that would not grow and multiply in the body under normal conditions. An important example of this is *C. difficile*–associated disease, an infection of the colon that is almost always caused initially by treatment with an antibiotic for another infection (Sunenshine & McDonald, 2006).

Any disease that lowers the body's defenses against infection places the client at risk. Examples are chronic pulmonary disease, which impairs ciliary action and weakens the mucous barrier; peripheral vascular disease, which restricts blood flow; burns, which impair skin integrity; chronic or debilitating

DEVELOPMENTAL CONSIDERATIONS   Infections

CHILDREN

Infections are a normal part of childhood, with most children experiencing some kind of infection from time to time. The majority of these infections is caused by viruses, and for the most part they are transient, relatively benign, and can be overcome by the body's natural defenses and supportive care. Otitis media, or ear infection, is one of the most frequent reasons parents take children to the doctor. It is an excellent example of a typically transient infection that can be overcome by the body's defenses and supportive care. In some cases, however, severe and even life-threatening infections occur. Considerations related to children include the following:

- Newborns may not be able to respond to infections due to an underdeveloped immune system. As a result, in the first few months of life, infections may not be associated with typical signs and symptoms (e.g., an infant with an infection may not have a fever).
- Newborns have some naturally acquired immunity that is transferred from the mother across the placenta at birth.
- Breast-fed infants enjoy higher levels of immunity against infections than infants fed with formula.
- Fevers of less than 39°C (102.2°F) in children should not be treated, except for comfort of the child.
- Children between 6 months and 5 years of age are at higher risk for fever-induced (febrile) seizures. Febrile seizures are not associated with neurological seizure disorders (e.g., epilepsy).
- Children who are immune compromised (e.g., leukemia, HIV) or have a chronic health condition (e.g., cystic fibrosis, sickle cell disease, congenital heart disease) need additional precautions to prevent exposure to infectious agents.
- Hand hygiene, comprehensive immunizations, proper nutrition, adequate hydration, and appropriate rest are essential to preventing and/or treating infections in children.
- Handwashing and good hygiene in day care and schools are important to prevent the spread of infections.
- Adolescents are at high risk for sexually transmitted diseases and should be well educated about how to prevent infections.

OLDER ADULTS

Normal aging may predispose older adults to increased risk of infection and delayed healing. As the body ages, changes take place in the skin, respiratory tract, gastrointestinal system, kidneys, and immune system. If unchallenged, these systems work well to maintain homeostasis for the individual, but if compromised by stress, illness, infections, treatments, or surgeries, these defense systems cannot provide adequate protection. Special considerations for older adults include the following:

- Nutrition is often poor in older adults. Certain nutritional components, especially adequate protein, are necessary to build up and maintain the immune system.
- Diabetes mellitus, which occurs more frequently in older adults, increases the risk of infection and delayed healing by causing an alteration in nutrition and impaired peripheral circulation, which in turn decrease the oxygen transport to the tissues.
- The immune system reacts slowly to the introduction of an antigen, allowing the antigen to reproduce itself several times before the immune system recognizes it.
- The normal inflammatory response is delayed, which often causes atypical responses to infections with unusual presentations. Instead of exhibiting the redness, swelling, and fever that are usually associated with infections, atypical symptoms, such as confusion and disorientation, agitation, incontinence, falls, lethargy, and general fatigue, are often seen first in the older adult.

Recognizing these changes in older adults is important for the early detection and treatment of infections and delayed healing. Nursing interventions to promote prevention include the following:

- Provide and teach ways to improve nutritional status.
- Use strict aseptic technique to decrease the risk of infections (especially nosocomial infections in health care facilities).
- Encourage older adults to have regular immunizations for flu and pneumonia.
- Be alert to subtle, atypical signs of infection and act quickly to diagnose and treat them.

---

diseases, which deplete protein reserves; and immune system diseases such as leukemia and aplastic anemia, which alter the production of white blood cells. Diabetes mellitus is a major underlying disease that predisposes clients to infection because compromised peripheral vascular status and increased serum glucose levels increase susceptibility.

Infectious Process in Older Adults

Older adults, particularly individuals over the age of 75 years, are at greater risk of acquiring an infection than younger people. Although the incidence of septicemia in the United States is increasing in all age groups, the greatest increase is among people over the age of 65 years (Baine, Yu, & Summe, 2001). Physiologic changes of aging that put older adults at increased risk for infection include the following:

- Cardiovascular changes: Decreased cardiac output, loss of capillaries, and decreased tissue perfusion, delaying inflammatory response and healing
- Respiratory system changes: Decreased mucociliary escalator, decreased elastic recoil, and a diminished cough reflex, leading to decreased clearance of respiratory secretions

- Genitourinary changes: Loss of muscle tone, reduced bladder contractility, altered bladder reflexes, and prostatic hypertrophy in men, leading to reduced bladder capacity and incomplete emptying
- Gastrointestinal system changes: Impaired swallow reflex, decreased gastric acidity, and delayed gastric emptying, increasing the risk of aspiration
- Skin and subcutaneous tissue changes: Thinning of skin, decreased cushioning, and decreased sensation, leading to increased risk of injury and ulceration
- Immune changes: Decreased phagocytosis, reduced inflammatory response, slowed or impaired healing processes, leading to reduced immunity

In addition to these physiologic changes, the following are other factors that can contribute to an older adult's increased risk for infectious disease:

- Decreased activity level related to musculoskeletal, neurologic, or balance problems
- Poor nutrition and an increased risk of dehydration

- Chronic diseases, such as diabetes mellitus, cardiac disease, and renal disease
- Chronic medication use
- Lack of recent immunizations against preventable infectious diseases
- Altered mentation and dementias
- Hospitalization or residence in a long-term care facility
- Presence of invasive devices, such as indwelling urinary catheters and gastric tubes

The thymus gland also atrophies, and by age 50–60 years, thymic hormone levels are undetectable. Although the exact relationship of these events to T-cell function is unclear, some T-cell populations decrease or decline in function as the person ages. The ability of T cells to proliferate following activation also declines with advancing age, and a portion of T cells cannot be activated in older adults (Porth, 2005). With these changes, cell-mediated immune function declines, and the client has reduced resistance to antigens, such as *M. tuberculosis,* influenza and varicella-zoster viruses, malignant cells, and tissue grafts.

Although immunoglobulin levels remain relatively stable, primary and secondary **antibody** responses decline with aging. This diminished antibody production has clinical implications in that immunizations (single-dose and booster) may not produce the expected protective immune response.

Older adults are not only at increased risk for infection, but also may not exhibit the classic manifestations of inflammation and infection. They are likely to take nonsteroidal anti-inflammatory drugs (NSAIDs) and corticosteroids, which interfere with inflammation and healing. The cardinal signs of inflammation—redness, heat, and swelling—tend to be diminished or absent in older adults. The classic signs of infection—fever and chills—may be absent altogether because of age-related changes in the immune system, loss of central temperature control mechanisms, decreased muscle mass, and loss of shivering ability. The older adult may have only subtle signs of sepsis, such as changes in mental status, disorientation, and tachypnea (Porth, 2005).

Supporting the Defenses of a Susceptible Host

People are constantly in contact with microorganisms in the environment. Normally a person's natural defenses ward off the development of an infection. Susceptibility is the degree to which an individual can be affected, that is, the likelihood of an organism causing an infection in that person. The following measures can reduce a person's susceptibility to infection:

- *Hygiene.* Intact skin and mucous membranes are one barrier against microorganisms entering the body. In addition, good oral care, including flossing the teeth, reduces the likelihood of an oral infection. Regular and thorough bathing and shampooing remove microorganisms and dirt that can result in an infection.
- *Nutrition.* A balanced diet enhances the health of all body tissues, helps keep the skin intact, and promotes the skin's ability to repel microorganisms. Adequate nutrition enables tissues to maintain and rebuild themselves and helps keep the immune system functioning well.

- *Fluid.* Fluid intake permits fluid output, which flushes out the bladder and urethra, removing microorganisms that could cause an infection.
- *Sleep.* Adequate sleep is essential to maintaining health and renewing energy.
- *Stress.* Excessive stress predisposes people to infections. Nurses can assist clients to learn stress-reducing techniques.
- *Immunizations.* The use of immunizations has dramatically decreased the incidence of infectious diseases. It is recommended that immunizations begin shortly after birth and be completed in early childhood (except for boosters). Immunizations may be given by injection, inhalation, oral solutions, or nasal sprays. They are frequently given in combination to minimize multiple injections. Because immunization schedules change frequently, it is advisable to update immunization schedules yearly.

PRECAUTIONS AND PRACTICES TO PREVENT AND MINIMIZE INFECTION
Disinfecting and Sterilizing

The first two links in the chain of infection, the etiologic agent and reservoir, are interrupted by the use of **antiseptics** (agents that inhibit the growth of some microorganisms) and **disinfectants** (agents that destroy pathogens other than spores), and by sterilization.

DISINFECTING A disinfectant is a chemical preparation, such as phenol or iodine compounds, used on inanimate objects. Disinfectants are frequently caustic and toxic to tissues. An antiseptic is a chemical preparation used on skin or tissue. Disinfectants and antiseptics often have similar chemical components, but disinfectants are more concentrated.

Both antiseptics and disinfectants have bactericidal or bacteriostatic properties. A **bactericidal agent** destroys bacteria, whereas a **bacteriostatic agent** prevents the growth and reproduction of some bacteria. An agent that is known to be effective against the specific bacteria should be selected. For example, spore-forming bacteria such as *C. difficile*, which is a frequent cause of nosocomial diarrhea, and *Bacillus anthracis* (anthrax) may be inhibited by only a few of the agents normally effective against other forms of bacteria. Table 8–4 lists commonly used antiseptics and disinfectants.

When disinfecting articles, nurses need to follow agency protocol and consider the following factors:

1. The type and number of infectious organisms. Some microorganisms are readily destroyed, whereas others require longer contact with the disinfectant.
2. The recommended concentration of the disinfectant and duration of contact.
3. The presence of soap. Some disinfectants are ineffective in the presence of soap or detergents.
4. The presence of organic materials. The presence of saliva, blood, pus, or excretions can readily inactivate many disinfectants.
5. The surface areas to be treated. The disinfecting agent must come into contact with all surfaces and areas.

TABLE 8–4 Commonly Used Antiseptics and Disinfectants, Effectiveness, and Use

	EFFECTIVE AGAINST					
AGENT	BACTERIA	TUBERCULOSIS	SPORES	FUNGI	VIRUSES	USE ON
Isopropyl and ethyl alcohol	X	X		X	X	Hands, vial stoppers
Chlorine (bleach)	X	X	X	X	X	Blood spills
Hydrogen peroxide	X	X	X	X	X	Surfaces
Iodophors	X	X	X	X	X	Equipment, intact skin and tissues if diluted
Phenol	X	X		X	X	Surfaces
Chlorhexidine gluconate (Hibiclens)	X				X	Hands
Triclosan (Bacti-Stat)	X					Hands, intact skin

Source: Berman, A., Snyder, S. J., Kozier, B., Erb, G. (2008). *Kozier & Erb's fundamentals of nursing: Concepts, process, and practice* (8th ed.). Upper Saddle River, NJ: Pearson Education.

STERILIZING Sterilization is a process that destroys all microorganisms, including spores and viruses. Four commonly used methods of sterilization are moist heat, gas, boiling water, and radiation.

- *Moist Heat.* To sterilize with moist heat (such as with an autoclave), steam under pressure is used to attain temperatures higher than the boiling point.
- *Gas.* Ethylene oxide gas destroys microorganisms by interfering with their metabolic processes. It is also effective against spores. Its advantages are good penetration and effectiveness for heat-sensitive items. Its major disadvantage is its toxicity to humans.
- *Boiling Water.* This is the most practical and inexpensive method for sterilizing in the home. The main disadvantage is that this method does not kill spores and some viruses. Boiling for a minimum of 15 minutes is advised to disinfect articles in the home.
- *Radiation.* Both ionizing (such as alpha, beta, and x-rays) and nonionizing (ultraviolet light) radiation are used for disinfection and sterilization. The main drawback to ultraviolet light is that the rays do not penetrate deeply. Ionizing radiation is used effectively in industry to sterilize foods, drugs, and other items that are sensitive to heat. Its main advantage is that it is effective for items difficult to sterilize, and its chief disadvantage is that the equipment is very expensive.

Isolation Precautions

Isolation refers to measures designed to prevent the spread of infection or potentially infectious microorganisms to health personnel, clients, and visitors. Several sets of guidelines have been used in hospitals and other health care settings.

Category-specific isolation precautions use seven categories: strict isolation, contact isolation, respiratory isolation, tuberculosis isolation, enteric precautions, drainage/secretions precautions, and blood/body fluid precautions.

Disease-specific isolation precautions do exactly that: provide precautions to protect against a specific disease. These precautions delineate use of private rooms with special ventilation, sharing of rooms only with other clients infected with the same organism, and gowning to prevent gross soilage of clothes for specific infectious diseases (Garner & Simmons, 1983).

Universal precautions (UP) are techniques to be used with all clients to decrease the risk of transmitting unidentified pathogens (CDC, 1987; U.S. Department of Health and Human Services [USDHHS], 1988). Universal precautions obstruct the spread of **bloodborne pathogens**, those microorganisms that are carried in blood and body fluids that are capable of infecting other persons with serious and difficult to treat viral infections, namely, hepatitis B virus, hepatitis C virus, and HIV. The CDC does not recommend that universal precautions replace disease-specific or category-specific precautions, but that they be used in conjunction with them.

The **body substance isolation (BSI)** system employs generic infection control precautions for all clients, except those with the few diseases transmitted through the air. The BSI system (Jackson, 1993) is based on three premises:

1. All people have an increased risk for infection from microorganisms entering through mucous membranes and nonintact skin.
2. All people are likely to have potentially infectious microorganisms in all of their moist body sites and substances.
3. An unknown portion of clients and health care workers will always be colonized or infected with potentially infectious microorganisms in their blood and other moist body sites and substances.

The term *body substance* refers to blood, some body fluids, urine, feces, wound drainage, oral secretions, and any other body product or tissue.

In addition to other actions and precautions discussed in this concept, significant emphasis is placed on avoiding injury from sharp instruments, taking measures in cases of exposure to bloodborne pathogens, and communicating information about biohazards to employees. In most cases, Federal regulations require that warning labels be affixed to containers of regulated waste and to refrigerators and freezers containing blood or other potentially infectious materials. The labels required are fluorescent orange or orange-red and feature the biohazard legend shown in Figure 8–2 ■.

CDC (HICPAC) ISOLATION PRECAUTIONS (1996)
The Hospital Infection Control Practices Advisory Committee (HICPAC) of the CDC presented new guidelines for isolation precautions in hospitals in 1996 (Garner & HICPAC, 1996). These guidelines designate two tiers of precautions:

1. Standard Precautions
2. Transmission-Based Precautions

Standard Precautions are used in the care of all hospitalized persons regardless of their diagnosis or possible infection status. They apply to blood; all body fluids, secretions, and excretions except sweat (whether or not blood is present or visible); nonintact skin; and mucous membranes. Thus, they combine the major features of UP and BSI. Box 8–1 lists recommended isolation precautions for use in hospitals.

Transmission-Based Precautions are used in addition to standard precautions for clients with known or suspected infections that are spread by contact or by airborne or droplet transmission. The three types of transmission-based precautions may be used alone or in combination, but always *in addition to* standard precautions. They encompass all of the conditions or diseases previously listed in the category-specific or disease-specific classifications developed by the CDC in 1983.

Airborne precautions are used for clients who are known to have or suspected of having serious illnesses transmitted by airborne droplet nuclei smaller than 5 microns. Examples of such illnesses are measles (rubeola), varicella (including disseminated zoster), and tuberculosis. The CDC has prepared special guidelines for preventing the transmission of tuberculosis. The most current information can be found on the CDC Division of Tuberculosis Elimination Web site.

Droplet precautions are used for clients who are known or suspected to have serious illnesses transmitted by particle droplets larger than 5 microns. Examples of such illnesses are diphtheria (pharyngeal); *Mycoplasma* pneumonia; pertussis; mumps; rubella; streptococcal pharyngitis, pneumonia, and scarlet fever in infants and young children; and pneumonic plague.

Contact precautions are used for clients who are known or suspected to have serious illnesses that are easily transmitted by direct client contact or by contact with items in the client's environment. According to the CDC (Garner & HICPAC, 1996),

such illnesses include gastrointestinal, respiratory, skin, or wound infections or colonization with multidrug-resistant bacteria; specific enteric infections, such as *C. difficile,* enterohemorrhagic *Escherichia coli 0157:H7, Shigella,* and hepatitis A, in diapered or incontinent clients; respiratory syncytial virus, parainfluenza virus, and enteroviral infections in infants and young children; and highly contagious skin infections, such as herpes simplex virus, impetigo, pediculosis, and scabies.

ISOLATION PRACTICES
The initiation of practices to prevent the transmission of microorganisms is generally a nursing responsibility that is based on a comprehensive assessment of the client. This assessment takes into account the status of the client's normal defense mechanisms, the client's ability to implement necessary precautions, and the source and mode of transmission of the infectious agent. The nurse then decides whether to wear gloves, gown, mask, and protective eyewear. *In all client situations, nurses must cleanse their hands before and after providing care.*

In addition to the precautions cited within this concept, nurses implement aseptic precautions when performing many specific therapies that are described in this textbook. The following are examples of aseptic precautions:

■ Use strict aseptic technique when performing any invasive procedure (e.g., inserting an intravenous needle or catheter) and when changing surgical dressings.
■ Change intravenous tubing and solution containers according to hospital policy (e.g., every 48–72 hours).
■ Check all sterile supplies for expiration date and intact packaging.
■ Prevent urinary infections by maintaining a closed urinary drainage system with a downhill flow of urine. Keep the drainage bag and spout off the floor.
■ Implement measures to prevent impaired skin integrity and accumulation of secretions in the lungs (e.g., encourage the client to move, cough, and breathe deeply at least every 2 hours).

PERSONAL PROTECTIVE EQUIPMENT
All health care providers must apply clean or sterile gloves, gowns, masks, and protective eyewear according to the risk of exposure to potentially infective materials.

Gloves Gloves are worn for three reasons:

1. They protect the hands when the nurse is likely to handle any body substances.
2. Gloves reduce the likelihood of nurses transmitting their own endogenous microorganisms to individuals receiving care. Nurses who have open sores or cuts on the hands must wear gloves for protection.
3. Gloves reduce the chance that the nurse's hands will transmit microorganisms or a fomite from one client to another client.

In all situations, gloves are changed between client contacts. Nurses should clean their hands each time they remove gloves for two primary reasons: The gloves may have imperfections or be damaged during wearing, allowing microorganism entry, and the hands may become contaminated during glove removal.

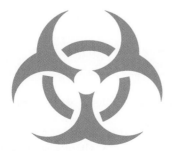

Figure 8–2 ■ Biohazard alert.

Box 8–1 Recommended Isolation Precautions in Hospitals

Standard Precautions
- Designed for all clients in hospital
- Apply to (a) blood; (b) all body fluids, excretions, and secretions except sweat; (c) nonintact (broken) skin; and (d) mucous membranes
- Designed to reduce the risk of transmission of microorganisms from recognized and unrecognized sources

1. Perform proper hand hygiene after contact with blood, body fluids, secretions, excretions, and contaminated objects, whether or not gloves are worn.
   a. Perform proper hand hygiene immediately after removing gloves.
   b. Use a nonantimicrobial product for routine hand cleansing.
   c. Use an antimicrobial agent or an antiseptic agent for the control of specific outbreaks of infection.
2. Wear clean gloves when touching blood, body fluids, secretions, excretions, and contaminated items (e.g., soiled gowns).
   a. Clean gloves can be unsterile unless their use is intended to prevent the entrance of microorganisms into the body. (See the following discussion of sterile gloves.)
   b. Remove gloves before touching noncontaminated items and surfaces.
   c. Perform proper hand hygiene immediately after removing gloves.
3. Wear a mask, eye protection, or a face shield if splashes or sprays of blood, body fluids, secretions, or excretions can be expected.
4. Wear a clean, nonsterile gown if client care is likely to result in splashes or sprays of blood, body fluids, secretions, or excretions. The gown is intended to protect clothing.
   a. Remove a soiled gown carefully to avoid the transfer of microorganisms to other individuals (e.g., clients or other health care workers).
   b. Cleanse hands after removing gown.
5. Carefully handle client care equipment that is soiled with blood, body fluids, secretions, or excretions to prevent the transfer of microorganisms to other individuals and the environment.
   a. Ensure reusable equipment is cleaned and reprocessed correctly.
   b. Dispose of single-use equipment correctly.
6. Handle, transport, and process linen that is soiled with blood, body fluids, secretions, or excretions in such a manner to prevent contamination of clothing and the transfer of microorganisms to other individuals and to the environment.
7. Prevent injuries from used scalpels, needles, and other equipment, and place in puncture-resistant containers.

Transmission-Based Precautions
Airborne Precautions
Use standard precautions, as well as the following:

1. Place client in a private room that has negative air pressure, 6–12 air changes per hour, and either discharge of air to the outside or a filtration system for the room air.
2. If a private room is not available, place client with another client who is infected with the same microorganism.
3. Wear a respiratory device (N95 respirator) when entering the room of a client who is known or suspected of having primary tuberculosis.
4. Susceptible people should not enter the room of a client who has rubeola (measles) or varicella (chickenpox). If they must enter, they should wear a respirator.
5. Limit movement of client outside the room to essential purposes. Place a surgical mask on the client during transport.

Droplet Precautions
Use standard precautions, as well as the following:

1. Place client in private room.
2. If a private room is not available, place client with another client who is infected with the same microorganism.
3. Wear a mask if working within 3 feet of the client.
4. Limit movement of client outside the room to essential purposes. Place a surgical mask on the client during transport.

Contact Precautions
Use standard precautions, as well as the following:

1. Place client in private room.
2. If a private room is not available, place client with another client who is infected with the same microorganism.
3. Wear gloves as described in standard precautions.
   a. Change gloves after contact with infectious material.
   b. Remove gloves before leaving the client's room.
   c. Cleanse hands immediately after removing gloves, using an antimicrobial agent. Note: If the client is infected with *C. difficile*, do *not* use an alcohol-based hand rub, as it may not be effective on these spores. Use soap and water.
   d. After hand cleansing, do not touch possibly contaminated surfaces or items in the room.
4. Wear a gown (see standard precautions) when entering a room if there is a possibility of contact with infected surfaces or items, or if the client is incontinent, has diarrhea, a colostomy, or wound drainage that is not contained by a dressing.
   a. Remove gown in the client's room.
   b. Make sure uniform does not contact possible contaminated surfaces.
5. Limit movement of client outside the room.
6. Dedicate the use of noncritical client care equipment to a single client or to clients with the same infecting microorganisms.

Source: Adapted from "Guidelines for Isolation Precautions in Hospitals," by J. S. Garner and the Hospital Infection Control Practices Advisory Committee (HICPAC), 1996, *Infection Control Hospital Epidemiology, 17*, pp. 53–80, and 1996, *American Journal of Infection Control, 24*, pp. 24–52.

Some of the gloves used in infection control are made of latex rubber, as are various other items used in health care (e.g., catheters, blood pressure cuffs, rubber sheets, intravenous tubing, stockings and binders, adhesive bandages, and dental dams). Because of the frequent use of gloves, health care workers and some clients with chronic illnesses have increasingly reported allergic reactions to latex. Latex gloves that are lubricated by powder or cornstarch are particularly allergenic because the latex allergen adheres to the powder, which is aerosolized during glove use and inhaled by the user.

Latex gloves that are labeled "hypoallergenic" still contain measurable latex and should not be used by or on persons with known latex sensitivity. Recent studies show some level of latex allergy in 8–12% of health care personnel (Occupational Safety and Health Administration, 2005). The people at greatest risk for developing latex allergies are those with other allergic conditions and those who have had frequent or long-term exposure to latex. Even though most hospitals have eliminated latex products wherever possible and established a "latex-free environment" goal, clients and health care workers should be assessed for possible allergies to latex.

Gowns Clean or disposable impervious (water-resistant) gowns or plastic aprons are worn during procedures when the nurse's uniform is likely to become soiled. Sterile gowns may be indicated when the nurse changes the dressings of a client with extensive wounds (e.g., burns). *Single-use gown technique* (using a gown only once before it is discarded or laundered) is the usual practice in hospitals. After the gown is worn, the nurse discards it (if it is paper) or places it in a laundry hamper. Before leaving the client's room, the nurse cleanses his or her hands.

PRACTICE ALERT
Wearing a client hospital gown over your uniform does not serve any infection control purpose.

Face Masks Masks are worn to reduce the risk of transmitting organisms by the droplet contact and airborne routes, and by splatters of body substances. The CDC recommends that masks be worn by the following persons:

1. Individuals close to the client if the infection (e.g., measles, mumps, or acute respiratory diseases in children) is transmitted by large-particle aerosols (droplets). Large-particle aerosols are transmitted by close contact and generally travel short distances (about 1 m, or 3 feet).
2. All persons entering the room if the infection (e.g., pulmonary tuberculosis and SARS-CoV) is transmitted by small-particle aerosols (droplet nuclei). Small-particle aerosols remain suspended in the air and thus travel greater distances by air. Special masks that provide a tighter face seal and better filtration may be used for these infections.

Various types of masks differ in their filtration effectiveness and fit. Single-use disposable surgical masks are effective for use while the nurse provides care to most clients, but they should be changed if they become wet or soiled. These masks are discarded in the waste container after use. Disposable particulate respirators of different types may be effective for droplet transmission, splatters, and airborne microorganisms. Some respirators now available are effective in preventing inhalation of tuberculin organisms. The National Institute for Occupational Safety and Health (NIOSH) tests and certifies such respirators. Currently, the category "N" respirator at 95% efficiency (referred to as an N95 respirator) meets tuberculosis and SARS control criteria.

During performance of certain techniques requiring surgical asepsis (sterile technique), masks are worn (a) to prevent droplet contact transmission of exhaled microorganisms to the sterile field or to a client's open wound, and (b) to protect the nurse from splashes of body substances from the client.

Eyewear Protective eyewear (goggles, glasses, or face shields) and masks are indicated in situations in which body substances may splatter the face. If the nurse wears prescription eyeglasses, goggles must still be worn over the glasses to extend around the sides of the glasses.

DISPOSAL OF SOILED EQUIPMENT AND SUPPLIES Many pieces of equipment are supplied for single use only and disposed of afterward. Some items, however, are reusable. Agencies have specific policies and procedures for handling soiled equipment (e.g., disposal, cleaning, disinfecting, and sterilizing), and nurses need to become familiar with these practices in the employing agency. Appropriate handling of soiled equipment and supplies is essential to prevent inadvertent exposure of health care workers to articles contaminated with body substances and contamination of the environment.

Bagging Articles that are contaminated or likely to have been contaminated with infective material such as pus, blood, body fluids, feces, or respiratory secretions need to be enclosed in a sturdy bag impervious to microorganisms before they are removed from the room of any client. Some agencies use labels or bags of a particular color that designates them as infective wastes.

CDC guidelines recommend the following methods:
- A single bag, if it is sturdy and impervious to microorganisms, and if the contaminated articles can be placed in the bag without soiling or contaminating its outside
- Double-bagging if the above conditions are not met

Follow agency protocol or use the following CDC guidelines to handle and bag soiled items:
- Place garbage and soiled *disposable* equipment, including dressings and tissues, in the plastic bag that lines the waste container. Some agencies separate dry and wet waste material and incinerate dry items, such as paper towels and disposable items. No special precautions are required for disposable equipment that is not contaminated.
- Place *nondisposable* or *reusable* equipment that is visibly soiled in a labeled bag before removing it from the client's room or cubicle, and then send it to a central processing area for decontamination. Some agencies may require that glass bottles or jars and metal items be placed in separate bags from rubber and plastic items. Glass and metal can be sterilized in an autoclave, but rubber and plastic are damaged by this process and must be cleaned by other methods, such as gas sterilization.
- Disassemble special procedure trays into component parts. Some components are disposable, whereas others need to be sent to the laundry or central services for cleaning and decontaminating.
- Bag soiled clothing before sending it home or to the agency laundry.

Linens Soiled linens should be handled as little as possible and with the least agitation possible before placing them in a laundry hamper. This prevents gross microbial contamination of the air and persons handling the linen. The bag is closed before sending it to the laundry in accordance with agency practice.

Laboratory Specimens Laboratory specimens, if placed in a leakproof container with a secure lid and labeled as a biohazard, need no special precautions. Care should be used when collecting specimens to avoid contaminating the outside of the container. Containers that are visibly contaminated on the outside should be placed inside a sealable plastic bag before they are sent to the laboratory to prevent personnel from having hand contact with potentially infective material.

Dishes Dishes require no special precautions. Soiling of dishes can largely be prevented by encouraging clients to cleanse their hands before eating. Some agencies use paper dishes for convenience, which are disposed of in the refuse container.

Blood Pressure Equipment Blood pressure equipment needs no special precautions unless it becomes contaminated with infective material. If it does become contaminated, the agency policy should be followed to decontaminate it. Cleaning procedures vary according to whether it is a wall or portable unit. In some agencies, a disposable cuff is used for clients placed on contact precautions.

Thermometers Nondisposable thermometers are generally disinfected after use. The nurse should check agency practice.

Disposable Needles, Syringes, and Sharps Place needles, syringes, and "sharps" (e.g., lancets, scalpels, and broken glass) into a puncture-resistant container. To avoid puncture wounds, use approved safety or needleless systems and do not detach needles from the syringe or recap before disposal.

PRACTICE ALERT

Federal rules protecting the privacy of personal health information may extend to the client labels placed on disposable supplies such as intravenous fluid containers. Agencies may require that these be returned to the pharmacy so that personal information can be removed before disposal. Check agency policy.

TRANSPORTING CLIENTS WITH INFECTION Avoid transporting clients with infections outside their own rooms unless it is absolutely necessary. If a client must be moved, the nurse follows agency protocol to implement appropriate precautions and measures to prevent soilage of the environment. For example, the nurse ensures that any draining wound is securely covered, or that the client who has an airborne infection wears a surgical mask during transport. In addition, the nurse notifies personnel at the receiving area of any infection risk so that they can maintain necessary precautions.

PSYCHOSOCIAL NEEDS OF ISOLATION CLIENTS Clients requiring isolation precautions can develop several problems as a result of the special precautions taken in their care and their separation from other people. Two of the most common are sensory deprivation and decreased self-esteem related to feelings of inferiority. Sensory deprivation occurs when the environment lacks normal stimuli for the client, such as communication with others. Nurses should therefore be alert to common clinical signs of sensory deprivation, such as boredom, inactivity, slowness of thought, daydreaming, increased sleeping, thought disorganization, anxiety, hallucinations, and panic.

A client's feeling of inferiority can stem from perception of the infection itself or from the required precautions and related isolation. In North America, many people place a high value on cleanliness, and the idea of being "soiled," "contaminated," or "dirty" can make clients feel as if they are at fault and substandard. Although this is obviously not true, infected individuals may feel "not as good" as others and blame themselves. An appropriate nursing diagnosis may be Risk for Situational Low Self-Esteem.

Nurses need to provide care that prevents or addresses sensory deprivation and feelings of inferiority. Related nursing interventions include the following:

1. Assess the individual's need for stimulation.
2. Initiate measures to help meet the need for stimulation, including regular communication with the client and diversionary activities, such as toys for a child and books, television, or radio for an adult. Provide a variety of foods to stimulate the client's sense of taste, and stimulate the client's visual sense by providing a view or an activity to watch.
3. Explain the infection and the associated procedures to help clients, their families, and caregivers understand and accept the situation.
4. Demonstrate warm, accepting behavior. Avoid conveying to the client any sense of annoyance about the precautions or any feelings of revulsion about the infection.
5. Do not use stricter precautions than are indicated by the diagnosis or the client's condition.

Sterile Technique

An object is sterile only when it is free of all microorganisms. It is well known that sterile technique is practiced in operating rooms and special diagnostic areas. Less well known, perhaps, is that sterile technique is also employed for many procedures in general care areas, such as administering injections, changing wound dressings, performing urinary catheterizations, and administering intravenous therapy. In these situations, all of the principles of surgical asepsis are applied, as in the operating and delivery rooms; however, not all of the sterile techniques that follow are always required. For example, before an operating room procedure, the "scrub" nurse generally puts on a mask and cap, performs a surgical hand scrub, and then dons a sterile gown and gloves. In a general care area, the nurse may only perform hand cleansing and don sterile gloves. The basic principles of surgical asepsis and practices that relate to each principle are outlined in Table 8–5.

STERILE FIELD A **sterile field** is a microorganism-free area. Nurses often establish a sterile field by using the innermost side of a sterile wrapper or by using a sterile drape. When the field is established, sterile supplies and sterile solutions can be placed on it. Sterile forceps are often used to handle and transfer sterile supplies.

So that sterility can be maintained, supplies may be wrapped in a variety of materials. Commercially prepared items are frequently wrapped in plastic, paper, or glass. Liquids are preferably packaged in amounts adequate for one use only. Any leftover liquid is discarded.

TABLE 8–5 **Principles and Practices of Surgical Asepsis**

PRINCIPLES	PRACTICES
All objects used in a sterile field must be sterile.	All articles are sterilized appropriately before use by dry or moist heat, chemicals, or radiation.
	Always check a package containing a sterile object for intactness, dryness, and expiration date. Sterile articles can be stored only for a prescribed time; after that, they are considered unsterile. Any package that appears already open, torn, punctured, or wet is considered unsterile.
	Storage areas should be clean, dry, off the floor, and away from sinks.
	Always check chemical indicators of sterilization before using a package. The indicator is often a tape used to fasten the package or contained inside the package. The indicator changes color during sterilization, indicating that the contents have undergone a sterilization procedure. If the color change is not evident, the package is considered unsterile. Commercially prepared sterile packages may not have indicators but may be marked with the word *sterile*.
Sterile objects become unsterile when touched by unsterile objects.	Handle sterile objects that will touch open wounds or enter body cavities only with sterile forceps or sterile gloved hands.
	Discard or resterilize objects that come into contact with unsterile objects. Whenever the sterility of an object is questionable, assume the article is unsterile.
Sterile items that are out of vision or below the waist or table level are considered unsterile.	Once left unattended, a sterile field is considered unsterile.
	Sterile objects are always kept in view. Nurses do not turn their backs on a sterile field.
	Only the front part of a sterile gown, from shoulder to waist (or table height, whichever is higher), and the cuff of the sleeves to 2 inches above the elbows are considered sterile.
	Always keep sterile gloved hands in sight and above waist/table level; touch only objects that are sterile.
	Sterile draped tables in the operating room or elsewhere are considered sterile only at surface level.
Sterile objects can become unsterile by prolonged exposure to airborne microorganisms.	Keep doors closed and traffic to a minimum in areas where a sterile procedure is being performed, because moving air can carry dust and microorganisms.
	Keep areas in which sterile procedures are carried out as clean as possible by frequent damp cleaning with detergent germicides to minimize contaminants in the area.
	Keep hair clean and short or enclose it in a net to prevent hair from falling on sterile objects. Microorganisms on the hair can make a sterile field unsterile.
	Wear surgical caps in operating rooms, delivery rooms, and burn units.
	Refrain from sneezing or coughing over a sterile field. Droplets containing microorganisms from the respiratory tract can travel 1 m (3 feet), making a sterile field unsterile. Some agencies recommend that masks covering the mouth and the nose should be worn by anyone working over a sterile field or an open wound.
	Nurses with mild upper respiratory tract infections should refrain from carrying out sterile procedures or wear masks.
	When working over a sterile field, keep talking to a minimum. Avert the head from the field if talking is necessary.
	To prevent microorganisms from falling over a sterile field, refrain from reaching over a sterile field unless sterile gloves are worn. Refrain from moving unsterile objects over a sterile field.

(continued)

TABLE 8–5 **Principles and Practices of Surgical Asepsis** (continued)

PRINCIPLES	PRACTICES
Fluids flow in the direction of gravity.	Unless gloves are worn, always hold wet forceps with the tips below the handles. When the tips are held higher than the handles, fluid can flow onto the handle and become contaminated by the hands. When the forceps are again pointed downward, the contaminated fluid can flow back down and contaminate the tips.
	During a surgical hand wash, hold the hands higher than the elbows to prevent contaminants from the forearms from reaching the hands.
Moisture that passes through a sterile object draws microorganisms from unsterile surfaces above or below the sterile surface by capillary action.	Sterile, moisture-proof barriers are used beneath sterile objects. Liquids (sterile saline or antiseptics) are frequently poured into containers on a sterile field. If they are spilled onto the sterile field, the barrier keeps the liquid from seeping beneath it. Keep the sterile covers on sterile equipment dry. Damp surfaces can attract microorganisms in the air. Replace sterile drapes that do not have a sterile barrier underneath when they become moist.
The edges of a sterile field are considered unsterile.	A 2.5-cm (1-in.) margin at each edge of an opened drape is considered unsterile because the edges are in contact with unsterile surfaces.
	Place all sterile objects more than 2.5 cm (1 in.) inside the edges of a sterile field.
	Any article that falls outside the edges of a sterile field is considered unsterile.
The skin cannot be sterilized and is unsterile.	Use sterile gloves or sterile forceps to handle sterile items.
	Prior to a surgical aseptic procedure, cleanse the hands to reduce the number of microorganisms on them.
Conscientiousness, alertness, and honesty are essential qualities in maintaining surgical asepsis.	When a sterile object becomes unsterile, it does not necessarily change in appearance. The person who sees a sterile object become contaminated must correct or report the situation. Do not set up a sterile field ahead of time for future use.

Source: Berman, A., Snyder, S. J., Kozier, B., Erb, G. (2008). *Kozier & Erb's fundamentals of nursing: Concepts, process, and practice* (8th ed.). Upper Saddle River, NJ: Pearson Education.

STERILE GLOVES   Sterile gloves may be donned by the open method or the closed method. The open method is most frequently used outside the operating room because the closed method requires that the nurse wear a sterile gown. Gloves are worn during many procedures to maintain the sterility of equipment and protect a client's wound.

Sterile gloves are packaged with a cuff of approximately 5 cm (2 in.) and with the palms facing upward when the package is opened. The package usually indicates the size of the glove (e.g., size 6 or 71/2).

Latex and latex-free (e.g., nitrile and vinyl) sterile gloves are available to protect nurses from contact with blood and body fluids. Latex and nitrile are more flexible than vinyl, mold to the wearer's hands, allow freedom of movement, and have the added feature of resealing tiny punctures automatically. Therefore, wear latex or nitrile gloves when performing tasks that (a) demand flexibility, (b) place stress on the material (e.g., turning stopcocks, handling sharp instruments or tape), and (c) involve a high risk of exposure to pathogens. Choose vinyl gloves for tasks that are unlikely to stress the

glove material, require minimal precision, and carry a minimal risk of exposure to pathogens.

STERILE GOWNS   Sterile gowning and closed gloving are carried out chiefly in operating and delivery rooms, where surgical asepsis is necessary. The closed method of gloving can be used only when a sterile gown is worn because the gloves are handled through the sleeves of the gown. Before these procedures, the nurse dons a hair cover and a mask and performs a surgical hand wash.

Infection Control for Health Care Workers

NIOSH is part of the CDC and is a research agency of the U.S. Department of Health and Human Services. It investigates potentially hazardous working conditions and publishes recommendations for preventing workplace illnesses and injuries. For example, in 1999 NIOSH published a study on preventing needlestick injuries in health care settings that found that the majority of needlestick injuries were preventable. This, in part, led to the Needlestick Safety and Prevention Act, which went into effect in April 2001.

The Occupational Safety and Health Administration (OSHA), an agency of the U.S. Department of Labor, publishes and enforces regulations to protect health care workers from occupational injuries, including exposure to bloodborne pathogens in the workplace. **Occupational exposure** is defined as skin, eye, mucous membrane, or parenteral contact with blood or other potentially infectious materials that may result from the performance of an employee's duties.

There are three major modes of transmission of infectious materials in the clinical setting:

1. Puncture wounds from contaminated needles or other sharps
2. Skin contact, which allows infectious fluids to enter through wounds and broken or damaged skin
3. Mucous membrane contact, which allows infectious fluids to enter through mucous membranes of the eyes, mouth, or nose

Using proper precautions with general medical asepsis, appropriately using personal protective equipment (PPE) (e.g., gloves, masks, gowns, goggles, special resuscitative equipment), and vigilance in the clinical area will place the caregiver at significantly less risk for injury. The chance of a health care worker becoming infected following exposure to pathogens varies widely— estimates range from 30% for hepatitis B (nonimmune workers), to 1.8% for hepatitis C, to 0.3% for HIV (CDC, 2003). Measures to be taken in cases of possible exposure to these viruses are delineated by the CDC. Hepatitis C, a worldwide epidemic greater than HIV, has become a significant concern to all health care workers, because there is currently no vaccine against the virus or postexposure prophylaxis. Prevention remains the primary goal.

OSHA requires that health care employers make the hepatitis B vaccine and vaccination series available to all employees. Other vaccinations may also be made available (e.g., nurses working in an obstetric area should be vaccinated against rubella to protect pregnant clients and their fetuses).

> **PRACTICE ALERT**
> Nurses should consider in advance whether they would want prophylaxis for HIV exposure, because it should optimally begin within 1 hour of exposure.

Role of the Infection Control Nurse

All health care organizations are required to have interdisciplinary infection control committees that may include representatives from the clinical laboratory, housekeeping, maintenance, dietary, and client care areas. One important member of this committee is the infection control nurse. This nurse is specially trained to be knowledgeable about the latest research and practices in preventing, detecting, and treating infections. All infections are reported to the infection control nurse in a manner that permits recording and analyzing statistics that can assist in improving infection control practices. In addition, the infection control nurse may be involved in employee education and implementation of the bloodborne pathogen exposure control plan mandated by OSHA.

ALTERATIONS

Microorganisms—including bacteria, viruses, fungi, and parasites—often invade the human body and proliferate when they are undetected, uncontrolled, or not eliminated by the inflammatory and immune responses. In most cases, contact between humans and microorganisms is incidental and may even be beneficial to both organisms. Resident bacteria of the skin, mucous membranes, and gastrointestinal tract are an important part of the body's defense system. However, many microorganisms are virulent; that is, they have the ability to cause disease. Pathogens are virulent organisms rarely found in the absence of disease. Some microorganisms, known as opportunistic pathogens, rarely, if ever, cause harm to people with intact immune systems, but are capable of producing infectious disease in immunocompromised hosts (Porth, 2005).

Modern medicine, antibiotic therapy, immunizations, and other public health measures to protect food and water supplies have significantly reduced the prevalence of infectious diseases in many parts of the world. In spite of these advances, many infections, including malaria, typhoid, and tuberculosis, remain prevalent in developing nations. Sexually transmitted infections rage through modern cities and industrialized populations. New varieties and strains of pathogens, such as HIV, evolve to cause disease.

To a certain extent, modern medicine has contributed to the development of infectious diseases caused by antibiotic-resistant strains of microorganisms. For example, tuberculosis is on the rise in the United States, partially because organisms have become resistant to standard therapies. Clients receive immunosuppressive therapy following organ or tissue transplant and in the treatment of neoplasms, making them more susceptible to infection. Metal and plastic prosthetic devices are implanted, providing potential sites for colonization of disease-producing organisms (Fauci et al., 1998). Many diseases that were long considered unrelated to microorganisms may also actually be infectious; for example, colonization of the gastric mucosa with *Helicobacter pylori* is the predominant cause of peptic ulcer disease, and oncogenic viruses are able to transform normal cells into malignant cells.

Poor hygiene behaviors of young children and their caregivers facilitate transmission of infectious diseases in child care settings and other environments, including hospitals, clinics, and physician offices. The fecal-oral and respiratory routes are the most common modes of transmission in children. Children often do not wash their hands after toileting unless they are closely supervised. They put toys and their hands in their mouths, and then rub their nose and eyes. They often are unable to care for a runny nose without help. Diapers may leak stool and provide exposure to fecal organisms. In addition, caregivers in child care centers, other persons caring for children, and health care professionals may not use proper hand hygiene techniques. All of these behaviors promote the transmission of infection.

Pathogens

Pathogens capable of infecting and causing disease in susceptible hosts include bacteria, viruses, *Mycoplasma, Rickettsia, Chlamydia,* fungi, and parasites, such as protozoa, helminths (worms), and arthropods (Box 8–2). Each organism causes a different specific reaction in the host.

A number of mechanisms have evolved in pathogens to facilitate their transmission and increase their ability to invade the host and cause disease. Factors influencing the transmission of an organism include its resistance to drying and to variations in environmental temperature. For example, spore-forming organisms are extremely resistant to drying.

Many microorganisms are capable of producing toxins or enzymes to facilitate their invasion of the host, increase their resistance to host defenses, and increase their ability to cause disease. Adhesion factors produced by or incorporated into the cell wall or membrane of the pathogen improve its ability to attach and colonize the host. Pathogens may also produce enzymes to enhance their spread to local tissues, chemicals to block specific immune processes or deplete neutrophils and macrophages, or extracellular capsules to discourage phagocytosis.

Pathogens are often capable of producing toxins that alter or destroy the normal function of host cells and promote colonization, proliferation, and invasion by the pathogen. Toxins often increase the disease-producing capability of the pathogen and, in some cases, are totally responsible for it. For example, cholera, tetanus, and botulism result from bacterial toxins, not from the direct effects of the infection. **Exotoxins** are soluble proteins that the microorganisms secrete into surrounding tissue. Exotoxins are highly poisonous, causing cell death or dysfunction. **Endotoxins** are found in the cell wall of Gram-negative bacteria and released only when the cell is disrupted. They have less specific effects than exotoxins, but can activate many human regulatory systems, producing fever, inflammation, and potentially clotting, bleeding, or hypotension when released in large quantities.

Stages of the Infectious Process

When infectious disease develops in a host, it typically follows a predictable course, with stages based on the progression and intensity of manifestations. Stages include

1. Incubation period
2. Prodromal stage
3. Acute stage
4. Convalescent stage

The initial stage is the *incubation period*, during which the pathogen begins active replication but does not yet cause symptoms. Depending on the organism and host factors, the incubation period may last from hours, as with *Salmonella*, to years, as with HIV infection.

In the *prodromal stage*, symptoms begin to appear. At this stage, symptoms are often nonspecific and include general malaise, fever, myalgias, headache, and fatigue.

Maximal impact of the infectious process occurs during the *acute stage* as the pathogen proliferates and disseminates rapidly. Toxic byproducts of microorganism metabolism and cell lysis, along with the immune response, produce tissue damage and inflammation during this stage (Porth, 2005). Manifestations are more pronounced and specific to the infecting organism and site. Fever and chills may be significant during this phase.

Box 8–2 **Pathogenic Organisms**

BACTERIA

Bacteria are single-celled organisms that are capable of autonomous reproduction. Bacteria have different characteristics and growth requirements: *Aerobes* require oxygen for survival, whereas *anaerobes* cannot survive in the presence of oxygen; *Gram-positive* bacteria stain purple when subjected to crystal violet stain, whereas *Gram-negative* bacteria do not stain with crystal violet stain, but turn red when subjected to safranin stain; and the colonies formed by replicating bacteria differ from one another.

VIRUSES

Viruses are obligate intracellular parasites that are incapable of reproducing outside of a living cell. Some viruses are shed continuously from infected cell surfaces; others, after inserting their genetic material into that of the infected cell, remain latent until they are stimulated to replicate. Viruses may or may not cause lysis and death of the host cell during replication. Oncogenic viruses are able to transform normal cells into malignant cells.

MYCOPLASMA

Although similar to bacteria, *Mycoplasma* are smaller and have no cell wall, making them resistant to antibiotics that inhibit cell wall synthesis, such as penicillins.

RICKETTSIA AND *CHLAMYDIA*

As obligate intracellular parasites with a rigid cell wall, *Rickettsia* and *Chlamydia* have some features of both bacteria and viruses. Rather than depending on the host cell for reproduction, they use vitamins, nutrients, and products of metabolism (e.g., ATP) from the host. *Chlamydia* are transmitted by direct contact, whereas many Rickettsiae infect the cells of arthropods (e.g., fleas, ticks, and lice) and are transmitted from these vectors to humans.

FUNGI

Fungi are prevalent throughout the world, but few are capable of causing disease in humans. Most fungal infections are self-limited, affecting the skin and subcutaneous tissue. Some fungi, such as *Pneumocystis carinii*, can cause life-threatening opportunistic infections in the immunocompromised host.

PARASITES

The term *parasite* is typically applied to members of the animal kingdom that infect and cause disease in other animals. Protozoa, helminths, and arthropods are considered parasites. Protozoa are single-celled organisms transmitted via direct or indirect contact or by an arthropod vector. Helminths are wormlike parasites: Roundworms, tapeworms, and flukes are examples. They gain entry into humans primarily through ingestion of fertilized eggs or penetration of larvae through the skin or mucous membranes. Arthropod parasites, such as scabies (mites), lice, and fleas, typically infest external body surfaces, causing localized tissue damage and inflammation. Transmission is by direct contact with the arthropod or its eggs.

Source: Data summarized from Porth, C. M. (2005). *Pathophysiology: Concepts of altered health states* (7th ed.). Philadelphia: Lippincott Williams & Wilkins.

However, alcoholic clients and the older adults may respond to severe infection by becoming hypothermic. A client in the acute stage of infection is often tachycardic and tachypneic because of increased metabolic demands. Localized manifestations include redness, heat, swelling, pain, and impaired function. When the infectious disease affects an internal organ, manifestations are related to inflammatory changes in that organ and surrounding tissue. The client may experience tenderness to palpation over the site or show signs of impaired function, such as the hematuria and proteinuria that are characteristic of renal infections.

If the infectious process is prolonged, manifestations of the continuing immune response may become apparent. Catabolic and anorexic effects of the infection can lead to loss of body fat and muscle wasting. Immune complexes may be deposited at sites other than the primary infection, resulting in an inflammatory process. Glomerulonephritis (e.g., following strep throat) and vasculitis are possible results. Another possible consequence of prolonged infection and immune response is the triggering of an autoimmune disease process, such as rheumatic cardiomyopathy or celiac disease. Type 1 diabetes mellitus is thought to be the result of such a response (Porth, 2005).

As the infection is contained and the pathogen eliminated, the *convalescent stage* of the disease occurs. During this stage, affected tissues are repaired and manifestations resolve. Resolution of the infection is total elimination of the pathogen from the body without residual manifestations.

If a balance between organism and host factors occurs, with neither predominating, chronic disease may develop, or the organism may be driven into a protected site, such as an abscess. A *carrier state* develops when host defenses eliminate the infectious disease, but the organism continues to multiply on mucosal sites (Fauci et al., 1998).

Complications of Infectious Diseases

Multiple and varied complications are associated with infectious diseases. They are typically specific to the infecting organism and the body system affected.

Acute invasion of the blood by certain microorganisms or their toxins can result in septicemia and septic shock. Although bacteremia, the presence of bacteria in the blood, may not have serious effects, in septicemia, systemic disease is associated with their presence or that of toxins. Septic shock indicates a state of hypotension and impaired organ perfusion resulting from sepsis. Unless treated aggressively, septic shock leads to diffuse cell and tissue injury, and potentially to organ failure.

Nosocomial Infections

Nosocomial infections, called health care–associated infections (HAIs), are classified as infections that are associated with the delivery of health care services in a facility such as a hospital or nursing home. HAIs add hospital days, reduce admissions by occupying available beds, and increase the cost of health care (Stone, Hedblom, Murphy, & Miller, 2005). Nosocomial infections can either develop during a client's stay in a facility or manifest after discharge. They typically manifest after 48 hours of hospitalization. Infections that manifest within 48 hours of hospitalization are attributed to community sources.

Urinary tract infection is the most common type of HAI and the most frequent cause of Gram-negative septicemia in hospitalized clients. Pneumonia is the second most common hospital-acquired infection, with a mortality rate of 20–50%. It is associated with mechanical ventilators, tracheostomies, and endotracheal intubation (Porth, 2005). Bacteremia is associated with intravascular and urinary catheters. Because of the risk of infection, insertion of central lines and urinary catheters is conducted as a sterile procedure with careful attention to preventing contamination. *Clostridium difficile*–associated diarrhea is a frequently acquired nosocomial infection. Associated with antibiotic use, the risk of acquiring this infection increases with length of hospital stay, especially in an intensive care unit (ICU). Nosocomial microorganisms can also be acquired by health care personnel working in the facility, which can cause significant illness and time lost from work.

Nosocomial infections have received increasing attention in recent years. They are believed to involve approximately 2 million clients per year, cause 90,000 deaths, and add $4.5 billion in excess health care costs annually. The Joint Commission (formerly known as The Joint Commission on Accreditation of Healthcare Organizations), an independent, not-for-profit organization that accredits and certifies health care organizations and programs in the United States, included reducing the risk of health care–associated infections as one of the 2006 National Patient Safety Goals. The most common settings where nosocomial infections develop are hospital surgical and medical ICUs. The microorganisms that cause nosocomial infections can originate from the clients themselves (an **endogenous** source) or from the hospital environment and hospital personnel (**exogenous** sources). Most nosocomial infections appear to have endogenous sources. *Escherichia coli, Staphylococcus aureus,* and enterococci are the most common infecting microorganisms.

A number of factors contribute to nosocomial infections. **Iatrogenic infections** are the direct result of diagnostic or therapeutic procedures. One example of an iatrogenic infection is the bacteremia that results from insertion of an intravascular line. Not all nosocomial infections are iatrogenic, nor are all nosocomial infections preventable.

Another factor that contributes to the development of nosocomial infections is the compromised host, that is, a client whose normal defenses have been lowered by surgery or illness. Clients entering hospitals are often the least able to mount immune defenses to infection. Immunologic responses may be compromised and normal defenses impaired in clients with, for example, cancer or chronic diseases, pressure ulcers, or organ transplants (Tierney, McPhee, & Papadakis, 2006). Nosocomial infections also occur when antibiotic therapy has altered the body's natural defenses and impaired resistance to harmful microorganisms. Endogenous organisms outside their normal habitats (such as in *E. coli* in the urinary tract) become a threat to the client.

Other pharmacologic and therapeutic procedures, such as chemotherapy, the use of corticosteroids, and radiation therapy, also contribute to nosocomial infections. Gram-negative enteric bacteria and Gram-positive *S. aureus* are the most common bacteria responsible.

Invasive procedures and altered immune defenses are the main factors that contribute to infection. Urinary catheterization is the number one cause; cardiac catheterization, insertion of peripheral and central intravenous lines, respiratory care procedures, and surgical procedures are also closely linked to nosocomial infection. Consequently, the urinary tract, surgical wounds, the respiratory tract, and invasive catheter sites on the skin are most often affected by hospital-acquired infection. Hospital-acquired pneumonia is the second most common nosocomial infection, accounting for 15–20% of these serious infections. Sopena and Sabria (2005) found hospital-acquired pneumonia, usually associated with ICU residency and mechanical ventilation, in non-ICU clients with severe underlying disease and a hospital stay greater than 5 days. Organisms causing the infection are often resistant to many drugs and may not respond to antibiotics that are usually effective in treating infections acquired outside the hospital.

The hands of personnel are a common vehicle for the spread of microorganisms. Insufficient hand cleansing is an important factor contributing to the spread of nosocomial microorganisms.

PRACTICE ALERT

Since October 2002, alcohol-based hand rub has been recommended by the CDC as the preferred method for hand hygiene (CDC, 2002a). Antiseptic soaps and detergents are the next most effective agents, and nonantiseptic soaps are the least effective. A soap and water wash is recommended for visibly soiled hands. Wearing gloves does not eliminate the need for handwashing.

Table 8–6 outlines the most common microorganisms responsible for nosocomial infections and their causes.

PREVENTING NOSOCOMIAL INFECTIONS Prevention is the most important control measure for nosocomial infections. The pathogens causing these infections are transmitted primarily by contact with hospital personnel and contaminated inanimate objects (Posani, 2004). *Effective handwashing is the single most important measure in infection control.* Although infections can also be transmitted by the airborne route, via contaminated equipment, and from the environment, these are less significant routes. Invasive procedures and equipment should be used only when absolutely necessary; for example, it is not appropriate to insert an indwelling catheter when the only indication is incontinence. Peripheral intravenous equipment and sites must be kept clean and changed regularly: intravenous bags and bottles every 24 hours, tubing every 24–96 hours, and sites every 2–3 days according to agency policy (CDC, 2002b; Evans-Smith, 2005).

Meticulous use of medical and surgical asepsis is necessary to prevent transport of potentially infectious microorganisms.

Many nosocomial infections can be prevented using proper hand hygiene techniques, environmental controls, sterile technique when warranted, and identification and management of clients at risk for infection. Many research studies have investigated the effectiveness of aseptic technique. Not all, however, show what might have been considered intuitive results. For example, no controlled studies have shown that removing nail polish or rings influences the rate of infection following surgical hand scrubbing and gloving (Arrowsmith, Maunder, Sargent, & Taylor, 2005). A number of studies have shown a link between artificial fingernails and infection transmission, especially fungal infections. In any case, nurses use critical thinking and agency policy in implementing infection control procedures.

Hand hygiene is important in every setting, including hospitals. It is considered one of the most effective infection control measures. Any client can harbor microorganisms that are currently harmless to the client yet potentially harmful to another person or to the same client if the microorganisms find a portal of entry. It is important that both the nurses' and clients' hands be cleansed at the following times to prevent the spread of microorganisms: before eating, after using the bedpan or toilet, and after the hands have come in contact with any

TABLE 8–6 **Nosocomial Infections**

MOST COMMON MICROORGANISMS	CAUSES
Urinary Tract	
Escherichia coli	Improper catheterization technique
Enterococcus species	Contamination of closed drainage system
Pseudomonas aeruginosa	Inadequate hand cleansing
Surgical Sites	
Staphylococcus aureus (including methicillin-resistant strains—MRSA)	Inadequate hand cleansing
Enterococcus species (including vancomycin-resistant strains—VRE)	Improper dressing change technique
Pseudomonas aeruginosa	
Bloodstream	
Coagulase-negative staphylococci	Inadequate hand cleansing
Staphylococcus aureus *Enterococcus* species	Improper intravenous fluid, tubing, and site care technique
Pneumonia	
Staphylococcus aureus	Inadequate hand cleansing
Pseudomonas aeruginosa	Improper suctioning technique
Enterobacter species	

Source: Berman, A., Snyder, S. J., Kozier, B., Erb, G. (2008). *Kozier & Erb's fundamentals of nursing: Concepts, process, and practice* (8th ed.). Upper Saddle River, NJ: Pearson Education.

body substances, such as sputum or drainage from a wound. In addition, health care workers should cleanse their hands before and after giving care of any kind.

For routine client care, the WHO (2005) recommends handwashing under a stream of water for at least 20 seconds using plain granule soap, soap-filled sheets, or liquid soap when hands are visibly soiled, after using the restroom, after removing gloves, before handling invasive devices (such as intravenous tubing), and after contact with medical equipment or furniture.

However, soap and water are inadequate to sufficiently remove pathogens. The CDC recommends use of alcohol-based antiseptic hand rubs (rinses, gels, or foams) before and after direct client contact. Recently, placement of alcohol-based antiseptic hand rub dispensers has been approved for agency corridors (Centers for Medicare and Medicaid Services, 2005). Previous concerns that this represented a fire hazard have been addressed in the regulations.

Antimicrobial soaps are usually provided in high-risk areas, such as the newborn nursery, and are frequently supplied in dispensers at the sink. Studies have shown that the convenience of antimicrobial foams and gels, which do not require soap and water, may increase health care workers' adherence to hand cleansing. The CDC recommends antimicrobial hand cleansing agents.

It is important to recognize that performing hand hygiene with either soap or alcohol-based cleansers can damage the skin through the drying effect of the detergents or chemicals. If the nurse develops dermatitis, the client may be at higher risk for infection, because handwashing does not decrease bacterial counts on skin with dermatitis. The nurse is also at higher risk because the normal skin barrier has been broken. Although lotions, moisturizers, and emollients have been tried, no research has yet confirmed their effectiveness in minimizing the problem.

Antibiotic-Resistant Bacteria

Antibiotic-resistant microorganisms are increasing at an alarming rate, primarily due to the prolonged and inappropriate use of antibiotic therapy. Although antibiotic therapy is expected to eradicate all targeted microorganisms, sometimes a few bacteria survive, leading to bacteria that reproduce with antibiotic resistance already encoded into their genetic makeup (Lehne, 2004). Other bacteria produce enzymes that inactivate drugs, change drug binding sites, or alter their cell membrane to prevent drug absorption.

Some of the current resistant strains include

- Methicillin-resistant *S. aureus* (MRSA)
- Multidrug-resistant tuberculosis (MDR-TB)
- Penicillin-resistant *Streptococcus pneumoniae* (PRSP)
- Vancomycin-resistant *Enterococcus* (VRE)
- Vancomycin-intermediate or -resistant *S. aureus* (VISA or VRSA)
- Extended-spectrum beta-lactamase (ESBL) (Kjonegaard & Myers, 2005).

MRSA is becoming more prevalent in community settings in which young people, such as children in day care and amateur and professional athletes, share equipment. MRSA colonizes in the nares and skin. Health care personnel often transmit *S. aureus* unknowingly on their hands, because it is transmitted primarily by direct physical contact, not through respiratory droplets (Kjonegaard & Myers, 2005). Most *S. aureus* strains resist treatment by methicillin and similar drugs, which are the treatment of choice for *S. aureus* infections. Vancomycin has been the only uniformly effective drug for hospital-acquired MRSA; however, community-acquired MRSA is sensitive to antibiotics such as tetracycline, doxycycline, clindamycin, sulfamethoxazole-trimethoprim, cephalexin, dicloxacillin, erythromycin, and quinolones. Soft-tissue infections with MRSA may manifest as abscesses, furuncles, or cellulites, and may be mistaken for spider bites.

In 1997, a new form of *S. aureus* emerged with resistance to vancomycin, known as vancomycin-intermediate or vancomycin-resistant *S. aureus.* (VISA or VRSA); both VISA and VRSA are resistant to methicillin. Clients with MRSA, VISA, or VRSA are isolated in a private room using contact precautions.

Enterococci are part of the normal flora of the gastrointestinal and female genital tracts. Frequent use of vancomycin caused *Enterococci* to develop resistance, leading to VRE.

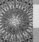 **EVIDENCE-BASED PRACTICE** **Does Frequency of Handwashing Vary According to Risk of Infection Transmission?**

In this Canadian study, all visits by nurses in an acute care hospital to selected client rooms were recorded for 3 days and 2 nights to assess compliance with handwashing. The highest level of infection transmission risk was contact with body fluids in 11% of visits and contact with skin in 40% of visits. The overall rate of handwashing was 46%; however, the rate for visits involving contact with body fluids was 81% and contact with skin was 61%. Nurses returned immediately to the same client 45% of the time. The rate of handwashing was higher for the last of a series of visits to a client's room. The researchers concluded that nurses adjusted their handwashing rates in accordance with the risk level of each visit.

Implications
Many studies have examined compliance with handwashing policies among health care workers. In almost every case, the compliance rates were far below what is recommended. This study suggests that raw data of compliance are less useful than examining the use and pattern of handwashing in those cases in which the care provider recognizes the highest risk of infection transmission. Education programs about hand hygiene may be more effective if patterns of care and levels of risk are incorporated into recommendations.

Source: Raboud J., Saskin, R., Wong, K., Moore, C., Parucha, G., Bennett, J., et al. (2004). Patterns of handwashing behavior and visits to patients on a general medical ward of healthcare workers. J. Raboud, R. Saskin, K. Wong, C. Moore, G. Parucha, J Bennett, et al. *Infection Control and Hospital Epidemiology, 25,* pp. 198–202.

EVIDENCE-BASED PRACTICE   Antibiotics and Infection

Nurses who discharge clients from outpatient and acute care settings frequently teach clients to take a complete prescribed dose of oral antibiotics to manage acute infectious illness. Ingesting less than complete doses exposes clients to the risk of resistant infections and can result in less than therapeutic outcomes. There are many potential barriers to the completion of antibiotic dosing: cost of purchase; difficulty swallowing the pills; multiple, frequent doses; and the potential for adverse, unpleasant side effects.

Aronson (2005) studied in depth the experience of 11 clients who had just completed a short-term antibiotic regimen to treat a variety of acute infectious illnesses with various antibiotic regimens. The 11 participants represented diverse gender and cultural backgrounds. They participated in 30-minute interviews within 2 weeks of completing their antibiotic regimen. The interviews were audiotaped and evaluated for themes. This qualitative study is the first part of a research program to evaluate an intervention that promotes adherence to taking antibiotics for a short-term period. The clients' descriptions, views, and experiences are the unique aspect of this research on adherence to antibiotic self-administration; most studies of adherence have been conducted from the prescribers' rather than the clients' perspective.

Aronson analyzed the client descriptions of their experiences taking their prescribed antibiotics by organizing the responses into categories of consistent themes. A second colleague experienced in qualitative research independently analyzed the data, and the results were compared until the categories were agreed upon. The central theme that emerged was successful antibiotic self-administration. The clients integrated the dosing into their daily schedules and adapted to any unplanned circumstances. The primary categories involved in self-administration were (1) medication-taking behaviors, (2) factors influencing adherence, and (3) attitudes and beliefs about the medication and the value of completing the prescribed dose. Subcategories were identified for each of these main categories.

Clients described methods for remembering to take the medication, methods of dealing with anticipated or experienced side effects, and factors that built trust in their relationship with the prescriber. Clients with a higher severity of symptoms leading to antibiotic prescription were more likely to report intention to adhere to the dosing regimen.

Implications for Nursing

Nurses teach clients about short-term antibiotic self-administration in outpatient and inpatient settings. The findings from this study can be used to guide educational interactions. Based on the findings in this study, nurses should encourage client involvement in the decision to take short-term antibiotic medications in order to strengthen the relationship with the prescriber. Nurses can ask clients to identify the method they will use to remind themselves to take each dose, and inquire about their knowledge of and plans to manage side effects from the medication.

Critical Thinking in Client Care

1. Identify methods that clients can use to remind themselves of dosing schedules.
2. An 86-year-old woman is being discharged to her home following a respiratory infection. Identify the information she will need to learn about short-term antibiotic medication when she is discharged.
3. Discuss potential side effects of short-term antibiotics on the gastrointestinal tract.
4. Discuss the interrelationship between malnutrition and immune system function.

Source: Data from Aronson, B. (2005). Medication management behaviors of adherent short-term antibiotic users. *Clinical Excellence for Nurse Practitioners, 9*(1), 23–30.

Direct transmission occurs on the hands of health care personnel and from contact with contaminated equipment. In cases of infection, stringent infection control measures are instituted, care is provided using contact precautions, and clients are placed either alone or with other VRE-infected clients.

Streptococcus pneumoniae, the most common cause of community-acquired pneumonia, has developed into its resistant form, penicillin-resistant *S. pneumoniae.* Unlike MRSA and VRE, PRSP is transmitted by droplets from the respiratory tract and requires transmission-based droplet precautions.

C. difficile is an organism that has developed very resistant and highly morbid strains associated with frequent use of broad-spectrum antibiotics in hospitals. A common cause of nosocomial diarrhea, it is usually treated with metronidazole or vancomycin (Rao & Bradley, 2003). An even more virulent strain has been identified that is resistant to both metronidazole and vancomycin (Warny et al., 2005).

Extended-spectrum beta-lactamase–producing microorganisms are resistant to third-generation cephalosporins and include Gram-negative *Klebsiella* and *E. coli.* These organisms colonize indwelling urinary catheters and gastrostomies,

as well as mechanical ventilators. They spread by direct and indirect contact.

Universal precautions, most importantly handwashing, and modest use of antibiotics are critical actions for stopping the spread of antibiotic-resistant bacteria. Equipment such as stethoscopes, blood pressure cuffs, and thermometers should be restricted to use by each client identified with one of these diseases. Personal protective gear that is used and disposed of appropriately is another important safeguard.

Certain antibiotics can also induce resistance in some strains of organisms. This resistance has become so widespread that the CDC has created a 12-step Campaign to Prevent Antimicrobial Resistance in Healthcare Settings, which consists of four strategies: preventing infection, diagnosing and treating infection effectively, using antimicrobials wisely, and preventing transmission.

Biological Threat Infections

Since the terrorist attacks on September 11, 2001, and the development of anthrax cases in the United States, there is an increased level of concern about the possible use of biological weapons. The most likely pathogens to be used for this purpose include anthrax, smallpox, botulism, pneumonic plague, and viral hemorrhagic fevers.

As with any potential large-scale infectious disease, state public health systems are charged with the responsibility of identifing cases, controlling the spread of infection, and preparing the local and state responses for caring for the potential large numbers of ill adults and children. As a part of this responsibility, public health authorities conduct **disease surveillance**, monitoring patterns of disease occurrence from the cases of infectious and communicable diseases reported by health care workers to state health officials. Disease surveillance procedures may be followed for any type of communicable and infectious disease, from *shigella* to H1N1 influenza to a biological threat infection.

Pediatric Infectious and Communicable Diseases

Reducing the number of preventable childhood illnesses is a major national goal in *Healthy People 2010*, and nurses are important partners in this effort. Specific objectives targeted at reducing or eliminating specific infectious diseases (USDHHS, 2000) include

- *Elimination.* Rubella and congenital rubella syndrome, diphtheria, *Haemophilus influenza* type b, measles, mumps, polio, and tetanus.
- *Reduction.* Pertussis, hepatitis B, varicella, food-borne pathogens, and HIV infection. Common preventable infectious diseases are a significant public health problem. The national health objectives are a reflection of how significant these preventable diseases are as a public health problem. Table 8–7 lists selected infectious and communicable diseases in children.

TABLE 8–7 Selected Infectious and Communicable Diseases in Children

DISEASE	CLINICAL MANIFESTATIONS	CLINICAL THERAPY	NURSING MANAGEMENT
Diphtheria⁺⁺ *Causal agent: Corynebacterium diphtheriae* *Epidemiology:* Occurs mostly in colder months in unimmunized or partially immunized children and immunized children with waning immunity. Cases of cutaneous and wound diphtheria occur sporadically in the tropics. Maternal immunity lasts up to 6 months after birth. The disease is endemic in areas where immunization is no longer routine, such as Russia. *Transmission:* Contact with nasal or eye discharge or skin lesion, or, less commonly, by indirect contact with contaminated items. Unpasteurized milk has served as a vehicle. *Incubation period:* 2–7 days or longer *Period of communicability:* Usually 2–4 weeks or until 4 days after antibiotics are started	Symptoms can be mild or severe with a gradual onset over 1–2 days. Low-grade fever, anorexia, malaise, rhinorrhea with a foul odor, cough, sore throat, hoarseness, stridor or noisy breathing, cervical lymphadenitis, and pharyngitis may be present. In more severe cases, the membranes of the tonsils, pharynx, and larynx are affected. The characteristic membranous lesion is a thick, bluish white to grayish black patch that covers the tonsils. It can spread to cover the soft and hard palates and the posterior portion of the pharynx. Attempts to remove the membrane result in bleeding. *Complications:* Produces an endotoxin that causes myocarditis and peripheral neuropathy (diplopia, slurred speech, difficulty swallowing, or paralysis of the palate) or ascending paralysis similar to Guillain-Barré syndrome.	Diagnostic tests include a culture from any mucosal or cutaneous lesion. Administer IV antitoxin and antibiotics within 3 days of onset of symptoms. The child must be tested for sensitivity to horse serum before giving the antitoxin. When diphtheria is suspected, antibiotic therapy (penicillin G or erythromycin) should be initiated without waiting for laboratory results. Removal of the membrane may be needed to treat airway obstruction. *Prognosis:* With treatment, prognosis is good. If untreated, death can occur due to airway obstruction. *Prevention:* Diphtheria is a vaccine-preventable disease. Booster doses are needed every 10 years after primary series. This is a reportable disease.	■ Use droplet precautions for pharyngeal disease and contact precautions for cutaneous disease. ■ Monitor closely for signs of increasing respiratory distress, as well as cardiac and neurologic complications. Provide humidified oxygen as necessary. ■ Have emergency airway equipment available. ■ Administer antibiotics. Give no medications containing caffeine or other stimulants. ■ Use oral suction gently as necessary. ■ Allow children to use mouthwash if desired. Gargling is not permitted because it can irritate the pharyngeal surfaces. ■ Encourage liquids as tolerated. Intravenous fluids may be necessary. ■ Provide emotional support to the family. ■ Initiate the search for client contacts to give antibiotics and immunization boosters.

(continued)

TABLE 8–7 Selected Infectious and Communicable Diseases in Children (continued)

DISEASE	CLINICAL MANIFESTATIONS	CLINICAL THERAPY	NURSING MANAGEMENT
Erythema Infectiosum (Fifth Disease) *Causal agent*: Human parvovirus B-19 *Epidemiology:* Occurs worldwide, most often in winter and spring. The disease also occurs in epidemics, with peak activity every 6 years. The incidence is highest in children between the ages of 5 and 14 years. *Transmission:* Respiratory secretions and blood *Incubation period:* 6–21 days *Period of communicability:* Believed to be highest the week before symptom onset 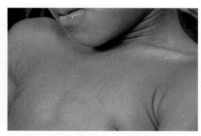 Lace-like, erythematous, maculopapular rash with erythema infectiosum. *Source:* Courtesy of Maura Connor.	Stage 1 begins as a flu-like illness (headache, chills, malaise, nausea, body ache) lasting 2–3 days. A symptom-free period of 1–7 days follows. Stage 2 occurs 1 week later with a fiery-red rash on the cheeks, giving a "slapped face" appearance. Circumoral pallor is seen. In 1–4 days a lace-like, symmetric, erythematous, maculopapular rash appears on the trunk and limbs, spreading proximal to distal, but sparing the palms and soles. Stage 3 lasts 1–3 weeks as the rash fades, but can reappear if the skin is irritated or exposed to sunlight. The rash can be mildly pruritic. *Complications*: Children with hemolytic conditions can have transient aplastic crisis. Arthritis and arthralgia can occur.	Diagnosis is made by physical signs or a serologic test for immunoglobulin M (IgM) parvovirus B-19–specific antibody. Medical treatment is supportive, and recovery is usually spontaneous. Children with hemolytic conditions may need blood transfusions if an aplastic crisis occurs. Immunodeficient clients may develop a chronic infection for which IV immune globulin therapy is often effective (American Academy of Pediatrics, 2006). *Prognosis*: Fetal infection can occur, resulting in fetal hydrops or spontaneous abortion. *Prevention*: Avoid contact with infected persons.	■ Children with aplastic crisis are often hospitalized. ■ Use standard and droplet precautions. Isolation is needed only for children with aplastic crisis or who are immunosuppressed. ■ Nonaspirin antipyretics may be given to control fever. ■ Use soothing oatmeal or Aveeno baths if the rash is pruritic. Antipruritics may also help to relieve itching. ■ Encourage rest and offer frequent fluids. ■ Keep children out of direct sunlight if possible. Provide protective, light, loose clothing if exposure to sunlight cannot be avoided. ■ Provide quiet diversionary activity. There is no reason to keep the immune-competent child out of school or day care once he or she is no longer infectious. ■ Explain the three stages of rash development to parents.
Haemophilus Influenzae, Type B[+] *Causal agent*: Coccobacilli *H. influenzae* bacteria, which has several serotypes and can be encapsulated or nonencapsulated *Epidemiology:* Occurs most often in the spring and summer. Most commonly affected are infants and young children in child care centers. Low-birth-weight children and children with chronic illnesses have an increased susceptibility. *Transmission:* Direct contact or droplet inhalation. The organism is frequently asymptomatically colonized in the respiratory tract. *Incubation period*: Unknown *Period of communicability:* Three days from onset of symptoms	Begins with a viral upper respiratory infection. The organism passes through the mucosal barrier to directly invade the bloodstream. It can cause several severe invasive illnesses, including meningitis, epiglottitis, pneumonia, septic arthritis, and cellulitis. It is also a cause of sepsis in infants. Other illnesses include sinusitis, otitis media, bronchitis, and pericarditis. Each disease has very specific clinical manifestations. Invasive disease has decreased 99% since the introduction of the vaccine (American Academy of Pediatrics, 2006). *Complications*: Illness caused by *H. influenzae* type B responds to antibiotic therapy. Left untreated, severe sequelae and death, especially in young infants, can occur from conditions such as meningitis, epiglottitis, sinusitis, pneumonitis, and cellulitis.	Diagnosis is made by culture of blood, cerebrospinal fluid, or middle ear aspirate. Treatment consists of antibiotic therapy. Rifampin may be given to unprotected household contacts (not pregnant women), if another child has not completed immunizations, within 1 week after diagnosis. *Prognosis:* With rapid diagnosis and treatment, recovery is good, but highly dependent on the disease the organism has caused. When treatment is delayed, the prognosis for full recovery becomes much more guarded. *Prevention*: Immunization for *H. influenzae* type B	■ Use droplet precautions until 24 hours after the initiation of antibiotics. ■ Antibiotic therapy is administered intravenously for severe infections. Infections such as otitis media can be managed with oral antibiotics. ■ Unimmunized children under the age of 4 years are at increased risk for developing disease from *H. influenzae*. Specific prophylactic measures for susceptible children may be ordered by the physician. ■ Administer antipyretics to help the child feel more comfortable. ■ Closely monitor IV sites for patency and infiltration. ■ Perform nursing care measures specific to the illness. ■ Inform family members that rifampin turns urine and other body fluids orange, and it will cause stains.

TABLE 8–7   Selected Infectious and Communicable Diseases in Children (continued)

DISEASE	CLINICAL MANIFESTATIONS	CLINICAL THERAPY	NURSING MANAGEMENT
Influenza *Causal agent:* Orthomyxoviridae, types A and B *Epidemiology:* Prevalent in the United States from October to March, but the virus is active in other parts of the world year-round. During annual epidemics, 10–40% of healthy children are infected, and 1% are hospitalized (American Academy of Pediatrics, 2006). *Transmission:* Spreads by aerosolized particles and direct contact with respiratory secretions. *Incubation period:* 1–4 days *Period of communicability:* One day before symptoms until 5 days after onset of illness	Abrupt onset of fever (38–40°C), chills, cough, runny nose, sore throat, malaise, aches, headache, and anorexia. Children can have nausea and vomiting, diarrhea, and abdominal pain. Children may also present with croup, bronchiolitis, conjunctivitis, or other nonspecific febrile illness. *Complications:* Otitis media, exacerbations of chronic lung conditions such as asthma and cystic fibrosis. Pneumonia, croup, bronchiolitis, and wheezing can occur in up to 25% of children. Myositis, myocarditis, encephalitis, transverse myelitis, Reye's syndrome, and Guillain-Barré syndrome are all potential complications.	Diagnostic tests may include viral culture, rapid antigen testing from throat or nasopharynx, polymerase chain reaction, and immuno-fluorescence. Treatment is supportive. Antiviral therapy (oseltamivir, and zanamivir) may be given to children 1 year of age or older at high risk of complications. Relenza is approved for children 5 years and older (Food and Drug Administration, 2006). Amantadine and rimantadine should not be used due to viral resistance (Centers for Disease Control, 2006c, pp. 2–3). Follow updated antiviral therapy guidelines on http://www.cdc.gov/flu. When antiviral medication is initiated within 2 days of symptoms, the duration of symptoms may be reduced by 1–1 1/2 days. *Prevention:* Influenza vaccine is now recommended for infants and children over 6 months of age.	■ Use droplet and contact precautions for hospitalized infants and children. ■ The child is usually cared for at home. Encourage parents to wash hands frequently and to reduce exposure of other family members to the infected child. ■ Provide fluids to keep nasal secretions moist and prevent dehydration. ■ Provide acetaminophen or ibuprofen for fever management and mild pain. ■ If antiviral medications are given, be alert for nausea and vomiting. Zanamivir can exacerbate asthma. ■ Provide rest and quiet diversional activities. ■ Teach parents to be alert to signs of complications from the viral infection. ■ Nurses should be familiar with pandemic influenza plans for the local area and state (http://www.pandemicflu.gov).
Measles (Rubeola) [*+] *Causal agent:* Morbillivirus, a member of the paramyxovirus group *Epidemiology:* Occurrence peaks in the late winter and early spring. In developed countries, measles occurs mostly in outbreaks among unimmunized children, or possibly those with declining immunity. Spreads by direct contact with droplets or by airborne route. Passive maternal immunity lasts 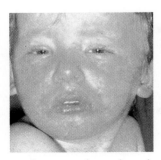 Confluent maculopapular rash with measles. *Source:* Courtesy of Centers for Disease Control and Prevention.	Children are quite ill in the 3–5 day prodromal phase, with symptoms including high fever, conjunctivitis, coryza, cough, anorexia, and malaise. Koplik's spots (small, irregular, bluish white spots on a red background) appear on the buccal mucosa about 2 days before and after the rash appears. The characteristic red, blotchy maculopapular rash that becomes confluent usually appears 2–4 days after onset of prodromal phase. The rash begins on the face and spreads to the trunk and extremities. Symptoms gradually subside in 4–7 days. Other symptoms include anorexia, malaise, fatigue, and generalized lymphadenopathy.	Diagnosis can be made by a serologic test for IgM measles antibody. Treatment is supportive. No antiviral therapy is available. Antibiotics are used for secondary bacterial infections. *Prognosis:* Recovery is generally good with supportive care. *Prevention:* Measles is a vaccine-preventable disease. Immune globulin, administered up to 6 days after exposure, can be helpful in preventing the disease in susceptible persons (immunocompromised children, infants less than 1 year of age, pregnant women). All health care workers should have documented immunity.	■ If the child is hospitalized, maintain airborne precautions during the contagious period. ■ Use a cool-mist vaporizer to help clear respiratory passages. ■ Suction nose and oral cavity very gently as necessary. ■ Give nonaspirin antipyretics for fever and antipruritics for itching. ■ Assess lungs carefully, especially in young children in whom pneumonias are a common complication. ■ Antitussives may be ordered to control coughing. ■ Keep lights dim and cover windows if the child has photophobia. ■ Elevate the head of the bed. Keep the room cool with good air circulation. Provide light and nonirritating blankets.

(continued)

TABLE 8–7 **Selected Infectious and Communicable Diseases in Children** (continued)

DISEASE	CLINICAL MANIFESTATIONS	CLINICAL THERAPY	NURSING MANAGEMENT
Measles (Rubeola) (continued) until the infant is age 12–15 months. In developing countries, measles remains an endemic disease and is a significant cause of infant and child morbidity and mortality. *Transmission:* Airborne, respiratory droplets and contact with infected persons *Incubation period:* Aproximately 8–12 days *Period of communicability:* Begins 3–5 days before the rash until 4 days after the rash appears	*Complications:* Diarrhea, otitis media, pneumonia, bronchitis, laryngotracheo-bronchitis, encephalitis, and death. Complications and sequelae occur most often in children who are malnourished, medically fragile, and immunosuppressed. The younger the child, the greater the risk for complications.	This is a reportable disease. A total of 37 cases were reported in the United States in 2004, and many were imported from another country or secondary exposures to these infected children (Centers for Disease Control, 2005b).	■ Keep skin clean and dry. No soaps should be used. ■ Maintain fluid intake. Offer cool liquids frequently in small amounts. Blended, pureed, and mashed foods are most easily tolerated. ■ Maintain bedrest. Visitors should be immune to measles. ■ Provide diversions such as music, stories, and favorite toys.
Meningococcus *Causal agent:* Neisseriameningitides, a Gram-negative diplococcus *Epidemiology:* Most often in winter or early spring. Spread by respiratory droplets from human carriers. Majority of infections in the United States are caused by serogroups B, C, and Y. Highest rates are in children under 2 years and 11 years and older (Bilukha & Rosenstein, 2005). African Americans and persons of low socioeconomic status are at higher risk. Outbreaks have occurred in child care centers, college dormitories, and military recruit camps. *Transmission:* Direct contact with droplet respiratory secretions *Incubation period:* 1–10 days *Period of communicability:* Until 24 hours after antibiotic started 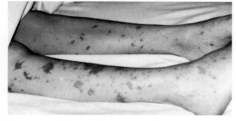 Purpura with meningococcemia *Source:* Used with permission of the America Academy of Pediatrics. Retrieved June 20, 2004, from http://www.vaccineinformation.org/photos/variaapoo3.jpg.	Abrupt onset of flulike symptoms of fever, chills, malaise, muscle aches, vomiting, and prostration (extreme exhaustion). Meningitis neurologic signs include drowsiness, disorientation, hallucinations, and convulsions. Meningococcemia: An urticarial, maculopapular, or petechial rash also appears that may progress to purpura. The condition may further deteriorate to shock, hypotension, disseminated intravascular coagulation, and coma. *Complications:* Loss of digits or limbs due to necrosis, hearing loss, arthritis, myocarditis, pericarditis, ataxia, seizures, hemiparesis, cranial nerve palsies, and obstructive hydrocephalus. Up to 10% of children and 25% of adolescents with invasive meningococcal disease die (American Academy of Pediatrics, 2006).	Diagnostic tests include cultures of the blood and cerebrospinal fluid. A Gram stain of petechial skin scrapings may also be done. *Treatment:* Penicillin G is given IV (cefotaxime, ceftriaxone, and ampicillin are alternate antibiotics). Chloramphenicol is used for children allergic to penicillin. The child is managed aggressively in the ICU to maintain the airway, assist ventilation, and manage shock with IV fluids and vasopressors. Plasma, blood, or platelets are used to treat the disseminated intravascular coagulation. *Prevention:* A vaccine has been approved for adolescents 11 years and older. A vaccine is available for children over 2 years old with asplenia and other high-risk conditions. Close contacts are given medication (rifampin, ceftriaxone, or ciprofloxacin) for prophylaxis. Health professionals exposed to oral secretions need prophylaxis (American Academy of Pediatrics, 2006). This is a reportable disease.	■ The child will be hospitalized. Use standard precautions and droplet precautions until the antibiotic has been administered for 24 hours. ■ Disease onset is abrupt and rapidly progresses to life threatening. Be alert for development of shock and respiratory compromise. Have emergency equipment available and be prepared to perform resuscitation. ■ When giving IV fluids and blood products, make sure the child does not get overloaded with fluids, and monitor for evidence of increased intracranial pressure. ■ Keep the family informed of the child's status and treatment as the disease progresses. Help the family to mobilize its support system. ■ The surviving child will likely need rehabilitation. Work with the social worker or case manager to transition the child to long-term care. ■ Help identify close contacts who should receive prophylactic antibiotics and educate them about the expected side effects (e.g., orange urine with rifampin). ■ Teach close contacts to be observant for signs of illness and to seek health care promptly if they occur.

TABLE 8–7 Selected Infectious and Communicable Diseases in Children (continued)

DISEASE	CLINICAL MANIFESTATIONS	CLINICAL THERAPY	NURSING MANAGEMENT
Mononucleosis *Causal agent*: Epstein-Barr virus (EBV), a member of the herpesvirus group *Epidemiology*: Occurs worldwide in no seasonal pattern. Infection commonly occurs early in life, and it often spreads among family members. *Transmission*: Direct contact with infected oropharyngeal and genital tract secretions. EBV can survive in saliva for several hours outside the body. EBV can also be transmitted by blood transfusion. *Incubation period*: Estimated to be 30–50 days *Period of communicability*: Indeterminate, asymptomatic carriage is common (American Academy of Pediatrics, 2006).	In very young children, mononucleosis can cause irritability, but be otherwise asymptomatic. A maculopapular rash may be seen in a few cases. In other children, the disease is characterized by malaise, headache, anorexia, abdominal pain, fatigue, and fever for 2–3 days, followed by lymphadenopathy and a sore throat. Hepatospleno-megaly can occur. Pain from swelling of the tonsils and lymph nodes may be significant. The syndrome typically lasts 2–3 weeks and is self-limited. Weakness and lethargy may continue for several months. *Complications*: Rare side effects include central nervous system symptoms, such as encephalitis, aseptic meningitis, and Guillain-Barré syndrome. Splenic rupture, respiratory failure, and hematologic complications such as thrombocytopenia can also occur. In immunodeficient children, fatal infections or lymphomas can develop.	Diagnostic tests include the serologic monospot test or a heterophil antibody response test. Greater than 10% atypical lymphocytes and a positive heterophil antibody response test are diagnostic (American Academy of Pediatrics, 2006). Treatment is supportive. Corticosteroids may be used to control tonsillar swelling and pain when there is impending airway obstruction, massive splenomegaly, myocarditis, or hemolytic anemia. Ampicillin and amoxicillin should be avoided, as a nonallergic rash often develops (American Academy of Pediatrics, 2006). *Prognosis*: After recovery, the virus remains latent in the lymphoid system. It can be reactivated during periods of immuno-suppression. *Prevention*: There is no known prevention.	■ Children are usually treated at home. Standard precautions should be used. ■ Give antipyretics and analgesics for fever and sore throat. Offer warm saltwater for gargling. Offer soft foods and encourage fluids. ■ Maintain bedrest during acute phase. ■ Give adolescents a sense of responsibility by involving them in decisions about care whenever possible. Be sure to include parents and adolescents in discussions. ■ Reassure adolescents who may be worried about keeping up with schoolwork that they can return to school when the fever is gone and swallowing is normal. ■ Teens should avoid kissing until the fever has been gone for several days. ■ Contact sports should be avoided until the liver and spleen are normal, usually in about 4 weeks. ■ If splenomegaly is present, alcohol should be avoided for 3 months after liver function test results return to normal.
Mumps (Parotitis)[+] *Causal agent:* Rubulavirus in the Paramyxoviridae family 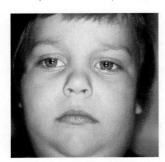 Parotid gland swelling with mumps. *Source:* Courtesy of Centers for Disease Control and Prevention.	Malaise, low-grade fever, earache, headache, pain with chewing, and decreased appetite and activity; followed by bilateral or unilateral parotid gland swelling. Swelling peaks around the third day. Meningeal signs (stiff neck, headache, and photophobia) occur in about 15% of clients. *Complications*: Orchitis (inflammation of the epididymis, pain on testicular palpation, and scrotal swelling—most often unilateral) may occur in postpubertal males; sterility is relatively rare (American Academy of Pediatrics, 2006). Oophoritis, pancreatitis, glomerulonephritis, myocarditis, thrombocytopenia, cerebellar ataxia, and hearing impairment are sometimes seen.	Diagnostic tests include a viral culture from a throat washing, urine, or cerebrospinal fluid. Serum mumps IgM antibody titer may also be performed. Therapy is supportive, focused on symptom relief. *Prognosis*: Mumps is usually self-limiting. *Prevention*: Mumps is a vaccine-preventable disease. This is a reportable disease. In 2006 an outbreak of more than 2,500 cases of mumps in 11 states occurred in the United States. The infection was originally imported from Britain (Centers for Disease Control, 2006d).	■ Use standard and droplet precautions for hospitalized children while contagious. ■ Children are usually cared for at home. They are generally uncomfortable, but are rarely very ill. ■ Avoid exposure to immunocompromised or susceptible individuals. ■ Give nonaspirin analgesics and antipyretics to control fever and pain. ■ Encourage fluid intake. Swallowing and chewing may be painful. Offer soft and blended foods. Avoid foods and beverages that increase salivary flow (citrus, spices, and candies), because they cause pain.

(continued)

TABLE 8–7 Selected Infectious and Communicable Diseases in Children (continued)

DISEASE	CLINICAL MANIFESTATIONS	CLINICAL THERAPY	NURSING MANAGEMENT
Mumps (Parotitis) (continued) *Epidemiology:* Occurs worldwide in unvaccinated children, most often in winter and spring. Infection and vaccination induce lifelong immunity. Maternal antibodies begin to disappear in infants at the age of 12–15 months. *Transmission:* Contact with respiratory tract secretions. *Incubation period:* 12–25 days *Period of communicability:* 1–2 days before parotid swelling until 9 days after swelling occurs			■ Talking may be painful. Provide a bell or other attention-getting device. ■ Apply warm or cool compresses, whichever is preferred, to the parotid area. ■ Be alert for signs of complications. Headache, stiff neck, vomiting, and photophobia may indicate meningeal irritation. ■ Provide scrotal supports if testicular swelling occurs. ■ Reassure children that the facial swelling will go away. ■ Keep children out of school or child care until 9 days after parotid swelling occurs. Encourage diversional activities.
Pertussis (Whooping Cough)[+] *Causal agent:* Bordetella pertussis *Epidemiology:* Occurs worldwide. Most common in children under 6 months of age. Epidemic cycles occur every 3–4 years. Pertussis can occur in health care workers, adolescents, and adults who have waning immunity, and these individuals can spread the disease to unimmunized children. Neither pertussis infection nor vaccine immunity is long lasting (Cherry, 2005). *Transmission:* Respiratory droplets and direct contact with discharge from the respiratory membranes *Incubation period:* 7–10 days *Period of communicability:* Begins about 1 week after exposure. Communicable for 5–7 days after antibiotic therapy is initiated. The disease is most contagious before the paroxysmal cough stage.	The onset is insidious. *Catarrhal stage:* The disease begins with nasal congestion, a runny nose, low-grade fever, and a mild nonproductive cough, lasting about 2 weeks. *Paroxysmal stage:* The cough is more severe at night, with coughing spasms when the child attempts to expel a thick mucoid plug. A forceful inspiration through a narrowed glottis and stridor, or "whooping," follows. Young infants may have apnea rather than the "whooping." Sucking on a bottle may trigger the coughing spell. Coughing may be accompanied by flushing; cyanosis; vomiting; and profuse drainage from the nose, eyes, and mouth. Paroxysmal coughing can last 1–6 weeks or more. Dehydration may result from decreased oral intake. *Convalescent stage:* Up to 6 weeks, when paroxysms gradually subside. Adolescents and adults often have symptoms of an upper respiratory infection with persistent coughing spasms lasting longer than 7 days. *Complications:* Pneumonia, atelectasis, otitis media, encephalopathy, seizures, and death. Highest mortality rate and complication rate is in infants under 1 year.	Diagnostic tests include culture and polymerase chain reaction (PCR) testing. Treatment with macrolide antibiotics (erythromycin, azithromycin, and clarithromycin); corticosteroids, if ordered; and supportive care. *Prognosis:* The disease is most severe in infants under 1 year of age, and most deaths occur in this age group. *Prevention:* Pertussis is a vaccine-preventable disease. Close contacts should be treated with macrolide antibiotics for prophylaxis (Tiwari, Murphy, & Moran, 2005). Vaccine protection wanes after 5–10 years. This is a reportable disease. An estimated 800,000–3.3 million cases occur in the United States per year in a cyclic pattern (Cherry, 2005).	■ Use droplet precautions until 5–7 days after antibiotics are initiated. Most hospitalized cases occur in children under the age of 5 years. ■ Use a cardiac monitor and pulse oximetry to continuously assess respirations and oxygen saturation. The smaller the child, the greater the risk for respiratory distress and apnea. ■ Remain with the child during coughing spells, when hypoxic and apneic episodes are most likely. Give oxygen if ordered. Have emergency equipment available. ■ Provide humidification. Gentle suctioning may be necessary. ■ Give nonaspirin antipyretics as needed for fever. ■ Encourage frequent rest periods. ■ Allow the child to eat desired foods in small, frequent feedings. ■ Encourage the child to take fluids. The child may need IV hydration if oral intake is not tolerated. ■ Provide emotional support to parents. ■ Teach parents to watch for signs of respiratory failure and dehydration if the child is managed at home.

TABLE 8–7 Selected Infectious and Communicable Diseases in Children (continued)

DISEASE	CLINICAL MANIFESTATIONS	CLINICAL THERAPY	NURSING MANAGEMENT
Pneumococcal infection[+] *Causative agent: Streptococcus pneumoniae,* a Gram-positive diplococcus *Epidemiology*: The organism is found in the nasopharynx of healthy people. Outbreaks occur in the winter and spring among people in crowded settings. In temperate climates, 8 of 90 serotypes account for most of the invasive pediatric infections. The disease is more common in infants, young children, African Americans, American Indians, and Alaskan Natives. Of particular concern is the development of penicillin- and multi-antibiotic-resistant strains. *Transmission*: Respiratory secretions and droplets *Period of communicability*: Unknown; probably less than 24 hours after beginning effective antibiotic therapy	The signs and symptoms are related to the focal area of infection. The organism causes otitis media, sinusitis, pharyngitis, laryngotracheo-bronchitis, pneumonia, meningitis, and bacteremia. In otitis media, upper respiratory infection, fever, ear pain, and decreased appetite are seen. In bacteremia, there is unexplained fever and no localized infection site. In pneumonia, fever, chills, chest pain, dyspnea, malaise, and a productive cough are seen. In meningitis, inconsolable crying, increased irritability, lethargy, refusal to eat, nausea, vomiting, diarrhea, myalgia, photophobia, and seizures are seen. *Complications*: Prior to the introduction of a vaccine, it caused 30–50% of acute otitis media, and was a major cause of sinusitis, meningitis, bacteremia, and pneumonia (Durbin, 2004). Other complications include septic arthritis, osteomyelitis, endocarditis, and brain abscess.	Diagnostic tests include bacterial culture from site of infection. Symptomatic care is provided. Antibiotic selection is based on susceptibility of organism to penicillin, macrolides, and other agents. Up to 50% of pneumococcal strains are penicillin resistant. Third-generation cephalosporins (cefotaxime or ceftriaxone) may be used. Vancomycin and rifampin are used in combination when strains are resistant to the antibiotics listed above (American Academy of Pediatrics, 2006). *Prevention*: Many serotypes are preventable with immunization. A significant reduction in invasive disease and antibiotic-resistant strains caused by serotypes in the vaccine has occurred since vaccination of infants was initiated (Durbin, 2004).	■ If the child is hospitalized, maintain standard precautions. ■ Provide nonaspirin antipyretics for control of fever and comfort. ■ Encourage fluids, and monitor intake and output. ■ Monitor vital signs and level of consciousness to identify signs of worsening condition. ■ Educate parents about the need for the vaccine, as the unimmunized child could become infected repeatedly with different serotypes. ■ Many children with mild disease are treated at home. Educate parents about signs indicating a need to seek additional medical care, the need for proper medication administration, and comfort measures for the child. ■ Individuals with congenital asplenia or traumatic splenectomy, malignancy, sickle cell disease, and nephrotic syndrome are at higher risk for invasive disease with this organism. ■ Additional factors that increase risk of pneumococcal disease include poverty, crowded housing, homelessness, and exposure to tobacco smoke.
Poliomyelitis[+] *Causal agent:* Poliovirus is an enterovirus with three serotypes. *Epidemiology*: Occurs worldwide. Polio primarily affects children and immuno-compromised or unimmunized adults caring for infants who received live poliovirus vaccine. The vaccine induces lifelong immunity. Since live poliovirus vaccine was discontinued in the United States, no vaccine-associated paralytic poliomyelitis has been reported since 2000 (American Academy of Pediatrics, 2006, p. 543). *Transmission*: Primarily by the fecal-oral route, but also the respiratory route *Incubation period*: Usually 7–10 days (range 3–21 days) *Period of communicability*: Greatest shortly before and right after clinical symptoms develop when the virus is in the throat; excreted in the feces for several weeks	Affects the central nervous system. Less severe infections may be limited to fever and stiffness in the neck and back, headache, vomiting, and sore throat. In other cases, fever, headache, stiff neck, Kernig or Brudzinski sign, decreased deep tendon reflexes, and progressive weakness occur. With cranial nerve involvement, there may be respiratory tract muscle paralysis. An increased respiratory rate may interfere with the ability to talk, because frequent pauses are needed. Onset of paralysis may be sudden, over hours, or gradual over 3–5 days. Paralysis results from damage to motor neurons. *Complications*: Permanent motor paralysis, respiratory arrest, myocardial failure, aseptic meningitis, and postpolio syndrome	Diagnosis is made by cell culture from stool or throat swabs. Treatment is supportive. No chemotherapeutic agents that directly kill the poliovirus are available. *Prognosis*: Respiratory complication is life threatening and involves 5–10% of all cases. Respiratory paralysis can lead to death, and motor paralysis can result in long-term disability. *Prevention*: Poliomyelitis is a vaccine-preventable disease. This is a reportable disease.	■ Use standard and contact precautions in the hospital and keep the child on strict bedrest. ■ Observe closely for respiratory paralysis (ineffective cough, talking with frequent pauses, shallow and rapid respiratory rate). Have emergency equipment at bedside. Assist ventilations as needed until mechanical ventilation is set up. ■ Administer sedatives and nonaspirin analgesics as ordered to allow for rest and comfort. Moist hot packs may relieve discomfort. ■ Encourage fluids. ■ Position the child to promote body alignment. ■ Perform range-of-motion exercises to prevent contractures after the acute phase. ■ Provide emotional support. ■ Clients are alert and aware. Tell them what is happening to them. ■ Long-term orthopedic (physical therapy) support may be needed by some children.

(continued)

TABLE 8–7 Selected Infectious and Communicable Diseases in Children (continued)

DISEASE	CLINICAL MANIFESTATIONS	CLINICAL THERAPY	NURSING MANAGEMENT
Roseola (Exanthem Subitum, Sixth Disease) *Causal agent:* Human herpesvirus type 6 (HHV-6) *Epidemiology:* Occurs worldwide, primarily in children 6–24 months of age (after maternal antibodies decline); no seasonal pattern *Transmission:* Likely to be from respiratory secretions of healthy individuals *Incubation period*: Appears to be 9–10 days *Period of communicability*: Lifelong persistent viral shedding in healthy individuals (American Academy of Pediatrics, 2006)	Sudden, high fever up to 40.5°C (105°F) for 3–8 days, during which the child does not appear toxic (normal appetite and behavior). The fever phase is followed by a characteristic pale pink, discrete, maculopapular rash that starts on the trunk and spreads to the face, neck, and extremities. The rash can last for 1–2 days. The child's appetite is normal. *Complications*: Children may have febrile seizures during high fever stage. Encephalopathy can develop in rare cases.	Roseola is self-limiting, and treatment is supportive. *Prognosis*: Roseola is benign in most cases. Nearly all children over 2 years of age have an antibody titer to HHV-6 (American Academy of Pediatrics, 2006).	■ Children are rarely hospitalized, but if they are, use standard precautions. ■ Give nonaspirin antipyretics to control fever. ■ Observe closely for any seizure activity, especially during the acute febrile periods. ■ Encourage fluids. ■ Reassure parents that the rash will disappear in a few days.
Rotavirus *Causal agent:* Group A, B, and C rotaviruses *Epidemiology:* Occurs during late fall to early spring in yearly diarrhea epidemics in the United States; it is the most common cause of severe diarrhea in children under 5 years. *Transmission:* Fecal-oral route *Incubation:* 2–4 days *Period of communicability:* Virus is present in stool before onset and may persist up to 21 days after onset of symptoms.	Acute onset of low-grade fever and vomiting followed by watery diarrhea 1–2 days later. Up to 10–20 diarrheal stools a day. Symptoms last 3–8 days. *Complications*: Dehydration and electrolyte disturbances. Death occurs in rare circumstances.	Diagnosis is by enzyme immunoassay or latex agglutination assay to detect group A rotavirus antigen. Treatment involves adequate fluid and electrolyte replacement with oral rehydration solution. Introducing a regular diet within a few hours of rehydration shortens the duration of the disease (Dennehy, 2005). In severe dehydration, IV fluid resuscitation is performed. No antiviral therapy is available. *Prevention*: Naturally acquired infection protects against reinfection that causes severe diseases. A new vaccine has been approved for infants.	■ Use standard and contact precautions. ■ Hand hygiene with soap and water removes 75% of virus from contaminated hands. Use of alcohol-based hand sanitizers after washing with soap and water increases effectiveness (Dennehy, 2005). ■ Clean contaminated surfaces followed by disinfection with an alcohol-containing disinfectant (Dennehy, 2005). ■ Assess hydration status frequently. ■ Breastfeeding is continued during oral rehydration therapy. Formula feeding can begin 12–24 hours after oral rehydration therapy is started. ■ Older children can be fed complex carbohydrates and lean meats, yogurt, fruits and vegetables 12–24 hours after oral rehydration therapy is started.
Rubella (German Measles)[+] *Causal agent:* An RNA virus, member of the family Togaviridae, genus *Rubivirus* *Epidemiology:* Occurs worldwide and is most prevalent in the winter and spring. Maternal antibodies disappear about 6–9 months after birth. Most U.S. cases occur among foreign-born children and adults from countries that do not have rubella vaccination programs. Congenital rubella syndrome is thought to occur due to lack of immunization. Four cases were reported from 2001–2004 in	Rubella is generally a mild disease with a characteristic pink, nonconfluent, maculopapular rash. The rash appears on the face; progresses to the neck, trunk, and legs; and disappears in the same order. Prodromal symptoms occur 1–5 days before the rash and include low-grade fever, headache, malaise, coryza, sore throat, and anorexia. Forchheimer spots (discrete, erythematous pinpoint or larger lesions on the soft palate) are seen during the prodromal phase. Generalized lymphadenopathy involving the	Diagnostic tests include cell culture from a nasal swab and detection of IgM or IgG antibodies. Treatment is supportive. Rubella is generally self-limiting in children. *Prognosis*: Disease is usually mild and benign. Major risk is for fetus if the mother is infected in the first trimester. Congenital rubella syndrome is associated with ophthalmologic, cardiac, auditory, and neurologic anomalies.	■ Maintain standard and droplet precautions for contagious children. ■ Maintain contact precautions for infants with congenital rubella syndrome until 1 year of age unless nasopharyngeal and urine cultures are repeatedly negative after 3 months of age (American Academy of Pediatrics, 2006). ■ Children are usually treated at home. They should be isolated from pregnant women.

TABLE 8–7 Selected Infectious and Communicable Diseases in Children (continued)

DISEASE	CLINICAL MANIFESTATIONS	CLINICAL THERAPY	NURSING MANAGEMENT
Rubella (German Measles) (continued) the United States (Centers for Disease Control, 2005a). *Transmission:* Droplet spread, direct contact with infected persons, or contact with articles soiled by nasal secretions *Incubation period:* 14–21 days (most commonly 16–18 days) *Period of communicability:* Seven days before until 7 days after the onset of rash. Infants with congenital rubella may shed the virus for months after birth.	postauricular, suboccipital, and posterior cervical areas is common up to 7 days before the rash. Many cases are asymptomatic. Neonatal signs of congenital rubella syndrome include growth retardation, radiolucent bone disease, hepatospleno-megaly, thrombocytopenia, and purpuric skin lesions (giving a "blueberry muffin" appearance). *Complications:* Complications are rare, but include arthritis in adolescents, and encephalitis.	*Prevention:* Rubella is a vaccine-preventable disease. Females of childbearing age need to be immunized to reduce the risk for congenital rubella syndrome. All health care workers should have documented immunity. 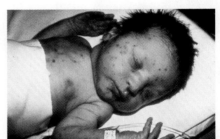 "Blueberry muffin" appearance in infant with congenital rubella syndrome. *Source:* Courtesy of Centers for Disease Control and Prevention.	■ Give nonaspirin analgesics and antipyretics for any pain and fever. ■ Allow children to choose what they would like to eat and drink. Encourage fluids. ■ Provide quiet activities. ■ Exclude children from child care or school for 7 days after onset of rash. School and child care facilities should be notified of the child's illness.
Streptococcus A *Causal agent:* Group A streptococci (GAS) *Epidemiology:* The illness is caused by various M-protein groups of group A beta-hemolytic streptococci. Different strains are associated with pharyngeal and pyodermal infections, and also rheumatic fever and acute glomerulonephritis (American Academy of Pediatrics, 2006). Pharyngeal infections tend to occur more in late fall, winter, and spring. Pyodermal infections tend to occur in warmer seasons because of the association with minor skin trauma and insect bites. *Transmission:* Contact with respiratory secretions for pharyngitis or skin lesions for pyoderma *Incubation period:* Pharyngeal: usually 2–5 days; Pyodermal: usually 7–10 days	*Pharyngeal:* Abrupt onset with a sore throat, dysphagia, malaise, high fever, chills, headache, abdominal pain, anorexia, and vomiting. A beefy red pharynx with exudate (strep throat) and tender cervical nodes are seen. Palatal petechiae may be seen. Cough and rhinitis are absent in most cases. *GAS respiratory tract infection:* Children under 3 years may develop serous rhinitis and a respiratory illness with moderate fever, irritability, and anorexia rather than pharyngitis. *Scarlet fever:* A characteristic erythematous, "sandpaper" rash that blanches with pressure appears in some cases 12–48 hours after onset of symptoms, concentrates in flexor skin creases, and spares the circumoral area. In 3–4 days, the rash begins to fade, and the tips of the toes and fingers begin to peel. The classic strawberry tongue is seen on days 4–5. *Pyodermal:* Lesions (impetigo) are honey-colored crusts at the site of open lesions.	Diagnosis can be made by a rapid strep antigen test or culture of secretions from the pharynx and tonsils. Cultures of skin lesions are not indicated (American Academy of Pediatrics, 2006). Prompt antibiotic treatment is effective. Penicillin V is the drug of choice. Erythromycin is used if the child is allergic to penicillin. Uncomplicated impetigo is treated with mupirocin ointment. Invasive strains causing necrotizing fasciitis or myositis need IV antibiotics and surgical intervention (exploration and debridement of dead tissue). *Prognosis:* Recovery is usually good with antibiotic therapy. Up to 15% of healthy children become chronic carriers (American Academy of Pediatrics, 2006).	■ Children with uncomplicated infections are usually cared for at home. ■ Promote bedrest during the febrile stage. ■ Give nonaspirin antipyretics to control fever. Teach parents important signs of a worsening condition. ■ For pharyngeal infections, offer warm saltwater for gargling, a soft diet, and nonacidic beverages. Encourage fluids. Provide cool, clear liquids. Swallowing may be difficult. ■ Explain to parents the importance of giving the child the full course of antibiotics. ■ Encourage family members with sore throats to have throat cultures taken. ■ For impetigo, teach the parents to wash the skin, remove crusts, and apply antibiotic ointment. ■ If the child is hospitalized, maintain droplet precautions for pharyngeal infections and contact precautions for skin lesions for 24 hours after beginning antibiotics. Monitor vital signs, especially temperature. Administer antibiotics as ordered.

(continued)

TABLE 8–7 Selected Infectious and Communicable Diseases in Children (continued)

DISEASE	CLINICAL MANIFESTATIONS	CLINICAL THERAPY	NURSING MANAGEMENT
Streptococcus A (continued) *Period of communicability:* Four weeks in untreated pharyngeal infections; noncontagious within 24 hours of starting antibiotics 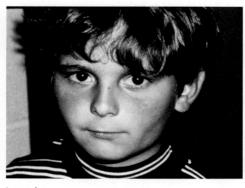 Impetigo.	*Complications:* If untreated, acute otitis media, sinusitis, peritonsillar or retropharyngeal abscess, cervical lymphadenitis, acute rheumatic fever, acute glomerulonephritis occur. Invasive disease with toxic shock syndrome, bacteremia, and necrotizing fasciitis or myositis can be fatal.	*Prevention:* None	■ If the child develops invasive streptococcal infection, use standard precautions. The child with toxic shock syndrome will need intensive care to manage shock and fluid and electrolyte imbalances.
Tetanus *Causal agent: Clostridium tetani* or tetanus bacillus *Epidemiology:* The bacillus is common and exists as a spore in soil, dust, and animal excretions. The organism produces an endotoxin that affects the central nervous system. *Transmission:* The organism is transmitted to humans through puncture wounds or broken skin. Newborns can acquire tetanus via the umbilical cord if they are born in an unclean area, a contaminated implement is used to cut the cord, or clay is applied to the umbilical cord as a ritual in some Middle Eastern cultures. *Incubation period:* 3 days to 3 weeks (average 8 days) *Period of communicability:* Not communicable to other individuals except through skin wounds	Stiffness of the neck and jaw, with painful facial spasms and difficulty chewing and swallowing over a few days, and headache. Noise and sudden movements can stimulate spasms. Spasms of facial muscles may produce a grinning expression (risus sardonicus). Localized prolonged and painful muscle contraction may occur at the site of the wound. Eventually rigidity of the abdomen and trunk produce *opisthotonos* (rigid hyperextension of the entire body). Spasms and fever occur, along with difficulty swallowing the increased oral secretions. Respiratory muscles can be affected and cause airway obstruction and suffocation. Newborns have difficulty with sucking, progressing to an inability to suck, irritability, and nuchal rigidity. *Complications:* Laryngospasm, respiratory distress, or death	Tetanus immune globulin is given to unimmunized persons as soon as possible. Tetanus toxoid is given at the same time at a separate site. Medications are provided to treat muscle spasms. Intensive care is provided with cardiorespiratory monitoring, assisted ventilation, IV metronidazole or penicillin G, nutrition, and supportive care. Wound cleansing and debriding are performed. Survival beyond 4 days indicates an increased chance of recovery. Paroxysms become less frequent, and complete recovery may take weeks. *Prognosis:* 30% mortality; much higher in newborns. Intensive care has improved mortality. *Prevention:* Tetanus is a vaccine-preventable disease. Tetanus boosters are updated every 10 years, or, if a potentially contaminated wound occurs, in 5 years. Proper surgical debridement of wounds decreases the chance of infection.	■ Prevent disease by checking immunization records and administering immunizations as necessary. ■ Give immune globulin to unimmunized persons. ■ Assist with wound debridement. ■ Use standard precautions, as the child with tetanus is hospitalized. ■ Monitor the child's condition. Handle as little as possible. Reduce stimulation by placing the child in a quiet, darkened room. ■ Offer skin and respiratory care. The child may need an endotracheal tube, suctioning, and supplemental oxygen for airway support. ■ Provide feedings via total parenteral nutrition or feeding tube. ■ Maintain hydration with intravenous fluids and electrolytes. ■ Try to reduce the child's anxiety, as mental status may be unaffected. ■ Prepare the family for a possible poor prognosis.

Note: *Indicates that a vaccine or antitoxin is available for use in high-risk or as-needed situations. †Indicates that the disease has a safe and effective vaccine.

Source: Adapted from Ball, J. W., Bindler, R. M. W., Cowen, K. J. (2010). *Child health nursing: Partnering with children and families* (2nd ed.). Upper Saddle River, NJ: Pearson Education.

ALTERATIONS AND TREATMENTS

The following summary table includes the most frequent infectious illnesses or diseases with which a nurse may come in contact. Others include, but are not limited to, bacterial meningitis, bacterial endocarditis, giardiasis, Chlamydia, tetanus, streptococcus A, shigella, hepatitis, and HIV.

Alteration	Description	Treatment
Cellulitis	Acute bacterial infection of the dermis and underlying connective tissue	▪ Antibiotics ▪ Antipyretics ▪ Palliative care ▪ Fluid administration
Urinary tract infection	Infection of any part of the urinary tract: kidneys, ureters, urinary bladder, or urethra	▪ Antibiotics per culture results ▪ Antipyretics ▪ Fluid management
Viral pneumonia	Infection of the lung, often causing fluid accumulation in one or more lobe	▪ Treatment based on symptoms ▪ Cough suppressant, expectorant ▪ Rest ▪ Encouraging breathing ▪ Support for respiratory effort may include oxygen, Fowler's position, respiratory toilet
Otitis Media	Inflammation of the middle ear	▪ Palliative care ▪ Antibiotics only if symptoms do not resolve after 48–72 hours
Influenza	Highly contagious viral respiratory disease	▪ Antipyretics ▪ Rest ▪ Fluid management ▪ Monitor for respiratory rate, pattern, and effective airway clearance ▪ Antiviral medications can reduce duration and severity of symptoms ▪ Prevention through vaccination of at-risk individuals
Conjunctivitis	Highly contagious inflammation of the conjunctiva	▪ Antibiotics ▪ Palliative care
Tuberculosis	Chronic, recurrent infectious disease caused by *Mycobacterium tuberculosis*	▪ Fluid management ▪ Monitoring vital signs, especially temperature, frequently ▪ Administering antipyretics and analgesics ▪ Antitubercular medications ▪ Respiratory support as dictated by symptoms ▪ Isolation
Sepsis	Whole body inflammatory process resulting in acute critical illness	▪ Reverse underlying cause ▪ Protect respiratory and cardiovascular systems ▪ Fluid management ▪ Monitor neurologic status, vital signs

ASSESSMENT

During the assessing phase of the nursing process, the nurse obtains the client's history, conducts the physical assessment, and gathers laboratory data.

Nursing History

During the nursing history, the nurse assesses the degree to which a client is at risk for developing an infection and any client complaints suggesting the presence of an infection. To identify clients at risk, the nurse reviews the client's chart and structures the nursing interview to collect data regarding the factors that influence the development of infection, especially existing disease process, history of recurrent infections, current medications and therapeutic measures, current emotional stressors, nutritional status, and history of immunizations (see the following Assessment Interview).

Physical Assessment

Signs and symptoms of an infection vary according to the body area involved. For example, sneezing, watery, or mucoid discharge from the nose and nasal stuffiness commonly occur with

EVIDENCE-BASED PRACTICE **Medicating for Fever**

A recent study in Israel of 464 children ages 6–36 months compared the treatment of fever with acetaminophen (12.5 mg/kg) every 6 hours, ibuprofen (5 mg/kg) every 8 hours, and alternating doses of acetaminophen (12.5 mg/kg) and ibuprofen (5 mg/kg) every 4 hours. The group of children receiving the alternating therapy had a more rapid reduction of fever and a lower mean temperature than the two other groups (Sarrell, Wielunsky, & Cohen, 2006). This study did not effectively compare alternating doses of antipyretics with single antipyretics because the alternating medications were given more frequently than the single medication, and more antipyretic medication was in the bloodstream at one time. More study is needed before parents are routinely encouraged to alternate acetaminophen and ibuprofen for treating a fever.

an infection of the nose and sinuses, and urinary frequency and cloudy or discolored urine often occur with a urinary infection. Commonly, the skin and mucous membranes are involved in a local infectious process, resulting in the following:

- Localized swelling
- Localized redness
- Pain or tenderness with palpation or movement
- Palpable heat at the infected area
- Loss of function of the body part affected, depending on the site and extent of involvement

In addition, open wounds may exude drainage of various colors. Signs of systemic infection include the following:

- Fever
- Increased pulse and respiratory rate if the fever is high
- Malaise and loss of energy
- Loss of appetite and, in some situations, nausea and vomiting
- Enlargement and tenderness of lymph nodes that drain the area of infection

Table 8–8 lists the clinical manifestation of infection in infants and children by body system.

TABLE 8–8 Clinical Manifestation of Infection in Infants and Children

BODY SYSTEM	INFANTS	CHILDREN
Central nervous system	Irritable	Irritable or combative
	Decreased responsiveness	Stiff neck
	Lethargy	Back pain
	Bulging anterior fontanel	Decreased responsiveness
	High-pitched cry	Photophobia
	Muscle weakness	Brudzinski sign
	Additional Signs in Newborns:	Kernig sign
	Seizures	Malaise
	Subtle changes in muscle tone or hypotonia	
Cardiovascular system	Tachycardia	Tachycardia
	Decreased perfusion	Decreased perfusion
	Weak peripheral pulses	Weak peripheral pulses
	Pallor or mottled skin	Pallor or flushed, dry skin
	Flushed, dry skin	Delayed capillary refill time
	Delayed capillary refill time	
	Additional Signs in Newborns:	
	Cyanosis	
	Hypotension	
	Bradycardia	
Respiratory system	Tachypnea	Tachypnea
	Increased work of breathing with retractions, nasal flaring	Dyspnea

TABLE 8–8 Clinical Manifestation of Infection in Infants and Children (continued)

BODY SYSTEM	INFANTS	CHILDREN
	Crackles	Retractions
	Cough	Nasal flaring
	Stridor	Crackles
	Decreased oxygen saturation	Cough
	Irregular breathing	Stridor
	Additional Signs in Newborns:	Decreased oxygen saturation
	Apnea (new onset or increased episodes)	
	Increased or new-onset oxygen requirement	
	Grunting	
Gastrointestinal system	Vomiting	Nausea and vomiting
	Diarrhea	Diarrhea
	Abdominal distention	Abdominal discomfort
	Poor feeding	Abdominal distention
	Additional Signs in Newborns:	Poor appetite
	Abdominal wall discoloration	
	Paralytic ileus	
	Bloody stool	
	Jaundice or hepatosplenomegaly	
Renal system	WBCs and bacteria in urine	WBCs and bacteria in urine
	Additional Signs in Newborns:	
	Decreased urine output	
	Hematuria, proteinuria	
Hematopoietic system	Neutropenia	Leukocytosis
	Increased immature WBCs (bands) in bacterial infections	Increased immature WBCs (bands) in bacterial infections
	Lymphocytosis in viral infections	Lymphocytosis in viral infections
	Additional Signs in Newborns:	
	Fraction of band cells >0.2	
	Thrombocytopenia	
Metabolic system	Hyperthermia or hypothermia	Hyperthermia
	Hypoglycemia or hyperglycemia	Chills
		Hypothermic in septic shock
Other systems	Rash	Rash
	Dry mucous membranes	Petechiae and/or purpura
	Poor skin turgor	Dry mucous membranes
	Sunken anterior fontanel	Poor skin turgor
	Petechiae and/or purpura	

Source: Ball, J. W., Bindler, R. M. W., Cowen, K. J. (2010). *Child health nursing: Partnering with children and families* (2nd ed.). Upper Saddle River, NJ: Pearson Education.

Assessment Interview   Client at Risk for Infections

- When were you last immunized for diphtheria, tetanus, poliomyelitis, rubella, measles, influenza, hepatitis, and pneumococcal pneumonia?
- When did you last have a tuberculin skin test?
- What infections have you had in the past, and how were these treated?
- Have any of these infections recurred?
- Are you taking any antibiotics, anti-inflammatory medications such as aspirin or ibuprofen, or medications for cancer?
- Have you had any recent diagnostic procedure or therapy that penetrated your skin or a body cavity?

- What past surgeries have you had?
- How would you describe your eating habits? Do you eat a variety of types of foods?
- Do you take vitamins?
- On a scale of 1–10, how would you rate the stress you have experienced in the past 6 months?
- Have you experienced any loss of energy, loss of appetite, nausea, headache, or other signs associated with specific body systems (e.g., difficulty urinating, urinary frequency, or a sore throat)?

Note: As with all history taking, the nurse must individualize the specific terms used, examples given to the client, and teaching techniques used to validate agreement on the meaning of words according to the client's culture, language spoken, and education or intellectual abilities.

DIAGNOSTIC TESTS

To assess the client's response to infection, identify the infecting organism, and monitor the progress of therapy, the following diagnostic tests may be ordered:

- *WBC count* provides clues about the infecting organism and the body's immune response to it (Table 8–9).
- *WBC differential* is also ordered (see Table 8–9). Neutrophilia, or increased numbers of circulating neutrophils (or PMNs), is a common response to infection, as the bone marrow responds to an increased need for phagocytes. Along with neutrophilia, a shift to the left is common in acute infection. This means that there are more immature neutrophils in circulation than normal (Figure 8–3 ■), indicating an appropriate bone marrow response.

- *Procalcitonin (CTpr)* is a precursor of the hormone calcitonin. Procalcitonin increases dramatically during infection and sepsis, and is accepted as both a marker of sepsis and a harmful mediator in lower respiratory tract and systemic infections (Christ-Crain et al., 2004; Müller & Becker, 2001).
- **Cultures** *of the wound, blood, or other infected body fluids* are used to identify probable microorganisms by their characteristics, such as shape, growth patterns, and Gram-staining qualities. After the organism is cultured, it is subjected to various antibiotics known to be effective against its particular strain to determine which antibiotic is likely to be most effective. This is known as sensitivity testing. Generally, 24–48 hours are required to grow the organism, potentially delaying initiation of therapy. Because antibiotics (and possibly oxygen therapy) can alter the ability to culture an organism, specimens should be obtained before instituting therapy.

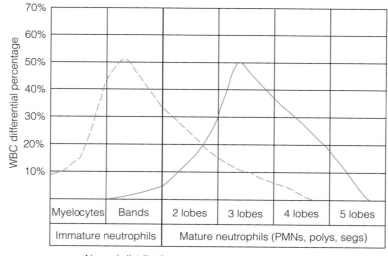

Type of WBC	Normal differential	Shift to left
Myelocytes	0%	Present
Band neutrophils (bands)	3–5%	Increased
Segmented neutrophils (segs, polys, PMNs)	50–65%	May be stable, increased, or decreased

Figure 8–3 ■ Neutrophils by stage of maturity and normal distribution in the blood.

TABLE 8–9 **White Blood Cell Count and Differential**

CELL TYPE AND NORMAL VALUE	INCREASED	DECREASED
Total WBCs: 4,000–10,000 per mm³	*Leukocytosis:* Infection or inflammation, leukemia, trauma or stress, tissue necrosis	*Leukopenia:* Bone marrow depression, overwhelming infection, viral infections, immunosuppression, autoimmune disease, dietary deficiency
Neutrophils (segs, PMNs, or polys): 55–70%	*Neutrophilia:* Acute infection or stress response, myelocytic leukemia, inflammatory or metabolic disorders	*Neutropenia:* Bone marrow depression, overwhelming bacterial infection, viral infection, Addison's disease
Eosinophils (eos): 1–4%	*Eosinophilia:* Parasitic infections, hypersensitivity reactions, autoimmune disorders	*Eosinopenia:* Cushing's syndrome, autoimmune disorders, stress, certain drugs
Basophils (basos): 0.5–1%	*Basophilia:* Hypersensitivity responses, chronic myelogenous leukemia, chickenpox or smallpox, splenectomy, hypothyroidism	*Basopenia:* Acute stress or hypersensitivity reactions, hyperthyroidism
Monocytes (monos): 2–8%	*Monocytosis:* Chronic inflammatory disorders, tuberculosis, viral infections, leukemia, Hodgkin's disease, multiple myeloma	*Monocytopenia:* Bone marrow depression, corticosteroid therapy
Lymphocytes (lymphs): 20–40%	*Lymphocytosis:* Chronic bacterial infection, viral infections, lymphocytic leukemia	*Lymphocytopenia:* Bone marrow depression, immunodeficiency, leukemia, Cushing's syndrome, Hodgkin's disease, renal failure

Source: Data from Corbett, J. V. (2004). *Laboratory tests and diagnostic procedures with nursing diagnoses* (6th ed.). Upper Saddle River, NJ: Prentice Hall; and Pagana, K. D., & Pagana, T. J. (1997). *Diagnostic and laboratory test reference* (3rd ed.). St. Louis, MO: Mosby-Year Book.

- *Serologic testing* provides an indirect means of identifying infecting agents by detecting antibodies to the suspected organism. When the antibody titer against a specific organism rises during the acute phase of an infectious disease and begins to fall during convalescence, the diagnosis is supported. Although it is not as accurate as culture, serology is particularly useful for organisms that cannot easily be cultured, such as hepatitis B and HIV (Porth, 2005).
- *Direct antigen detection methods* are in the process of being developed. These tests use monoclonal antibodies, which are purified antibody forms, to detect antigens in specimens from a diseased host (Porth, 2005). See Box 8–3. These tests offer rapid and accurate identification of the offending microorganism.
- *Antibiotic peak and trough levels* monitor therapeutic blood levels of the prescribed medication(s). The therapeutic range, that is, the minimum and maximum blood levels at which the drug is effective, is known for a given drug. By measuring blood levels at the predicted peak (1–2 hours after oral administration, 1 hour after intramuscular administration, and 30 minutes after intravenous administration) and trough (lowest level, usually a few minutes before the next scheduled dose), health care personnel can determine that the client is maintaining a level within the therapeutic range at all times, ensuring maximal effect from the drug. Measuring blood levels of a prescribed medication also helps determine whether the drug is reaching a toxic or harmful level during therapy, an unintended result that can increase the likelihood of adverse effects.

- *Radiologic examination of the chest, abdomen, or urinary system* may be ordered to detect organ abnormalities that indicate an inflammatory response or tissue damage.
- *Lumbar puncture* is performed to obtain cerebrospinal fluid (CSF) for examination and culture if a central nervous system (CNS) infection, such as meningitis or encephalitis, is suspected.
- *Ultrasonic examination, such as an echocardiogram or renal ultrasonography,* is a noninvasive diagnostic test to evaluate organ function.
- *Urinalysis* is a noninvasive test to assess for the presence of bacteria or blood in the urine.

THERAPEUTIC MANAGEMENT INTERVENTIONS

The goals of care for the client with an infection are to identify the organ system affected by the infection, identify the causative agent, and achieve a cure by the least toxic, least expensive, and most effective means. Fortunately, most infectious diseases are self-limiting and will resolve with little or no medical care. However, medical treatment may be required for an overwhelming infection or immunocompromised host.

The body part or organ system affected by the infection is often obvious from the client's history and presenting signs and symptoms. Identifying the system allows the range of possible infecting organisms to be narrowed to those known to affect that system. The manner of presentation provides further

Box 8–3 **Monoclonal Antibodies**

Antigens typically have numerous antigenic determinant sites, each capable of stimulating a different subset of B cells. Each clone secretes a slightly different antibody from the others. The resulting immunoglobulin produced is therefore *polyclonal,* with multiple different antibodies. In 1975, researchers devised a technique for making a single clone of "immortal" B cells that could be maintained indefinitely in a laboratory and would produce a single antibody to a specific antigen (see figure below). This pure antibody, known as a *monoclonal* antibody, offers the following advantages:

- It can target specific antigens.
- It has a single, constant binding affinity for the antigen.
- It can be diluted to a specific titer or concentration, because it is not mixed with other antibodies.
- It can be purified to avoid adverse responses (McCance & Huether, 2002).

In addition to providing passive protection from disease, monoclonal antibodies are being used in a variety of other ways, including the diagnosis and treatment of cancer, immunosuppression to prevent rejection of transplanted tissue or organs, immune response analysis, imaging techniques for diagnostic uses, and the early detection of viral infections (Lehne, 2004; McCance & Huether, 2002).

Source: Figure adapted from Becker, W., & Deane, D. (1986). *The world of the cell.* Redwood City, CA: Benjamin Cummings; Mahon, C. R., & Manuselis, G. Jr. (1995). *Textbook of diagnostic microbiology.* Philadelphia: W.B. Saunders. Reprinted with permission.

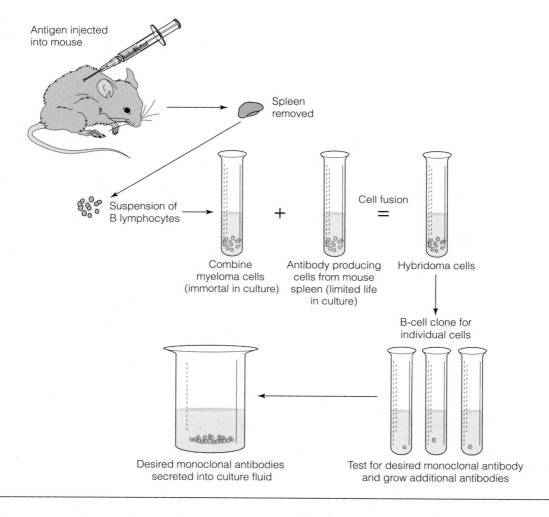

Antigen injected into mouse — Spleen removed — Suspension of B lymphocytes — Combine myeloma cells (immortal in culture) + Antibody producing cells from mouse spleen (limited life in culture) = Cell fusion — Hybridoma cells — B-cell clone for individual cells — Test for desired monoclonal antibody and grow additional antibodies — Desired monoclonal antibodies secreted into culture fluid

clues as to the diagnosis. For example, pneumococcal pneumonia typically presents with the acute onset of chills, fever, and cough in a previously healthy adult, whereas a client with viral pneumonia relates a gradual onset of symptoms, with systemic manifestations such as muscle aches and headache often predominant. A history of recent activities also provides

clues. Family members who all vomit and have diarrhea within 12 hours after a picnic probably do not have the flu.

Once the infecting agent has been identified, either positively or by probability, therapy can be specifically tailored to the client's needs. Viral infections often resolve without treatment other than supportive care, such as providing rest and fluids.

Skin infections may respond to a topical agent, avoiding the potential adverse effects of one administered systemically.

All skills and treatments, whether administering medications (see the following Medications feature) or preparing a client for discharge, are performed in a manner that prevents possible infection of clients. Some skills are specific to preventing infection, diagnosing infection, and treating the client with a diagnosed infection. Nursing skills used in preventing infection and caring for clients diagnosed with infection can be found in the skills manual and include the following:

- Hand hygiene
- Basic medical asepsis
- Use of standard precautions
- Isolation techniques
- Sterile field
- Culture specimen collection
- Use of personal protective equipment and decontamination

MEDICATIONS Antimicrobial Agents

Once the infecting organism and affected body system have been identified, specific therapy to cure the infectious disease can begin. The number of antimicrobial agents available makes choosing the appropriate one seem overwhelming. The perfect anti-infective agent would destroy pathogens while preserving host cells, be effective against many organisms while not promoting the development of resistance, distribute to necessary tissues, and remain in the body for relatively long periods.

Because no available antimicrobial meets all these criteria, physicians look for an agent that will be effective, has little toxicity, can be administered with relative convenience, and is cost effective. Characteristics of both the host and the infecting organism are considered in making the selection.

Classification	Mechanism of Action	Generic Drug Examples	Nursing Considerations
Antibiotics - Amino-glycosides - Macrolides - Tetracyclines - Cephalosporins - Penicillins - Sulfonamides - Fluoro-quinolones	May be used prophylactically to prevent infection or treat existing bacterial infection. Specific antibiotic is chosen based on pathogen causing infection.	Cefaclor, erythromycin, penicillin, tobramycin, trimethoprim-sulfamethoxazole	- Teach clients importance of taking the entire prescribed amount. - Encourage adequate fluid intake. - Monitor for signs of allergic reaction. - Assess renal and hepatic function and vital signs.
Antifungal	Selective for fungal plasma membranes, they inhibit ergosterol synthesis.	Amphotericin B, anidulafungin, caspofungin acetate, flucytosine, micafungin, fluconazole, nystatin	- Carefully monitor client's condition. - Use cautiously in clients with renal impairment, severe bone marrow suppression, and pregnancy. - Closely monitor kidney function (intake and output, BUN, creatine, daily weights). - Monitor serum electrolytes.
Antipyretic/Analgesic	Relieves pain and reduces fever.	Acetaminophen	- Monitor temperature. - Assess pain level. - Teach proper administration.
Antipyretic, Analgesic, Anti-inflammatory	Reduces fever and inflammation, in addition to relieving pain.	Aspirin, ibuprofen	- Monitor temperature. - Assess pain level. - Teach proper administration.
Antimalaria	Interrupts the complex lifecycle of plasmodium, with greater success early in the course of the disease.	Atovaquone, proguanil, chloroquine, hydroxychloro-quine sulfate, mefloquine, primaquine phosphate, pyrimethamine, quinine	- Carefully monitor client's condition. - Provide education about prescribed drug treatment. - Contraindicated in clients with hematological disorders or severe skin disorders such as psoriasis, and during pregnancy. - Assess lab results (complete blood cell count [CBC], liver and renal function tests, G5PD deficiency). - Obtain a baseline electrocardiogram. - Monitor for gastrointestinal side effects and changes in cardiac rhythm.

(continued)

MEDICATIONS Antimicrobial Agents (continued)

Classification	Mechanism of Action	Generic Drug Examples	Nursing Considerations
Antihelminthic	Is targeted at killing the parasites locally in the intestine and systemically in the tissues and organs they have invaded.	Albendazole, diethyl-carbamazine, ivermectin, mebendazole, praziquantel, pyrantel	■ Monitor vital signs, CBC, and liver function studies after obtaining a baseline. ■ Specific worm or parasite must be identified before initiating therapy. ■ Educate on nature of parasite infestation to prevent future reinfestation. ■ Warn clients if bowel elimination of worm is anticipated. ■ Assess for GI symptoms. ■ Monitor for CNS side effects.
Antiretroviral ■ Nonnucleoside reverse transcriptase inhibitors ■ Nucleoside and nucleotide reverse transcriptase inhibitors ■ Protease inhibitors ■ Fusion and integrase inhibitors	Target specific phases of the HIV replication cycle, requiring multiple drugs taken concurrently.	Delavirdine, efavirenz, abacavir, didanosine, amprenavir, atazanavir, darunavir, enfuvirtide, raltegravir, acyclovir, cidofovir, docosanol, idoxuridine, penciclovir	■ Clients require extensive teaching regarding pharmacotherapy, disease process, and prevention of contaminating others. ■ Psychosocial issues must be addressed to improve compliance with treatment regimen. ■ Use nonjudgmental approach. ■ Assess for side effects that can dramatically affect the client's life. ■ Assess T-cell count and client response to pharmacotherapy.

8.1 CELLULITIS

KEY TERMS
Cellulitis, *258*
Erythema, *258*
Inflammation, *258*
Lymphadenopathy, *258*
Lymphangitis, *260*
Septicemia, *259*
Tinea pedis, *259*
White blood cell, *258*

Basis for Selection of Exemplar
Centers for Disease Control and Prevention (CDC)
Joint Commission (JCAHO)
Institute for Healthcare Improvement (IHI)

LEARNING OUTCOMES
After reading about this exemplar, you will be able to do the following:
1. Describe the pathophysiology, etiology, and clinical manifestations of cellulitis.
2. Identify the risk factors associated with cellulitis.
3. Illustrate the nursing process in providing culturally competent care across the life span for individuals with cellulitis.
4. Formulate priority nursing diagnoses appropriate for an individual with cellulitis.
5. Create a plan of care for an individual with cellulitis.
6. Employ evidence-based caring interventions (or prevention) for an individual with cellulitis.
7. Assess expected outcomes for an individual with cellulitis.
8. Describe therapies used in the collaborative care of an individual with cellulitis.

OVERVIEW

Infection can occur in a small localized area, affect an entire organ system, or attack the entire body, as in the case of septicemia. Cellulitis is an example of an infection that can be small and well contained, but, if not treated promptly, it can develop into a life-threatening septicemia.

Cellulitis is an acute bacterial infection of the dermis and underlying connective tissue. It is characterized by red or lilac, tender, warm, edematous skin that may have an ill-defined, nonelevated border. Cellulitis usually occurs on the face and lower extremities as a result of trauma or a compromised skin barrier. Its chief symptom is **inflammation**, which includes intense pain, heat, redness, and swelling. It may appear in a localized area as a complication of a wound infection, or it may involve an entire limb. In severe infections, fever may be present, as well as an increase in **white blood cells** (WBCs) and tender lymph nodes (**lymphadenopathy**). Elevated WBCs and fever, although common signs of infection, may not be present in frail, older clients.

PATHOPHYSIOLOGY AND ETIOLOGY

Normal flora gain entry into the dermis through a break in the skin. There, they multiply, causing an inflammatory response with classic signs of inflammation, including **erythema** (redness), pain, warmth at the site, and edema. The wound is generally irregular in shape with well-defined borders. As the organisms grow in number, they can overwhelm the immune response that normally contains and localizes inflammation. This allows cellular debris to accumulate, resulting in enlarged areas of involvement.

Erysipelas, a superficial cellulitis of the skin caused by group A *Streptococcus*, usually affects the lower extremities or the face (Figure 8–4 ■). The involved area is bright red and raised with well-defined borders. Skin infections such as this can predispose the individual to **septicemia** and septic shock. Although antibiotic therapy is effective, the most important method of therapy is prevention.

If treated promptly, the prognosis is generally very good. However, delays in treatment can result in septicemia as bacteria enter the circulating blood system.

Etiology

Common causative organisms are *Staphylococcus aureus, hemolytic Streptococci (group g Streptococci and Streptococcus pyogenes), Streptococcus pneumoniae, Haemophilus influenzae,* and beta-hemolytic and group A *Streptococcus* (Curtis, 2007). Cellulitis can also result from a nearby abscess or sinusitis. Onset is usually rapid.

Risk Factors

Children with cellulitis often have a history of trauma, impetigo, folliculitis, untreated tooth decay, or recent otitis media. As the skin becomes thinner and less elastic with age, older adults become more susceptible to injury and breakdown of tissue, which can result in cellulitis. Peripheral neuropathy with decreased sensation and circulation can lead to abrasions, burns, and stasis ulcers that can become infected. Reduced physical activity, malnutrition, dehydration, and other systemic illnesses are also predisposing factors. Any interruption of skin integrity can lead to infection, especially with organisms that are part of the normal skin flora.

Other factors that increase the risk of infection include any illness that compromises skin integrity, such as diabetes mellitus; obesity; a previous history of cellulitis; peripheral vascular disease; tinea pedis; and alcohol abuse (Mayo Foundation for Medical Education and Research, 2006). Clients with **tinea pedis** (fungal infection of the feet) or lymphatic obstruction are most vulnerable to cellulitis and may experience recurrent infections over time.

Clinical Manifestations and Therapies

Clients with cellulitis experience a rapid onset and appear ill. Classic signs and symptoms include erythema, edema of the face or infected limb, warmth, and tenderness around the infected site (Figure 8–5 ■). Other symptoms include fever,

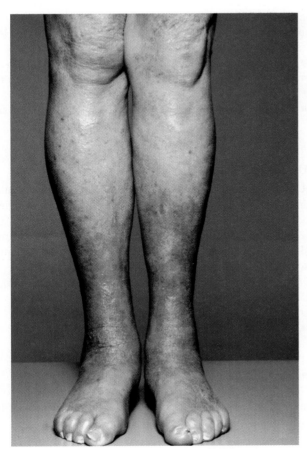

Figure 8–4 ■ Erysipelas, a superficial cellulitis of the skin caused by group A streptococcus.
© Custom Medical Stock Photography.

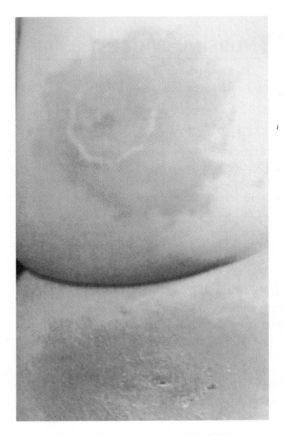

Figure 8–5 ■ Characteristic appearance of cellulitis.

CLINICAL MANIFESTATIONS AND THERAPIES

ETIOLOGY	CLINICAL MANIFESTATIONS	CLINICAL THERAPIES
Fever	Tachycardia, tachypnea, elevated temperature, lethargy	■ Maintain adequate hydration. ■ Administer antipyretics. ■ Treat underlying cause.
Skin inflammation	Redness, pain, warmth, edema	■ Administer antibiotics. ■ Maintain bedrest. ■ Provide adequate nutrition to promote healing. ■ Manage pain using both pharmacologic and nonpharmacologic therapies.
Septicemia	Whole-body inflammation manifested by fever, altered WBC count (may be high or low), and hemodynamic alterations (tachycardia, tachypnea, decreased cardiac output)	■ Monitor hemodynamic status. ■ Administer antibiotic therapy. ■ Provide fluid management. ■ Provide supportive care based on symptoms. ■ Measure vital signs frequently.

chills, malaise, and enlargement and tenderness of regional lymph nodes (also see the preceding Clinical Manifestations and Therapies). **Lymphangitis** (inflammation of a lymph vessel) may be present. In some cases, a rapidly progressive lesion can lead to septicemia.

NURSING PROCESS

The nurse plays an important role in assessing the status of the client and teaching self-care to prevent complications.

Assessment

Assessment centers on recognition of infection, documentation of location and related symptoms, and monitoring of vital signs. The nurse assesses the wound frequently (at least every 2 hours), including tracing along the border with a marker to allow for any change in size to be clearly recognized. In the event of change, the nurse places a new mark so that future care providers can clearly see if the wound enlarges.

Diagnosis

Nursing diagnoses that may be appropriate for a client with cellulitis include the following:

- Impaired skin integrity related to mechanical factors (injury, the inflammatory process, and presence of infection)
- Acute pain related to destruction of tissue due to infection
- Interrupted family processes related to home care needs of the child with acute illness

Planning

Planning care for the client with cellulitis is directed at pain management, client teaching related to self-care, and infection resolution without progression to systemic infection. Potential outcomes may include the following:

- Client will report pain of 3 or lower, on a scale of 1–10.
- Client will describe situations requiring contact with the provider.
- Client will explain how to take antibiotics and analgesics properly.

Implementation

Because of the risk of sepsis, cellulitis is managed carefully. Administer prescribed oral or intravenous antibiotics as scheduled. Supportive care includes warm compresses to the affected area four times daily, elevation of the affected limb, and bedrest. Outpatient follow-up is crucial to ensure positive response to therapy.

Advise clients about possible complications, such as abscess formation, and to contact their health care provider if any of the following signs develop:

- Spread of the infected area in the 24- to 48-hour period after the start of treatment
- Temperature over 38.3°C (101°F)
- Increased lethargy

Reinforce to clients and caregivers the importance of compliance with the treatment regimen and the seriousness of the possible complications.

NURSING CARE PLAN   A Client With Cellulitis

Maria Gonzalez is a 74-year-old widow who lives in an assisted living facility in a small town in central Pennsylvania. Her family includes three daughters and two sons who live out of state and a son who lives within 5 miles of Ms. Gonzalez's home. While visiting his mother, he notices a red area on her lower leg and asks her about it. She says it developed earlier today and is very painful. She's been treating it with wet compresses, but that does not seem to be helping much. Her son takes her to the local emergency department, where the nurse admits her to one of the examination rooms.

ASSESSMENT

Ms. Gonzalez speaks Spanish and is able to communicate only minimally in English. Her son acts as an interpreter when necessary. Ms. Gonzalez's history reveals diabetes mellitus with complications of peripheral vascular disease and neuropathy in the right leg, hypertension, coronary artery disease with angina, and cataracts in both eyes. She says she is allergic to penicillin and sulfa drugs. She denies ever having had a similar wound and describes the pain as a 7 on a 1–10 scale.

Physical examination of the painful right leg reveals an irregularly shaped, flat area that is red, warm, and painful, extending from just below the knee to mid-shin, and wrapping medially from midline to the back of the leg. The wound measures 6 in. by 5 in. at its widest point. Her vital signs are temperature 100.8°F oral, pulse 88 beats/min, respirations 16 breaths/min. and BP 122/74 mmHg.

The physician orders laboratory studies that reveal an elevated WBC count. Because of her age and medical history, the physician orders blood cultures and admits her to the facility for IV antibiotics and monitoring.

DIAGNOSES

- Altered skin integrity related to infectious process
- Acute pain related to the inflammatory process secondary to cellulitis
- Deficient knowledge of the cause of the skin disorder and recommended treatment
- Anxiety related to the need to be admitted to the hospital and inability to communicate with staff
- Impaired verbal communication related to the inability to speak English

EXPECTED OUTCOMES

- Skin will heal without evidence of a secondary infection or complication of sepsis.
- Client will obtain relief of pain with the proper use of medications.
- Client will verbalize an understanding of the disease process and participate in the treatment plan.
- Client will describe proper home care, including self-administration of medication after discharge.
- Client anxiety will be reduced after orientation to the hospital environment and speaking with staff members who also speak Spanish.
- Communication will be improved after assigning a Spanish-speaking nurse and using translation services in the hospital.

PLANNING AND CARING INTERVENTIONS

- Provide orientation to facility and treatment plan (IV therapy, warm soaks) in Spanish.
- Keep right leg elevated and explain the need to stay in bed.
- Trace outer border of wound with black marker and avoid washing off marks to allow for assessment every 2 hours. Report any increase in size to provider.
- Provide verbal and written instructions (in Spanish) for self-care after discharge, including the following:
  a. Take all antibiotics prescribed until they are gone.
  b. Take medications as prescribed for pain.
  c. Take the antibiotic for your wound every 6 hours, even during nighttime hours, for 10 days.
  d. Monitor the size of the wound and notify physician if there is any increase or if fever returns.
  e. Apply warm, moist heat to wound four times a day.
  f. Wash hands carefully before applying warm, moist compresses.
  g. Reduce activity to bathroom privileges only and keep right leg elevated.
  h. Monitor oral temperature and take two acetaminophen (Tylenol) for temperature higher than 100°F orally.

EVALUATION

Ms. Gonzalez's wound decreased in size over the next 48 hours. She was discharged with a prescription for antibiotics to be taken orally for 10 days and pain medication, although she reported that the pain was almost gone by the time she went home. Her fever subsided within 36 hours of beginning treatment. Mrs. Gonzalez will see her physician at the completion of oral antibiotics and says she will call the office sooner if the wound increases in size or her fever returns.

CRITICAL THINKING IN THE NURSING PROCESS

1. Identify barriers to care in this case. What nursing interventions can be initiated to overcome these barriers?
2. What further assessments and interventions might have been indicated had the wound shown little improvement or the pain remained severe?
3. If Ms. Gonzalez were unable to provide self-care after discharge, what options might the nurse have recommended for this client?

Evaluation

Outcomes developed in collaboration with the client will be evaluated to determine the client's progress. The nurse should trace the outer edges of the wound with a black marker to allow for better evaluation of changes in the size and area covered by the wound. The provider should be notified if the cellulitis enlarges or spreads.

COLLABORATION

Treatment of cellulitis is aimed at reducing the infection, promoting comfort, and preventing complications such as septicemia. Care is provided in collaboration with family members and other members of the health care team. Recovery from an extensive wound that impairs use of an extremity or limb for an extended period of time may require consultation with an occupational or respiratory therapist. If the face is involved, referral to a dentist may be necessary.

Diagnostic Tests

Blood studies may show an increase in WBCs. Cultures are taken to identify the causative organisms. Blood cultures are taken if the client has a toxic (very ill) appearance.

Clinical Therapy

If the face is involved, antibiotic therapy is administered to avoid serious complications such as periorbital cellulitis. Clients with severe cases or a large affected surface area are treated with systemic antibiotics and analgesics in the hospital to prevent sepsis. Clients with cellulitis on the trunk, limbs, or perianal area may be treated on an outpatient basis with oral antibiotics. Recovery begins within 48 hours, but therapy should continue for at least 10 days. Untreated cellulitis or cellulitis that does not respond to treatment can lead to osteomyelitis, arthritis, or serious systemic infection.

REVIEW **Cellulitis**

RELATE: LINK THE CONCEPTS

Linking the concept of Inflammation with the concept of Infection:
1. What role does inflammation play in cellulitis?

READY: GO TO COMPANION SKILLS MANUAL

1. Administering medication
2. Preventing skin breakdown
3. Preparing a client for discharge
4. Assessing body temperature
5. Physical assessment
6. Managing pain
7. Applying compresses and moist packs
8. Collecting a blood culture
9. Obtaining a wound drainage specimen

REFLECT: CASE STUDY

Norma James is a 65-year-old widow who lives alone. Although she has lived in the neighborhood for years, she is somewhat 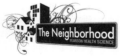 socially isolated. She has two adult sons with whom she has limited contact, because they live out of state and rarely call. She has only a few individuals she considers friends; she does not particularly like many people and prefers the company of her six cats.

Mrs. James has a long history of type 2 diabetes mellitus and hypertension. In more recent years, she has been diagnosed with atrial fibrillation. She has multiple physicians and takes multiple medications, including the following:

- Glucotrol: 10 mg, twice a day
- Captopril, 50 mg, twice a day
- Digoxin, 125 mcg, once a day
- Coumadin, 5 mg, once a day

Mrs. James has a known drug allergy to penicillin.

Mrs. James does not work; she has very limited savings and relies on Social Security benefits for income. She smokes about half a pack of cigarettes a day and has been a smoker since she was in her 20s. She drinks alcohol "a couple times a year, usually a glass of wine at a special dinner."

She does not drive and relies on her friends, neighbors, or the city bus for transportation. She lives near a grocery store and prides herself in being able to get most things she needs without assistance. She spends most of her time alone at home and occupies herself by watching television, reading, and doing crossword and jigsaw puzzles.

Mrs. James noticed a small, tender area on her upper thigh yesterday and, remembering what the cashier at the convenience store told her, decided to apply butter and put a bandage over it. This morning when she woke up, her leg was extremely painful, and the bandage she had applied over the tiny red spot yesterday was in the center of a large red spot that now covers her entire left thigh, front and back. She felt feverish and took her temperature, getting a reading of 101.4°F orally. She calls her doctor's office and is told that she needs to come right in, but she says she cannot do that; she does not feel well enough to take the bus, and all of her neighbors are at work right now. She says she will come to the doctor's office tomorrow when she feels better.

1. If you were the nurse speaking with Mrs. James, what would you say?
2. What options might you offer to get her to the health care facility—whether a provider's office or the local hospital?
3. What will likely happen if Mrs. James continues to refuse to be seen?

8.2 URINARY TRACT INFECTION

BASIS FOR SELECTION OF EXEMPLAR

Centers for Disease Control and Prevention (CDC)

Joint Commission (JCAHO)

Institute for Healthcare Improvement (IHI)

LEARNING OUTCOMES

After reading about this exemplar, you will be able to do the following:

1. Describe the pathophysiology, etiology, and clinical manifestations of urinary tract infection.

2. Identify the risk factors associated with urinary tract infection.

3. Illustrate the nursing process in providing culturally competent care across the life span for individuals with urinary tract infection.

4. Formulate priority nursing diagnoses appropriate for an individual with urinary tract infection.

5. Create a plan of care for an individual with urinary tract infection.

6. Employ evidence-based caring interventions (or prevention) for an individual with urinary tract infection.

7. Assess expected outcomes for an individual with urinary tract infection.

8. Describe therapies used in the collaborative care of an individual with urinary tract infection.

OVERVIEW

The urinary tract includes the kidneys, ureters, urinary bladder, and urethra. Any part of this system can be affected by pathogens. A severe infection may involve multiple components of the urinary tract. Kidney infections can affect urine production and waste elimination, resulting in renal failure (explained in the Fluids and Electrolytes concept). Infection can interrupt the **urinary drainage system** (those organs required to drain urine from the kidneys, including the ureters, urinary bladder, and urethra), obstructing urine flow and affecting elimination.

■ When caring for clients with urinary tract infections, it is important to consider the client's modesty in voiding, possible difficulty in discussing the genitals, potential embarrassment about being exposed for examination and testing, and fear of changes in body function. These psychosocial issues can interfere with the client's willingness to seek help, discuss treatment, and learn about preventive measures.

■ Nursing interventions for clients with urinary tract infections are directed toward primary prevention, early detection, and management of the disorder through health teaching and nursing care.

■ Bacterial infections of the urinary tract are a common reason for seeking health services, second only to upper respiratory infections. More than 8 million people are treated annually for urinary tract infection (UTI) (Porth, 2005). Community acquired UTIs are common in young women, but unusual in men under the age of 50.

■ Most community-acquired UTIs are caused by *Escherichia coli*, common Gram-negative enteral bacteria. Approximately 10–15% of symptomatic UTIs are caused by *Staphylococcus saprophyticus*, a Gram-positive organism. Catheter-associated UTIs often involve other Gram-negative bacteria, such as *Proteus*, *Klebsiella*, *Serratia*, and *Pseudomonas*.

PATHOPHYSIOLOGY AND ETIOLOGY

The urinary tract is normally sterile above the urethra. Adequate urine volume, a free flow from the kidneys through the urinary meatus, and complete bladder emptying are the most important mechanisms of maintaining sterility. Pathogens that enter and contaminate the distal urethra are washed out during voiding. Other defenses for maintaining sterile urine include the normal acidity of urine itself and the bacteriostatic properties of the bladder and urethral cells.

The peristaltic activity of the ureters and a competent vesicoureteral junction help to maintain sterility of the upper urinary tract. As the ureter enters the bladder, the distal portion tunnels between the mucosa and muscle layers of the bladder wall (Figure 8–6 ■). During voiding, increased intravesicular (within the bladder) pressure compresses the ureter, preventing **reflux**, or the backflow of urine toward the kidneys. In males, a long urethra and the antibacterial effect of zinc in prostatic fluid also help prevent contamination of this normally sterile environment.

UTIs can be bacterial, viral, or fungal, and may be categorized in several ways. Anatomically, UTIs may affect the lower or the upper urinary tract. Lower urinary tract infections include *urethritis*, inflammation of the urethra; *prostatitis*, inflammation of the prostate gland; and **cystitis**, inflammation of the urinary bladder. The most common upper urinary tract infection is pyelonephritis, inflammation of the kidney and renal pelvis. The infection can involve superficial tissues, such as the bladder mucosa, or invade other tissues, such as prostate or renal tissues.

Epidemiologically, UTIs are identified as community acquired or **nosocomial** (often associated with catheterization). UTIs can be further categorized as acute or chronic, with the latter being either recurrent or persistent.

Cystitis is the most common UTI. This infection tends to remain superficial, involving the bladder mucosa. The mucosa becomes hyperemic (red) and may hemorrhage. The inflammatory response causes pus to form, a process that causes the classic manifestations associated with cystitis.

Pyelonephritis is inflammation of the renal pelvis and parenchyma, the functional kidney tissue. *Acute pyelonephritis* is a bacterial infection of the kidney, and *chronic pyelonephritis* is associated with nonbacterial infections and inflammatory processes that can be metabolic, chemical, or immunologic in origin (see the Inflammation concept).

Acute pyelonephritis usually results from an infection that ascends to the kidney from the lower urinary tract.

Asymptomatic bacteriuria or cystitis can lead to acute pyelonephritis. Risk factors include pregnancy (due to slowed ureteral peristalsis), urinary tract obstruction, and congenital malformation. Urinary tract trauma, scarring, calculi (stones), kidney disorders such as polycystic or hypertensive kidney disease, and chronic diseases such as diabetes can also contribute to pyelonephritis. **Vesicoureteral reflux**, a condition in which urine moves from the bladder back toward the kidney, is a common risk factor in children who develop pyelonephritis that is also seen in adults when bladder outflow is obstructed.

The infection spreads from the renal pelvis to the renal cortex. The pelvis, calyces, and medulla of the kidney are primarily affected, with WBC infiltration and inflammation. The kidney becomes grossly edematous. Localized abscesses may develop on the cortical surface of the kidney. As with cystitis, *E. coli* is the organism responsible for 85% of the cases of acute pyelonephritis. Other organisms commonly found include *Proteus* and *Klebsiella*, bacteria that normally inhabit the intestinal tract.

The onset of acute pyelonephritis is typically rapid, with chills and fever, malaise, vomiting, flank pain, costovertebral tenderness, and urinary frequency. Symptoms of cystitis also may be present. The older adult may present with a change in behavior, acute confusion, incontinence, or a general deterioration in condition.

Etiology

UTIs are the second most common infections in children, after otitis media. An estimated 3% of girls and 1% of boys will have a UTI by age 11 years (National Kidney and Urological Diseases Information Clearinghouse, 2003). Most UTIs among newborns and young infants occur in boys, as obstructive structural defects that predispose infants to infection have a higher incidence in males. The incidence of UTIs in older infants and children is higher in girls because the shorter female urethra (2 cm [1 in.] in young girls) has closer proximity to the anus and vagina, increasing the risk of contamination by fecal bacteria.

Pathogens usually enter the urinary tract by ascending from the mucous membranes of the perineal area into the lower urinary tract. Bacteria that have colonized the urethra, vagina, or perineal tissues are the usual source of infection (Porth, 2005). From the bladder, bacteria can continue to ascend the urinary tract, eventually infecting the *parenchyma* (functional tissue) of the kidneys (Kasper et al., 2005). Hematogenous spread of infection to the urinary tract is rare; infections introduced in this manner are usually associated with previous damage or scarring of the urinary tract. Bacteria introduced into the urinary tract can cause asymptomatic bacteriuria or an inflammatory response with manifestations of UTI.

At least 10–15% of hospitalized clients with indwelling urinary catheters develop bacteriuria. The longer the catheter remains in place, the greater the risk for infection. Bacteria, including *E. coli*, *Proteus*, *Pseudomonas*, and *Klebsiella*, reach the bladder either by migrating through the column of urine

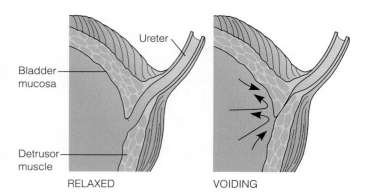

Figure 8–6 ■ A competent vesicoureteral junction. Note how increased intravesicular pressure during voiding occludes the distal portion of the ureter, preventing reflux.

within the catheter or moving up the mucous sheath of the urethra outside the catheter (Kasper et al., 2005). Bacteria enter the catheter system at the connection between the catheter and drainage system or through the emptying tube of the drainage bag. Colonization of perineal skin by bowel flora is a common source of infection in catheterized women.

Another cause of UTI is vesicoureteral reflux, the backflow of urine from the bladder into the ureters during voiding. Bacteria in the urine can be swept up to the kidneys, leading to pyelonephritis. Vesicoureteral reflux also prevents complete emptying of the bladder and, because urine returns to the bladder, it creates a reservoir for bacterial growth (Huether, 2006). Vesicoureteral reflux can also result from a structural anomaly in which the ureters insert into the bladder in an abnormal position.

Renal scarring can result from **hydronephrosis** (accumulation of urine in the renal pelvis as a result of obstructed outflow) or pyelonephritis, due to the inflammatory and ischemic effects of the infection. Scars have been associated with hypertension, proteinuria, and kidney failure. The risk of kidney damage increases in the following cases:

- UTI in an infant less than 1 year of age
- Delay in diagnosis and effective antibacterial treatment for an upper UTI
- Anatomic obstruction or nerve supply interruption
- Recurrent episodes of upper UTIs

Risk Factors

Clients can be predisposed to UTI by a variety of factors (Box 8–4). Some risk factors cannot be changed (e.g., aging and a female's short urethra). Cystitis occurs most frequently in adult females, usually because of colonization of the bladder by bacteria that are normally found in the lower gastrointestinal tract. These bacteria gain entry by ascending the short, straight female urethra. Wiping from back to front after urination can transfer bacteria from the anorectal area to the urethra.

In women, sexual activity increases the risk for UTI, because bacteria can be introduced into the bladder via the urethra during sexual intercourse. Use of spermicidal compounds with a diaphragm, cervical cap, or condom alters the normal bacterial flora of the vagina and perineal tissues and further increases the risk for UTI. Diaphragms are not recommended for women with a history of UTIs because pressure from the diaphragm on the urethra can interfere with complete bladder emptying and lead to recurrent UTIs.

Some females lack a normally protective mucosal enzyme and have decreased levels of cervicovaginal antibodies to enterobacteria, further increasing their risk. Personal hygiene practices and voluntary urinary retention can contribute to the risk for UTI in women. Up to three UTIs annually is considered to be within normal limits for sexually active women and does not usually warrant additional diagnostic tests beyond urine culture.

Prostatic hypertrophy and bacterial prostatitis are risk factors among males. Circumcision appears to have a protective effect. Anal intercourse also is a risk factor for men. In healthy adult men, UTIs are unusual and may prompt additional diagnostic testing.

Urinary stasis increases the risk of UTI. Stasis may be caused by abnormal anatomic structures or abnormal function (e.g., a **neurogenic bladder** in which an interrupted nerve supply from meningomyelocele or spinal cord trauma impairs bladder voiding function and leads to incomplete bladder emptying). Children typically void five to six times a day. Infrequent voiding, which is common in school-age children, results in incomplete emptying of the bladder and urinary stasis. Voluntarily suppressing the desire to urinate is a predisposing factor, as retention overdistends the bladder and can lead to an infection. Other factors associated with increased risk of UTI include an irritated perineum, uncircumcised male in the first 6 months of life, constipation, masturbation, sexual abuse, and sexual activity in adolescent females (Dulczak & Kirk, 2005).

Asymptomatic bacteriuria (ASB) (bacteria in the urine that actively multiply without accompanying clinical symptoms) is a condition that becomes significant if a woman is pregnant, because about 30% of pregnant women with untreated ASB will develop symptomatic UTIs (Smail, 2007). ASB is almost always caused by a single organism, typically E. coli. If more than one type of bacteria is cultured, the possibility of urine-culture contamination must be considered.

A woman who has had a UTI is susceptible to recurrent infection. If a pregnant woman develops an acute UTI, especially with a high temperature, amniotic fluid infection can develop and retard the growth of the placenta.

Box 8–4 **Risk Factors for UTI**

FEMALE
- Short, straight urethra
- Proximity of urinary meatus to vagina and anus
- Sexual intercourse
- Use of diaphragm and spermicidal compounds for birth control
- Pregnancy

MALE
- Uncircumcised
- Prostatic hypertrophy
- Anal intercourse

BOTH MALES AND FEMALES
- Aging
- Urinary tract obstruction
- Neurogenic bladder dysfunction
- Vesicoureteral reflux
- Genetic factors
- Catheterization

Source: LeMone, P., & Burke, K. (2008). *Medical-surgical nursing: Critical thinking in client care* (4th ed.). Upper Saddle River, NJ: Pearson Education.

Congenital and acquired factors that contribute to the risk of infection include urinary tract obstruction by tumors or calculi, structural abnormalities such as strictures, impaired bladder innervation, bowel incontinence, and chronic diseases such as diabetes mellitus. Instrumentation of the urinary tract (e.g., catheterization or cystoscopy) is a major risk factor for UTI. Even when performed under strict aseptic conditions, catheterization can result in bladder infection. Research indicates that the risk for catheter-associated UTI is reduced when anesthetic lubricating gels are inserted into the urethra prior to catheter insertion (Bardsley, 2005). The placement of the catheter prevents the flushing action of voiding, and bacteria can ascend to the bladder through the catheter lumen or via exudate between the urethral mucosa and the catheter.

Older clients have an increased incidence of UTI. The greatest increase is seen in men, as the ratio of female-to-male UTI in older adults changes from 50:1 to less than 5:1. Although the bacteriostatic effect of prostatic fluid and a longer urethra provide an effective barrier to bladder infection for adult males, the hypertrophy of the prostate that is commonly associated with aging increases the risk of cystitis in older males. An enlarged prostate can impede urine flow, leading to incomplete bladder emptying and urinary stasis. Bacteria are not completely flushed with voiding, allowing colonization of the bladder. An increased risk of urinary stasis, chronic disease states (such as diabetes mellitus), and an impaired immune response also contribute to the higher incidence of UTI in older adults. In older women, loss of tissue elasticity and weakening of perineal muscles often contribute to the development of a cystocele or rectocele. Resulting changes in bladder and urethral position increase the risk of incomplete bladder emptying.

The risk for UTI increases during pregnancy, particularly during the second trimester, secondary to the pressure of the fetus, which causes urinary stasis and incomplete bladder emptying. The diagnosis of UTI in the pregnant client carries significant risks for the mother and fetus. UTIs are associated with an increased risk of preeclampsia (Conde-Agudelo, Villar, & Lindheimer, 2008). An increased risk of premature birth and intrauterine growth restriction is associated with acute pyelonephritis, which is often caused by asymptomatic bacteriuria (ASB). Although the exact cause is unknown, there is an increased risk of premature rupture of membranes associated with UTI. If urine stasis exists, the risk of UTI increases, because of bacteriuria and the presence of dilated ureters and renal pelves, which persist for about 6 weeks after delivery.

The postpartal woman is at increased risk of developing urinary tract problems caused by the normal postpartal diuresis, increased bladder capacity, and decreased bladder sensitivity from stretching or trauma. Possible inhibited neural control of the bladder following the use of general or regional anesthesia and contamination from catheterization also put the postpartal woman at risk for UTIs. These factors make it essential that the mother empty her bladder completely with each voiding. UTI in the newborn predisposes the neonate to hyperbilirubinemia (elevated serum bilirubin).

Clinical Manifestations and Therapies

The symptoms of UTI depend on the infection's location as well as the client's age. Symptoms in a newborn tend to be nonspecific—unexplained fever, failure to thrive, poor feeding, vomiting and diarrhea, strong-smelling urine, and irritability. Any child younger than 2 years of age with a fever of unknown origin should be tested for a UTI. The more "classic" symptoms of lower UTI are not seen until the toddler years, as shown in the following Clinical Manifestations and Therapies. Approximately 40% of UTIs are asymptomatic.

Typical presenting symptoms of cystitis include **dysuria** (painful or difficult urination), urinary frequency and **urgency** (a sudden, compelling need to urinate), and **nocturia** (voiding two or more times at night). In addition, the urine may have a foul odor and appear cloudy (**pyuria**) or bloody (**hematuria**) because of mucus, excess white cells in the urine, and bleeding of the inflamed bladder wall. Suprapubic pain and tenderness also may be present. See Box 8–5 for manifestations of cystitis.

Older clients may not experience the classic symptoms of cystitis. Instead, they often present with nonspecific manifestations, such as nocturia, incontinence, confusion, behavior change, lethargy, loss of appetite, or "just not feeling right." Fever may be present; however, hypothermia also may develop in an older adult. Particularly in a long-term care setting, a change in behavior may be the only indicator of a UTI (Bentley et al., 2001). This can be frustrating for the family members and health care team, who may easily suspect any number of other possible causes when an older adult presents with these symptoms.

The symptoms usually seen in younger adults with UTIs—urgency and frequency—are common age-related changes in the older adult and therefore lack diagnostic usefulness. If, however, an older adult has not previously experienced urinary urgency, and presents with a shortened period of time between the urge to void and actual urination, or urinary frequency of more than seven voids per 24-hour period, his or her symptoms should be thoroughly investigated.

The majority of UTIs in older adults are asymptomatic (Nicolle, 2003). Some authors term this condition *asymptomatic UTI*, whereas others apply the term *UTI* only to those older adults with symptoms, and use *bacteriuria* to define the presence of bacteria in the urine with no concomitant symptoms (Nicolle, 2003). Asymptomatic UTI does not require treatment. In fact, treatment does not improve the morbidity or

---

Box 8–5 **Manifestations of Cystitis**

- Dysuria
- Pyuria
- Frequency
- Hematuria
- Urgency
- Suprapubic discomfort
- Nocturia

Source: LeMone, P., & Burke, K. (2008). *Medical-surgical nursing: Critical thinking in client care* (4th ed.). Upper Saddle River, NJ: Pearson Education.

CLINICAL MANIFESTATIONS AND THERAPIES

ETIOLOGY	CLINICAL MANIFESTATION	CLINICAL THERAPY
Lower UTI—cystitis	Frequency, dysuria, urgency, enuresis, strong-smelling urine, cloudy urine, hematuria, abdominal or suprapubic pain	Administer 5- to 7-day course of trimethoprim or sulfamethoxazole or antibiotic matching organism sensitivity, encourage oral fluids, administer analgesic such as acetaminophen or Pyridium.
Upper UTI—pyelonephritis	High fever, chills, abdominal pain, flank pain, costovertebral angle tenderness, persistent vomiting, moderate to severe dehydration Infants may have nonspecific signs such as poor appetite, failure to thrive, lethargy, irritability. Older children may have signs of cystitis.	Administer antipyretics and intravenous antibiotics initially, and then transition to oral antibiotics matching organism sensitivity for a total of 7–10 days. Rehydration is essential.

mortality in affected older persons (Gandhi, 2006; Krogh & Bruskewitz, 1998; McCue, 1999; Nicolle, 2003; Steers, 1999). Routine urinalysis for older adults without symptoms is neither appropriate nor cost effective.

Cystitis is usually uncomplicated and readily responds to treatment. When left untreated, the infection can ascend to involve the kidneys. Severe or prolonged infection can lead to sloughing of bladder mucosa and ulcer formation. Chronic cystitis can lead to bladder stones.

Catheter-associated UTIs often are asymptomatic. Gram-negative bacteremia is the most significant complication associated with these UTIs. Most catheter-associated UTIs resolve quickly when the catheter is removed and a short course of antibiotic is administered. Intermittent catheterization carries a lower risk of infection than does an indwelling catheter, and is preferred for clients who are unable to empty their bladder by voiding. UTIs in catheterized older adults tend to be polymicrobial and difficult to eradicate. Before an indwelling catheter is used, the potential benefits to the older adult must be carefully weighed against the serious risks posed.

Instillation of anesthetic lubricating gel into the urethra prior to catheter insertion further reduces the risk by dilating the urethra and reducing trauma to fragile urethral tissues (Bardsley, 2005).

NURSING PROCESS

The nursing process for UTI generally focuses on returning the client to maximum health. In order to maintain optimum urinary health, nurses should be alert for opportunities to provide health promotion. Teach measures to prevent UTI to all clients, particularly to young, sexually active women. Encourage clients to maintain a generous fluid intake of 2.0–2.5 quarts per day, increasing intake during hot weather and strenuous activity. Discuss the need to avoid voluntary urinary retention, emptying the bladder every 3–4 hours. Instruct women to cleanse the perineal area from front to back after voiding and defecating. Teach to void before and after sexual intercourse to flush out bacteria introduced into the urethra and bladder. Teach measures to maintain the integrity of perineal tissues, such as avoiding bubble baths, feminine hygiene sprays, and vaginal douches; wearing cotton briefs; and avoiding synthetic materials. Unless contraindicated, suggest the following measures to maintain acid urine: Drink two glasses of low-sugar cranberry juice daily, take ascorbic acid (vitamin C), and avoid excess intake of milk and milk products, other fruit juices, and sodium bicarbonate (baking soda).

Assessment

Focused assessment data for the client with a suspected UTI includes the following:

- *Health history:* Current symptoms, including frequency, urgency, burning on urination, and number of voidings per night; color, clarity, and odor of urine; other manifestations, such as lower abdominal, back, or flank pain, nausea or vomiting, or fever; duration of symptoms and any treatment attempted; history of previous UTIs and their frequency; possibility of pregnancy and type of birth control used; chronic diseases such as diabetes; current medications; and any known allergies.
- *Physical examination:* General health; vital signs including temperature; abdominal shape, contour, and tenderness to palpation (especially suprapubic); and percuss for costovertebral tenderness.

Nursing assessment for a child with a suspected UTI involves assessing the infant or child for signs of acute or chronic illness, examining the genitourinary system, and collecting a urine specimen for culture. Assess the infant for toxic (very ill) appearance, fever, and oral fluid intake. Evaluate the child's oral fluid intake. Assess for quality, quantity, and frequency of voiding. Measure the child's height and weight, and plot the data on a growth curve to identify any change in growth pattern associated with a chronic illness. Take the infant's or child's blood pressure. Palpate the abdomen and suprapubic and costovertebral areas for masses, tenderness, and distention.

Sexually active adolescents may deny having symptoms for fear of disclosing their sexual activity to their parents. Careful questioning may be necessary to elicit a response despite these concerns. The nurse should be open and approachable, and give the client and family the chance to address their concerns.

Diagnosis

Priority nursing diagnoses focus on comfort, urinary elimination, and teaching/learning needs and may include the following:

- Acute pain related to dysuria, systemic discomforts, or renal pain secondary to upper UTI
- Impaired urinary elimination related to UTI
- Deficient knowledge related to self-care, medication administration, and/or knowledge of preventative measures
- Risk for disproportionate growth (pediatric clients) related to chronic infection and renal damage
- Urinary retention related to infrequent voiding habits or vesicoureteral reflux
- Risk for deficient fluid volume related to fever and inadequate intake
- Fear related to the possible long-term effects of the disease

Planning

The client's general health, abilities for self-care, and risk factors that may contribute to UTI are considered when planning and implementing nursing care for the client with a UTI. Outcomes, developed in collaboration with the client, may include the following:

- Describes pain as a 3 or lower on a 1–10 scale.
- Regains normal voiding pattern and produces normal urine without blood, bacteria, or protein.
- Verbalizes understanding of disease process, proper method of taking medications, and required follow-up care.
- Provides strategies for reducing the risk of another UTI.

Implementation

Nursing care for the hospitalized client with a complicated UTI focuses on administering prescribed medications, promoting rehydration, assessing renal function, and teaching the client and family how to minimize the risk of future infection.

Pain

Pain is a common manifestation of both lower and upper UTIs. Urinary tract pain is caused primarily by distention and increased pressure within the urinary tract. The severity of the pain is related to the rate at which inflammation and distention develop, not their degree.

> **PRACTICE ALERT**
> The older adult with a UTI may not complain of dysuria. Be alert for other manifestations of UTI, such as incontinence or cloudy or malodorous urine. Inflammatory and immune responses tend to diminish with aging, reducing the irritative symptoms of UTI.

In cystitis, inflammation causes a sensation of fullness; dull, constant suprapubic pain; and possibly low back pain. The inflamed bladder wall and urethra cause dysuria, pain, and burning on urination. Bladder spasms may develop, causing periodic severe, stabbing discomfort. Pain associated with pyelonephritis is often steady and dull, localized to the outer abdomen or flank region. Urologic disorders rarely cause central abdominal pain.

Nursing interventions for the client experiencing pain include the following:

- Assess pain: timing, quality, intensity, location, duration, and aggravating and alleviating factors. A change in the nature, location, or intensity of the pain could indicate an extension of the infection or a related but separate problem.
- Teach or provide comfort measures, such as warm sitz baths, warm packs or heating pads, and balanced rest and activity. Systemic analgesics, urinary analgesics, or antispasmodic medication should be used as ordered. Warmth relaxes muscles, relieves spasms, and increases local blood supply. Because pain can stimulate a stress response and delay healing, it should be relieved when possible.
- Increase fluid intake unless contraindicated. Increased fluid dilutes urine, reducing irritation of the inflamed bladder and urethral mucosa.
- Instruct the client to notify the primary care provider if pain and discomfort continue or intensify after therapy is initiated. Pain and discomfort in voiding typically are relieved within 24 hours of initiating antibiotic therapy. Continued discomfort may indicate a complicated UTI or other urinary tract disorder.

Impaired Urinary Elimination

Inflammation of the bladder and urethral mucosa affects the normal process and patterns of voiding, causing frequency, urgency, and burning on urination, as well as nocturia. Urine may be blood tinged, cloudy, and malodorous. The client with short- or long-term urinary retention requires additional measures to assess for and prevent UTI.

Because bladder training is such an important milestone for young children, any disorder that affects voiding can have developmental implications. A toddler who has been toilet trained may regress and require diapers temporarily due to incontinence related to the UTI. An older child may develop **enuresis** (the involuntary passage of urine after control has been established) after a prolonged period of being dry at night. A preschooler may perceive the infection as punishment for an imagined wrong, such as masturbation. Reassure parents that this temporary period of urinary incontinence is normal when associated with UTI and emphasize that they should offer the child support rather than disapproval.

> **PRACTICE ALERT**
> Nurses who work with clients in hospitals and other institutional settings should provide easy access to a bedpan, urinal, commode, or bathroom. Make sure that lighting is adequate and that pathways are free from obstacles for clients getting up to use the bathroom. Frequency, urgency, and nocturia increase the risk of urinary incontinence and injury due to falls, particularly in older or debilitated clients.

PRACTICE ALERT

Unless contraindicated, instillation of an anesthetic lubricating gel into the urethra (10 mL for a male and 6 mL for a female) promotes comfort during the procedure, protects fragile urethral tissues from trauma, and reduces the risk for catheter-associated UTI (Bardsley, 2005).

Nursing interventions for clients with impaired urinary elimination include the following:

- Monitor (or instruct the client to monitor) color, clarity, and odor of urine. Urine should return to clear yellow within 48 hours, unless drug therapy causes a change in the color of urine. If clarity does not return, further investigation may be necessary.
- Instruct clients with impaired urinary elimination to avoid caffeinated drinks, including coffee, tea, and cola; citrus juices; drinks containing artificial sweeteners; and alcoholic beverages. Caffeine, citrus juices, and artificial sweeteners irritate bladder mucosa and the detrusor muscle, and can increase urgency and bladder spasms.
- Use strict aseptic technique and a closed urinary drainage system when inserting a straight or indwelling urinary catheter. Insert indwelling catheters to the full recommended length (4 inches or more in women and to the bifurcation in men) before inflating the balloon. Bacteria colonizing the perineal tissues or on the nurse's hands can be introduced into the bladder during catheterization. Aseptic technique reduces this risk. Inflating the balloon while it is in the urethra damages urethral tissues and can cause significant discomfort for the client.
- When possible, use intermittent straight catheterization to relieve urinary retention. Remove indwelling urinary catheters as soon as possible. Using intermittent straight catheterization allows the bladder to fill and completely empty in a more normal manner, maintaining physiologic function. The risk of infection associated with an indwelling catheter is about 3–5% per day of catheterization (Kasper et al., 2005).
- Maintain the closed urinary drainage system, and use aseptic technique when emptying the catheter drainage bag. Maintain gravity flow to prevent reflux of urine into the bladder from the drainage system. Bacteria can enter the drainage system when its integrity is interrupted (e.g., disconnecting the catheter from the drainage system) or during emptying of the drainage bag. These bacteria can ascend the column of urine to the bladder, causing UTI.
- Provide perineal care on a regular basis and following defecation. Use antiseptic preparations only as ordered. Regular cleansing of perineal tissues reduces the risk of colonization by bowel or other bacteria. Although antiseptic solutions may be ordered for catheter care, they can dry perineal tissues and reduce normal flora, increasing the risk of colonization by pathogens, and should not be used routinely.

Ineffective Health Maintenance

Because clients with UTIs are at increased risk for future UTIs, they need to understand the disease process, risk factors, measures to prevent recurrent infection, diagnostic procedures, and best practices for home care. In addition, clients need to understand that, even when the manifestations of UTI are relieved, the treatment plan needs to continue. Failure to complete the full course of therapy and recommended follow-up can lead to continued bacteriuria and recurrent infections.

 EVIDENCE-BASED PRACTICE   Male Catheterization

Insertion of an indwelling (retention) catheter is a commonly performed procedure in hospitals and long-term care facilities. Although the location of the female urethral meatus presents a challenge to maintaining catheter sterility during insertion, the anatomy of the male urethra presents a different set of challenges. Little research is available to support evidence-based practice for male urethral catheterization. In addition, reports of urethral injury in men related to catheter insertion and balloon inflation are not uncommon.

A multidisciplinary team of researchers at the University of Colorado Hospital conducted a study to determine the correct urethral catheter placement in male adults (Daneshgari, Krugman, Bahn, & Lee, 2002). Their research showed that inserting the catheter to the bifurcation (attachment of the arm for balloon inflation) always placed the retention balloon well within the urinary bladder prior to its inflation. Insertion to any lesser distance was inadequate to ensure safe balloon inflation without potential damage to the urethra.

Implications for Nursing

Nursing fundamentals and skills texts recommend inserting the retention catheter from 6–10 inches into the male urethra before inflating the balloon. Some texts recommend inserting the catheter 1–2 inches beyond the point at which urine is obtained before inflating the balloon. This study (Daneshgari et al., 2002) showed that these recommendations could result in an attempt to inflate the balloon while that portion of the catheter is still in the urethra, not fully into the bladder. To ensure safe practice and reduce the risk for injury and discomfort, insert a retention catheter to the bifurcation before inflating the balloon.

Critical Thinking in Client Care

1. Why is insertion of a urinary catheter frequently a more uncomfortable and difficult procedure for a male client than a female client? What nursing measures or techniques can be used to reduce this discomfort?
2. Sterile technique generally is used when catheterizing clients in acute care settings. However, clients who require intermittent catheterization to empty their bladder typically use clean technique. Would clean technique be appropriate in an acute or long-term care setting? Why or why not?

Source: Daneshgari, F., Krugman, A., Bahn, A., & Lee, R. S. (2002). Evidence-based multidisciplinary practice: Improving the safety and standards of male bladder catheterization. *Medsurg Nursing, 11*(5), 236–241, 246.

NURSING CARE PLAN A Client With Cystitis

Miija Waisanen is a 25-year-old second-year nursing student. She was recently married, and she and her husband live in an apartment near the college she attends. Mrs. Waisanen has never been pregnant, and she is using a diaphragm for birth control. She presents at the local urgent care clinic complaining of low back pain, frequency, urgency, and burning on urination, which began the day before.

ASSESSMENT

Patrice Ramiros, RN, admits Mrs. Waisanen to the clinic. Mrs. Waisanen denies having had similar symptoms in the past or ever having been diagnosed with a urinary tract infection. She describes her pain as a constant, dull ache that does not change with movement. She feels the need to urinate almost constantly, but experiences difficulty in starting her stream, and burning pain, and cramping when voiding. She reports getting up four times the night before to urinate. She denies painful intercourse and states that her last menstrual period began only 2 weeks ago. Physical examination reveals: BP 112/68 mmHg; pulse 90 beats/min and regular, and afebrile. Suprapubic tenderness is noted, but there is no flank or costovertebral angle tenderness. Clean-catch urine specimen shows hematuria, multiple WBCs, and a bacteria count greater than 10^5 /mL.

The nurse practitioner prescribes trimethoprim-sulfamethoxazole (TMP-SMZ) 160 mg/800 mg po two times a day for 3 days, and aspirin or acetaminophen gr × po every 4 hours as needed for pain. Mrs. Waisanen is instructed to return to the clinic in 7 days for a follow-up urine culture, or sooner if her symptoms do not improve.

DIAGNOSES

- Pain related to infection and inflammatory process in the urinary tract
- Impaired urinary elimination related to inflammation, as evidenced by frequency, urgency, nocturia, and dysuria
- Deficient knowledge related to lack of information about risk factors for UTI

EXPECTED OUTCOMES

- Client reports relief of low back pain and burning on urination.
- Client reports a normal voiding pattern without frequency, urgency, nocturia, and abnormal urine characteristics.
- Client verbalizes understanding of the disease process, related risk factors, follow-up instructions, and symptoms of recurrence that indicate the need for medical attention.

PLANNING AND IMPLEMENTATION

- Teach comfort measures: warm sitz baths, a heating pad on low heat applied to the lower back or abdomen, rest, increased fluid intake, avoiding caffeinated beverages, and aspirin or acetaminophen as ordered.
- Advise client to refrain from sexual intercourse until infection and inflammation have cleared to avoid further irritation of inflamed tissues.
- Discuss the possible relationship between using a diaphragm for birth control and UTIs in women.
- Discuss dietary and hygiene practices to prevent UTI symptoms.
- Discuss symptoms indicating the need for further intervention and the risks of undertreatment.

EVALUATION

Six months later, Mrs. Waisanen rotates through the urgent care clinic for her community-based nursing experience. When Ms. Ramiros asks how she is doing, Mrs. Waisanen reports that her symptoms and urine cleared within about a day after starting the antibiotic, and she has had no further problems. She has seen her women's health care nurse practitioner to change her birth control to oral contraceptives, increased her intake of fluid and vitamin C, and no longer puts off urinating until she "has time to go!"

CRITICAL THINKING IN THE NURSING PROCESS

1. What physiologic and psychosocial factors put Mrs. Waisanen at risk for UTI?
2. Compare the benefits and drawbacks to short-course therapy versus conventional therapy for UTI.
3. Why was it appropriate for the nurse practitioner to use short-course therapy with the advice to return if symptoms did not clear?
4. Develop a care plan for Mrs. Waisanen for the nursing diagnosis Ineffective Health Maintenance.

Nurses who work with clients with ineffective health maintenance should do the following:

- Teach clients how to obtain a midstream clean-catch urine specimen. Cleansing of the urinary meatus and perineal area reduces contamination of the specimen by external cells and bacteria. Ninety percent of urethral bacteria are cleared in the first 10 mL of voided urine, so a midstream specimen is representative of urine in the bladder.

- Assess knowledge about the disease process, risk factors, and preventive measures. The client may have little understanding of UTI, its causes, and contributing factors.
- Discuss the prescribed treatment plan and the importance of taking all prescribed antibiotics.
- Help the client develop a plan for taking medications, such as taking them with meals (unless contraindicated) or setting out all doses for the day in the morning. Missed

doses of antibiotic can result in subtherapeutic blood levels and reduced effectiveness. Taking medication in association with a regular daily activity such as meals helps clients remember doses.

■ Instruct clients to keep appointments for follow-up and urine culture. Follow-up urine culture, often scheduled 7–14 days after completion of antibiotic therapy, is vital to ensure complete eradication of bacteria and prevent relapse or recurrence.

■ Teach measures to prevent future UTI, as discussed at the beginning of this exemplar. Keeping urine dilute and acidic and voiding regularly help to flush bacteria out of the bladder and urethra. The proximity of the female urethral meatus to the vagina and anus increases the risk of bacterial contamination, especially during intercourse. Bubble baths, feminine hygiene sprays, synthetic fibers, and douches can dry and irritate perineal tissues, promoting bacterial growth.

See Box 8–6 for information about avoiding cystitis for women.

Evaluation

The outcome of treatment for UTI may be determined by follow-up urinalysis and culture. Cure, as evidenced by the absence of pathogens in the urine, is the desired outcome. When therapy fails to eradicate bacteria in the urine, it is known as **unresolved bacteriuria**. **Persistent bacteriuria**, or *relapse*, occurs when a persistent source of infection causes repeated infection after the initial cure. **Reinfection** is the development of a new infection with a different pathogen following successful UTI treatment (Tierney, McPhee, & Papadakis, 2005). Clients are generally required to submit a urinalysis for culture 7–10 days after completing a course of antibiotics to ensure that bacteria have been eliminated.

Box 8–6 Key Facts to Remember

Information for Women About Ways to Avoid Cystitis

■ If you use a diaphragm for contraception, try changing methods or using another size of diaphragm.

■ Avoid bladder irritants such as alcohol, caffeine products, and carbonated beverages.

■ Increase fluid intake, especially water, to a minimum of six to eight glasses per day.

■ Make regular urination a habit; avoid long waits.

■ Practice good genital hygiene, including wiping from front to back after urination and bowel movements.

■ Be aware that vigorous or frequent sexual activity may contribute to UTI.

■ Urinate before and after intercourse to empty the bladder and cleanse the urethra.

■ Complete medication regimens even if symptoms decrease.

■ Do not use medication left over from previous infections.

■ Drink cranberry juice to acidify the urine. This has been found to relieve symptoms in some cases.

Source: Ball, J. W., Bindler, R. M. W., Cowen, K. J. (2010). *Child health nursing: Partnering with children and families* (2nd ed., p. 129). Upper Saddle River, NJ: Pearson Education.

Expected outcomes of nursing care include the following:

■ The client increases fluid intake and number of voidings each day.

■ Client completes prescribed course of antibiotic therapy.

■ Urine is free from bacteria following treatment.

■ Client experiences no recurrent UTIs for 1 year.

■ Client incorporates preventative self-care measures into daily regimen.

COLLABORATION

Collaborative treatment of UTI focuses on eliminating the causative organism, preventing relapse or reinfection, and identifying and correcting any contributing factors. Drug treatment with antibiotics and urinary anti-infectives is commonly used. In some cases, surgery may be indicated to correct contributing factors.

Diagnostic Tests

■ Urinalysis to assess for pyuria, bacteria, and blood cells in the urine. A bacteria count greater than 100,000 (10^5) per milliliter is indicative of infection. Rapid tests for bacteria in the urine include using a *nitrite dipstick* (which turns pink in the presence of bacteria) and the *leukocyte esterase test*, an indirect method of detecting bacteria by identifying lysed or intact WBCs in the urine.

■ Urine should be a midstream clean-catch specimen; if necessary, straight catheterization or "mini-cath," with strict aseptic technique, may be used. Catheterization is avoided if possible to reduce the risk of further infection. Routine urinalysis for older adults without symptoms is neither appropriate nor cost effective.

PRACTICE ALERT

Urine obtained from infants using urine collection bags may be used for urinalysis and to screen for UTI, but the specimen collection procedure is not sterile. Confirmation of a UTI must be made with urine collected by a clean-catch or catheterization procedure (Raszka & Khan, 2005).

■ **Gram stain** of the urine may be done to identify the infecting organism by shape and characteristic (Gram-positive or Gram-negative).

■ Urine culture and sensitivity tests may be ordered to identify the infecting organism and the most effective antibiotic. Culture requires 24–72 hours, so treatment to eliminate the most common organisms often is initiated without culture.

EVIDENCE-BASED PRACTICE

Cleansing with nonsterile gauze, moistened with tap water and soap, is as effective for clean-catch specimen collection as prepackaged sterile towelettes, and is gentler to the mucous membranes (Ünlü, Sardan, & Ülker, 2007).

CARE SETTINGS Community-Based Care for Prevention of UTIs

Because both upper and lower urinary tract infections are usually managed in the community, teaching is the most important nursing intervention. Provide instruction on the following topics:

- Risk factors for UTI and how to minimize or eliminate these factors through increased fluid intake, regular elimination, and personal hygiene measures
- Early manifestations of UTI and the importance of seeking medical intervention promptly
- Maintaining optimal immune system function by attending to physical and psychosocial stressors, such as lack of adequate rest, poor nutrition, and high levels of emotional stress
- The importance of completing the prescribed treatment and keeping follow-up appointments

- Minimizing the risk of UTI when an indwelling urinary catheter is necessary:
  a. Use alternatives to an indwelling catheter when possible. For urinary incontinence, try scheduled toileting, incontinence pads or diapers, and external catheters if possible. For urinary retention, teach the client or a family member to perform straight catheterization every 3–4 hours using clean technique.
  b. When an indwelling catheter is necessary, teach care measures such as perineal care, managing and emptying the collection chamber, maintaining a closed system, and bladder irrigation or flushing if ordered.

Urine cultures do not distinguish between upper and lower UTIs (Raszka & Khan, 2005). UTI in an older person with an indwelling catheter is considered to be complicated and may include a variety of microorganisms.

PRACTICE ALERT

Urine specimens collected for culture must be delivered to the laboratory within 1 hour or the specimen must be refrigerated to prevent the growth of organisms that occur with prolonged room temperature exposure.

- WBC with differential may be done to detect the typical changes associated with infection, such as leukocytosis (elevated WBC) and increased numbers of neutrophils.

In clients with recurrent infections or persistent bacteriuria, additional diagnostic testing may be ordered to evaluate for structural abnormalities, renal scarring, and other contributing factors. These tests include the following:

- **Intravenous pyelography (IVP)**, also known as *excretory urography,* is used to evaluate the structure and excretory function of the kidneys, ureters, and bladder. As the kidneys clear an intravenously injected contrast medium from the blood, the size and shape of the kidneys, their calyces and pelvises, the ureters, and the bladder can be evaluated, and structural or functional abnormalities, such as vesicoureteral reflux, can be detected.

- **Voiding cystourethrography** involves instilling contrast medium into the bladder, and then using x-rays to assess the bladder and urethra when filled and during voiding. This study can detect structural and functional abnormalities of the bladder and urethral strictures. This test has a lower risk of allergic response to the contrast dye than IVP.

- **Cystoscopy**, direct visualization of the urethra and bladder through a cystoscope, can be used to diagnose conditions such as prostatic hypertrophy, urethral strictures, bladder calculi, tumors, polyps, diverticula, and congenital abnormalities. A

tissue biopsy may be obtained during the procedure, and other interventions may be performed (e.g., stone removal or stricture dilation).

- *Manual pelvic* or *prostate examinations* are done to assess for structural changes of the genitourinary tract, such as prostatic enlargement, cystocele, or rectocele.

- *Renal and bladder ultrasound and DMSA scanning* are used to detect pyelonephritis and renal scarring (Dulczak & Kirk, 2005).

Pharmacologic Therapy

Most uncomplicated infections of the lower urinary tract can be treated with a short course of antibiotic therapy. Upper urinary tract infections, in contrast, usually require longer treatment (2 or more weeks) to eradicate the infecting organism. Treatment should be initiated as soon as the diagnosis of UTI is made.

Antibiotics are selected based on the age of the client, sensitivity of the cultured organism, renal function, and the client's signs and symptoms. Gender is a consideration in treatment choices, because men require longer periods of treatment than women. The longer urethra in men makes it less likely that bacteria can ascend into the bladder. When bacteria do reach the older man's bladder, the infection is considered to be complicated and requires a longer course of treatment. The antibiotic is changed if necessary after culture sensitivity is determined.

Follow-up cultures may be obtained 48–72 hours after drug therapy is started in the pediatric client who is still febrile (Raszka & Khan, 2005). Children with pyelonephritis should be maintained on antibiotic prophylaxis until radiologic tests are performed to detect any structural defects.

Short-course therapy (either a single antibiotic dose or a 3-day course of treatment) reduces treatment cost, increases compliance, and has a lower rate of side effects. Single-dose therapy is associated with a higher rate of recurrent infection and continued vaginal colonization with *E. coli*, making a

EVIDENCE-BASED PRACTICE VUR and Prophylactic Antibiotics

A randomized control trial of 218 children, ages 3 months to 18 years, who were diagnosed with pyelonephritis and mild or moderate vesicoureteral reflux (VUR), evaluated the effect of prophylactic antibiotics on outcomes. One-half of the children received antibiotics, and the remainder did not. Children were seen every 3 months for the year of the study, and each had a urine culture at each visit.

Results indicated that the presence of mild or moderate VUR did not increase the incidence of UTI, pyelonephritis, or renal scarring following an acute episode of pyelonephritis. The children who did not receive prophylactic antibiotics had no more infections or renal scarring than the children who did receive antibiotics (Garin, Olavarria, Nieto et al., 2006).

3-day course of treatment the preferred option for uncomplicated cystitis. Oral TMP-SMZ, TMP, or a quinolone antibiotic such as ciprofloxacin (Cipro) or enoxacin (Penetrex) may be ordered.

Men and women with pyelonephritis, urinary tract abnormalities or stones, or a history of previous infections with antibiotic-resistant infections require a 7- to 10-day course of TMP-SMZ, ciprofloxacin, ofloxacin (Floxin), or an alternative antibiotic. The client with severe illness may need hospitalization. Intravenous ciprofloxacin, gentamicin, ceftriaxone (Rocephin), or ampicillin may be prescribed for severe illness or sepsis associated with UTI.

Children who appear ill and cannot tolerate oral antibiotics are often hospitalized because they need rehydration and parenteral antibiotic treatment until they have been afebrile for 24 hours. Infants can develop permanent kidney damage or generalized sepsis if the UTI is not treated aggressively. If a structural defect is identified, surgical correction may be necessary to prevent recurrent infections that could lead to renal damage.

Clients who experience frequent symptomatic UTIs may be treated with prophylactic antibiotic therapy. Drugs such as TMP-SMZ, TMP, and nitrofurantoin (Furadantin, Macrodantin, Macrobid) do not achieve effective plasma concentrations at recommended doses, but do reach effective concentrations in the urine. Nitrofurantoin also may be used to treat UTI in pregnant women.

Antibiotics and urinary anti-infectives generally are not recommended to treat asymptomatic bacteriuria in catheterized clients. The preferred treatment for catheter-associated UTI is removal of the indwelling catheter, followed by a 10- to 14-day course of antibiotic therapy to eliminate the infection.

Surgery

Surgery may be indicated for recurrent UTI if diagnostic testing indicates calculi, structural anomalies, or strictures that contribute to the risk of infection. Stones, or *calculi,* in the renal pelvis or bladder are an irritant and provide a matrix for bacterial colonization. Treatment may include surgical removal of a large calculus from the renal pelvis or cystoscopic removal of bladder calculi. *Percutaneous ultrasonic pyelolithotomy* or *extracorporeal shock wave lithotripsy* (see the Elimination concept) may be used instead of surgery to crush and remove stones.

Ureteroplasty, the surgical repair of a ureter, may be indicated for structural abnormality or stricture of a ureter. This may be combined with a ureteral reimplantation if vesicoureteral reflux is present. The client returns from these surgeries with an indwelling urinary catheter (Foley or suprapubic) and a **ureteral stent** (a thin catheter inserted into the ureter to provide for urine flow and ureteral support), which remains in place for 3–5 days. Box 8–7 describes nursing care of the client with a ureteral stent in place.

Follow-up urine cultures should be obtained according to the frequency specified by agency guidelines. Clients with pyelonephritis may have repeat urine cultures monthly for 3 months, every 3 months for 6 months, and then annually. Most reinfections occur within 1 year, and subsequent infections may be asymptomatic. For children with VUR or recurrent infections, a long-term, suppressive dose of an antibiotic may be ordered in an attempt to keep the urine sterile and prevent subsequent pyelonephritis and renal scarring, but there is limited evidence that this is effective (Raszka & Khan, 2005). Children with renal scarring should have their blood pressure monitored.

Complementary Therapies

Complementary therapies, such as aromatherapy or herbal preparations, may be used in conjunction with antibiotics to treat UTI. Low-sugar cranberry juice or extract and blueberry juice also are commonly used to prevent and treat UTI. Adding bergamot, sandalwood, lavender, or juniper oil to bath water may help relieve the discomfort of UTI. Herbal supplements such as saw palmetto have a urinary antiseptic effect, and may be beneficial in treating or preventing UTI. Consult a qualified herbologist for recommended doses and appropriate use. Some aromatherapy and herbal preparations are contraindicated in clients with allergies; those clients should check with their allergist before participating in these types of therapies.

HEALTH CARE

Research indicates the best practice is not to treat asymptomatic bacteriuria. If you were caring for a client with bacteria in the urine who denied any symptoms or problems, how would you explain the decision not to treat this? Would best practice change if the client wanted a prescription for an antibiotic? What would you tell the client who adamantly demands a prescription for an antibiotic after being informed that it is not in his or her best interest?

Box 8–7 **Ureteral Stent**

Ureteral stents are used to maintain patency and promote healing of the ureters (see figure below). A stent may be temporary, used during and after a surgical procedure, or it may be used for longer periods in clients with ureteral obstruction due to tumors, strictures, or other causes.

Stents may be positioned during surgery or cystoscopy. They are made of a nontoxic material such as silicone or polyurethane, with side drainage holes placed along the length of the stent. Stents are radiopaque for easy radiographic identification. One or both ends of the stent may be pigtail or J shaped to prevent migration.

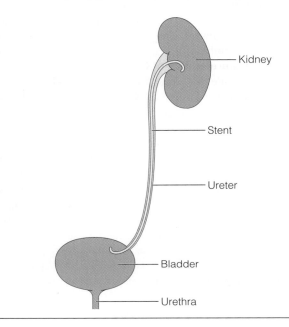

- Kidney
- Stent
- Ureter
- Bladder
- Urethra

In caring for a client with a ureteral stint, the nurse should do the following:

- Label all drainage tubes, including stents, for easy identification. Attach each catheter and stent to a separate closed drainage system. Careful labeling allows close monitoring of output from all sources and reservoirs. Separate drainage systems minimize the risk of infection.
- If the stent has been brought to the surface, secure it and maintain its position. The stent is usually placed in the renal pelvis. It is important to secure it well to prevent trauma to the kidney, inadvertent removal of the stent, and ureter obstruction.
- Monitor urine output, including color, consistency, and odor. Monitor for signs of infection or bleeding, including fever, tachycardia, pain, hematuria, and cloudy or malodorous urine. The stent facilitates urine flow, but can become obstructed due to bleeding, calculi, or sediment. Obstruction can result in hydronephrosis and kidney damage. The stent itself is a foreign body in the urinary tract and can increase the risk of UTI.
- Maintain fluid intake, encouraging fluids that acidify urine, such as low-sugar apple, cranberry, and blueberry juice. The stent can precipitate calculus formation as well as UTI. Increasing fluid intake and acidifying the urine help prevent these complications.
- For an indwelling stent, stress the need for regular follow-up to monitor for and prevent complications such as UTI and calculi. The client with an indwelling stent may tend to forget that the stent is in place and become noncompliant with follow-up and preventive measures.

Source: LeMone, P., & Burke, K. (2008). *Medical-surgical nursing: Critical thinking in client care* (4th ed.). Upper Saddle River, NJ: Pearson Education.

REVIEW **Urinary Tract Infection**

RELATE: **LINK THE CONCEPTS**

Linking the concept of Inflammation with the concept of Infection:
1. The topic of nephritis is covered under the Inflammation concept. Why is nephritis not covered under the concept of Infection?

READY: **GO TO COMPANION SKILLS MANUAL**

1. Providing perineal-genital care
2. Managing pain
3. Administering medication
4. Collecting a midstream urine specimen
5. Collecting urine externally
6. Performing urinary catheterization

REFLECT: **CASE STUDY**

Mrs. James, who was introduced under the exemplar of cellulitis within this concept, wakes up one day and does not feel well. She is taken by ambulance to the Neighborhood Hospital, where a diagnosis of stroke is made. She has a feeding tube and indwelling catheter placed, and later develops a fever and confusion. Urine in the drainage bag is cloudy. A urine specimen is collected and sent to the laboratory for urinalysis and culture and sensitivity. Results confirm the diagnosis of UTI.

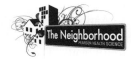

1. How will Mrs. James' history of diabetes mellitus affect her risk for and response to UTI?
2. What risk factors does Mrs. James have that place her at increased risk for UTI?
3. After removing the indwelling catheter and treating the UTI with antibiotics for 7 days, urine culture reveals the bacteria remain in the urine. What does the nurse anticipate will be done next if the client still experiences symptoms? How would the treatment differ if the client did not have symptoms?

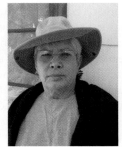

REFERENCES

American Academy of Pediatrics Committee on Infectious Disease. (2006). *Red book: 2006 Report of the Committee on Infectious Disease* (27th ed.). Elk Grove Village, IL: American Academy of Pediatrics.

Aronson, B. (2005). Medication management behaviors of adherent short-term antibiotic users. *Clinical Excellence for Nurse Practitioners, 9*(1), 23–30.

Arrowsmith, V. A., Maunder, J. A., Sargent, R. J., & Taylor, R. (2005). Removal of nail polish and finger rings to prevent surgical infection. *The Cochrane Library* (Oxford) (ID #CD003325).

Baine, W. B., Yu, W., & Summe, J. P. (2001). The epidemiology of hospitalization of elderly Americans for septicemia or bacteremia in 1991–1998. Application of Medicare claims data. Annals of Epidemiology, 11(2), 118–126.

Barbacane, J. L. (2004). Back to the basics: Handwashing. *Geriatric Nursing, 25*(2), 90–92.

Bardsley, A. (2005). Use of lubricant gels in urinary catheterization. *Nursing Standard, 20*(8), 41–46.

Becker, W., & Deeane, D.(1986) *The world of the cell*, Redwood City, CA: Benjamin Cummings.

Bentley, D. W., Bradley, S., High, K., Schoenbaum, S., Taler, G., & Yoshikawa, T. (2001). Practice guidelines for evaluation of fever and infection in long-term care facilities. *Journal of the American Geriatrics Society, 49*, 210–222.

Bilukha, O. O., & Rosenstein, N. (2005). Prevention and control of meningococcal disease. *Morbidity and Mortality Weekly Report, 54*(RR-7), 1–21.

Boyce, J. M., & Pittet, D. (2002). Guideline for hand hygiene in health-care settings: Recommendations of the Healthcare Infection Control Practices Advisory Committee and the HICPAC/SHEA/APIC/IDSA Hand Hygiene Task Force. *Morbidity and Mortality Weekly Report, 51*(RR-16), 1–44.

Carr, M. P. (2004). Waterless hand washing: A new era in hand hygiene. *Journal of Practical Hygiene, 13*(2), 33–36.

Centers for Disease Control and Prevention. (1987). Recommendations for prevention of HIV transmission in health-care settings. *Morbidity and Mortality Weekly Report (suppl.), 36*(2s), 1S–18S.

Centers for Disease Control and Prevention. (1997). 1997 USPHS/IDSA guidelines for the prevention of opportunistic infections in persons infected with human immunodeficiency virus. *Morbidity and Mortality Weekly Report, 46*(RR-12), 1–46.

Centers for Disease Control and Prevention. (2001). Updated U.S. Public Health Service guidelines for the management of occupational exposures to HBV, HCV, and HIV and recommendations for postexposure prophylaxis. *Morbidity and Mortality Weekly Report 50*(RR-11), 1–67.

Centers for Disease Control and Prevention. (2002a). Guidelines for hand hygiene in health-care settings. *Morbidity and Mortality Weekly Report, 51*(RR-16), 1–56.

Centers for Disease Control and Prevention. (2002b). Immunization registry use and progress—United States, 2001. *Morbidity and Mortality Weekly Report, 51*(3), 53–56.

Centers for Disease Control and Prevention. (2003). *Exposure to blood: What healthcare personnel need to know*. Atlanta, GA: CDC.

Centers for Disease Control and Prevention. (2004a). *Sequence for donning and removing personal protective equipment*. Retrieved July 16, 2006, from www.cdc.gov/ncidod/dhqp/ppe.html

Centers for Disease Control and Prevention. (2004b). Vaccines for Children program. Retrieved May 12, 2006, from http://www.cdc.gov/PROGRAMS/IMMUN10.HTM

Centers for Disease Control and Prevention. (2005a). Achievements in public health: Elimination of rubella and congenital rubella syndrome—United States, 1969–2004. *Morbidity and Mortality Weekly Report, 54*(11), 279–282.

Centers for Disease Control and Prevention. (2005b). Measles—United States, 2004. *Morbidity and Mortality Weekly Report, 54*(48), 1229–1231.

Centers for Disease Control and Prevention. (2005c). National, state, and urban area vaccination coverage among children aged 19–35 months—United States, 2004. *Morbidity and Mortality Weekly Report, 54*(29), 717–721.

Centers for Disease Control and Prevention. (2005d). *Public health guidance for community-level preparedness and response to severe acute respiratory syndrome (SARS) version 2: Supplement I: Infection control in healthcare, home, and community settings*. Retrieved June 3, 2006, from http://www.cdc.gov/ncidod/sars/guidance/I/healthcare.htm

Centers for Disease Control and Prevention. (2006a). CDC's advisory committee recommends changes in varicella vaccinations. Retrieved July 5, 2006, from http://cdc.gov/od/media/pressrel/r060629-b.htm

Centers for Disease Control and Prevention. (2006b). Preventing tetanus, diphtheria, and pertussis among adolescents: Use of tetanus toxoid, reduced diphtheria toxoid, and acellular pertussis vaccines. *Morbidity and Mortality Weekly Report, 55*, 1–34.

Centers for Disease Control and Prevention. (2006c). Prevention and control of influenza: Recommendations of the Advisory Committee on Immunization Practices (ACIP). *Morbidity and Mortality Weekly Report, 55*, 1–44.

Centers for Disease Control and Prevention. (2006d). *Recommended childhood and adolescent immunization schedule, United States, 2005*. Retrieved June 1, 2006, from http://www.cdc.gov/nip/recs/child-schedule.htm#printable

Centers for Disease Control and Prevention. (2006e). *Recommended adult immunization schedule, United States, 2006*. Retrieved June 1, 2006, from http://www.cdc.gov/nip/recs/adult-schedule.htm#print

Centers for Disease Control and Prevention. (2006f, May 18). Update: Multistate outbreak of mumps—United States, January 1-May 2, 2006, *Morbidity and Mortality Weekly Dispatch 55*, 1–5.

Centers for Medicare and Medicaid Services. (2005). Alcohol based hand rub solutions TIA 00-1 (101). *Federal Register, 70*(57), 15229–15239.

Cherry, J. D. (2005). The epidemiology of pertussis: A comparison of the epidemiology of the disease pertussis with the epidemiology of *Bordatella pertussis* infection. *Pediatrics, 115*(5), 1422–1427.

Christ-Crain, M., Jaccard-Stolz, D., Bingisser, R., Gencay, M. M., Huber, P. R., Tamm, M., et al. (2004). Effect of procalcitonin-guided treatment on antibiotic use and outcome in lower respiratory tract infections: Cluster-randomised, single-blinded intervention trial. *Lancet, 363*(9409), 600–607.

Conde-Agudelo, A., Villar, J., & Lindheimer, M. (2008). Maternal infection and risk of preeclampsia: Systematic review and metaanalysis. *American Journal of Obstetrics & Gynecology, January*, 7–22.

Curtis, D. (2007). Cellulitis. Retrieved October 2007 from http://www.emedicine.com/EMERG/topic88.htm

Daneshgari, F., Krugman, M., Bahn, A., & Lee, R. S. (2002). Evidence-based multidisciplinary practice: Improving the safety and standards of male bladder catheterization. *Medsurg Nursing, 11*(5), 236–241, 246.

Dennehy, P. H. (2005). Update on a high-morbidity infection: Rotavirus. *Contemporary Pediatrics, 22*(12), 34–40.

Department of Health and Human Services, Office of Disease Prevention and Promotion. (2000). *Healthy People 2010*. Washington, D.C., http://www.healthypeople.gov

Dulczak, S., & Kirk, J. (2005). Overview of the evaluation, diagnosis, and management of urinary tract infections in infants and children. *Urologic Nursing, 25*(3), 185–191.

Durbin, W. J. (2004). Pneumococcal infections. *Pediatrics in Review, 25*(12), 418–423.

Evans-Smith, P. (Ed.). (2005). *Taylor's clinical nursing skills: A nursing process approach*. Philadelphia: Lippincott Williams & Wilkins.

Fauci, A. et al. (1998). *Harrison's principles of internal medicine* (14th ed.). New York: McGraw-Hill.

Food and Drug Administration. (2006). FDA approves a second drug for prevention of influenza A and B in adults and children. Accessed April 3, 2006, from http://www.fda.gov/bbs/topics/news/2006/new01231.html

Gandhi, M. (2006). *Asymptomatic bacteriuria*. Retrieved July 1, 2008, from http://www.nlm.nih.gov/medlineplus/ency/article/000520.htm

Garcia-Martin, M., Lardelli-Claret, P., Jimenez-Moleon, J. J., Bueno-Cavanillas, A., de Dios Luna del Castillo, J., & Galvez-Vargas, R. (2001). Proportion of hospital deaths potentially attributable to nosocomial infection. *Infection Control and Hospital Epidemiology, 22*, 708–714.

Garin, E. H., Olavarria, F., Nieto, V. G., Valenciano, B., Campos, A., & Young, L. (2006). Clinical significance of primary vesicoureteral reflux and urinary antibiotic prophylaxis after acute pyelonephritis: A multicenter, randomized controlled study. *Pediatrics, 117*(3), 626–632.

Garner, J. S., & Hospital Infection Control Practices Advisory Committee. (1996). Guidelines for isolation precautions in hospitals. *Infection Control Hospital Epidemiology, 17*, 53–80; and *American Journal of Infection Control, 24*, 24–52.

Garner, J. S., & Simmons, B. P. (1983). *CDC guideline for isolation precautions in hospitals* (HHS Publication No. CDC 83-8314). Atlanta, GA: U.S. Department of Health and Human Services, Public Health Service, Centers for Disease Control.

Goldrick, B. A. (2003). Adult respiratory infections. *American Journal of Nursing, 103*(10), 65–66.

Goldrick, B. A. (2004a). 21st century emerging and reemerging infections. *American Journal of Nursing, 104*(1), 67–70.

Goldrick, B. A. (2004b). MRSA, VRE, and VRSA: How do we control them in nursing homes? *American Journal of Nursing, 104*(8), 50–51.

Hospital Infection Control Practices Advisory Committee. (1995). Recommendations for preventing the spread of vancomycin resistance. *American Journal of Infection Control, 23*, 87–94; *Infection Control and Hospital Epidemiology, 16*, 105–113; and *Morbidity and Mortality Weekly Report, 44* (RR-12), 1–13.

Houghton, D. (2006). HAI prevention: The power is in your hands. *Nursing Management, 37*(Suppl.), 1–7.

Huether, S. E. (2006). Alterations of renal and urinary tract function in children. In K. L. McCance & S. E. Huether, *Pathophysiology: The biologic basis for disease in adults and children* (5th ed., pp. 1337–1352). St. Louis: Elsevier Mosby.

Jackson, M. M. (1993). Infection precautions: What works and what does not. *CRNA: The Clinical Forum for Nurse Anesthetists, 4*(2), 77–82.

Jarvis, J. R. (2001). Infection control and changing health-care delivery systems. *Emerging Infectious Diseases, 7*, 170–173.

Joint Commission on Accreditation of Healthcare Organizations. (2006). *National patient safety goals*. Oakbrook Terrace, IL: JCAHO. Retrieved June 3, 2006, from http://www.jointcommission.org/Standards/NationalPatientSafetyGoals/

Kasper, D. L., Braunwald, E., Fauci, A. S., Hauser, S. L., Longo, D. L., & Jameson, J. L. (Eds.). (2005). *Harrison's principles of internal medicine* (16th ed.). New York: McGraw-Hill.

Kjonegaard, R., & Myers III, F. E. (2005). Arresting drug-resistant organisms. *Nursing 2005, 35*(6), 48–50.

Krogh, R. H., & Bruskewitz, R. C. (1998). Disorders of the lower genitourinary tract. *Clinical Geriatrics, 6*(13), 19–25.

Lehne, R. A. (2004). *Pharmacology for nursing care* (4th ed.). St. Louis, MO: Saunders/Elsevier.

Mahon, C. R. & Manuselis Jr, G. (1995). *Textbook of diagnostic microbiology*. Philadelphia: W.B. Saunders.

Markenson, D. (2005). The treatment of children exposed to pathogens linked to bioterrorism. *Infectious Diseases of North America, 19*, 731–745.

Mayo Foundation for Medical Education and Research. (2006). *Recurrent cellulitis: What causes it?* Retrieved October 15, 2007, from http://www.nlm.nih.gov/medlineplus/cellulitis.html

McCance, K., & Huether, S. (2002). *Pathophysiology: The biologic basis for disease in adults and children* (4th ed.). St. Louis, MO: Mosby.

McCue, J. D. (1999). Treatment of urinary tract infections in long-term care facilities: Advice, guidelines, and algorithms. *Clinical Geriatrics, 7*(8), 11–17.

Müller, B., & Becker, K. L. (2001). Procalcitonin: How a hormone became a marker and mediator of sepsis. *Swiss Medical Weekly, 131*, 595–602.

National Center for HIV, STD, and TB Prevention, Division of Tuberculosis Elimination. (2004). *Self-study modules on tuberculosis.* Retrieved July 16, 2006, from http://www.phppo.cdc.gov/phtn/tbmodules/Default.htm

National Institute for Occupational Safety and Health. (1999). *Preventing needlestick injuries in health care settings.* (DHHS Publication No. 2000-108) Cincinnati, OH: U.S. Department of Health and Human Services, Public Health Service, Centers for Disease Control and Prevention, National Institute for Occupational Safety and Health.

National Kidney and Urological Diseases Information Clearinghouse. (2003). Urinary tract infections in children. NIH Publication No. 04-4246. Retrieved December 13, 2004 from, http://www.kidney.niddk.nih.gov/kudiseases/pubs/uitchildren/index.htm

Nicolle, L. E. (2003). Urinary tract infections in the elderly. In W. R. Hazzard, J. P. Blass, J. B. Halter, J. G. Ouslander, & M. E. Tinetti (Eds.), *Principles of geriatric medicine and gerontology* (5th ed., pp. 1107–1116). New York: McGraw-Hill.

Occupational Safety & Health Administration. (2005). *Latex allergy.* Retrieved June 3, 2006, from http://www.osha.gov/SLTC/latexallergy/

Pagana, K. D., & Pagana, T. J. (2002). *Mosby's manual of diagnostic and laboratory tests* (2nd ed.). St. Louis, MO: Mosby.

Peate, I. (2004). Infection control. Occupational exposure of staff to HIV and prophylaxis therapy. *British Journal of Nursing, 13,* 1146–1150.

Porth, C. (2005). *Pathophysiology: Concepts of altered health states* (6th ed.). Philadelphia: Lippincott Williams & Wilkins.

Posani, T. (2004). *Clostridium difficile:* Causes and interventions. *Critical Care Nursing Clinics of North America, 16*(4), 547–551.

Raboud, J., Saskin, R., Wong, K., Moore, C., Parucha, G., Bennett, J., et al. (2004). Patterns of handwashing behavior and visits to patients on a general medical ward of healthcare workers. *Infection Control and Hospital Epidemiology, 25,* 198–202.

Rao, A. S., & Bradley, S. F. (2003). *Clostridium difficile* in older adults and residents of long-term care facilities. *Annals of Long-Term Care, 11*(5), 42–47.

Raszka, W. V., & Khan, O. (2005). Pyelonephritis. *Pediatrics in Review, 26*(10), 364–369.

Sarrell, E. M., Wielunsky, E., & Cohen, H. A. (2006). Antipyretic treatment in young children with fever. *Archives of Pediatric and Adolescent Medicine, 160*(2), 197–202.

Sehulster, L. M., Chinn, R. Y. W., Arduino, M. J., Carpenter, J., Donlan, R., Ashford, D., et al. (2004). *Guidelines for environmental infection control in health-care facilities. Recommendations from CDC and the Healthcare Infection Control Practices Advisory Committee (HICPAC).* Chicago: American Society for Healthcare Engineering/American Hospital Association.

Smail, F. (2007). Asymptomatic bacteriuria in pregnancy. *Best Practice & Research Clinical Obstetrics and Gynaecology, 21*(3), 439–450.

Sopena, N., & Sabria, M. (2005). Multicenter study of hospital-acquired pneumonia in non-ICU patients. *Chest, 127*(1), 213–219.

Srinivasan, A., McDonald, L. C., Jernigan, D., Helfand, R., Ginsheimer, K., Jernigan, J., et al. (2004). Foundations of the severe acute respiratory syndrome preparedness and response plan for healthcare facilities. *Infection Control and Hospital Epidemiology, 25,* 1020–1025.

Steers, W. D. (1999). Meeting the urologic needs of the aging population. *Clinical Geriatrics, 7*(5), 62–64, 73.

Stirling, B., Littlejohn, P., & Willbond, M. L. (2004). Nurses and the control of infectious disease: Understanding epidemiology and disease transmission is vital to nursing care.

Stone, P. W., Hedblom, E. C., Murphy, D. M., & Miller, S. B. (2005). The economic impact of infection control: Making the business case for increased infection control resources. *American Journal of Infection Control, 33*(9), 542–547.

Sunenshine, R. H., & McDonald, L. C. (2006). *Clostridium difficile*-associated disease: New challenges from an established pathogen. *Cleveland Clinical Journal of Medicine, 73,* 187–197.

Tierney, L. M., Jr., McPhee, S. J., & Papadakis, M. A. (Eds.). (2005). *Current medical diagnosis & treatment 2006.* New York: McGraw-Hill.

Tierney, L., McPhee, S., & Papadakis, M. (Eds). (2006). *Current medical diagnosis & treatment 2007.* Stamford, CT: Appleton & Lange.

Tiwari, T., Murphy, T. V., & Moran, J. (2005). Recommended antimicrobial agents for the treatment and postexposure prophylaxis of pertussis: 2005 CDC guidelines. *Morbidity and Mortality Weekly Report, 54*(RR-14), 1–16.

Ünlü, H., Sardan, Y. C., & Ülker, S. (2007). Comparison of sampling methods for urine cultures. *Journal of Nursing Scholarship, 39*(4), 325–329.

U.S. Department of Health and Human Services, Public Health Service. (1988). Update: Universal precautions for prevention of transmission of human immunodeficiency virus, hepatitis B virus, and other bloodborne pathogens in health care settings. *Morbidity and Mortality Weekly Report, 37*(24), 377–388.

Warny, M., Pepin, J., Fang, A., Killgore, G., Thompson, A., Brazier, J., et al. (2005). Toxic production by an emerging strain of *Clostridium difficile* associated with outbreaks of severe disease in North America and Europe. *Lancet, 366,* 1079–1083.

World Health Organization. (2005). *WHO guidelines on hand hygiene in health care.* Geneva, Switzerland: WHO.

Yetman, R. J., Parks, D., & Taft, E. (2002). Management of patients exposed to biologic weapons. *Journal of Pediatric Health Care, 16*(5), 256–261.

Inflammation

9

Concept at-a-Glance

Concept Learning Outcomes

After reading about this concept you will be able to do the following:

1. Summarize the physiologic process required to mount an inflammatory response and describe the response's contribution to homeostasis.

2. List factors affecting inflammation.

3. Identify commonly occurring alterations in inflammatory response and related treatments.

4. Explain common physical assessment procedures used to examine inflammation in clients across the life span.

5. Outline diagnostic and laboratory tests and expected findings to determine the individual's inflammatory response.

6. Explain management of inflammatory disorders aimed at limiting the response and supporting the helpful effects.

7. Demonstrate nursing process in providing culturally competent and caring interventions across the life span for individuals with inflammatory disorders.

8. Identify pharmacologic interventions in caring for the individual with inflammatory disorders.

Concept Key Terms

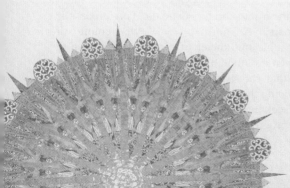

About Inflammation

Inflammation is a nonspecific but complex response to reduce the effects of what the body sees as harmful. Inflammation may result from an injury such as an ankle sprain. It may also result from an underlying infection. Autoimmune diseases frequently cause inflammation sufficient to result in tissue damage. Other harmful agents include pathogens, damaged cells, and irritants.

Under normal circumstances, inflammation acts as a protective process that stimulates healing and prevents further damage or progressive deterioration. The occasional uncomfortable symptoms of normal inflammation are usually successfully treated with palliative care. However, the inflammatory process can get carried away, leading to problems such as autoimmune disorders (e.g., rheumatoid arthritis, psoriasis, asthma, and allergies). These conditions may require more aggressive care, including pharmacotherapy. ●

NORMAL PRESENTATION

Inflammation is an adaptive response to injury or illness that brings fluid, dissolved substances, and blood cells into the interstitial tissues where the invasion or damage has occurred. The response is called *nonspecific* because the same events occur regardless of the cause of the inflammatory process. Through the inflammatory reaction, the invader is neutralized and eliminated, destroyed tissue is removed, and the process of healing and repair is initiated. Inflammation is the first phase of the healing process. During the inflammatory process, particulate matter, bacteria, damaged cells, and inflammatory exudate are removed through phagocytosis. This process, called **debridement**, prepares the wound for healing. Adequate nutrition is essential for inflammation and healing to proceed. Through the process of inflammation, a large number of potentially damaging chemicals and microorganisms may be neutralized.

Inflammation is an adaptive mechanism that destroys or dilutes the injurious agent, prevents further spread of the injury, and promotes the repair of damaged tissue. It is characterized by five signs: (a) pain, (b) swelling, (c) redness, (d) heat, and (e) impaired function of the part, if the injury is severe. Commonly, words with the suffix *-itis* describe an inflammatory process. For example, *appendicitis* means inflammation of the appendix; *gastritis* means inflammation of the stomach.

Injurious agents can be categorized as physical agents, chemical agents, and microorganisms. *Physical agents* include mechanical objects causing trauma to tissues, excessive heat or cold, and radiation. *Chemical agents* include external irritants (e.g., strong acids, alkalis, poisons, and irritating gases) and internal irritants (substances manufactured within the body, such as excessive hydrochloric acid in the stomach). Microorganisms that can cause inflammation include bacteria and viruses.

The Function of Inflammation

The human body has developed many complex ways to defend itself against injury and invasion by microorganisms. Inflammation is one of these defense mechanisms. The central purpose of inflammation is to contain the injury or destroy the microorganism. By neutralizing the foreign agent and removing cellular debris and dead cells, inflammation allows repair of the injured area to proceed at a faster pace.

Signs of inflammation include swelling, pain, warmth, and redness of the affected area.

Inflammation may be classified as *acute* or *chronic*. During acute inflammation, such as that caused by minor physical injury, 8–10 days are normally needed for the symptoms to resolve and repair to begin. If the body cannot contain or neutralize the damaging agent, inflammation may continue for long periods and become chronic. In chronic autoimmune disorders, such as lupus and rheumatoid arthritis, inflammation may persist for years with symptoms becoming progressively worse. Other disorders such as seasonal allergies occur at predictable times during each year, and the resulting inflammation may produce only minor, annoying symptoms.

Stages of Inflammation

A series of dynamic events is commonly referred to as the three stages of the inflammatory response:

First stage: Vascular and cellular responses
Second stage: Exudate production
Third stage: Reparative phase

VASCULAR AND CELLULAR RESPONSES At the start of the first stage of inflammation, blood vessels at the site of injury or infection constrict. The injured tissues release histamines, kinins, and prostaglandins in response to the injury or infection. These substances serve as chemical mediators to dilate blood vessels and contract smooth muscle, causing more blood to flow to the injured area. This marked increase in blood supply is referred to as **hyperemia** and is responsible for the characteristic sign of redness and the heat that accompanies inflammation.

Vascular permeability increases at the site with dilation of the vessels. Fluid, proteins, and **leukocytes** (white blood cells) leak into the interstitial spaces, causing the signs of inflammatory swelling (edema) and pain to appear. Pain is caused by the pressure of accumulating fluid on nerve endings and the irritating chemical mediators. Fluid pouring into areas such as the pleural or pericardial cavity can seriously affect organ function. In other areas, such as joints, mobility is impaired by accumulating fluid.

Blood flow slows in the dilated vessels, allowing more leukocytes to arrive at the injured tissues. The leukocytes aggregate or line up along the inner surface of the blood vessels. This process is known as **margination**. Leukocytes then move through the blood vessel wall into the affected tissue spaces, a process called **emigration**.

In response to the exit of leukocytes from the blood, the bone marrow produces more leukocytes in even larger numbers and releases them into the bloodstream. This process is called **leukocytosis**. A normal leukocyte count of 4,500–11,000 per cubic millimeter of blood can increase to 20,000 or more when inflammation occurs.

All conditions that cause inflammation will result in an individual experiencing this first stage of inflammation. Often individuals do not seek medical treatment for an inflammatory response unless it progresses to the second stage and exudate results. Typical injuries for which an individual will seek treatment for stage 1 inflammation include sprained ankles and wrists, broken bones, and minor blunt force injuries (e.g., two children running into each other on a playground).

EXUDATE PRODUCTION In the second stage of inflammation, inflammatory **exudate** is produced. The term *exudate* comes from the Latin word meaning "exude" or "to ooze." Exudate consists of fluid that escaped from the blood vessels, dead phagocytic cells, and dead tissue cells and the products they release.

The nature and amount of exudate vary according to the tissue involved and the intensity and duration of the inflammation. The major types of exudate are serous, purulent, and hemorrhagic (sanguineous). Serous exudate typically accompanies mild inflammation and presents as clear or straw colored with a thin, watery consistency. Purulent exudate is usually opaque, or milky. Commonly referred to as "pus," purulent exudate normally indicates the presence of infection and contains a large quantity of cells and necrotic debris. Because hemorrhagic exudate contains blood from ruptured blood vessels, it is red and thick. This type of exudate exudes from tissue or its capillaries as a result of infection or injury.

Whether the presence of exudate should be reported depends primarily on the underlying cause and the amount and degree of the exudate. A minor cut that exhibits either serous or hemorrhagic exudate may resolve with simple first aid. Exudate over a larger surface or that appears in conjunction with other symptoms, such as fever, will warrant a greater degree of medical care.

REPARATIVE PHASE The third stage of the inflammatory response involves the repair of injured tissues by regeneration or replacement with fibrous tissue (scar) formation. **Regeneration** is the replacement of destroyed tissue cells by cells that are identical or similar in structure and function. Damaged cells are replaced one by one, and new cells are organized so that the architectural pattern and function of the tissue are restored. The ability to regenerate cells varies considerably from one type of tissue to another. For example, epithelial tissues of the skin and the digestive and respiratory tracts have a good regenerative capacity, as long as their underlying support structures are intact. The same holds true for osseous, lymphoid, and bone marrow tissues. Tissues that have little regenerative capacity include nervous, muscular, and elastic tissues.

When regeneration is not possible, repair occurs by fibrous (scar) tissue formation. The inflammatory exudate with its interlacing network of fibrin provides the framework for this tissue to develop. Damaged tissues are replaced with the connective tissue elements of collagen, blood capillaries, lymphatics, and other tissue-bound substances. In the early stages of this process, the tissue is called **granulation tissue**. It is a fragile, gelatinous tissue that appears pink or red because of the many newly formed capillaries. Later in the process, the tissue shrinks (the capillaries are constricted, even obliterated) and the collagen fibers contract, leaving a firmer fibrous tissue. This is called cicatrix, or scar tissue.

Histamine is a key chemical mediator of inflammation (Table 9–1). It is stored primarily within mast cells located in tissue spaces under epithelial membranes such as the skin, bronchial tree, and digestive tract and along blood vessels. **Mast cells** detect foreign agents or injury and respond by releasing histamine, which initiates the inflammatory response within seconds. In addition to its role in inflammation, histamine also directly stimulates pain receptors. Both mast cells and histamine are important components of the allergic process.

When released at an injury site, histamine dilates nearby blood vessels, causing capillaries to become more permeable. Plasma, complement proteins, and phagocytes can then enter the area to neutralize foreign agents. The affected area may become congested with blood, which can lead to significant swelling and pain. Figure 9–1 ■ illustrates the fundamental steps in acute inflammation.

Rapid release of the chemical mediators of inflammation on a large scale throughout the body is responsible for **anaphylaxis**, a life-threatening allergic response that may result in shock and death (Box 9–1). A number of chemicals, insect stings, foods, and some therapeutic drugs can cause this widespread release of histamine from mast cells if the person has an allergy to any of these substances.

TABLE 9–1 Chemical Mediators of Inflammation

MEDIATOR	DESCRIPTION
Bradykinin	Present in an inactive form in plasma and mast cells; vasodilator that causes pain; effects are similar to those of histamine
Complement	Series of at least 20 proteins that combine in a cascade fashion to neutralize or destroy an antigen
Histamine	Stored and released by mast cells; causes dilation of blood vessels, smooth-muscle constriction, tissue swelling, and itching
Leukotrienes	Stored and released by mast cells; effects are similar to those of histamine
Prostaglandins	Present in most tissues and stored and released by mast cells; increase capillary permeability, attract white blood cells to site of inflammation, and cause pain

Source: Adams, M.P., Holland, Jr., L.N., & Bostwick, P.M. (2008). *Pharmacology for nurses: A pathophysiologic approach* (2nd ed.). Upper Saddle River, NJ: Pearson, Inc.

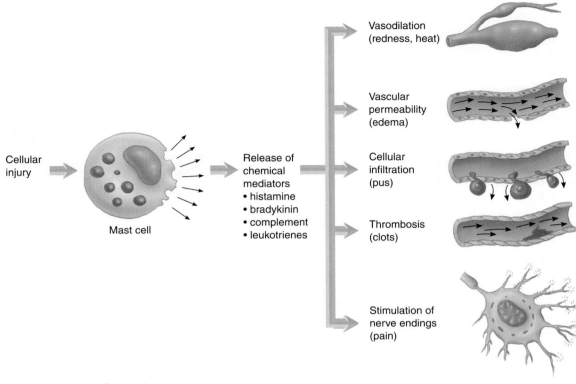

Figure 9–1 ■ Steps in acute inflammation.

Histamine Receptors

Histamine works by combining with specific cellular histamine receptors. There are four classified receptors, with the H_1 receptors and H_2 receptors participating in the inflammatory process. **H_1 receptors** are present in the smooth muscle of the vascular system, the bronchial tree, and the digestive tract. Stimulation of these receptors results in itching, pain, edema, vasodilation, bronchoconstriction, and the characteristic symptoms of inflammation and allergy. In contrast, **H_2 receptors** are present primarily in the stomach, and their stimulation results in the secretion of large amounts of hydrochloric acid.

Box 9–1 Symptoms and Treatment of Anaphylaxis

Anaphylaxis is a life-threatening allergic reaction that necessitates immediate emergency medical treatment. Anaphylaxis develops extremely rapidly—in seconds to minutes—and requires immediate initiation of the Emergency Medical System (EMS). Signs and symptoms of anaphylaxis include the following:

- Wheezing sounds, labored breathing
- Nausea, vomiting, or diarrhea
- Weakness, light-headedness, dizziness
- Blue skin as a result of oxygenation impairment or pale skin resulting from shock (advanced signs)
- Inflammation of the airways, swelling of the throat (this can become severe enough to block the airway)
- Hives, itching
- Low blood pressure
- Abnormal heart rhythm

Epinephrine is the first line of treatment for an individual experiencing an anaphylactic reaction. Given by subcutaneous or intramuscular injection, epinephrine dilates the airways and narrows the blood vessels, essentially counteracting the allergic response. Some allergic individuals carry Epi-pens, self-injectors with epinephrine, to use in the case of an anaphylactic response. EMS should be called for an individual having an anaphylactic reaction even if he or she is carrying and uses an Epi-pen. During and immediately following an anaphylactic response, airway protection is critical, so adjunctive medications may include beta-agonists, antihistamines, and corticosteroids. A severe reaction resulting in laryngeal swelling sufficient to close the airway may require a tracheotomy.

ALTERATIONS

Inflammation can occur in virtually any tissue, organ, or system. The suffix -*itis* indicates inflammation such as in appendic*itis*, arth*ritis* or pancreat*itis*. Many autoimmune disorders involve the inflammatory response and result from the body misinterpreting its own tissues as harmful and needing to be destroyed or limited. Rheumatoid arthritis, systemic lupus erythematosus, and Guillain Barré syndrome are a few examples of autoimmune responses involving inflammation. The following are some common diseases that have an inflammatory component:

- Allergic rhinitis
- Anaphylaxis
- Ankylosing spondylitis
- Appendicitis
- Arthritis (the most common inflammatory disorder, and the leading cause of disability in the United States)
- Contact dermatitis
- Crohn's disease
- Gall bladder disease
- Hashimoto's thyroiditis
- Inflammatory bowel disease (affecting 300,000–500,000 Americans each year)
- Nephritis
- Peptic ulcers
- Rheumatoid arthritis
- Systemic lupus erythematosus
- Ulcerative colitis

ALTERATIONS AND TREATMENTS Inflammation

Alteration	Description	Treatment
Allergic rhinitis	Commonly known as hay fever, it is caused by a variety of particulate matter, including dust mites, molds, and pollens of specific seasonal plants. Exposure to these allergens can cause antibody production with the release of histamine, triggering the inflammatory response in the allergic individual.	Antihistamines, decongestants, and antileukotrienes are common treatments for mild to moderate allergic rhinitis. Allergy desensitization therapy to reduce the body's response to allergens may be helpful to the more allergic individual.
Anaphylaxis	A severe and acute systemic allergic reaction proceeds to anaphylactic shock after large quantities of immunological mediators are released. Acute inflammation can result in edema of the airways and anoxia.	Epinephrine, dexamethasone, and diphenhydramine are usually the medications of choice. Nursing care includes maintaining a patent airway, removing allergens causing reaction if possible, and reducing client anxiety. If treatment is not initiated quickly enough, a tracheostomy may be performed to open the airway and prevent or treat respiratory arrest.
Ankylosing spondylitis	Chronic painful inflammatory arthritis primarily affects the spine and sacroiliac joints, causing fusion of the spine.	No cure is available but treatments include physical therapy, exercise, and medications including NSAIDs, immunosuppressants, and biologicals that are tumor necrosis factor (TNF) blockers.
Appendicitis	The appendix is inflamed.	The inflamed appendix is surgically removed.
Arthritis (osteoarthritis, gout, rheumatoid arthritis, or psoriatic arthritis)	Inflammation of the joint or joints that eventually results in damage to the joint.	Common treatments include heat, physical therapy, gentle exercise of the joint, anti-inflammatory medications (most commonly NSAIDs). Severe deterioration may lead to the need for joint replacement.
Contact dermatitis	Skin reaction results from exposure to an allergen causing skin irritation.	Treated with hydrocortisone cream (0.5–1%), removing contact to allergen if possible, cool soaking of skin to reduce discomfort/itching, diphenhydramine.
Crohn's disease	Inflammatory disease of the GI tract can affect any part of the digestive tract from mouth to anus.	No cure is known. Exacerbations can be treated and prevented with changes to lifestyle (changes in diet, smoking cessation, and proper hydration), antibiotics for infections, aminosalicylate, and anti-inflammatory drugs. If exacerbations do not respond to medical treatment, surgical removal of the inflamed area may be required.

(continued)

ALTERATIONS AND TREATMENTS Inflammation (continued)

Alteration	Description	Treatment
Glomerulonephritis	The glomeruli in the kidneys are inflamed.	Acute form may improve spontaneously with treatment of cause, often antibiotics for strep infection. Other treatments for acute and chronic form may include diuretics, ACE inhibitors, calcium channel blockers, and beta blockers. Temporary dialysis may be needed to support kidney function if kidney failure occurs.
Hashimoto's thyroiditis	T-cells attack the thyroid gland in this autoimmune disease believed to be most common cause of primary hypothyroidism.	Treatment is thyroid hormone replacement.
Systemic lupus erythematosus	Chronic autoimmune disorder attacks the body's cells and tissues, resulting in inflammation and tissue damage. Can occur anywhere in the body but most often affects the heart, joints, skin, lungs, blood vessels, liver, kidneys, and nervous system.	There is no known cure, but palliative treatment combined with NSAIDs, antimalarials, and disease-modifying antirheumatic drugs can reduce the frequency and severity of flare-ups. When flares occur, treatment with corticosteroids and immunosuppressants in combination with antimalarials has proven successful; often requires analgesics for pain.
Ulcerative colitis	Inflammatory bowel disease usually affects the large bowel and is characterized by ulcerated areas causing bloody diarrhea.	Treatment depends on extent of bowel involvement and disease severity. Aminosalicylates, corticosteroids, immunosuppressive drugs, and surgery are the most common treatments. Oatmeal and fiber from Brassica may be recommended because they seem to reverse ulceration.

PHYSICAL ASSESSMENT

During the assessment phase of the nursing process, the nurse obtains the client's history, conducts the physical assessment, and gathers laboratory data. Assessment for inflammation, which can impact any of the body's tissues, will be guided by the area of the body involved. Classic signs to assess for are indicated in the Inflammation Assessment feature.

History

When taking the patient's medical history, the nurse assesses (a) the degree to which a client is at risk of developing inflammation and (b) any client self-reports that suggest the presence of inflammation. To identify clients at risk, the nurse reviews the client's chart and structures the nursing interview to collect data regarding the factors influencing the development of inflammation, especially existing conditions. Because inflammation can involve any organ or organ system, a thorough history of the patient's systems is required.

Signs and symptoms of inflammation vary according to the body area involved. Appendicitis may involve abdominal pain, rigid abdomen, and elevated white blood cell count. Arthritis may involve joints that are warm, red, edematous, and painful. As a result, physical assessment may be focused on any area of the body, depending on where the inflammation is suspected or noted. Localized inflammation requires assessment for localized edema, pain or tenderness with palpation or movement, redness or palpable heat at the inflamed area, and reduced or absent function in the body part involved. Conditions causing more widespread inflammation, such as nephritis or allergies, may cause more diverse symptoms.

Inflammation Assessment

Local Manifestations	Systemic Manifestations
■ Erythema	■ T > 100.4°F (38°C) or < 96.8°F (36°C)
■ Warmth	■ P > 90 beats/min
■ Pain	■ R > 20 breaths/min (tachypnea)
■ Edema	■ WBC > 12,000/mm^3 or >10% bands
■ Functional impairment	

Source: LeMone, P., & Burke, K. (2008). *Medical-surgical nursing: Critical thinking in client care* (4th ed.). Upper Saddle River, NJ: Pearson, Inc.

Assessment Interview Inflammation

- Do you have any pain? If the client reports pain, the nurse should assess the pain for location, intensity, type, severity, current treatments, and effectiveness of treatment.
- Are you taking any anti-inflammatory medications such as aspirin or ibuprofen, or medications for chronic conditions?
- Have you had any recent diagnostic procedure or therapy that penetrated your skin or a body cavity?
- What past surgeries have you had?

- How would you describe your eating habits? Do you eat a variety of types of foods?
- Do you take vitamins or dietary supplements?
- On a scale of 1–10, how would you rate the stress you have experienced in the last 6 months?
- Have you experienced any loss of energy, loss of appetite, nausea, headache, or other signs associated with specific body systems (e.g., difficulty urinating, urinary frequency, or a sore throat)?

Note: As with all history taking, the nurse must individualize the specific terms used; give examples to the client; and use teaching techniques to validate agreement on the meaning of words according to the client's culture, language spoken, and education or intellectual abilities.
Source: Berman, A., Snyder, S.J., Kozier, B., & Erb, G. (2008). *Kozier & Erb's fundamentals of nursing: Concepts, process, and practice* (8th ed.). Upper Saddle River, NJ: Pearson, Inc.

DIAGNOSTIC TESTS

A primary laboratory test ordered to detect the presence of inflammation is the erythrocyte sedimentation rate (ESR). ESR measures how far the erythrocyte settles in a tube over a given period of time, usually 1 hour. Normal sedimentation rate for males is 0–15 mm/h, 0–20 mm/h for women. It is not unusual to see the sedimentation rate slightly elevated in older adults. When an inflammatory process is active, the increased proportion of fibrinogen causes red blood cells to stick to one another and settle faster, resulting in a higher reading.

Another important diagnostic laboratory test is the C-reactive protein (CRP). CRP is a protein found in the blood that is produced by the liver and fat cells in response to the inflammatory process. In the absence of liver failure, a rise in CRP levels indicates an inflammatory process is occurring somewhere in the body. CRP can also be used to evaluate the effectiveness of treatment for inflammation. Research also indicates the CRP can be used to assess risk for cardiac disease, as it elevates in response to arterial damage.

Other laboratory tests for inflammation are ordered based on the cause, location, and type of inflammation suspected. A WBC with differential may be ordered to determine the presence of an infection; serum protein electrophoresis may reveal increased gamma globulin and decreased albumin, indicating systemic lupus erythematosus; and routine chemistry panels may reveal kidney involvement, abnormal liver function, or increased muscle enzymes if the muscle is involved.

DIAGNOSTIC TESTS The White Blood Cell Count and Differential

CELL TYPE AND NORMAL VALUE	INCREASED	DECREASED
Total white blood cells (WBCs): 4,000–10,000 per mm³	*Leukocytosis:* Infection or inflammation, leukemia, trauma or stress, tissue necrosis	*Leukopenia:* Bone marrow depression, overwhelming infection, viral infections, immunosuppression, autoimmune disease, dietary deficiency
Neutrophils (segs, PMNs, or polys): 55–70%	*Neutrophilia:* Acute infection or stress response, myelocytic leukemia, inflammatory or metabolic disorders	*Neutropenia:* Bone marrow depression, overwhelming bacterial infection, viral infection, Addison's disease
Eosinophils (eos): 1–4%	*Eosinophilia:* Parasitic infections, hyper-sensitivity reactions, autoimmune disorders	*Eosinopenia:* Cushing's syndrome, autoimmune disorders, stress, certain drugs
Basophils (basos): 0.5–1%	*Basophilia:* Hypersensitivity responses, chronic myelogenous leukemia, chickenpox or smallpox, splenectomy, hypothyroidism	*Basopenia:* Acute stress or hypersensitivity reactions, hyperthyroidism
Monocytes (monos): 2–8%	*Monocytosis:* Chronic inflammatory disorders, tuberculosis, viral infections, leukemia, Hodgkin's disease, multiple myeloma	*Monocytopenia:* Bone marrow depression, corticosteroid therapy
Lymphocytes (lymphs): 20–40%	*Lymphocytosis:* Chronic bacterial infection, viral infections, lymphocytic leukemia	*Lymphocytopenia:* Bone marrow depression, immunodeficiency, leukemia, Cushing's syndrome, Hodgkin's disease, renal failure

Source: Data from Corbett, J. V. (2004). Laboratory tests and diagnostic procedures with nursing diagnoses (6th ed.), Upper Saddle River, NJ: Prentice Hall and *Diagnostic and Laboratory Test Reference* (3rd ed.) by K. D. Pagana and T. J. Pagana, 1997, St. Louis, MO: Mosby-Year Book.

CARING INTERVENTIONS

Management of inflammation due to injury is generally aimed at reducing mobility of the involved area, elevation to reduce edema, antipyretics if fever is involved, and anti-inflammatory medications. Other causes of inflammation will necessitate other, more specific treatments. For example, surgery will be indicated in most cases for appendicitis and gallbladder disease, antibiotics may be required to treat inflammation caused by infection, and steroids may be indicated for severe systemic inflammation. A client's diet should be evaluated to ensure that he or she is receiving adequate nutrients to support healing, including adequate protein, carbohydrates, and vitamins. Vitamins important in cellular repair include vitamin C.

Nurses working with clients experiencing inflammation should be sure to emphasize the importance of preventing further injury, taking medications as prescribed to treat or prevent illness, and maintaining adequate intake of liquids and nutrients. Family teaching may be necessary if the client needs assistance with changing dressings, preventing the inflamed area from exposure to water while bathing, or any other aspects of daily living until healing occurs. Additional client teaching during the reparative phase may be necessary to ensure that the client does not resume activity too quickly and that the client continues treatment until healing is complete and the client is released by the physician.

PHARMACOLOGIC THERAPIES

Pharmacological therapies are aimed at reducing the inflammatory response and reducing pain associated with the symptoms of inflammation. Common medications include nonsteroidal anti-inflammatory drugs (NSAIDs), which have fewer adverse effects than the more powerful anti-inflammatory corticosteroids. Corticosteroids are normally administered when inflammation is more severe or is life threatening. NSAIDs, in addition to their anti-inflammatory actions, are also analgesics and antipyretics that help not only to reduce inflammation but also to minimize its effects.

MEDICATIONS

Classification	Actions	Common drugs	Nursing considerations
NSAIDs	Analgesic, antipyretic, and anti-inflammatory properties act by inhibiting the synthesis of prostaglandins (lipids found in all tissues with potent physiological effects in addition to promoting inflammation depending on the tissue where they are found). NSAIDs block inflammation by inhibiting cyclooxygenase (COX), the key enzyme in the biosynthesis of prostaglandins.	Ibuprofen, naproxen sodium, aspirin, indomethacin, celecoxib	■ Give on an empty stomach if tolerated or with food if nausea, vomiting, or abdominal pain occurs. ■ Give for pregnancy category B. ■ Do not administer to clients with peptic ulcer disease. ■ Avoid NSAIDs with anticoagulants. ■ Actions of some diuretics can be reduced with NSAIDs. ■ May increase bleeding time. ■ Monitor client response to treatment. ■ Use with caution in the elderly because of potential reduction in kidney and liver function.
Glucocorticoids	Natural hormones are released by the adrenal cortex with potent anti-inflammatory actions on nearly every cell in the body that can suppress severe cases of inflammation. Generally reserved for short-term treatment due to serious potential side effects.	Betamethasone, cortisone, dexamethasone, hydrocortisone	■ If administered im, administer deep im to avoid atrophy or abscesses. ■ Do not use in presence of systemic infection due to reduced immune response. ■ Do not discontinue abruptly. ■ Use in pregnancy category C. ■ Carefully monitor condition, blood glucose levels, WBC count, changes in mood, or signs of Cushing's syndrome if used long term. ■ Use cautiously in clients with gastrointestinal ulcers, renal disease, hypertension, osteoporosis, varicella, diabetes mellitus, heart failure, mental instability, or any disease that reduces immune response (HIV, cancer, etc.).
Analgesics	Give to treat the pain associated with inflammation if NSAID analgesic effect is not sufficient alone.	Morphine, oxycodone	■ Monitor pain status for adequate relief of pain. ■ If administering a narcotic, monitor respiratory rate. ■ See concept of pain for further information about analgesics.
Natural therapies	Eicosapentaenoic acid (EPA) and docosahexaenoic acid (DHA) have anti-inflammatory actions in addition to their triglyceride-lowering activity.	Fish oils	■ Interactions may occur between fish oil supplements and aspirin and other NSAIDs. While rare, interactions may be manifested by increased susceptibility to bruising, nosebleeds, hemoptysis, hematuria, and blood in the stool.

Source: Adams, M.P., Holland, Jr., L.N., & Bostwick, P.M. (2008). *Pharmacology for nurses: a pathophysiologic approach* (2nd ed.). Upper Saddle River, NJ: Pearson Inc.

REFERENCES

Adams, M.P., Holland, Jr., L.N., & Bostwick, P.M. (2008). *Pharmacology for nurses: A pathophysiologic approach* (2nd ed.). Upper Saddle River, NJ: Pearson Education.

Berman, A., Snyder, S.J., Kozier, B., & Erb, G. (2008). *Kozier & Erb's fundamentals of nursing: Concepts, process, and practice* (8th ed.). Upper Saddle River, NJ: Pearson Education.

LeMone, P., & Burke, K. (2008). *Medical-surgical nursing: Critical thinking in client care* (4th ed.). Upper Saddle River, NJ: Pearson Education.

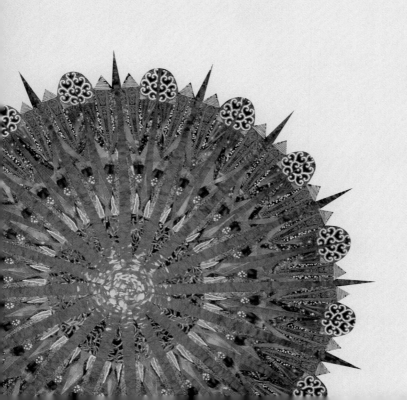

Oxygenation

Concept at-a-Glance

Concept Learning Outcomes

After reading about this concept, you will be able to do the following:

1. Summarize the structure and physiologic processes of the respiratory system related to oxygenation.

2. List factors affecting oxygenation.

3. Identify commonly occurring alterations in oxygenation and their related treatments.

4. Explain common physical assessment procedures used to evaluate respiratory health of clients across the life span.

5. Outline diagnostic and laboratory tests and expected findings to determine the individual's oxygenation status.

6. Explain management of respiratory health and prevention of respiratory illness.

7. Demonstrate the nursing process in providing culturally competent care across the life span for individuals with common alterations in oxygenation.

8. Identify pharmacologic interventions in caring for the individual with alterations in respiratory function.

Concept Key Terms

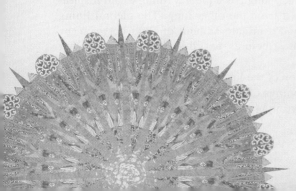

About Oxygenation

Oxygenation can be defined as the mechanisms that facilitate or impair the body's ability to supply oxygen to all cells of the body. The function of the respiratory system is to obtain oxygen from atmospheric air, to transport this air through the respiratory tract into the alveoli, and ultimately to diffuse oxygen into the blood that carries oxygen to all the cells of the body. The respiratory system achieves all this through **respiration**, the act of inhaling (**inspiration**) and exhaling (**expiration**) air to transport oxygen to the alveoli so that oxygen may be exchanged for carbon dioxide, and the carbon dioxide expelled from the body. The actual exchange of oxygen and carbon dioxide is called **ventilation**.

The respiratory system is divided into two parts: the upper respiratory tract and the lower respiratory tract. The upper respiratory tract begins with the nose and ends in the pharynx. The lower respiratory tract begins at the epiglottis and ends in the alveoli. The alveoli are the functional portion of the respiratory system where the exchange of oxygen and carbon dioxide occurs by diffusion at the alveoli-pulmonary capillary bed interface. Adequate oxygenation within the body depends on a healthy, intact respiratory system. ●

Breathing is often an unnoticed activity that contributes to vital oxygenation of the cells and tissues. When oxygen status changes, breathing usually compensates to bring more air into the lungs. Changes in breathing patterns should be taken seriously and acted upon promptly because alterations in oxygen delivery can cause serious consequences.

Mrs. Lee presents at the emergency room where she reports that she has been breathing rapidly and deeply for the past 2 hours. She reports, "I cannot breathe. Get some fresh air in here." While still being interviewed by the triage nurse, her respiratory rate goes from 40 breaths per minute to 30 breaths per minute. Her respiratory quality changes from deep to shallow. The triage nurse follows protocol, summoning additional registered nurses, a respiratory therapist, a physician, a radiology technologist, and a phlebotomist to the room.

Although other indicators of hemodynamic instability also existed for Mrs. Lee, the sudden change in breathing was most important in determining whether a more aggressive approach to her care was necessary.

NORMAL PRESENTATION

Adequate oxygenation of the body depends on a healthy, intact respiratory system. The respiratory system obtains oxygen from atmospheric air and transports it into the alveoli, where oxygen diffuses into a capillary and is carried by the blood to all the cells of the body. The respiratory system also passes carbon dioxide from the body.

The upper respiratory system is the inlet for air into the body. The nose is the typical inlet. The nose is midline on the face, with the same color as facial skin. The nose is divided into two nares that are moist, pink, mucosa-lined passageways. The purpose of the nares is to warm, humidify, and filter air as it is breathed into the nose. The upper respiratory tract has two protective mechanisms to prevent foreign matter from entering the lower respiratory tract: sneezing and cilia. Foreign matter that enters the nose irritates the nasal passages and induces sneezing. Sneezing is a reflexive action that clears the upper airway. This reflexive action is active even in the neonatal period. Cilia are microscopic fine hairs within the posterior portion of the nares that

trap small particles of foreign matter to prevent their entry into the lower respiratory tract. The cilia propel foreign matter into the pharynx to be coughed out or swallowed.

Breathing also happens through the mouth, which allows air to enter the respiratory system through the pharyngeal cavity. The respiratory system shares this cavity with the gastrointestinal system, providing passage for air during breathing and for food or drink during swallowing.

A protective mechanism within the pharyngeal cavity prevents food or drink from entering the lower respiratory tract. The glottis is the opening into the lower respiratory tract. The epiglottis is pendulous tissue that covers the tracheal opening during swallowing or any time foreign matter contacts the glottis. The closure of the epiglottis is a reflexive response.

The lower respiratory tract is enclosed in the musculoskeletal structures of the neck and thoracic cavity. The trachea, which sits midline in the neck, is the entrance way for air into the lungs. During normal breathing, the muscular structures of the neck are relaxed and the larynx easily rises and falls with a swallow. The chest wall effortlessly and symmetrically rises and falls with each equally spaced breath. Inspiration is half the rate of expiration. **Eupnea** describes breathing within the expected respiratory rates. **Auscultation**, listening to the body's sounds with a stethoscope, is an important diagnostic tool. Auscultation of the trachea will reveal a **tubular** sound of air movement, as if produced through a tube, when airways are clear and functioning.

The trachea bifurcates (divides in two) into two bronchi to access the right and left lungs (Figures 10–1 ■ and 10–2 ■). The right bronchus is shorter and wider than the left. Each bronchus further divides into bronchioles that terminate in the alveoli sacs. These passageways for air dilate and contract. The trachea and larger bronchi are supported by C-shaped cartilage rings, as well as by smooth muscle. The smaller bronchioles are supported by smooth muscles only. Bronchioles deliver air to the alveoli. These air passageways dilate and contract as the autonomic nervous system regulates the smooth muscles supporting them. The movement of air within the bronchial tree creates a mixture of sounds of air flowing through a tube and the breeziness of the open alveolar lung fields. This is termed **bronchovesicular** sound.

The lungs are also described in terms of their lobes. The lobes lie obliquely in the thoracic cavity. The right lung has three lobes; the left lung has two lobes. The inferior lobes are the largest. Most of the inferior lobes lie in the posterior thoracic cavity. Each lung has a pleural lining to aid respiration and separate it from the other lung. The pleural lining has two layers, and a minute amount of fluid between the layers allows the structures to glide across one another during respiration.

The final portion of the lower respiratory system is the air sacs. The outcroppings of the air sacs are called alveoli. The alveoli are the portion of the lungs that fulfill the function of

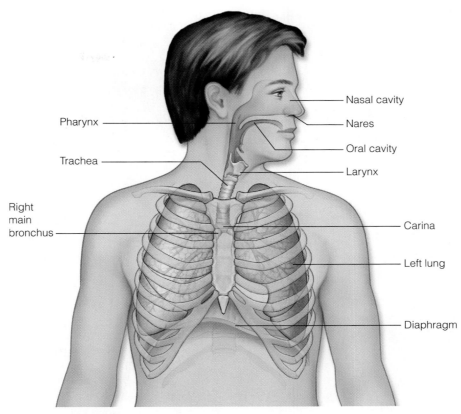

Pharynx

Trachea

Right
main
bronchus

Nasal cavity

Nares

Oral cavity

Larynx

Carina

Left lung

Diaphragm

Figure 10–1 ■ Anatomy of the respiratory system.

the respiratory system. Alveoli are not directly connected to a specific bronchiole, but are interconnected to the terminal airways and to each other. This facilitates the filling of each alveoli with air. The sounds of air moving into and out of the lobes at the alveolar level are soft and breezy, defined as **vesicular**.

The alveoli have specialized cells that produce surfactant. **Surfactant** controls surface tension and keeps the alveoli from collapsing and sticking to itself. Surfactant is produced only with adequate oxygenation. Alveolar macrophages keep the alveoli region free of microbes and are swept upward from the alveolar region by cilia in the airway passages. Macrophages are large cells of the immune system that remove waste and harmful microorganisms from the alveoli and from other areas of the body. Mast cells in the alveoli mediate the immune response within the airways.

Alveoli have a simple squamous epithelial lining and basement that interface with the basement and epithelial lining of pulmonary capillaries. This interface is where oxygen and carbon dioxide diffusion occurs. The concentration of oxygen is greater in the alveoli than in the blood in the capillaries, so oxygen diffuses across the membranes into the blood. The concentration of carbon dioxide is greater in the blood, so it diffuses into the alveoli. Figure 10–3 ■ shows the alveolar-capillary membrane interface.

The typical drive to breathe occurs due to **hypercarbia**. Hypercarbia is an increased level of carbon dioxide in the blood. Receptor sites within the medulla and pons are sensitive to carbon dioxide levels in the blood. Elevated levels of carbon dioxide induce inhalation of air into the lungs. Yawns and sighs are induced after periods of shallow breathing or breath holding. Exhalation is a passive response to relaxation of the muscles of respiration. The typical breathing rate is regularly spaced, with inspiration half as long as expiration (I:E = 1:2).

TABLE 10–1 Respirations Throughout the Life Span

VALUE RANGES BY AGE GROUP	RATE (BREATHS/MIN)
Newborns	30–60
Infants	20–40
Toddlers	20–30
Preschooler	20–26
School aged	12–24
Adolescence	14–20
Adults	10–20
Older adults	12–24

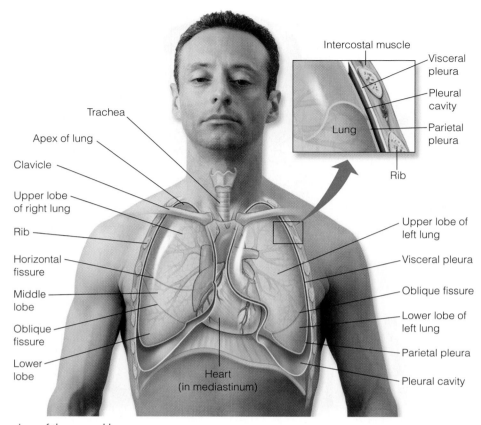

Figure 10–2 ■ Anterior view of thorax and lungs.

The normal respiratory rate in an adult ranges from 10 to 20 breaths per minute. Table 10–1 shows normal ranges for various age groups. Depth of normal inspiration is about 500 mL of air with each breath. The expansion of the chest wall is observable, but is neither shallow nor great. Quality of breathing refers to the effort involved in taking a breath and the sounds that may occur with inspiration or expiration. Quality of breathing requires a **patent airway**, one that is open and free of obstruction.

Receptor sites in the aortic arch and carotid arteries monitor oxygen. These receptors will induce inspiration with low enough levels of oxygen. Stretch receptors with the lungs control the volume of air inhaled with each breath. During relaxed states, the lungs will fill to approximately one half a liter. Strenuous activities of exercise result in deeper breaths of increasing volume to meet the oxygen demands of skeletal muscles.

The ability of the respiratory system to deliver oxygen to the blood depends on an inflated and well-oxygenated alveolus and an associated capillary with freely flowing blood at an adequate blood pressure. The movement of oxygen across the alveolar-capillary membrane into a well-perfusing capillary is defined as the **ventilation-perfusion** (V-Q) ratio. The concentration levels of oxygen and carbon dioxide dictate the movement of each gas across the alveolar-capillary membrane.

ALTERATIONS

The typical drive to breathe occurs due to hypercarbia. Hypercarbia interferes with the body's ability to respond appropriately to increased levels of carbon dioxide. When this happens, instead of hypercarbia initiating the breathing response, decreased levels of oxygen initiate the drive to breathe. This is commonly seen in individuals with **chronic obstructive pulmonary disease (COPD)**, resulting from prolonged cigarette smoking, as smoking is the primary cause of prolonged elevated levels of carbon dioxide.

Hypoxemia is defined as a decreased level of oxygen. Chest wall in-drawing is an early indicator of hypoxemia. **Cyanosis** is a late sign of hypoxemia and is seen as a blue tinge to the skin in fair individuals. In individuals with darker pigmentation, cyanosis may present as gray coloration of the skin. An indicator of chronic hypoxemia is clubbed nail beds. Clubbed nail beds have an angle of 180°

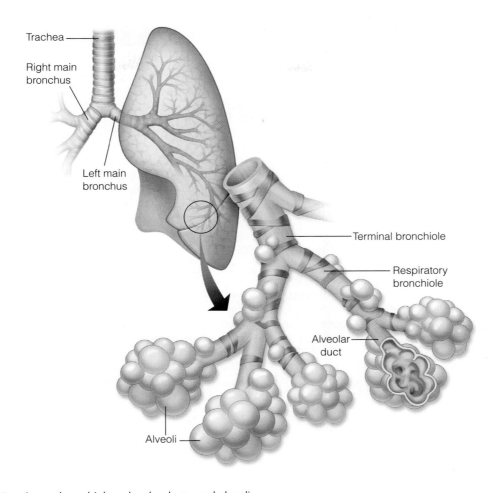

Figure 10–3 ■ Respiratory bronchioles, alveolar ducts, and alveoli.

or greater, depending on the duration of time an individual has had hypoxemia.

A number of factors affect a healthy respiratory system. The air an individual breathes, either indoors or outdoors, may be polluted. Exposure to airborne irritants may produce an inflammatory response within the airways. Infectious illnesses of the respiratory tract and hemoglobin disorders such as sickle cell anemia interfere with effective respiratory function. Lifestyle behaviors may affect respiratory health. Some medications affect respiratory rate and depth. Generally, inflammation, infection, sputum production, and compromised airflow contribute to alterations in respiratory health. *Healthy People 2010* has several directives related to maintaining or attaining respiratory health. These include the following:

■ Management of environmental air quality is necessary to decrease the concentration of respiratory irritations affecting asthma and COPD in the United States. Environmental air quality includes interior and external air sources. A decrease in the use of tobacco products is necessary to stop the unnecessary damage to the health of tobacco users and those exposed secondhand to tobacco smoke. Tobacco smoking is the primary cause of COPD in Western countries such as the United States. Exposure to polluted air in homes and workplaces and to tobacco smoke exacerbates COPD, asthma, and respiratory synctial virus and is associated with sudden infant death syndrome.

■ Vaccination is encouraged to decrease transmission of preventable diseases, many of which are transmitted by respiratory secretions. Many illnesses historically seen in children now are prevented by immunization. Immunization for influenza and pneumonia protects adults from serious respiratory illness. Respiratory syncytial virus (RSV) is a highly contagious respiratory infection that affects all age groups, but that is most serious for children younger than 2 years of age. Sudden infant death syndrome (SIDS) is the major cause of death with unknown cause for infants older than 1 month of age.

ALTERATIONS AND TREATMENTS Respiratory System

Alteration	Description	Treatment
Chronic obstructive pulmonary disease (COPD)	COPD is a preventable, treatable disease of compromised airflow within the respiratory system. COPD is a progressive disorder that alters the structures of the respiratory system over time. Inflammation of the mucous membranes of the bronchial tubes occurs as well as loss of elasticity in lung parenchyma.	■ Smoking cessation ■ Avoidance of secondhand smoke ■ Administration of bronchodilators ■ Administration of corticosteroids ■ Use of breathing exercises ■ Respiratory therapy consult ■ Administration of pulmonary function tests ■ Spirometry ■ Complete blood count (CBC), chemistries, and arterial blood gases ■ Taking sputum specimen ■ Administration of oxygen ■ Physical therapy consult ■ Nutritional consult
Asthma	Asthma is a chronic inflammatory disease of the airways. Asthma presents with coughing, wheezing, shortness of breath, chest tightness, and sputum production. Asthma is defined in relation to severity and control as well as to impairments and risk.	■ Smoking cessation ■ Avoidance of secondhand smoke ■ Avoidance of aggravating factors ■ Respiratory therapy consult ■ Measuring daily peak expiratory flow rate ■ Administration of maintenance bronchodilators ■ Administration of maintenance corticosteroids ■ Exercise planning by physical therapy ■ Administration of short-acting bronchodilators for exercise ■ Measuring CBC, chemistry panels, and arterial blood gases ■ Taking a sputum specimen
Respiratory syncytial virus (RSV)	RSV is a highly contagious lower respiratory infection that affects nearly 100% of children younger than 2 years of age. Repeated infections of RSV occur throughout the life span, though subsequent infections tend to be milder.	■ Smoking cessation by caregivers ■ Avoidance of secondhand smoke ■ Separating sick individuals from well individuals ■ Observation of breathing pattern including, rate, rhythm, and quality ■ Teaching the parents or caregiver how to observe breathing patterns ■ Maintaining adequate fluid volume and calories ■ Oral and nasal suctioning ■ Possible use of bronchodilators and corticosteroids
Sudden infant death syndrome (SIDS)	SIDS is the leading cause of death of infants beyond the neonatal period. SIDS occurs most often between the first and the fourth months of life, but may occur up to 1 year of age. The cause of SIDS is not known. Infants who appear healthy are found dead by parents or caregivers. Preventive measures have reduced the incidence of SIDS in developed countries, including the United States.	■ Placing infant on his or her back to sleep ■ Smoking cessation by caregivers ■ Avoidance of secondhand smoke ■ Ensuring a totally smoke-free environment ■ Co-sleeper or same-room sleeping of infant and parents ■ Avoiding bed sharing ■ Maintaining adult-comfort room temperature ■ Breastfeeding ■ Using a pacifier
Acute respiratory distress syndrome (ARDS)	ARDS is a disorder with rapid onset of progressive malfunction of the lungs' ability to take in oxygen. Extensive lung tissue inflammation and small blood vessel injury occurs, followed by malfunction of other organs.	■ Measuring CBC, chemistry panels, and arterial blood gases ■ Taking sputum specimen ■ Administration of oxygen ■ Providing ventilator support ■ Administration of hemodynamic intravenous drugs

Alterations in oxygenation can be described in relation to changes in breathing patterns, patency of airway, or interference with gas exchange. Damage to the supporting thoracic structure, either by injury or disease, can contribute to interference in effective respiration. Irritation or inflammation of the respiratory mucosa also affects the ability of the respiratory system to obtain adequate oxygenation for the cells within the body.

The airway of an infant is very small in diameter. It can be occluded with minimal amounts of sputum or swelling from inflammation. Infants are obligatory nose breathers; therefore, even stuffy noses can interfere with the infant's breathing process. Children, especially infants and toddlers, learn about their world by placing things into their mouths and noses. Small objects may become caught in their airways, interfering with breathing.

Adults also may be at risk of catching a foreign object in their airways. Large bites of food that are improperly chewed and swallowed can become lodged in the throat, interfering with the passage of air into the lungs. Older adults are at even greater risk of choking on food because their cough reflex response is decreased. The incidence of gastroesophageal reflux disease increases with age, increasing the risk of aspiration of food into the lower respiratory tract.

Loss of airway patency can result from increased sputum production from upper and lower respiratory infection or irritation. Thick sputum secretions are of special concern in relation to blocking large and small airways. Inflammation of airways due to infections or irritants narrows airways, decreasing the movement of air through the respiratory system.

Respiratory rate, rhythm, depth, and quality determine adequate oxygenation to the cells. A respiratory rate greater than 20 breaths per minute in adults is called **tachypnea**. Anxiety or stress may cause an individual to breathe very rapidly, inhaling and exhaling deeply. Hyperventilation is rapid and deep inhalation and exhalation of air from the lungs. In hypoventilation, a reduced amount of air enters the alveoli, resulting in a decrease of oxygen and an increase of carbon dioxide. A respiratory rate of less than 10 breaths per minute in adults is called **bradypnea**. **Apnea** is the absence of breathing. Continuous apnea is termed *respiratory arrest* and is life-threatening.

Dyspnea, labored breathing or shortness of breath that is uncomfortable or painful, also occurs when breathing is insufficient to meet oxygen demand. Exertional dyspnea occurs with activity. **Orthopnea** is difficulty breathing when a person is supine. The nurse's ability to differentiate changes in respiratory rate is critical when working with any individual, but particularly critical when working with elder patients because pulmonary function declines with age. Chest walls and airways become more rigid, losing their elasticity, and musculoskeletal strength decreases and the effort to breathe increases.

Several breathing patterns with irregular rates, rhythms, depth, and quality indicate abnormalities within other body systems. Kussmaul's breathing occurs in the presence of metabolic acidosis and results in very deep and rapid breaths. These deep, rapid exhalations rid the body of large amounts of carbon dioxide, which affects the acid–base balance. Cheyne-Stokes respirations exhibit as deep, rapid breathing and slow, shallow breathing with periods of apnea. Cheyne-Stokes is seen in individuals with congestive heart failure, increased intracranial pressure, and drug overdoses. Biot's respirations are seen in individuals with central nervous system disorders. Biot's presents as shallow breathing with periods of apnea. Benzodiazepines, barbiturates, and opioids may cause decreased depth and rate of breathing due to their oxygenation-compromising central nervous system effects.

Abnormalities within the alveolar-capillary bed system alter V-Q ratios. Airflow in an alveolus blocked by sputum, inflammation with its complementary swelling, atelectasis, or fluid volume excesses can cause decreased ventilation. Blood clots, plaque buildup, and emphysemic adjacent alveolus interfere with capillary blood flow. Each of these V-Q mismatches results in inadequate oxygenation of body cells. Any and all of these types of V-Q mismatch may occur simultaneously (Figure 10–4 ■).

Any alteration that impairs the oxygenation process can be life-threatening. In addition to determining and then treating the presenting alteration, it is critical to determine its cause. A mild case of exercise-induced asthma may only require administration of an albuterol inhaler prior to the individual participating in exercise or sports activities. By contrast, COPD is much more difficult to treat.

In addition to the exemplars detailed in this concept, other diseases and some injuries, such as a fractured pleural rib, can cause impairment in oxygenation. One disease that presents multiple problems for clients and their physicians is sickle cell anemia. An inherited blood disorder, sickle cell anemia impairs the transport of oxygen through the blood. Sickle cell can cause a variety of complications, including organ failure.

Pneumothorax, or a partial lung collapse resulting from air or gas collecting in the lung or in the pleural space that surrounds the lungs, is a respiratory emergency. A pneumothorax that appears without any known cause is termed a *spontaneous pneumothorax*. Risk factors for this type of pneumothorax include emphysema, cystic fibrosis, and tuberculosis. A tension pneumothorax results from injury (e.g., a fractured rib) or as a result of a progressive lung disease, such as asthma or emphysema. Tension pneumothorax is more difficult to treat than pneumothorax and can result in heart failure. Signs and symptoms of a pneumothorax include sudden sharp pleuritic pain, worsened by movement such as breathing and coughing; asymmetrical chest wall movement; shortness of breath; and cyanosis.

Impaired oxygenation can be frightening and frustrating. It is frightening in that it may be life-threatening. It is frustrating in that shortness of breath and other symptoms common to impairment of oxygenation cause fatigue and can affect so many other bodily processes, which in turn affect quality of life.

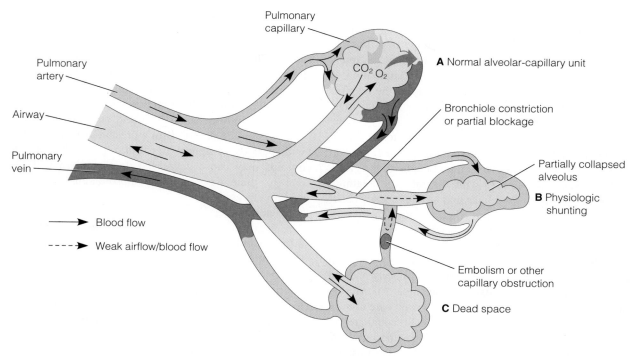

Figure 10–4 ■ Ventilation-perfusion relationships. *A,* Normal alveolar-capillary unit with an ideal match of ventilation and blood flow. Maximum gas exchange occurs between alveolus and blood. *B,* Physiologic shunting: A unit with adequate perfusion but inadequate ventilation. *C,* Dead space: A unit with adequate ventilation but inadequate perfusion. In the latter two cases, gas exchange is impaired.

PHYSICAL ASSESSMENT

The respiratory system health history and physical assessment include subjective and objective data. Lifestyle behaviors and current problems with breathing, including the presence of a cough and sputum, are determined. Any risk factors associated with compromised respiratory health are noted.

The assessment of any body system requires a systematic approach to ensure that no area or aspect of the body system is missed. The nurse uses all five senses to assess an individual. With inspection the nurse uses his or her eyes to observe expected and unexpected findings. Then with **palpation**, the nurse uses the hands to feel the areas related to the body system for **symmetry**, equality of the size, shape, or condition of opposite sides of the body. Next, the nurse uses **percussion**, a method of tapping the chest or back to assess underlying structures; tones heard during percussion determine solid-filled or air-filled spaces at the area percussed. Finally, the nurse uses auscultation to hear the sounds within the respiratory system (Box 10–1). Use of a stethoscope facilitates the hearing of sounds within the body. Any assessment is best supported by obtaining a full set of vital sign measurements with pulse oximetry.

An individual presenting with breathing problems may provide a number of objective and subjective indicators that confirm the report. Self-posturing (leaning forward or against a

Box 10–1 Adventitious Breathing Sounds

A number of adventitious sounds can be heard while auscultating the lower respiratory tract.
- **Stridor** is a high-pitched sound within the trachea and larynx that suggests narrowing of the tracheal passage.
- **Crackles** are high-pitched popping sounds, much like when one pours milk over crisped rice cereal. Crackles are heard on inspiration, due to fluid associated with or resulting from inflammation, or exudates, within the lung fields or localized atelectasis. **Atelectasis** is the collapse of lung tissue affecting all or part a lung, impacting the exchange of oxygen and carbon dioxide. The primary cuase of atelectasis is the obstruction of the bronchus serving the affected area.
- **Rhonchi** is a long, low-pitched sound that continues throughout inspiration. Rhonchi suggests blockage of large airway passages, which can sometimes be cleared with coughing.
- **Wheezing** is a high-pitched whistling sound most often heard on expiration and caused by the narrowing of bronchi, but wheezes can also be heard on inspiration.
- When inflamed pleural surfaces rub together, they can make a low-pitched, grating sound. This occurs more during inspiration, but can also occur during expiration.

Oxygenation Assessment

Technique/Normal Findings	Abnormal Findings

Nasal assessment

Inspect the nose symmetry.
Inspect the nasal cavity using a flashlight. The septum should fall midline and intact. The mucosa of the nares is pink and moist without drainage. Both nares should be patent.
(see Figure 10–5 ■)

- Asymmetry indicates trauma or surgery.
- Redness and/or swelling is observed.
- Deviated septum narrows or occludes one naris.
- Foreign bodies may be found in the nares, especially of infants, toddlers, and preschoolers.
- Purulent drainage occurs.
- Watery nasal drainage occurs.
- Pale turbinates are seen.

Thoracic assessment

Measure respiratory rate:

- Bradypnea
- Tachypnea
- Apnea

Assess quality of breathing:
 Determine regularity in timing
 I:E ratio is 1:2.
Assess depth of inspiration.
Observe effort to breath.

- Shortness of breath
- Dyspnea
- Orthopnea

Inspection of thoracic cavity

Anteroposterior diameter is half the transverse diameter. *Normal ratio is 1:2.* (see Figures 10–6 ■ and 10–7 ■)

- Anteroposterior equals transverse thoracic diameter measurements, called a barrel chest.

Inspection of the muscles of breathing

The chest walls gently rise and fall with each breath. The muscles in the neck are relaxed. The trachea is midline. The intercostal muscles raise the chest upward and outward with inhalation, then calmly relax with exhalation.

- Retraction of the intercostals occurs.
- Sternocleidomastoid muscles of the neck contract.
- Posturing occurs.

Inspection and palpation of the thoracic wall for symmetry

Symmetrical movement of the hands is observed with symmetrical hand placement on the chest wall. The trachea is midline.

- Asymmetry of movement occurs.
- Decreased expansion occurs.
- The trachea shifts from midline.

Skin assessment in relation to the respiratory system

Pink skin indicates adequate oxygenation of the cell throughout the body.
Nail beds are an extension of the finger and are normally curved with a 160° angle of the nail bed to the finger.

Cyanosis is a blue tinge to the skin in fair individuals and gray coloration of the skin in darker pigmented individuals.
Clubbed nail beds have an angle of 180° or greater, depending on the duration of time an individual has had hypoxemia.

---

table or wall to breathe) may be evident. A client may have difficulty speaking, taking breaths in the middle of sentences. The individual's voice may be raspy. In the absence of a productive cough, repeated throat clearing may indicate the presence of phlegm. Individuals who cannot breathe well often become frustrated when answering questions because the effort to answer further impairs breathing, and the effort to breathe quickly brings on fatigue. When working with any individual, as well as with someone with impaired breathing, the nurse should be patient and sympathetic. A pulse oximetry reading above 90% may not be a true indicator of the level of respiratory distress if the client has used an albuterol inhaler within 30–60 minutes of presenting at the clinic or emergency room. Increased frequency of use of albuterol inhalers or nebulizer treatments indicates a severe respiratory episode.

Clients who present with impairment at or near respiratory failure will not be able to respond to questions. Assessment questions should be tailored and asked of any

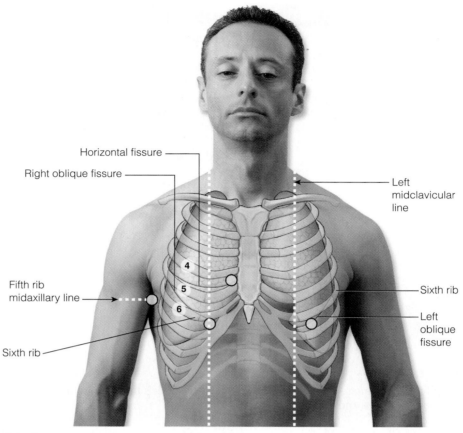

Figure 10–5 ■ Lobes of the lungs: anterior view.

Assessment Interview Oxygenation

CURRENT RESPIRATORY PROBLEMS

- Have you noticed any changes in your breathing pattern (e.g., shortness of breath, difficulty in breathing, need to be in upright position to breathe, or rapid and shallow breathing)?
- If so, which of your activities might cause these symptoms to occur?
- How many pillows do you use to sleep at night?

HISTORY OF RESPIRATORY DISEASE

- Have you had colds, allergies, asthma, tuberculosis, bronchitis, pneumonia, or emphysema?
- How frequently have these occurred? How long did they last? And how were they treated?
- Have you been exposed to any pollutants?

LIFESTYLE

- Do you smoke? If so, how much? If not, did you smoke previously, and when did you stop?
- Does any member of your family smoke?
- Is there cigarette smoke or other pollutants (e.g., fumes, dust, coal, asbestos) in your workplace?
- Do you drink alcohol? If so, how many drinks (mixed drinks, glasses of wine, or beers) do you usually have per day or per week?
- Describe your exercise patterns. How often do you exercise and for how long?

PRESENCE OF COUGH

- How often and how much do you cough?
- Is it productive, that is, accompanied by sputum, or nonproductive, that is, dry?
- Does the cough occur during certain activity or at certain times of the day?

DESCRIPTION OF SPUTUM

- When is the sputum produced?
- What is the amount, color, thickness, and odor of the sputum?
- Is it ever tinged with blood?

PRESENCE OF CHEST PAIN

- How does going outside in the heat or the cold affect you?
- Do you experience any pain with breathing or activity?
- Where is the pain located?
- Describe the pain. How does it feel?
- Does it occur when you breathe in or out?
- How long does it last, and how does it affect your breathing?
- Do you experience any other symptoms when the pain occurs (e.g., nausea, shortness of breath or difficulty breathing, lightheadedness, palpitations)?
- What activities precede your pain?
- What do you do to relieve the pain?

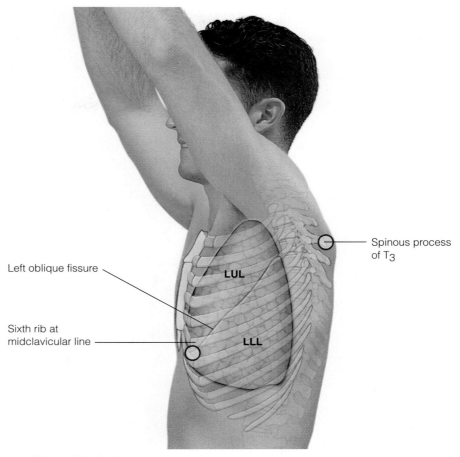

Left oblique fissure

Sixth rib at
midclavicular line

LUL

LLL

Spinous process
of T$_3$

Figure 10–6 ■ Lateral view of lobes of the left lung.

Assessment Interview Oxygenation (continued)

PRESENCE OF RISK FACTORS

■ Do you have a family history of lung cancer, cardiovascular disease (including strokes), or tuberculosis?

■ The nurse should also note the client's weight, activity pattern, and dietary assessment. Risk factors include obesity, sedentary lifestyle, and diet high in saturated fats.

MEDICATION HISTORY

■ Have you taken or do you take any over-the-counter or prescription medications for breathing (e.g., bronchodilator, inhalant, narcotic)?

■ If so, which ones? And what are the dosages, times taken, and results, including side effects? Are you taking them exactly as directed?

Source: Berman, A., Snyder, S. J., Kozier, B., & Erb, G. (2008). *Kozier & Erb's fundamentals of nursing: Concepts, process, and practice* (8th ed., p. 1365). Upper Saddle River, NJ: Pearson Education.

family member or friend accompanying the client to the emergency room. The client's physician should be notified immediately on the client's arrival at the hospital. The immediate concern is, of course, to return respiratory status as close to normal as possible. Adrenaline may be given in the case of respiratory failure related to anaphylaxis or allergic reaction. Chest tubes and ventilators may be necessary. Support for family care is also important at this time, as is an understanding of the client's religious and cultural preferences. The Roman Catholic Church, as well as other

denominations, have prayers that are said over those who are very sick. Jehovah's Witnesses have some prohibitions against blood transfusion, and this must be addressed if surgery should be necessary.

PRACTICE ALERT

Remember, the greatest area of inferior lobes is heard on the posterior chest. If the nurse skips listening to the back, much of the lung assessment data remain unknown.

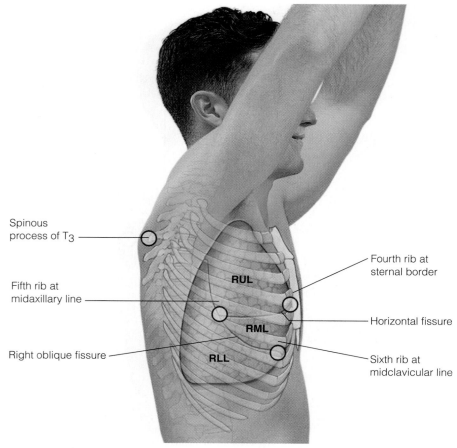

Figure 10–7 ■ Lateral view of lobes of the right lung.

DIAGNOSTIC TESTS

Specific diagnostic tests are used to assess for abnormalities of the respiratory system and to monitor for changes in individuals with chronic oxygenation impairment. Tests include those that determine the presence of inflammation or infection and changes in acid–base balance, and tests for viewing thoracic structures.

A sputum specimen may be used to identify the presence of microbes, metabolites of inflammation, and immunoglobulins. A sputum culture is used to identify specific microbes within the lower respiratory tract. Sputum is expectorant matter that may contain all or some mucus, cellular debris, blood, microorganisms, and purulent matter from the respiratory tract. It is important to ensure that the liquid obtained from an individual is from the lung fields and not from spit from his or her mouth. The proper identification of the microbe facilitates the selection of the appropriate antibiotic, antiviral, or antifungal agents to treat the inflammation. Excessive use of antibiotics for inflammatory processes that do not respond to the prescribed antibiotic has contributed to the emergence of drug-resistant microbes.

Arterial blood gas (ABG) provides a direct indication of oxygen and carbon dioxide exchange and the acid–base balance within the blood. The major chemical components monitored by ABG are hydrogen ions (pH), carbon dioxide (CO_2), oxygen (O_2), and bicarbonate (HCO_3). See Table 10–2 for normal ABG laboratory values. Each ABG component is reviewed in turn.

Initial assessment focuses on the oxygen values of the ABG. The oxygen value is defined by the amount of oxygen bound to hemoglobin (SaO_2) and the amount of oxygen dissolved in blood serum (PaO_2). An oxygen saturation value (SaO_2) in a healthy individual without any respiratory abnormalities is greater than 95%. The values of oxygen dissolved in blood serum (PaO_2) ranges from 80 to 100 mmHg. Oxygen levels that indicate hypoxemia should be treated by administering oxygen. Mild hypoxemia ranges from 60 to 79 mmHg, moderate hypoxemia ranges from 40 to 59 mmHg, and severe hypoxemia is less than 40 mmHg (Pruitt & Jacobs, 2004).

TABLE 10–2 Arterial Blood Gas Values

pH	7.35–7.45
CO_2	35–45
O_2	80–100
HCO_3	22–26

DEVELOPMENTAL CONSIDERATIONS Respiratory Development

INFANTS

- Respiratory rates are highest and most variable in newborns. The respiratory rate of a neonate is 40–80 breaths per minute.
- Infant respiratory rates average about 30 breaths per minute.
- Because of the structure of the ribcage infants rely almost exclusively on diaphragmatic movement for breathing. This is seen as abdominal breathing, as the abdomen rises and falls with each breath.

CHILDREN

- The respiratory rate gradually decreases, averaging around 25 breaths per minute in the preschooler and reaching the adult rate of 12–18 breaths per minute by late adolescence.
- During infancy and childhood, upper respiratory infections are common but usually not serious. Infants and preschoolers also are at risk for airway obstruction by foreign objects, such as coins and small toys. Cystic fibrosis, a chronic disease usually identified in early childhood, is a congenital disorder that affects the lungs, causing them to become congested with thick, tenacious (sticky) mucus. Asthma is another chronic disease often identified in childhood. The airways of the asthmatic child react to stimuli such as allergens, exercise, or cold air by constricting, becoming edematous, and producing excessive mucus. Airflow is impaired, and the child may wheeze as air moves through narrowed air passages.

OLDER ADULTS

- Older adults are at increased risk for acute respiratory diseases such as pneumonia and chronic diseases such as emphysema and chronic bronchitis. COPD may affect older adults, particularly after years of exposure to cigarette smoke or industrial pollutants.
- Pneumonia may not present with the usual symptom of a fever, but may present with atypical symptoms, such as confusion, weakness, loss of appetite, and increased heart rate and respiration.

Nursing interventions should be directed toward achieving optimal respiratory effort and gas exchange:

- Always encourage wellness and prevention of disease by reinforcing the need for good nutrition, exercise, and immunizations, such as for influenza and pneumonia.
- Increase fluid intake, if not contraindicated by other problems such as cardiac or renal impairment.
- Encourage proper positioning and frequent changing of position to allow for better lung expansion and air and fluid movement.
- Teach the client to use breathing techniques for better air exchange.
- Pace activities to conserve energy.
- Encourage the client to eat more frequent, smaller meals to decrease gastric distention, which can cause pressure on the diaphragm.
- Teach the client to avoid extreme hot or cold temperatures that will further tax the respiratory system.
- Teach actions and side effects of drugs, inhalers, and treatments.

Source: Berman, A., Snyder, S. J., Kozier, B., & Erb, G. (2008). *Kozier & Erb's fundamentals of nursing: Concepts, process, and practice* (8th ed., p. 1362). Upper Saddle River, NJ: Pearson Education.

The pH level is then assessed. The normal pH range is narrow, from 7.35 to 7.45; pH values less than 7.35 indicate acidosis and values greater than 7.45 indicate alkalosis.

Carbon dioxide values are assessed. Carbon dioxide is an acid expired from the lungs; changes in carbon dioxide are regulated by respiratory patterns. Carbon dioxide values range from 35 to 45 mmHg; values less than 35 mmHg indicate alkalosis and values greater than 45 mmHg indicate acidosis (Pruitt & Jacobs, 2004).

Bicarbonate is a base excreted via the kidneys; changes in bicarbonate are metabolic responses of the kidneys. Bicarbonate values range from 22 to 26 mEq/L. Values less than 22 mEq/L indicate acidosis and values greater than 26 mEq/L indicate alkalosis (Pruitt & Jacobs, 2004).

The body's natural inclination is to maintain a homeostatic balance. In relation to ABGs or acid–base, this means that the body will alter the carbon dioxide and bicarbonate levels to return the pH level to within normal range. Altering the individual components within acid–base balance is called *compensation*. A blood gas that has a pH greater than 7.45 indicates acidosis. If the same blood gas has a carbon dioxide greater than 45 mmHg, it indicates respiratory acidosis. The next value to be assessed is the bicarbonate level. If the value is in the normal range, the blood gas has not compensated. If the bicarbonate level is elevated, and the pH remains elevated the blood gas is partially compensated. A compensated blood gas will have carbon dioxide levels and bicarbonate levels that cause the pH to be in its normal range (Pruitt & Jacobs, 2004). A pH within normal range allows the body to achieve homeostasis.

Pulse oximetry is a noninvasive method of assessing arterial blood oxygenation. A clip or adhesive device with an infrared probe analyzes blood as it perfuses past the view of the two opposing sensors of the probe. Expected SaO_2 values in a healthy individual (one who has no alterations in pulmonary function) are greater than 95%.

Diagnosis of and differentiation of reactive airway diseases necessitates the use of **pulmonary function tests (PFTs)**. PFTs provide information about ventilation airflow, lung volume, and capacity and the diffusion of gas, and PFTs incorporate spirometry, peak flow meters, and the body plethysmograph. PFTs include measurement of inspired and expired air, as well as the diffusion ability of the alveolar-capillary membrane. A spirometer is used to measure airflow and lung volumes. **Incentive spirometry** measures the forced emptying of alveolar gas. Simply put, spirometry measures air exhaled from the lungs. Spirometry tests may be carried out in a primary care provider office or clinic. Levels for forced expiratory volume over 1 second (FEV1) and the ratio of forced expiratory volume over 1 second compared to forced expiratory volume (FEV1/FCV) are used to screen for pulmonary function deficits. Box 10–2 diagrams all the pulmonary function tests.

Peak expiratory flow rate (PEFR) is used to monitor the ability of an individual to exhale a specific volume of air related to the individual's age, gender, height, and weight.

DIAGNOSTIC TESTS Respiratory System

NAME OF TEST Sputum studies

- Culture and sensitivity
- Acid-fast smear and culture
- Cytology

PURPOSE AND DESCRIPTION Culture and sensitivity of a single sputum specimen is done to diagnose bacterial infections, identify the most effective antibiotic, and evaluate treatment.

Sputum is examined for presence of acid-fast bacillus, specifically tuberculosis. A series of three early morning sputum specimens is used.

Sputum is examined for presence of abnormal (malignant) cells. A single sputum specimen is collected in a special container of fixative solution.

NURSING CONSIDERATIONS Sputum specimens may also be obtained during bronchoscopy (described later) if the client is unable to provide a specimen. If collecting a specimen from client with infectious disease, such as tuberculosis, the nurse should wear personal protective equipment, and the specimen may be collected outdoors to dilute droplet nuclei if negative airflow is not available in the client's room.

Developmental Considerations Sputum may be collected from infants and young children, who cannot cooperate enough to expectorate into a cup, by performing deep suctioning of the pharynx to induce a cough reflex and produce sputum.

NAME OF TEST Arterial blood gases (ABGs)

PURPOSE AND DESCRIPTION This test of arterial blood is done to assess alterations in acid–base balance caused by a respiratory disorder, a metabolic disorder, or both. A pH of less than 7.35 indicates acidosis, and a pH of more than 7.45 indicates alkalosis. To determine a respiratory cause, assess the $PaCO_2$: If pH is decreased and $PaCO_2$ is increased, respiratory acidosis is indicated.

Normal values:

pH: 7.35–7.45

$PaCO_2$: 35–45 mmHg

PaO_2: 75–100 mmHg

HCO_3: 24–28 mEq/L

BE: ± 2 mEq/L

NURSING CONSIDERATIONS Arterial blood is collected in a heparinized needle and syringe. Sample is placed on an icebag and taken immediately to the laboratory. If client is receiving oxygen, indicate on laboratory slip. Apply pressure to puncture site for 2–5 minutes, or longer if needed. Do not collect blood from the same arm used for an intravenous (IV) infusion.

Developmental Considerations When performing arterial puncture on infants and young children, only the radial artery should be used after verifying ulnar perfusion via an Allen's test. The Allen's test is performed by having the client elevate the hand and make a fist for 30 seconds. Pressure is applied to the ulnar and radial artery, the client opens the hand, which should appear blanched from lack of perfusion, and then pressure is removed from the ulnar artery while pressure on the radial artery is maintained. If the hand does not become pink and perfused, it indicates damage to the ulnar artery and the radial artery in that arm should not be used for arterial puncture.

NAME OF TEST Pulse oximetry

PURPOSE AND DESCRIPTION

This noninvasive test is used to evaluate or monitor oxygen saturation of the blood. A device that uses infrared light is attached to an extremity (most commonly the finger, but can also be used on the toe, earlobe, or nose) and light is passed through the tissues or reflected off bony structures.

Normal values: 90–100%

NURSING CONSIDERATIONS Assess for factors that may alter findings, including faulty placement, movement, diminished perfusion (such as cool skin), dark skin color, and acrylic nails.

Developmental Considerations Fingers and toes are not appropriate sites for young infants because they are so small. Probes are available that wrap around the palm of the hand or sole of the foot with a piece of tape to hold them in place, and they work well.

NAME OF TEST Chest x-ray

PURPOSE AND DESCRIPTION Chest x-ray is used to identify abnormalities in chest structure and lung tissue, for diagnosis of diseases and injuries of the lungs, and to monitor treatment.

NURSING CONSIDERATIONS No special preparation is needed.

NAME OF TEST Computed tomography (CT)

PURPOSE AND DESCRIPTION CT of the thorax may be performed when x-rays do not show some areas well, such as the pleura and mediastinum. It is also done to differentiate pathologic conditions (such as tumors, abscesses, and aortic aneurysms), to identify pleural effusion and enlarged lymph nodes, and to monitor treatment. Images are shown in cross-section.

NURSING CONSIDERATIONS No special preparation is needed. Caution should be provided to cover the genitals of young children and avoid radiation of any type with pregnant women whenever possible. If x-rays must be obtained, a lead shield should be placed over the abdomen.

DIAGNOSTIC TESTS Respiratory System (continued)

NAME OF TEST Magnetic resonance imaging (MRI)

PURPOSE AND DESCRIPTION MRI of the thorax is used to diagnose alterations in lung tissue more difficult to visualize by CT scan and to identify abnormal masses and fluid accumulation.

NURSING CONSIDERATIONS Assess for any metallic implants (such as pacemaker, pacemaker wires, or implant). Test will not be performed if present.

Developmental Consideration Because the infant and young child are unable to cooperate, sedation may be required to keep them still enough for the test to be performed. If sedation is used, the child should be placed on a cardiorespiratory monitor throughout the examination so the nurse can monitor breathing.

NAME OF TEST Positron emission tomography (PET)

PURPOSE AND DESCRIPTION This relatively noninvasive test, when used to examine the lungs, is performed to identify lung nodules (cancers). The client is given a radioactive substance and cross-sectional images are displayed on a computer. Radiation from PET is only 25% of that from CT.

NURSING CONSIDERATIONS No alcohol, coffee, or tobacco is allowed for 24 hours prior to the test. Encourage increased fluid intake post-test to help eliminate the radioactive material.

Developmental Consideration Same as MRI.

NAME OF TEST Pulmonary angiography

PURPOSE AND DESCRIPTION This test is done to identify pulmonary emboli, tumors, aneurysms, vascular changes associated with emphysema, and pulmonary circulation. A catheter is inserted into the brachial or femoral artery and

threaded into the pulmonary artery, and dye is injected. ECG leads are applied to the chest for cardiac monitoring. Images of the lungs are taken.

RELATED NURSING CARE Monitor injection site and pulses distal to the site after the test.

NAME OF TEST Pulmonary ventilation/perfusion scan (V/Q scan)

PURPOSE AND DESCRIPTION This test is performed with two nuclear scans to measure breathing (ventilation) and circulation (perfusion) in all parts of the lungs. A perfusion scan is performed by injecting radioactive albumin into a vein and scanning the lungs. A ventilation scan is performed by scanning the

lungs as the client inhales radioactive gas. A decreased uptake of radioisotope during the perfusion scan indicates a blood flow problem, such as from a pulmonary embolus or pneumonitis. A decreased uptake of gas during the ventilation scan may indicate airway obstruction, pneumonia, or chronic pulmonary obstructive disease (COPD).

NURSING CONSIDERATIONS No special preparation is needed.

NAME OF TEST Bronchoscopy

PURPOSE AND DESCRIPTION Bronchoscopy is the direct visualization of the larynx, trachea, and bronchi through a bronchoscope to identify lesions, remove foreign bodies and secretions, obtain tissue for biopsy, and improve tracheobronchial drainage (Figure 10–8 ■). During the test, a catheter brush or biopsy forceps can be passed to obtain secretions or tissue for examination for cancer.

RELATED NURSING CARE

■ Provide routine preoperative care as ordered. *Bronchoscopy is an invasive procedure requiring conscious sedation or anesthesia. Care provided prior to the procedure is similar to that provided before many minor surgical procedures.*

■ Provide mouth care just prior to bronchoscopy. *Mouth care reduces oral microorganisms and the risk of introducing them into the lungs.*

■ Bring resuscitation and suction equipment to the bedside. *Laryngospasm and respiratory distress may occur following the procedure. The anesthetic suppresses the cough and gag reflexes, and secretions may be difficult to expectorate.*

■ Following the procedure, closely monitor vital signs and respiratory status. *Possible complications of bronchoscopy include laryngospasm, bronchospasm, bronchial perforation with possible pneumothorax or subcutaneous emphysema, hemorrhage, hypoxia, pneumonia or bacteremia, and cardiac stress.*

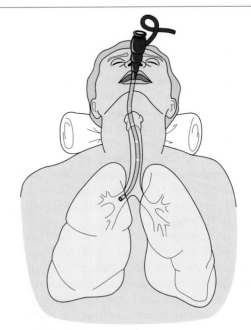

Figure 10–8 ■ Fiberoptic bronchosopy.

(continued)

DIAGNOSTIC TESTS Respiratory System (continued)

- Instruct to avoid eating or drinking for approximately 2 hours or until fully awake with intact cough and gag reflexes. *Suppression of the cough and gag reflexes by systemic and local anesthesia used during the procedure increases the risk for aspiration.*
- Provide an emesis basin and tissues for expectorating sputum and saliva. *Until reflexes have returned, the client may be unable to swallow sputum and saliva safely.*
- Monitor color and character of respiratory secretions. Secretions normally are blood tinged for several hours following bronchoscopy, especially if biopsy has been obtained. Notify the physician if sputum is grossly bloody. *Grossly bloody sputum may indicate a complication such as perforation.*
- Collect postbronchoscopy sputum specimens for cytologic examination as ordered. *Cells in the sputum may be examined if a tumor is suspected.*

Health Education for the Client and Family

- Fiberoptic bronchoscopy requires 30–45 minutes to complete. It may be done at the bedside, in a special procedure room, or in the surgical suite.
- The procedure usually causes little pain or discomfort, because an anesthetic is given. You will be able to breathe during the bronchoscopy.
- Some voice hoarseness and a sore throat are common following the procedure. Throat lozenges or warm saline gargles may help relieve discomfort.
- You may develop a mild fever within the first 24 hours following the procedure. This is a normal response.
- Persistent cough, bloody or purulent sputum, wheezing, shortness of breath, difficulty breathing, or chest pain may indicate a complication. Notify your physician if they develop.

NAME OF TEST Lung biopsy

PURPOSE AND DESCRIPTION Lung biopsy is done to obtain tissue to differentiate benign from malignant tumors of the lungs. It may be done during a bronchoscopy, or by surgical procedure.

NURSING CONSIDERATIONS Same as bronchoscopy or the same as a thoracotomy (incision through the chest wall) if a surgical biopsy is performed.

NAME OF TEST Thoracentesis

PURPOSE AND DESCRIPTION Thoracentesis is done to obtain a specimen of pleural fluid for diagnosis (and used as a procedure to remove pleural fluid or instill medication). A large-bore needle is inserted through the chest wall and into the pleural

space. Following the procedure, a chest x-ray is taken to check for a pneumothorax.

NURSING CONSIDERATIONS Same as care following a bronchoscopy or thoracotomy.

Source: LeMone, P., & Burke, K. (2008). *Medical-surgical nursing: Critical thinking in client care* (4th ed.). Upper Saddle River, NJ: Pearson Education.

PEFR allows individuals with asthma to monitor the reactivity of their lungs and adjust asthma treatments by the plan developed by the primary care provider and the individual. PEFR is not diagnostic for reactive airway diseases such as asthma and COPD.

Anterior-posterior **chest x-ray** (CXR) allows for two-dimensional visualization of the contents of the thoracic cavity. Thoracic computed tomography (CT) produces cross-sectional images of the contents of the chest. Thoracic CT may be used with dye to determine the presence of pulmonary embolism. Magnetic resonance imaging (MRI) allows for assessment of pulmonary embolism without the use of dye and is best for visualizing soft tissue and vascular structures. MRI is contraindicated in the individual who has implanted metal devices.

A pulmonary angiogram is used to identify structural changes in the pulmonary vasculature. Structural changes that cause occlusions may include blood clots, tumors, aneurysms, and overinflated alveoli. A pulmonary ventilation-perfusion scan (V-Q scan) uses radioactive isotopes to identify defects of ventilation and perfusion. Injected radioactive albumin helps identify defects of perfusion, whereas inhaled radioactive gas identifies defects of ventilation.

Bronchoscopy, a procedure that allows direct visualization of the lungs, is usually performed by a pulmonologist but may be performed by a primary care or emergency care physician.

A bronchoscope is inserted orally into the trachea and advanced to the bronchi bifurcation. Biopsies, clearing of mucus plugs, and photographic identification of internal lung structures can be carried out. Sedation is necessary for client comfort.

Thoracentesis is both an intervention and a test. Thoracentesis is performed to drain excessive pleural fluid from between the pleural linings. The fluid drained is often analyzed for blood, fiber, and microbe content.

PHARMACOLOGIC THERAPIES

Therapeutic management related to maintaining or attaining the health of the respiratory system focuses on the individual's ability to maintain a patent airway through the automatic protective mechanisms in the upper and lower respiratory tracts. The ability of the individual to maintain breathing patterns within the acceptable rates and quality for his or her particular age group is also assessed. Inspiration and expiration must provide adequate ventilation of the lung fields. Individuals also must demonstrate an ease of breathing without the use of positioning or accessory muscles. Individuals demonstrate their respiratory patterns to define adequate gas exchange. A collaborative assessment with the health care team helps support the indication of excessive increases or decreases in oxygen or carbon dioxide levels.

The care of an individual who has or is at risk for respiratory illness is a collaborative effort involving many types of

Box 10–2 **Pulmonary Function Tests**

Pulmonary function tests (PFTs) are performed in a pulmonary function laboratory. After preparing the client, a nose clip is applied and the unsedated client breathes into a spirometer or body plethysmograph, a device for measuring and recording lung volume in liters versus time in seconds. The client is instructed how to breathe for specific tests: for example, to inhale as deeply as possible and then exhale to the maximal extent possible. Using measured lung volumes, respiratory capacities are calculated to assess pulmonary status. The specific values determined by PFT and illustrated in the figure include the following:

- *Total lung capacity (TLC)* is the total volume of the lungs at their maximum inflation. Four values are used to calculate TLC.
    a. *Total volume (TV)*, the volume inhaled and exhaled with normal quiet breathing (also called tidal volume)
    b. *Inspiratory reserve volume (IRV)*, the maximum amount that can be inhaled over and above a normal inspiration
    c. *Expiratory reserve volume (ERV)*, the maximum amount that can be exhaled following a normal exhalation
    d. *Residual volume (RV)*, the amount of air remaining in the lungs after maximal exhalation
- *Vital capacity (VC)* is the total amount of air that can be exhaled after a maximal inspiration. It is calculated by adding together the IRV, TV, and ERV.

- *Inspiratory capacity* is the total amount of air that can be inhaled following a normal quiet exhalation. It is calculated by adding the TV and IRV.
- *Functional residual capacity (FRC)* is the volume of air left in the lungs after a normal exhalation. The ERV and RV are added to determine the FRC.
- *Forced expiratory volume (FEV1)* is the amount of air that can be exhaled in 1 second.
- *Forced vital capacity (FVC)* is the amount of air that can be exhaled forcefully and rapidly after maximum air intake.
- *Minute volume (MV)* is the total amount or volume of air breathed in 1 minute.

In older clients, residual capacity is increased, and vital capacity is decreased. These age-related changes result from the following:
- Calcification of the costal cartilage and weakening of the intercostal muscles, which reduce movement of the chest wall
- Vertebral osteoporosis, which decreases spinal flexibility and increases the degree of kyphosis, further increasing the anterior-posterior diameter of the chest
- Diaphragmatic flattening and loss of elasticity

Source: LeMone, P., & Burke, K. (2008). *Medical-surgical nursing: Critical thinking in client care* (4th ed., p. 1214). Upper Saddle River, NJ: Pearson Education.

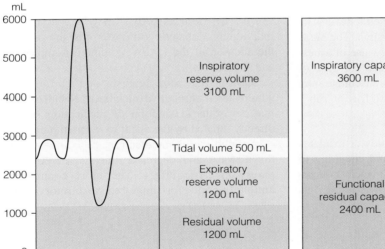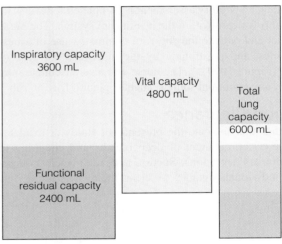

The relationship of lung volumes and capacities. Volumes (mL) shown are for an average adult male.

health care providers. Physicians, nurse practitioners, or physician assistants provide primary preventive and maintenance care for many individuals. Care for individuals with respiratory system alterations is often managed by a pulmonologist. Education of respiratory therapists (RTs) focuses on the cardiopulmonary system, along with acid–base balance, kidney function, and airway management. Physical therapists (PTs) provide maintenance and improvement of musculoskeletal system function. In relation to breathing, PTs teach exercises to improve endurance and strength for better oxygenation. Pharmacists use medications to improve airway patency and oxygen uptake, and reduce pulmonary secretions. Collaborating with the pharmacist in selecting medications may improve the individual's control of chronic diseases and prevent uncomfortable side effects. Individuals with respiratory alterations often have greater caloric need but lack the endurance to consume adequate nutrition. Nutritionists have the knowledge of caloric need and demand, as well as the best ways to provide the individual's dietary needs, to maintain health or support a return to health.

Nurses collaborate with the full health care team to develop a plan of care for the individual at risk for declining respiratory function related to respiratory illnesses. Therapeutic management of individuals at risk for respiratory compromise uses the knowledge and skills of other health care providers to support actual client functioning or provide aid to improve client respiratory function. Many collaborative interventions are needed to reestablish effective breathing patterns.

Temperature, Pulse, Respiration, and Pulse Oximetry

With each interaction between an individual and someone in the health care system, temperature, pulse, respiration, blood pressure, and pulse oximetry measurements should be obtained for baseline data. Baseline data alert health care providers to changes in an individual's overall status. An individual should be afebrile, with a regular rate and rhythm in heart sounds. Respiratory rate, rhythm, and quality are the focus of pulmonary assessment. Health care goals related to the respiratory system include regular rate, even rhythm, normal depth, and an easy respiratory effort. Dyspnea, diaphoresis, dusky skin, irritability, nasal flaring, restlessness, somnolence, tachycardia, and abnormal rates, rhythms, and depth are indicators of increased respiratory effort.

Respiratory Assessment

An individual respiratory assessment is completed for everyone who presents for care within the health care system. The nurse will inspect and palpate the chest for symmetry, use of accessory muscles, and positioning by the individual for ease of breathing (Figure 10–9 ■). The nurse will also auscultate lung sounds for any abnormal sounds, such as pleural friction rub.

Secretion Clearance

Lung sounds that indicate the presence of fluids or exudates necessitate encouragement of deep breaths and coughing to clear pulmonary secretions. Suction is needed to clear secretions in individuals unable to clear their own secretions.

Individuals who are producing sputum with a cough may require the collection of a sputum specimen. They may benefit from postural drainage to clear secretions from various lung fields. (See Companion Skills Manual text for these skills.)

Medication Administration

An individual whose lung sounds indicate narrowing of the airways will benefit from a bronchodilator and possibly an anti-inflammatory agent to improve airway patency. The administration of bronchodilators, as ordered by the primary care provider relaxes the muscles around the airway, improving airflow. Common bronchodilators of short duration (short-acting beta-agonists, or SABAs) are levalbuterol (Xenopenex). Inflammation of the airways also contributes to impairment of oxygenation. The administration of corticosteroids (various adrenal cortex steroids, such as prednisone) in the presence of inflammation, as ordered by the primary care provider, aids in opening the air passageways by reducing the inflammation. Because oral steroids have a number of side effects, they are usually administered for a short period of time. Dosages are tapered, with the individual slowly decreasing the amount taken over the course of the prescription.

Individuals with chronic respiratory problems such as COPD and asthma usually benefit from use of a long-acting beta agonist (LABA) in combination with an inhaled corticosteroid (ICS). Commonly prescribed preparations include Symbicort and Advair. Because LABAs may be contraindicated in some individuals, inhaled corticosteroids are available without the addition of the LABA; common examples are Pulmocort and Asmanex.

Short-acting beta agonists and corticosteroids can be administered through a nebulizer. Nebulizers are machines that aerosolize a solution of medication so that it can be directly inhaled by the client by a mouthpiece or mask.

Anticholinergic medications relax the smooth muscles of the airways and decrease mucous secretions by blocking parasympathetic effect. The most commonly prescribed anticholinergic for impaired respiratory function is an

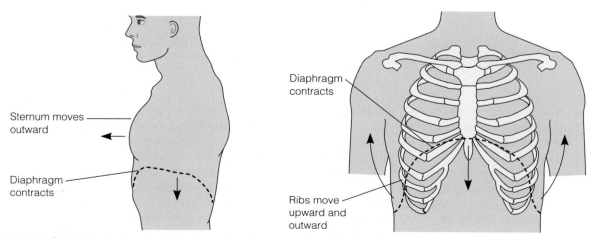

Figure 10–9 ■ Respiratory inspiration: Lateral and anterior views. Note the volume expansion of the thorax as the diaphragm flattens.

Sternum moves outward

Diaphragm contracts

Diaphragm contracts

Ribs move upward and outward

ipatromium bromide inhaler (e.g., Atrovent). Inhaled anticholinergics are a good alternative for patients who cannot tolerate beta-agonists, and can be effective in relieving bronchospasm resulting from use of beta-blocker medications. Xanthines are another type of drug sometimes used to treat asthma, chronic bronchitis, and emphysema. Xanthines cause small airway dilation and increase heart rate and renal blood flow. Theophylline (Slo-Bid) is one of the more generic names used for this type of medication. Because of the narrow therapeutic range of this type of medication and the potential for serious side effects, patients taking xanthines should have periodic blood tests to ensure they are maintaining optimal therapeutic levels and to guard against risk of toxicity.

Additional medications may be prescribed. These can vary depending on the nature of the respiratory impairment. Allergic asthmatic individuals, for example, may take immunotherapy (allergy shots) or other medications for allergies to prevent attacks.

Medication compliance in individuals with chronic or recurrent respiratory impairment is critical. Some medications used for treating respiratory diseases are fairly expensive. Although albuterol and corticosteroids are reasonably inexpensive, LABAs usually are more expensive and are associated with higher insurance copayments. For individuals who require multiple prescription medications to maintain respiratory health, the combined costs of these medications may be overwhelming. Most pharmaceutical companies have programs to assist clients who lack health insurance or whose standard of living is at or close to the poverty level. Most free clinics are able to provide free medication to qualifying individuals. Usually, individuals are not required to see the doctor at the free clinic to receive free medication; a prescription from the treating physician is sufficient.

Teenagers often do not take medications as prescribed, either because they are embarrassed to be seen taking medication or because their hectic schedules do not make it possible for them to be home at certain times to take medication. Additional client teaching may be necessary when working with teenagers.

Older adults may be at risk for accidental noncompliance with medication administration schedules. A nurse working with an older adult exhibiting signs of confusion or early dementia should consult with the client or family members to determine whether additional support is available regarding medication administration.

Alternative therapies that may assist individuals with respiratory impairment include yoga, which is a form of exercise that teaches deep breathing and relaxation. Adequate nutrition and fluids are essential to maintaining lung health, and fluid intake helps keep sputum thin so that it can be more easily expelled through coughing. Walking, swimming, and other forms of moderate exercise also help maintain lung volume, not to mention heart health and appropriate weight. Individuals with chronic respiratory ailments should consult with their treating physicians before beginning any exercise program.

Laboratory and Diagnostic Testing

Laboratory and diagnostic tests provide a baseline indication of respiratory health and guide the treatment plans for individuals who have respiratory illness. An overall laboratory assessment of the respiratory system includes ABG, complete blood count (CBC), **chemistry panels**, and antigen-antibody markers. ABGs reveal the acid–base balance and oxygen levels in arterial blood. Often the respiratory therapist completes the collection of an ABG, but collection may be performed by a registered nurse (RN) skilled in this procedure. CBC indicates oxygen-carrying capacity and presence of infection. CBC shows perfusion issues related to anemia or allergic responses. Individual behaviors that look like hypoxia could be related to abnormal chemistry levels. A chemistry panel will aid in the differentiation of hypoxemia from chemistry abnormalities.

Chest x-rays reveal the presence of fluids, exudates, or masses within the thoracic cavity. CT and MRIs provide more information about the structures within the thoracic cavity. Pulmonary angiography and pulmonary V-Q scans demonstrate the ventilation and perfusion activities of the respiratory system. Individuals who respond poorly to bronchodilators may benefit from assessment of their pulmonary function. PFTs demonstrate changes in pulmonary health. Results outside the anticipated range for the individual's age, gender, height, and weight may indicate the need to alter care interventions. The respiratory therapist carries out PFTs. Bronchoscopy may be used for direct visualization of pulmonary structures, suctioning of mucus plugs from larger bronchials, and collection of lung tissue biopsy specimens.

Encouraging Smoking Cessation

Individuals are assessed for tobacco use. Tobacco smoke exposure causes increased mucus production and reduced cilia action within the airway passages. Individuals who smoke present with a chronic cough and sputum production in the early years of tobacco use. Prolonged exposure to tobacco smoke yields a decline in pulmonary function. Because the capacity of the respiratory system to compensate is great, the sense of pulmonary decline occurs well after irreversible damage has occurred. All health care providers should encourage smoking cessation and advise nonsmoking individuals to avoid secondary smoke.

Cessation of smoking and use of spit tobacco contributes to an individual's overall health. Individuals who would like to quit should be offered nicotine replacement therapies, as ordered by the primary care provider. Box 10–3 lists strategies to decrease tobacco use. Reducing secondhand exposure of children to tobacco smoke within their homes and decreasing the exposure to secondhand smoke in public buildings will diminish the detrimental effects of tobacco for nonsmoking individuals.

Oxygen Administration

Decreases in oxygen saturation in arterial blood indicate a need for supplemental oxygen. A variety of devices can be used to administer oxygen to an individual. The selection of a device depends on the amount of oxygen needed to relieve hypoxemia. Noninvasive devices require patent airways to be effective.

Box 10–3 **Interventions for Tobacco Cessation**

ASK	ADVISE	ASSESS	ASSIST	ARRANGE
Identify and document tobacco use status for every individual at every health care interaction.	Urge every tobacco user to quit in a clear, strong, and personalized manner.	Determine if the tobacco user is willing to attempt to quit tobacco use at this time.	Request tobacco cessation medication order from primary care provider. Provide resources for counseling and support groups for the individual willing to attempt to quit tobacco use.	Establish a plan for follow-up contact for the individual willing to attempt to quit tobacco use within one week of quit date. Continue to ask tobacco users about quitting tobacco use at each visit.
Nurses document tobacco use with admission history and physical assessment.	Nurses provide tobacco cessation publications and teach about physiologic consequences of tobacco use with daily care interactions such as taking vital signs.	Nurses ask if individuals have attempted quitting tobacco before, what was effective, what did not work, and encourage trying with present visit.	Nurses seek nicotine replacement during hospitalizations and encourage individuals who have had nicotine replacement during hospitalization that they are on their way to quitting.	Nurses collaborate with individuals who desire to quit to arrange tobacco cessation support group contacts and request in-hospital tobacco cessation teaching.

Source: Adapted from the Tobacco Cessation Clinical Practice Guidelines as established by the U.S. Department of Health and Human Services. Used with permission.

The most common and comfortable device is the nasal cannula (Figure 10–10 ■). The nasal cannula delivers flow rates from 2 to 6 L/min that administers 24–44% fraction of inspired oxygen (FiO_2). An Oxymizer also entrails air through the nasal passage, but it has an added reservoir for oxygen (Figure 10–11 ■). This additional reservoir increases the amount of oxygen inhaled with each breath. A Vapotherm delivers oxygen via a nasal cannula, but it warms and filters oxygen and increases the positive end expiratory pressure of oxygen delivery via the cannula (Figure 10–12 ■). A simple mask covers the mouth and nose. It is fitted to the individual's face size. The mask itself provides an additional gas reservoir

to that provided by the nasopharynx alone (Figure 10–13 ■). Flow rates may be set from 5 to 10 L/min. The FiO_2 delivered is from 30 to 50%. To attain FiO_2 levels of 60% or more, masks that have an attached reservoir are necessary to provide adequate oxygen. The nonrebreather mask has a one-way valve between the attached reservoir and the face mask (Figure 10–14 ■). This ensures that appropriate levels of oxygen are inhaled, with no carbon dioxide from exhaled gases.

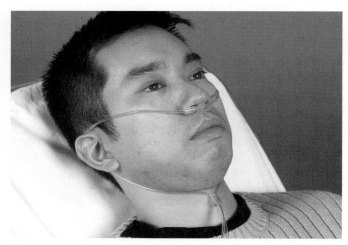

Figure 10–10 ■ A nasal cannula.

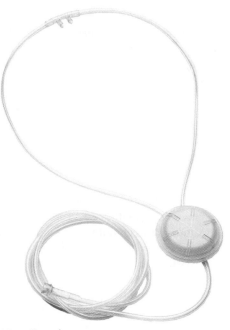

Figure 10–11 ■ Oxymizer.

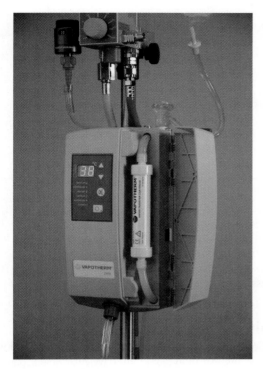

Figure 10–12 ■ Vapotherm.

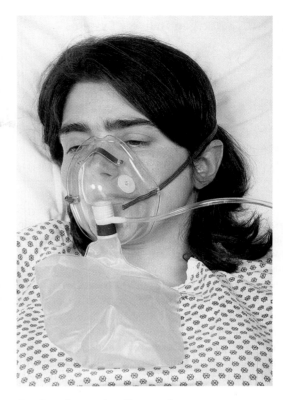

Figure 10–14 ■ A nonrebreather mask.
Photographer: Elena Dorfman

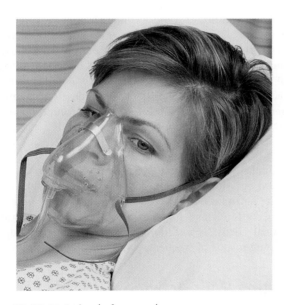

Figure 10–13 ■ A simple face mask.
Photographer: Jenny Thomas

Oxygen delivery at a specified flow rate requires the use of a venturi mask (Figure 10–15 ■). Venturi masks are set with a specific oxygen flow rate and specific jet adaptor device. Flow rates of 24–40% may be set with the venturi mask. Table 10–3 summarizes the types of oxygen devices, along with flow rates and oxygen delivery amounts.

Nursing care for the client receiving supplemental oxygen includes ensuring that flow is sufficient as required, that the client

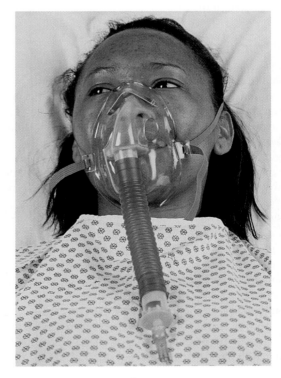

Figure 10–15 ■ A Venturi mask.
Photographer: Jenny Thomas

TABLE 10–3 Oxygen Delivery Systems

DEVICE	FLOW RATE SETTING	OXYGEN CONCENTRATION (FIO$_2$)
Nasal cannula	1–6 L/min	24–44%
Oxymizer	1–6 L/min	24–88%
Vapotherm	1–40 L/min	24–100%
Face mask	5–10 L/min	30–50%
Nonrebreather	10–15 L/min	Greater than 60%
Venturi mask	Set with jet adaptor for flow rate and FiO$_2$	

is reasonably comfortable with the manner of oxygen administration, and that indwelling catheters (lines) remain clear. For the client being discharged to home with supplemental oxygen, both the nurse and the respiratory therapist delivering the oxygen to the home must teach the client how to use the devices properly, the importance of checking oxygen levels in tanks, the need for a portable device for trips outside of the house, and the need to maintain the lines and keep them clear of obstruction.

Individuals prescribed supplemental oxygen for the first time may feel as though they have lost their quality of life. The nurse can assist the individual in understanding that supplemental oxygen will help him or her maintain quality of life, and that the individual can still participate in any number of activities. The nurse should be alert to any possible signs of depression in a client whose oxygen impairment is sufficient to warrant supplemental oxygen. Frustration, rising medical costs, and other issues can contribute to depression in a client with respiratory impairment.

Thoracic Catheter

A chest tube, or thoracic catheter, is used to treat conditions in which fluid enters the pleural cavity, causing lung collapse. Inserted under emergency conditions, and treated as a surgical procedure, a chest tube will typically remain in place for 2–5 days, until the client's x-rays indicate that all fluid from the pleural cavity has been removed.

There are many nursing considerations in working with a client who has a thoracic catheter, some of which will be specific to the underlying cause of the lung collapse. Typically, however, the nurse will need to do the following:

- Ensure oxygen therapy is immediately available at all times, if not already ordered and in place.
- Monitor dressings for drainage and air leakage; follow agency protocol for replacing or securing dressings.
- Monitor tubing to make sure it is free of kinks or other impediments.
- Monitor and record client vital signs as ordered.
- Monitor for and report any decrease in oxygen saturation, any changes in breath sounds, or any tympany or hollow sound with chest percussion.

- Assess for pain; administer pain medications as needed (PRN), notifying physician of any increase in client restlessness or anxiety.
- Monitor and report any changes in respiration or any excessive bleeding.

Monitoring Activity Tolerance

Alterations in the respiratory system can affect an individual's activity levels. An individual may have insufficient physiologic or psychologic energy to endure or complete required or desired daily activities. For the individual with poor oxygenation, fatigue or weakness can occur from scheduling too many activities too close together. Dyspnea or shortness of breath occurs at varying points in the exercise program, depending on the individual's endurance level. Periods of activity should be spaced with periods of rest if the individual is unable to carry out many consecutive activities. A physical therapist will develop an exercise program to improve musculoskeletal function and endurance.

Improving Nutrition

Individuals with respiratory alterations often need an increased calorie intake but lack the endurance to consume adequate nutrition. A nutritionist is able to aid the individual in choosing foods and supplements to meet daily caloric and nutritional needs. A nutritionist can guide the individual in developing menus of frequent, small, nutritious meals.

Assisting With Activities of Daily Living

Individuals who are too weak to provide their own care may need assistance in activities of daily living (ADLs). An individual with compromised oxygenation may have very poor endurance for activities. Personal care must be provided for individuals too weak or too fatigued to carry out their own ADLs. The family and the health care team must collaborate to provide sufficient support to the individual with compromised oxygenation, while encouraging the individual to do as much as possible to maintain appropriate physical strength and prevent deteriorating mental condition.

REFERENCES

American Academy of Pediatrics. (2006). *Diagnosis and management of bronchiolitis*. Retrieved from www.pediatrics.org/cdl/10.1542/peds.2006-2223

American Lung Association. (2008) Acute respiratory distress syndrome (ARDS) in *Lung Disease Data: 2008*. Retrieved December 25, 2008, from www.lungusa.org

Boyle, A. H., & Locke, D. L. (2004). Update on chronic obstructive pulmonary disease. *Medical-Surgical Nursing.*, 13(1).

Center for Disease Control and Prevention. (2003). Respiratory diseases. *Healthy People 2010*. (chapter 24). Retrieved from http://www.healthypeople.gov/Data

Center for Disease Control and Prevention. (2003). Tobacco Use. *Healthy People 2010*. (chapter 27). Retrieved from http://www.healthypeople.gov/Data

Cooper, A. C., Banasiak, N. C., & Allen, P. J. (2003). Management and prevention strategies for respiratory syncytial virus (RSV) bronchiolitis in infants and young children: A review of evidenced based practice interventions. *Pediatric Nursing*. 29(6), 452–456.

Corbridge, S. J. & Berry, J. K. (2007). Chronic obstructive pulmonary disease. *AAOHN Journal*. 55(5).

Cui, D. J. (2007). Key messages in the new asthma guidelines. *Clinician Reviews*, 17(11).

Cui, D. J. (2007). The new asthma guidelines: What primary care clinicians need to know. *Clinician Review*, 17(5).

Doherty, D. E., Gross, N. J., & Briggs, D. D. (2004). Today's approach to the diagnosis and management of COPD. *Clinician Reviews*, 14(1), 97–105.

Fiore MC, Jaen CR, Baker TB, et al. (2008). *Treating Tobacco Use and Dependence: 2008 Update*. Clinical Practice Guideline. Rockville, MD: U.S. Department of Health and Human Services. Public Health Service. May 2008.

George, K. J. (2008). A systemic approach to care: Adults Respiratory Distress Syndrome. *Journal of Trauma Nursing*, 15(1), 19–24.

GOLD committee. (2007). *Global Initiative for Chronic Obstructive Lung Disease*. Retrieved from www.goldcopd.org

Goldmann, D. A. (2001). Center for Disease Control. Epidemiology and prevention of pediatric viral respiratory infections in health-care institutions. Retrieved August 4, 2008, from http://www.cdc.gov/ncidod/eid/vol7no2/goldmann.htm

Holland, L. N., & Adams, M. P. (2007). *Core concepts in pharmacology* (2nd ed.). Upper Saddle River, NJ: Prentice Hall.

Kahdi, F. U., & Touijer, K. (2003). *Acute respiratory distress syndrome*. Retrieved December 25, 2008, from American Family Physician Web site: www.aafp.org/afp/20030115/315.html

Kara, M. (2005 Second quarter). Preparing nurses for the global pandemic of chronic obstructive pulmonary disease. *Journal of Nursing Scholarship*.

Key, J. L., Hayes, E. R., & McCuision, L. E. (2006). *Pharmacology: A nursing process approach* (5th ed.). St. Louis: Elsevier.

Kuebler, K. K., Buchsel, P.C., & Balkstra, C. R. (2008). Differentiating chronic obstructive pulmonary disease from asthma. *Journal of the American Academy of Nurse Practitioners*, 20, 445-454.

Mareib, E. N. (2001). The respiratory system. *Human anatomy and physiology* (5th ed.). San Francisco: Benjamin Cummings.

Martini, F. H. & Nath, J. L. (2009). The respiratory system. *Fundamentals of Anatomy & Physiology* (8th ed.). San Francisco: Pearson-Benjamin Cummings.

National Heart, Lung and Blood Institute. (2007). Expert panel report 3: Guidelines for the diagnosis and management of asthma. National Asthma Education and Prevention Program. Retrieved July 7, 2009, from http://www.nhlbi.nih.gov/guidelines/asthma/asthgdln.pdf.

Patrick, H. (2007). Is spirometry used too little in COPD patients? *Focus Journal* (Sept/Oct).

Pinkerton, K. E. & Joad, J. P. (2006). Influence of air pollution on respiratory health during perinatal development. Clinical and Experimental Pharmacology and Physiology. Vol. 33. pp 269–272.

Plopper, C. G., Smiley-Jewell, S. M., Miller, L. A., Fanucchi, M. V., Evans, M. J., Buckpitt, A. R. et al. (2007). Asthma/allergic airway disease: Does postnatal exposure to environmental toxicants promote airway pathobiology? *Toxicologic Pathology*, 35, 97–110.

Pruitt, W. C. & Jacobs, M. (2004). Interpreting arterial blood gases: Easy as A B C. *Nursing*, 34(8), 50–53.

Rebmann, T. (2005). Severe acute respiratory syndrome: Implications for perinatal and neonatal nurses. *Journal of Perinatal Nursing*, 19(4), 332–345.

Sole, M. L., Klein, D. G., & Mosely, M. J. (2005). Ventilatory assistance. *Introduction to Critical Care* (4th ed.). St. Louis: Elsevier-Saunders.

Schmid, T., Miskin, H., Schlesinger, Y., Argaman. Z., Kleid, D. (2005). Respiratory failure and hypercoagulability in a toddler with Lemierre's Syndrome. *Pediatrics*, 15(5), 620–622. Retrieved from www.pedicatrics.org/cgi/doi/10.1542/peds.2004-2005

Spratto, G. R., & Woods, A. L. (2009). *Delmar Nurse's Drug Handbook*. Clifton Park: Delmar-Cengage Learning.

Stedman's Medical Dictionary for Health Professionals and Nursing: Illustrated (5th ed.). (2005). Baltimore: Lippincott, Williams, & Wilkins:.

Verbrugge, S. J., Lachmann, B., & Kesecioglu, J. (2007). Lung protective ventilatory strategies in acute lung injury and acute respiratory distress syndrome: From experimental findings to clinical application. *Clinical Physiology and Functional Imaging*, 27(2), 67–90.

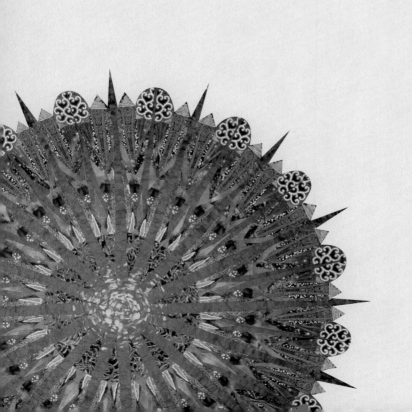

Sensory Perception

Concept at-a-Glance

Concept Learning Outcomes

After reading about this concept, you will be able to do the following:

1. Summarize the structure and physiologic processes of the sensory organs related to sensory perception.
2. List factors affecting sensory perception.
3. Identify commonly occurring alterations in sensory perception and their related treatments.
4. Explain common physical assessment procedures used to examine sensory perception health of clients across the life span.
5. Outline diagnostic and laboratory tests to determine the individual's sensory perception status.
6. Explain management of sensory perception health and prevention of illness related to sensory perception.
7. Demonstrate the nursing process in providing culturally competent and caring interventions across the life span for individuals with common alterations in sensory perception.
8. Identify pharmacologic interventions in caring for the individual with alterations in sensory perception function.

Concept Key Terms

Accommodation, *315*
Auditory, *312*
Awareness, *313*
Cataracts, *322*
Cerumen, *316*
Convergence, *316*
Corneal reflex, *314*
Cultural deprivation, *318*
Esotropia, *319*
Glaucoma, *322*
Gustatory, *312*
Hyperopia, *323*
Hypogeusia, *319*
Hyposmia, *319*
Impulse conduction, *312*
Kinesthetic, *312*
Macular degeneration, *322*

Myopia, *323*
Nystagmus, *319*
Olfactory, *312*
Perception, *313*
Presbycusis, *320*
Presbyopia, *323*
Ptosis, *325*
Pupillary light reflex, *315*
Receptor, *312*
Refraction, *315*
Sensory perception, *312*
Sensory reception, *312*
Stereognosis, *312*
Stimulus, *312*
Tactile, *312*
Visceral, *312*
Visual, *312*

About Sensory Perception

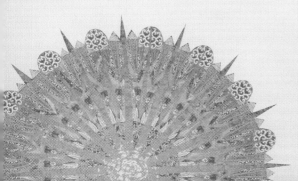

An individual's senses are essential for growth, development, and survival. Sensory stimuli give meaning to events in the environment. Any alteration in sensory functions can affect one's ability to operate within the environment. For example, many clients have impaired sensory functions that put them at risk in an institutional setting such as a school or assisted living facility; nurses can help these clients find ways to function safely in these often confusing environments. ●

The sensory process involves two components: reception and perception. **Sensory reception** is the process of receiving stimuli or data. These stimuli are either external or internal to the body. External stimuli are **visual** (sight), **auditory** (hearing), **olfactory** (smell), **tactile** (touch), and **gustatory** (taste). Gustatory stimuli can be internal as well. Other types of internal stimuli are kinesthetic and visceral. **Kinesthetic** refers to awareness of the position and movement of body parts. For example, a person walking is aware of which leg is forward. A related sense is **stereognosis**, the ability to perceive and understand an object through touch by its size, shape, and texture. A person holding a tennis ball is aware of its size, round shape, and soft surface without seeing it. **Visceral** means of or relating to any large organ within the body. Visceral organs may produce stimuli that make a person aware of them (e.g., a full stomach).

Sensory perception involves the conscious organization and translation of the data or stimuli into meaningful information.

For an individual to be aware of his or her surroundings, four aspects of the sensory process must be present: a stimulus, a receptor, impulse conduction, and perception.

- **Stimulus.** This is an agent or act that stimulates a nerve receptor.
- **Receptor.** A nerve cell acts as a receptor by converting the stimulus to a nerve impulse. Most receptors are specific, that is, sensitive to only one type of stimulus, such as visual, auditory, or touch.
- **Impulse conduction.** The impulse travels along nerve pathways to the spinal cord or directly to the brain. The cranial nerves (listed in Table 11–1 along with their functions) are important nerves controlling many actions required for

TABLE 11–1 Cranial Nerves and Their Functions

NAME	FUNCTION
I Olfactory	Sense of smell
II Optic	Vision
III Oculomotor	Eyeball movement Raising of upper eyelid Constriction of pupil Proprioception
IV Trochlear	Eyeball movement
V Trigeminal	Sensation of the upper scalp, upper eyelid, nose, nasal cavity, cornea, and lacrimal gland Sensation of the palate, upper teeth, cheek, top lip, lower eyelid, and scalp; sensation of the tongue, lower teeth, chin, and temporal scalp Chewing
VI Abducens	Lateral movement of the eyeball
VII Facial	Movement of facial muscles Secretions of lacrimal, nasal, submandibular, and sublingual glands Sensation of taste
VIII Acoustic	Sense of equilibrium Sense of hearing
IX Glossopharyngeal	Swallowing Gag reflex Secretions of parotid salivary gland Sense of taste Touch, pressure, and pain from pharynx and posterior tongue Pressure from carotid arteries Receptors to regulate blood pressure
X Vagus	Swallowing Regulation of cardiac rate Regulation of respirations Digestion Sensation from thoracic and abdominal organs Proprioception Sense of taste
XI Accessory	Movement of head and neck Proprioception
XII Hypoglossal	Movement of tongue for speech and swallowing

Source: LeMone, P., & Burke, K. (2008). *Medical-surgical nursing: Critical thinking in client care* (4th ed., p. 1511). Upper Saddle River, NJ: Pearson Education.

sensory perception (Figure 11–1 ■). For example, auditory impulses travel to the organ of Corti in the inner ear. From there, the impulses travel along the eighth cranial nerve to the temporal lobe of the brain.

■ **Perception.** Perception, or awareness and interpretation of stimuli, takes place in the brain. Specialized brain cells interpret the nature and the quality of the sensory stimuli. The level of consciousness affects the perception of the stimuli.

The brain has the capacity to adapt to sensory stimuli. For example, a person living in a city may not notice traffic noise that someone from a rural area finds loud and disturbing. Not all sensory stimuli are acted on; some are stored in the memory to be used at a later date. Sensory processing is not the same as cognition or awareness. Cognition is the process by which an individual learns, stores, retrieves, and uses information. **Awareness** is the ability to perceive environmental stimuli and body reactions and to respond appropriately through thought and action. The normal, alert person can assimilate many kinds of information at one time.

NORMAL PRESENTATION

Our sensory organs provide pathways for stimuli to reach the brain, allowing us to experience the world in which we live. Deficits in sensory perception may limit self-care, mobility, safety, independence, communication, and relationships with others.

Eyes

The eyes are complex structures, containing 70% of the body's sensory receptors. Both extraocular and intraocular structures are considered parts of the eye. Each eye is a sphere measuring about 1 in. (2.5 cm) in diameter, surrounded and protected by a bony orbit and cushions of fat. The primary functions of the eye are to encode the patterns of light from the environment through photoreceptors and to carry the

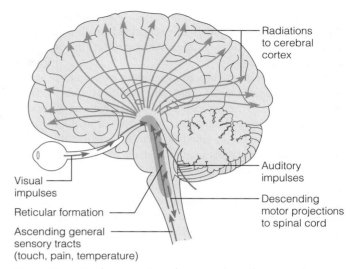

Figure 11–1 ■ The nerve impulses run along the ascending sensory tracts to reach the reticular activating system (RAS); then certain impulses reach the cerebral cortex where they are preceived.

From *Human Anatomy & Physiology*, 7th ed., by Elaine N. Marieb and Katja Hoehn. Copyright ® 2007 (p. 455) by Benjamin Cummings Publishing Company. Reprinted by permission of Pearson Education, Inc.

coded information from the eyes to the brain. The brain gives meaning to the coded information, allowing us to make sense of what we see.

EXTRAOCULAR STRUCTURES Although the extraocular structures of the eye are outside the eyeball, they are vital to its protection. These structures are the eyebrows, eyelids, eyelashes, conjunctiva, lacrimal apparatus, and extrinsic eye muscles (Figure 11–2 ■).

The eyebrows shade the eyes and keep perspiration away from them. The eyelids are thin, loose folds of skin covering the anterior eye. They protect the eye from foreign bodies, regulate the entry of light into the eye, and distribute tears by blinking.

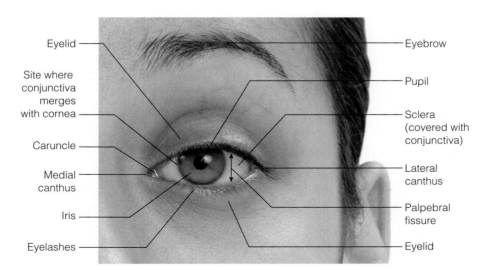

Figure 11–2 ■ Structures of the external eye.

The eyelashes are short hairs that project from the top and bottom borders of the eyelids. An unexpected touch to the eyelashes initiates the blinking reflex, which protects the eyes from foreign objects.

The conjunctiva is a thin, transparent mucus membrane that lines the inner surfaces of the eyelids and also folds over the anterior surface of the eyeball. The conjunctiva also lubricates the eyes. The lacrimal apparatus is composed of the lacrimal gland, the puncta, the lacrimal sac, and the nasolacrimal duct. Together, these structures secrete, distribute, and drain tears to cleanse and moisten the eye's surface.

Six extrinsic eye muscles control movement of the eye, allowing it to follow a moving object and move precisely. These muscles also help maintain the shape of the eyeball. The cranial nerves control the extrinsic muscles (Figure 11–3 ■).

INTRAOCULAR STRUCTURES The intraocular structures transmit visual images and maintain homeostasis of the inner eye. Those in the anterior portion of each eyeball are the sclera and the cornea, the iris, the pupil, and the anterior cavity (Figure 11–4 ■).

Sclera and Cornea The white sclera lines the outside of the eyeball, protecting it and giving it shape. The sclera gives way to the cornea over the iris and pupil. The cornea is transparent, avascular, and sensitive to touch. The cornea forms a window that allows light to enter the eye and is a part of its light-bending apparatus. When the cornea is touched, the eyelids blink (**corneal reflex**) and tears are secreted.

Iris and Pupil The iris is a disc of muscle surrounding the pupil and lying between the cornea and the lens. The iris gives the eye its color and regulates light entry by controlling the

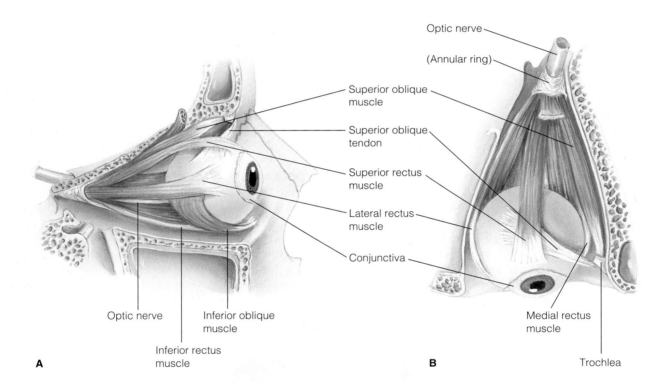

Name	Controlling cranial nerve	Action
Lateral rectus	VI (abducens)	Moves eye laterally
Medial rectus	III (oculomotor)	Moves eye medially
Superior rectus	III (oculomotor)	Elevates eye or rolls it superiorly
Inferior rectus	III (oculomotor)	Depresses eye or rolls it inferiorly
Inferior oblique	III (oculomotor)	Elevates eye and turns it laterally
Superior oblique	IV (trochlear)	Depresses eye and turns it laterally

Figure 11–3 ■ Extraocular muscles, *A*, Lateral view of the right eye. *B*, Superior view to the right eye. *C*, Innervation of the extraocular by the cranial nerves.

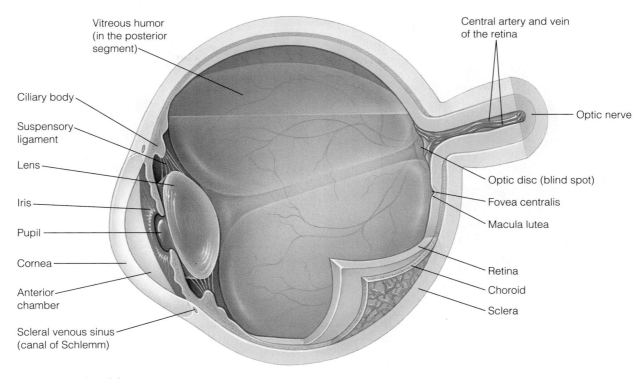

Figure 11–4 ■ Interior of the eye.

size of the pupil. The pupil is the dark center of the eye through which light enters. The pupil constricts when bright light enters the eye and when it is used for near vision; it dilates when light conditions are dim and when the eye is used for far vision. In response to intense light, the pupil constricts rapidly in the **pupillary light reflex**.

Anterior Cavity   The anterior cavity is made of the anterior chamber (the space between the cornea and the iris) and the posterior chamber (the space between the iris and the lens). The anterior cavity is filled with aqueous humor. Aqueous humor, a clear fluid, is constantly formed and drained to maintain a relatively constant pressure in the eye of from 15 to 20 mmHg. The canal of Schlemm, provides the drainage system for fluid moving between the anterior and posterior chambers. Aqueous humor provides nutrients and oxygen for the cornea and the lens.

Internal Chamber   The intraocular structures that lie in the internal chamber of the eye are the lens, the posterior cavity and vitreous humor, the ciliary body, the uvea, and the retina.

■ The lens is a biconvex, avascular, transparent structure located directly behind the pupil. It can change shape to focus and refract light onto the retina.

■ The posterior cavity lies behind the lens. It supports the posterior surface of the lens, maintains the position of the retina, and transmits light.

■ The uvea is the middle layer of the eyeball. This pigmented layer has three components: the iris, ciliary body, and choroid.

■ The ciliary body encircles the lens and, along with the iris, regulates the amount of light reaching the retina by controlling the shape of the lens. Blood vessels of the choroid nourish the layers of the eyeball. Its pigmented areas absorb light, preventing it from scattering within the eyeball.

■ The retina is the innermost lining of the eyeball. It has an outer pigmented layer and an inner neural layer. The outer layer, next to the choroid, serves as the link between visual stimuli and the brain. The transparent inner layer is made up of millions of light receptors in structures called rods and cones. Rods enable peripheral vision and vision in dim light. Cones enable vision in bright light and the perception of color.

REFRACTION   **Refraction** is the bending of light rays as they pass from one medium to another medium of different optical density. As light rays pass through the eye, they are refracted at several points: as they enter the cornea, as they leave the cornea and enter the aqueous humor, as they enter the lens, and as they leave the lens and enter the vitreous humor. At the lens, light is bent so that it converges at a single point on the retina. This focusing of the image is called **accommodation**. Because the lens is convex, the image projected onto the retina (the real image) is upside down and reversed from left to right. This real image is coded as electric signals that are sent to the brain. The brain decodes the image so that the person perceives it as it occurs in space (Figure 11–5 ■).

The eyes are best adapted to see distant objects. Both eyes fix on the same distant image and do not require any change in accommodation. For people with normal vision, the distance

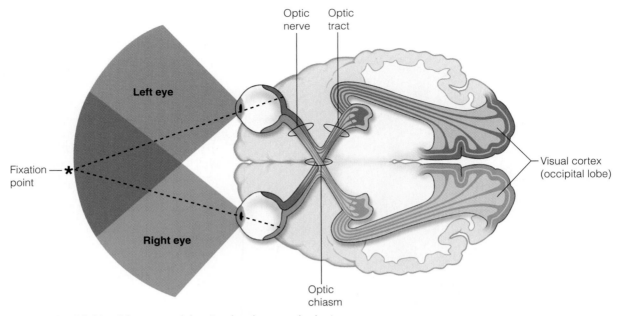

Optic nerve   Optic tract

Left eye

Fixation point

Right eye

Optic chiasm

Visual cortex (occipital lobe)

Figure 11–5 ■ Visual fields of the eye and the visual pathway to the brain.

from the viewed object at which the eyes require no accommodation is 20 ft (6 m). This point is called the far point of vision. To focus for near vision, the eyes must instantly accommodate the lens, constrict the pupils, and converge the eyeballs. The closest point on which a person can focus is called the near point of vision; in young adults with normal vision this is usually 8–10 in. (20–25 cm). Pupillary constriction helps eliminate most of the divergent light rays and sharpens focus. **Convergence** (the medial rotation of the eyeballs so that each is directed toward the viewed object) allows the image to be focused on the retinal fovea of each eye.

Ears

As a sensory organ, the ears have two primary functions, hearing and maintaining equilibrium. Anatomically, each ear is divided into three areas: the external ear, the middle ear, and the inner ear (Figure 11–6 ■). Each area has a unique function. All three are involved in hearing, but only the inner ear is involved in equilibrium.

EXTERNAL EAR The external ear consists of the auricles (or pinna), the external auditory canal, and the tympanic membrane.

The auricles are elastic cartilage covered with thin skin. They contain sebaceous and sweat glands and sometimes hair. Each auricle has a rim (the helix) and a lobe. The auricle serves to direct sound waves into the ear.

The external auditory canal serves as a resonator for the range of sound waves typical of human speech and increases the pressure that sound waves in this frequency range place on the tympanic membrane. The canal's ceruminous glands (modified apocrine glands) secrete a yellow to brown waxy substance called **cerumen** (earwax). Cerumen traps foreign bodies; it also has bacteriostatic properties, protecting the tympanic membrane and the middle ear from infections.

The tympanic membrane lies between the external ear and the middle ear. It is a thin, semitransparent, fibrous structure covered with skin on the external side and mucosa on the inner side. The membrane vibrates as sound waves strike it; these vibrations are transferred as sound waves to the middle ear.

MIDDLE EAR The middle ear is an air-filled cavity in the temporal bone. The posterior wall of the middle ear contains the mastoid antrum. This cavity communicates with the mastoid sinuses, which help the middle ear adjust to changes in pressure. The mastoid antrum also opens into the eustachian tube, which connects with the nasopharynx. The eustachian tube helps to equalize the air pressure in the middle ear by opening briefly in response to differences between middle ear pressure and atmospheric pressure. This action also ensures that vibrations of the tympanic membrane remain adequate. The mucous membrane lining the middle ear is continuous with the mucous membranes lining the throat.

The middle ear contains three auditory ossicles: the malleus, the incus, and the stapes. The malleus attaches to the tympanic membrane and articulates with the incus, which in turn articulates with the stapes. The stapes fits into the oval window. Vibrations of the tympanic membrane are conducted across the middle ear to the oval window by the ossicles. The vibrations then set in motion the fluids of the inner ear, which in turn stimulate the hearing receptors. Two small muscles attached to the ossicles contract reflexively in response to sudden loud noises, decreasing the vibrations and protecting the inner ear.

INNER EAR The inner ear is a maze of bony chambers located deep within the temporal bone just behind the eye socket. Within the inner ear the cochlea houses the organ of Corti, the receptor organ for hearing. The organ of Corti is a series of sensory hair cells, arranged in a single row of inner hair cells and three rows of outer hair cells. The hair cells are

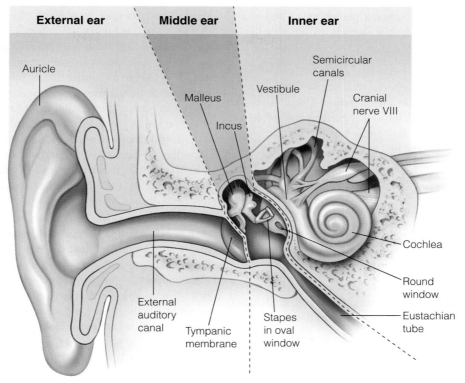

Figure 11–6 ■ The three parts of the ear.

innervated by sensory fibers from cranial nerve VIII. The organ of Corti is supported in the cochlea by the flexible basilar membrane, which has fibers of varying lengths that respond to different sound wave frequencies.

SOUND CONDUCTION Hearing is the perception and interpretation of sound. Sound is produced when the molecules of a medium are compressed, resulting in a pressure disturbance evidenced as a sound wave. The intensity or loudness of sound is determined by the amplitude (height) of the sound wave, with greater amplitudes causing louder sounds. The frequency of the sound wave in vibrations per second determines the pitch or tone of the sound, with higher frequencies resulting in higher sounds.

Sound waves enter the external auditory canal and cause the tympanic membrane to vibrate at the same frequency. The ossicles not only transmit the motion of the tympanic membrane to the oval window, but also amplify the energy of the sound wave.

Several brainstem auditory nuclei transmit impulses to the cerebral cortex. Fibers from each ear cross, with each auditory cortex receiving impulses from both ears. Auditory processing is so finely tuned that a wide variety of sounds of different pitch and loudness can be heard at any one time. In addition, the sources of the sounds can be localized.

EQUILIBRIUM The inner ear also provides information about the position of the head. This information is used to coordinate body movements so that equilibrium and balance are maintained. The types of equilibrium are static balance

(affected by changes in the position of the head) and dynamic balance (affected by the movement of the head).

Receptors called maculae detect changes in the position of the head. Maculae are groups of hair cells in the inner ear that have protrusions covered with a gelatinous substance. Embedded in this gelatinous substance are tiny particles of calcium carbonate called otoliths (ear stones) which sense gravity and movement.

Taste and Smell

The sense of taste is mediated by taste buds located on the dorsal surface of the tongue, in the lateral folds on the side of the tongue, on the epiglottis, on the larynx, and even on the first third of the esophagus. Many nerves are responsible for transmitting taste information to the brain, including cranial nerves VII, IX, and X. Taste buds are continually bathed in secretions from the salivary glands.

Taste is not the same thing as flavor. Traditionally five tastes have been identified: sour, sweet, bitter, salty, and umami. Taste combines with texture, temperature, and the perception of odor from the olfactory senses to produce the perception of flavor. Flavor is greatly regulated by sense of smell. Someone with a bad head cold, for example, may repeatedly complain that he or she cannot taste anything (National Institutes of Health, 2009).

The olfactory cells, located in the roof of the nasal cavity, form filaments that connect to the olfactory nerve (cranial nerve I) and are primarily responsible for the sense of smell. Nerve endings in the ear, throat, and mouth also play a part in the sense of smell, participating in our perception of and reaction to smells such as rancid milk or peppermint (National Institutes of Health, 2009).

Touch

Touch is the tactile sense that is perceived by nerve endings and transmits signals to the brain for interpretation. Touch orients a person to the environment and allows the exchange of information and sensation. The psychological benefits of touch are many and include the ability to be soothed, comforted, and held. Individuals in some cultures rely heavily on touching others during routine communication and find it difficult to refrain from touching others when they are unable to use their hands. Touch can also be protective by stimulating movement or withdrawal from hot, sharp, or unpleasant stimuli.

While all areas of the body are sensitive to touch, some are more sensitive than others due to having a greater number of receptors. Anyone who has ever burned his or her tongue or sliced a finger tip against the edge of a piece of paper understands this. In addition to the tongue and fingertips, the hands, feet, face and neck are particularly sensitive to touch.

Factors Affecting Sensory Perception

A number of factors affect the amount and quality of sensory stimulation, including a person's genetic make-up, developmental stage, culture, level of stress, isolation, medications and illness, and lifestyle.

CONGENITAL AND HEREDITARY CONDITIONS Many conditions lead to temporary or permanent impairment of sensory perception. Infants who are premature; whose mothers were infected prenatally with rubella, toxoplasmosis, or other viruses; or who have certain congenital and hereditary conditions are at a high risk for visual problems. Fetal alcohol syndrome (FAS) is a major cause of prenatal visual disturbance. Auditory Processing Disorder, a condition in which the individual has difficulty differentiating individual sounds in words, is one of several hearing disorders with which a child may be born. It creates difficulty for individuals in some environments, including and especially school. Its cause is unknown. Some people are born with impairment of the senses of smell and taste, but these can also be acquired from exposure to insecticides or radiation and through other means.

CULTURE An individual's culture often determines the amount of stimulation the person considers usual or "normal." For example, a child reared in a big-city Latino neighborhood, where extended families share responsibilities for

all the children, may be accustomed to more stimulation than a child reared in a European-American suburb of scattered single-family homes. In addition, the normal amount of stimulation associated with ethnic origin, religious affiliation, and income level, for example, also affects the amount of stimulation an individual desires and believes to be meaningful. A sudden change in cultural surroundings experienced by immigrants or visitors to a new country—specially where language, dress, and cultural behaviors differ—may also result in sensory overload or cultural shock.

Cultural deprivation, or cultural care deprivation, is a lack of culturally assistive, supportive, or facilitative acts. It is important that nurses be sensitive to what stimulation is culturally acceptable to a client. For example, in some cultures touching is comforting, whereas in others it is offensive.

STRESS During times of increased stress, people may find their senses overloaded and seek to decrease sensory stimulation. For example, a client dealing with physical illness, pain, hospitalization, and diagnostic tests may wish to have only close support people visit. The client may also need the nurse's help in reducing unnecessary stimuli (e.g., noise) as much as possible. On the other hand, clients may seek sensory stimulation during times of low stress.

ISOLATION Much research has been done to document the importance of touch in early life. Infants in incubators who are not touched will stop eating and fail to thrive. The same may be true for older people, especially those with cognitive or sensory impairments. Institutionalized older persons deprived of caring touch and nurturing physical contact experience a diminishing quality of life, a lessening of their desire to relate to others, and a weakening of what may already be a fragile relationship with physical reality (Nelson, 2001).

MEDICATION AND ILLNESS Certain medications can alter an individual's awareness of environmental stimuli. Narcotics and sedatives, for example, can decrease awareness of stimuli. Some antidepressants can alter perceptions of stimuli. Anyone taking several medications concurrently may show alterations in sensory function. Elders are especially at risk and need to be monitored carefully, particularly if they are simultaneously taking multiple medications for a variety of conditions. Certain medications, if taken over a long period of time, become ototoxic, injuring the auditory nerve and causing hearing loss that may be irreversible. (See Hearing Impairment Exemplar below.)

Diseases such as atherosclerosis restrict blood flow to the receptor organs and the brain, thereby decreasing awareness and slowing responses. Uncontrolled diabetes mellitus can

---

FOCUS ON DIVERSITY AND CULTURE   Otitis Media

Native American and Alaska Native (NA/AN) children have a very high rate of otitis media, perhaps related to culture-specific bony structure of the ear, nose, and mouth. One study found that NA/AN children are seen about three times more frequently in outpatient clinics for otitis media than are other children in the United States

(Curns et al., 2002). Nurses should be alert for the high incidence in these population groups, plan prevention programs, and ensure prompt care and teaching about treatments for families of children affected. What prevention measures would you emphasize with these families?

impair vision and is a leading cause of blindness in the United States. Some central nervous system diseases cause varying degrees of paralysis and sensory loss.

LIFESTYLE AND PERSONALITY Lifestyle influences the quality and quantity of stimulation to which an individual is accustomed. A client who is employed in a large company may be accustomed to diverse stimuli, whereas a client who is self-employed and works in the home is exposed to fewer, less diverse stimuli. People's personalities also differ in terms of the quantity and quality of stimuli with which they are comfortable. Some people delight in constantly changing stimuli and excitement, whereas others prefer a more structured life with few changes.

Age-Related Changes in Sensory Perception

The eyes of neonates differ from the eyes of adults in several ways. Visual acuity in neonates ranges between 20/100 and 20/400. Because the optic nerve is not yet completely myelinated, the ability to distinguish color and other details is decreased. The rectus muscles that control binocular vision may be somewhat uncoordinated at birth. By the age of 3 months, the eyes should be aligned and movement coordinated. Transient **nystagmus** (involuntary rapid eye movement) and **esotropia** (momentary turning inward of eyes) are common in neonates, but decrease in incidence during the first few months of life.

The cornea occupies a larger portion of the orbit in the infant and young child than in the adult; the infant's eyeball is about three-fourths of its adult size (Chamley, Carson, Randall, & Sandwell, 2005). Because the infant's eyeball is relatively unprotected laterally, it is more easily injured. The sclera of the neonate is thin and translucent with a bluish tinge, and the iris is blue or gray. Eye color changes during the first 6 months of life. By the age of 2 or 3 years, most children have a visual acuity of 20/50, and by the age of 6 or 7 years, visual acuity reaches 20/20.

Why do infants and young children have more ear problems than adults? The eustachian tube, which connects the nasopharynx to the middle ear, is proportionately shorter, wider, and more horizontal in infants than in older children or adults (see Figure 11–6). During sucking, yawning, and other movements, the tube opens for milliseconds, allowing free passage of air between the nasopharynx and the middle ear. These factors predispose young children to development of otitis media or middle ear infection.

Although auditory nerve function is not fully mature until about 5 months of age, the fetus begins to hear at about 20 weeks' gestation. Before 34 weeks' gestation, the external ear is soft, with little cartilage apparent. The external ear canal is small at birth, although the internal ear and middle ear are relatively large. As a result, the tympanic membrane is close to the surface and can be easily injured.

Newborns should be screened for hearing loss prior to hospital discharge. Universal screening of all newborns is mandated in at least 30 states, and in all states screening is done for children who are at high risk (e.g., have a history of infection during gestation, or are born with anomalies of the head or face). If a hearing loss is detected early, treatment can begin early and complications such as speech impairment or loss can be prevented. If an infant is found to have a hearing loss, it is recommended that treatment begin before 6 months of age (Joint Committee on Infant Hearing, 2000).

Changes in vision, hearing, smell, taste, and touch occur naturally throughout the aging process (Tables 11–2 and 11–3). The greatest declines in accommodation occur between 45 and 55 years of age, making this more a problem for middle-aged adults than for older adults. There is usually no change in accommodation after 60 years of age (Burke, 2002). However, normal physiologic changes in older adults put them at higher risk for altered sensory function, particularly hearing loss. Hearing loss is the third most common condition reported by the elderly. Approximately 40–45% of people over age 65 and more than 83% over the age of 70 have a hearing impairment (Gordon-Salant, 2005).

Although normal age-related changes in vision occur gradually, over time these changes can limit the functional ability of the older adult. Approximately 1.8 million community-dwelling older people report some difficulty with basic activities such as bathing, dressing, and walking around the house, in part because they are visually impaired. Unfortunately, visual impairment increases with age. Visual impairment is defined as visual acuity of 20/40 or worse while wearing corrective lenses, and legal blindness or severe visual impairment is 20/200 or more as measured by a Snellen wall chart at 20 ft.

The prevalence of blindness also increases with age, reaching its peak at about the age of 85. Fortunately, the prevalence of blindness in both eyes in the United States is low, about 1% among persons 70–74 years of age and 2.4% in persons 85 and older (Centers for Disease Control and Prevention, 2002). Visual impairment and blindness in the older person has four main causes: cataracts, age-related macular degeneration (ARMD), glaucoma, and diabetic retinopathy.

A diminished sense of taste, **hypogeusia**, is a normal sensory change usually occurring after the age of 70. The exact pathophysiology behind age-related gustatory changes remains unclear. However, studies have shown that both taste discrimination and sensitivity significantly change with age.

Olfactory dysfunction is more common than taste dysfunction. The three most common causes of loss of smell are nasal and sinus disease, upper respiratory infection, and head trauma (Bromley, 2000). Normal age-related changes influencing olfactory function are attributed to injury of the olfactory mucosa and reduction in both the number of sensory cells and neurotransmitters. Structural alterations of the upper airway, olfactory tract and bulb, hippocampus, amygdaloid complex, and hypothalamus have also been observed as contributing factors for diminished sense of smell, or **hyposmia**, in older adults (Schiffman, 1997).

Older persons with one or more sensory impairments are at risk for injury, weight loss, falls, malnutrition, and social isolation. Intact senses allow the older person to accurately

TABLE 11–2 Age-Related Changes in the Eye

AGE-RELATED CHANGE	SIGNIFICANCE
The lens: ■ ↓ elasticity, decreasing focus and accommodation for near vision (presbyopia) ■ ↑ density and size, making lens more stiff and opaque ■ Yellowing of the lens and changes in the retina affecting color perception	Most older adults require corrective lenses to accommodate close and detailed work. Increased opacity leads to the development of cataracts. As cataracts develop, they increase sensitivity to glare and interfere with night vision.
The cornea: ■ Fat deposits around the periphery and throughout the cornea ■ ↓ corneal sensitivity	A partial or complete white circle may form around the cornea (*arcus senilis*). Lipid deposits in the cornea cause vision to be blurred. Decreased sensitivity increases the risk of injury to the eye.
The pupil: ■ ↓ size and responsiveness to light pupil; sphincter hardening	Increased light perception threshold and difficulty seeing in dim light or at night means increased light is needed to see adequately.
The retina and visual pathways: ■ Visual fields narrow ■ Photoreceptor cells lost ■ Rods working less effectively ■ Macular degeneration ■ Depth perception distortion ■ Adaptation to dark and light taking longer	Peripheral vision is decreased and central vision may be lost due to macular degeneration. Increased risk of falls results from changes in depth perception and adaptation to changes in light. Vision progressively declines with age.
The lacrimal apparatus: ■ ↓ reabsorption of intraocular fluid ■ ↓ production of tears	Increased risk of developing glaucoma; eyes feel and look dry.
The posterior cavity: ■ Debris and condensation becoming visible ■ Vitreous body maybe pulling away from the retina	Vision is blurred and distorted. "Floaters" are often seen by the older person.

perceive the environment and remain appropriately involved with other people, places, and objects. Safety is compromised when the older person cannot see fall hazards on the floor, cannot smell a natural gas leak from a stove, cannot recognize the taste of spoiled milk, cannot hear a signaling fire alarm, and cannot feel a pebble in the shoe that could lead to

TABLE 11–3 Age-Related Changes in the Ear

AGE-RELATED CHANGE	SIGNIFICANCE
Inner ear: ■ Loss of hair cells, ↓ blood supply, less flexible basilar membrane, degeneration of spiral ganglion cells, and ↓ production of endolymph resulting in progressive hearing loss with age **(presbycusis)** ■ High-frequency sounds lost; middle- and low-frequency sounds maybe also lost or decreased ■ Vestibular structures degenerating, organ of Corti and cochlea	Older adults may require hearing aids to hear well. With loss of high-frequency sounds, speech may be distorted, contributing to a risk for problems with communication. Degeneration and atrophy of inner ear structures concerned with balance and equilibrium increase the risk for falls, atrophy.
Middle ear: ■ Muscles and ligaments weakening and stiffening, decreasing the acoustic reflex	Sounds made from one's own body and speech are louder and may further interfere with hearing, speech, and communications.
External ear: ■ Higher keratin content of cerumen, contributing to increased cerumen in the ear canal	Accumulated cerumen may impair hearing.

a blister or foot ulcer. Older persons with sensory dysfunction may suffer functional impairment, injury, social isolation, and depression.

ALTERATIONS

Common problems related to sensory impairment include injury, cataracts, glaucoma, and macular degeneration. Chronic use of certain medications and chronic diseases such as Alzheimer's can cause impairment of smell. Hearing impairment is discussed later in this concept.

Injuries

Children are particularly at risk for eye injury. In the United States, eye injuries are common in boys 11–15 years of age and in all children ages 9–11 years. Boys from 11 to 15 years have four times more eye injuries than girls. Approximately half of the 42,000 sports injuries that occur annually involve children (Committee on Sports Medicine and Fitness, 2004). Sports, darts, fireworks, air-powered BB guns, blunt and sharp objects, chemical and thermal burns, physical irritants, and abuse all may cause eye trauma (Behrman, Kliegman, & Jenson, 2004). Older children may be injured by chemicals in school science laboratories. Athletes, particularly those involved in sports that do not require use of a helmet, are at risk for eye injuries, whether they play professionally or recreationally. Use of projectile toys of any kind increases the risk of eye injury. Professional such as contractors, woodworkers, welders, and electricians are also at risk of eye injury and should wear protective goggles at all times.

Many eye injuries are minor, but without timely and appropriate intervention even a minor injury can threaten vision. For this reason, all eye injuries should be considered medical emergencies requiring immediate evaluation and intervention.

PRACTICE ALERT
Linking the Concepts – Sensory Perception, Family, Violence
External eye injuries are very common in children and by themselves will rarely indicate some form of abuse or nonaccidental trauma. Two black eyes, however, rarely occur by accident and raccoon eyes accompanied by swelling and skin injury are more likely to accompany nonaccidental fracture at the base of the skull (National Criminal Justice Reference Service, 2009). Ruptured tympanic membranes in combination with conjunctival and retinal hemorrhage are indicative of shaken baby syndrome. Retinal hemorrhage rarely occurs with any other type of injury. A nurse who suspects child abuse should follow his or her agency's protocol for reporting to Child Protective Services.

Ear injuries of many types are common in children. Lacerations, infections, and hematomas may occur in the external ear structures, especially the pinna. Children may place foreign objects in the ear, and insects may enter the ear canal.

Rupture of the tympanic membrane may result from head injuries, blows to the ear, or insertion of objects into the ear canal. Serous drainage from the ear can indicate a basilar skull fracture. Any injury resulting in earache, decreased hearing, persistent bleeding, or other discharge should be evaluated by a physician.

ALTERATIONS AND TREATMENTS Sensory Perception

ALTERATION	DESCRIPTION	TREATMENTS
Eye Injury	Damage to the structure of the eye; a common cause of vision loss in children. Often caused by sports injury or chemicals.	▪ All eye injuries should be considered medical emergencies requiring immediate evaluation and intervention ▪ Treatment varies due to type and severity of injury; treatments may include irrigation, foreign body removal and surgery
Cataracts	Opacification of eye that prevents refraction of light rays onto the retina; may be congenital or acquired	▪ Surgical removal of lens; lens may be implanted

Glaucoma	Optic neuropathy with gradual loss of peripheral vision; there are two main types, open-angle and angle-closure glaucoma	▪ Medications to control intraocular pressure and preserve vision in open-angle glaucoma
		▪ Surgery
		  ▪ Laser trabeculoplasty
		  ▪ Trabulectomy
		  ▪ Photocoagulation
		  ▪ Gionioplasty
		  ▪ Laser iridotomy

Macular degeneration (AMD)	Progressive disorder involving loss of central vision due to damage to the retina; there are two types, nonexudative and exudative	▪ High-dose antioxidants and zinc (early-to-intermediate dry AMD) ▪ Laser surgery or photodynamic therapy (wet AMD)

Cataracts

A **cataract** is an opacification (clouding) of the lens of the eye. This opacification can significantly interfere with light transmission to the retina and the ability to perceive images clearly. Cataracts are a common and significant cause of visual deficits, affecting nearly 20.5 million people over age 40 in the United States. By age 80, nearly half of the population is affected.

Glaucoma

Glaucoma is a condition characterized by optic neuropathy with gradual loss of peripheral vision and, usually, increased intraocular pressure of the eye. Glaucoma is a silent thief of vision. The client typically experiences no manifestations other than narrowing of the visual field, which occurs so gradually that it often goes unnoticed until late in the disease process.

Macular Degeneration

The leading cause of legal blindness and impaired vision in people over the age of 65 is age-related **macular degeneration** (AMD) (Prevent Blindness America, 2002).

SENSORY ASSESSMENT

Nursing assessment of sensory-perceptual functioning includes six components: (a) nursing history, (b) mental status examination, (c) identification of clients at risk, (d) the client's environment, (e) social support network, and (f) physical assessment.

Nursing History

During the nursing history, the nurse assesses present sensory perceptions, usual functioning, sensory deficits, and potential problems. In some instances, significant others or family members can provide data the client cannot. For example, family members may reveal signs of recent changes in the client's hearing ability, such as inattention to others, recent mood swings, difficulty following clear instructions, frequent requests to have something repeated, and unusually loud radio or television volumes. Assessment should include questions to obtain information related to noise exposure—loud, constant sounds from any type of equipment, for example—as well as hobbies or work that can cause burns or injuries. The nurse should always assess for chronic diseases or illness as well as medications taken by the client, regardless of the type of impairment suspected. The following Assessment Interview provides examples of interview questions to elicit data about the client's sensory-perceptual functioning.

Assessment Interview   Sensory-Perceptual Functioning

VISUAL
- How would you rate your vision (excellent, good, fair, or poor)?
- Do you wear eyeglasses or contact lenses?
- Describe any recent changes in your vision.
- Do you have any difficulty seeing near or far objects?
- Do you have any difficulty seeing at night? Have you ever experienced blurred vision, double vision, spots moving in front of your eyes, blind spots, light sensitivity, flashing lights, or halos around objects?
- When did you last visit an eye doctor?

AUDITORY
- How would you rate your hearing (excellent, good, fair, or poor)?
- Do you wear a hearing aid?
- Describe any recent changes in your hearing.
- Can you locate the direction of sounds and distinguish various voices?
- Are you having any trouble with balance?
- Do you experience any dizziness or vertigo? Do you experience any ringing, buzzing, humming, crackling noises, or fullness in the ears?
- Do you listen to loud music on a regular basis?
- Are you exposed to any loud noises at work? If so, what are they? How much or how often?

GUSTATORY
- Have you experienced any changes in taste (e.g., difficulty in differentiating sweet, sour, salty, and bitter tastes)?
- Do you enjoy the taste of foods as you did previously?

OLFACTORY
- Have you experienced any changes in smell?
- Do things (foods, flowers, perfumes, and so on) smell the same as previously?
- Can you distinguish foods by their odors and tell when something is burning?
- Have you experienced any changes in appetite? (Changes in appetite may be related to an impaired sense of smell.)

TACTILE
- Are you experiencing any pain or discomfort?
- Have you experienced any decrease in your ability to perceive heat, cold, or pain in your limbs?
- Do you have any numbness or tingling in your extremities?

KINESTHETIC
- Have you noticed any difficulty in perceiving the position of parts of your body?
- Do you need any assistance standing or sitting down?

Source: Berman, A., Snyder, S. J., Kozier, B., & Erb, G. (2008). *Kozier & Erb's fundamentals of nursing: Concepts, process, and practice* (8th ed., p. 984). Upper Saddle River, NJ: Pearson Education.

Mental Status and Cognition

Mental status is critical to any evaluation of the sensory-perceptual process. The nurse should assess for any recent history of mood swings or delirium. The nurse should also assess for any problems with cognitive function, including level of consciousness, orientation, memory, and attention span. It is important to note that sensory alterations can cause changes in mental status and cognitive functioning (adapted from Wahl & Heyl, 2003).

Client Environment

The nurse assesses the client's environment for quantity, quality, and type of stimuli. The client's environment may produce insufficient stimuli, placing the client at risk for sensory deprivation, or excessive stimuli, placing the client at risk for sensory overload. Nonstimulating environments include those that (a)

severely restrict physical activity and (b) limit social contact with family and friends. Because appropriate or meaningful stimuli decrease the incidence of sensory deprivation, the nurse must consider the client's health care environment for the presence of the following stimuli:

- Radio or other auditory device (e.g., cassette or CD player), including television and use of earphones with portable devices
- Clock or calendar
- Reading material (or toys for children)
- Number and compatibility of roommates (which may affect number of auditory devices used at one time, level of overall noise in the environment)
- Number of visitors.

In the client's home, the nurse may also note the presence of a video/DVD recorder, pets, bright colors, and adequate lighting.

Eye and Vision Assessment

Vision Assessment

Visual acuity is assessed with an eye chart such as the Snellen chart or the E chart for testing distance vision and the Rosenbaum chart for testing near vision. The Snellen chart contains rows of letters in various sizes, with standardized numbers at the end of each row. The number at the end of the row indicates the visual acuity of a client who can read the row at a distance of 20 feet. (If the client is unable to read or does not read English, you can use the E chart to test visual acuity.) The top number at the end of the row is always 20, representing the distance between the client and the chart. The bottom number is the distance (in feet) at which a person with normal vision can read the line. A person with normal vision can read the row marked 20/20. To conduct the

assessment, ask the person to stand 20 feet from the chart in a well-lit area. Ask the client to cover one eye with an opaque cover (Figure 11–7 ■). Then ask the client to read each row of letters, moving from largest letters to the smallest ones that the client can see. Measure visual acuity in the other eye in the same way, and then assess visual acuity while the client has both eyes uncovered. You may test the client who wears corrective lenses with and without the lenses.

The Rosenbaum chart is held at a distance of from 12 to 14 inches from the eyes, with visual acuity measured in the same manner as with the Snellen chart (Figure 11–8 ■). A gross estimate of near vision may also be assessed by asking the person to read from a magazine or newspaper.

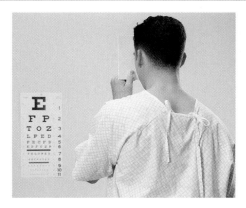

Figure 11–7 ■ Testing distant vision using the Snellen eye chart.

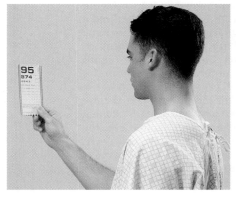

Figure 11–8 ■ Testing near vision using Rosenbaum eye chart.

Technique/Normal Findings	Abnormal Findings
Assess distant vision, using the Snellen or E chart. *When standing 20 feet from the chart, the client can read the smallest line of letters with or without corrective lenses (recorded as 20/20).*	■ Changes in distant vision are most commonly the result of **myopia** (nearsightedness). For example, a reading of 20/100 indicates impaired distance vision. A person has to stand 20 feet from the chart to read a line that a person with normal vision could read 100 feet from the chart.
Assess near vision, using a Rosenbaum chart or a card with newsprint held 12–14 inches from the client's eyes. *Normal near visual acuity is 14/14 with or without corrective lenses.*	■ Changes in near vision, especially in clients over age 45, can indicate **presbyopia**, impaired near vision resulting from a loss of elasticity of the lens related to aging. In younger clients, this condition is referred to as **hyperopia** (farsightedness).

Eye and Vision Assessment (continued)

Technique/Normal Findings	Abnormal Findings

Eye Movement Assessment

Assess the cardinal fields of vision to gain information about extraocular eye movements. Ask the client to follow a pen or your finger while keeping the head stationary. Move the pen or your finger through the six fields one at a time, returning to the central starting point before proceeding to the next field (Figure 11–9 ■). *The eyes should move through each field without involuntary movements.*

- Failure of one or both eyes to follow the object in any given direction may indicate extraocular muscle weakness or cranial nerve dysfunction.
- An involuntary rhythmic movement of the eyes, nystagmus, is associated with neurologic disorders and the use of some medications.

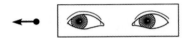

1 Penlight is to nurse's extreme left.

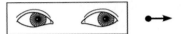

4 Penlight is to nurse's extreme right.

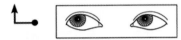

2 Penlight is left and up.

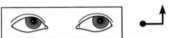

5 Penlight is right and up.

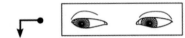

3 Penlight is left and down.

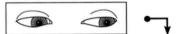

6 Penlight is right and down.

Figure 11–9 ■ The six cardinal fields of vision.

The cover–uncover test is a test for strabismus, a weakening of a muscle that causes one eye to deviate from the other when the person is focusing on an object. To conduct the test, hold a pen or your finger about 1 foot from the eyes and ask the person to focus on that object. Cover one of the client's eyes and note any movement in the uncovered eye; as you remove the cover, assess for movement in the eye that was just uncovered. Repeat the procedure with the other eye. *The uncovered eye should remain fixed straight ahead. The covered eye should remain fixed straight ahead after being uncovered.*

Assess convergence. *Ask the client to follow an object as you move it toward the client's eyes. Normally both eyes converge toward the center.*

- Failure of the eyes to converge equally on an approaching object may indicate a neuromuscular disorder or improper eye alignment.

Assess the corneal light reflex. *Direct a light source onto the bridge of the nose from 12 to 15 inches. Observe for equal reflection of the light from each eye.*

- Reflections of the light from different sites on the eyes reveal improper alignment.

Pupillary Assessment

Observe pupil size and equality. *Pupils should be of equal size, 3–5 mm.*

- Pupils that are unequal in size may indicate a severe neurologic problem, such as increased intracranial pressure.

Eye and Vision Assessment (continued)

Technique/Normal Findings	Abnormal Findings

Assess direct and consensual pupil response. *Ask the client to look straight ahead. Shine a light obliquely into one eye at a time. Observe for constriction of the pupil in the illuminated eye. Test both eyes. To test consensual pupil response, again shine a light obliquely into one eye at a time as the client looks straight ahead. Observe constriction of the pupil in the opposite eye. The normal direct and consensual pupillary response is constriction.*

- Failure of the pupils to respond to light may indicate degeneration of the retina or destruction of the optic nerve.
- A client who has one dilated and unresponsive pupil may have paralysis of the oculomotor nerve.
- Some eye medications may cause unequal dilation, constriction, or inequality of pupil size. Morphine and narcotic drugs may cause small, unresponsive pupils, and anticholinergic drugs such as atropine may cause dilated, unresponsive pupils.

Test for accommodation. Hold an object at a distance of a few feet from the client. The pupils should dilate. Ask the client to follow the object as you bring it to within a few inches of the client's nose. The pupils should constrict and converge as they change focus to follow the object.

- Failure of accommodation along with lack of pupil response to light may signal a neurologic problem.
- Lack of response to light with appropriate response to accommodation is often seen in clients with diabetes.

External Eye Assessment

Inspect the eyelids. *Eyelids should be the color of the client's facial skin, without redness, discharge, or drooping. The sclera should not be visible.*

- Unusual redness or discharge may indicate an inflammatory state due to trauma, allergies, or infection.
- Drooping of one eyelid, called **ptosis**, may be the result of a stroke, indicate a neuromuscular disorder, or be congenital (Figure 11–10 ■).
- Unusual widening of the lids may be due to exophthalmos, protrusion of the eyeball. Exophthalmos is often associated with hyperthyroid conditions.
- Yellow plaques noted on or near the lid margins are referred to as xanthelasma and may indicate high lipid levels.

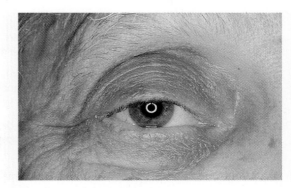

Figure 11–10 ■ Ptosis.
Source: Leonard Lessen/Peter Arnold, Inc. Custom Medical Stock Photo, Inc.

- An acute localized inflammation of a hair follicle is known as a hordeolum (sty) and is generally caused by staphylococcal organisms.
- A chalazion is an infection or retention cyst of the meibomian glands.

Inspect the puncta. *The puncta should be free of redness or discharge.*

- Unusual redness or discharge from the puncta may indicate an inflammation due to trauma, infection, or allergies.

Inspect the bulbar and palpebral conjunctiva. *The conjunctiva should be clear, moist, and smooth. The upper and lower palpebral conjunctiva should be clear, without redness or swelling.*

- Increased erythema or the presence of exudate may indicate acute conjunctivitis.
- A cobblestone appearance is often associated with allergies.
- A fold in the conjunctiva, called a pterygium, may be seen as a clouded area that extends over the cornea. This is an abnormal growth of the bulbar conjunctiva, usually seen on the nasal side of the cornea. It may interfere with vision if it covers the pupil.

Inspect the sclera. *The sclera is white in Caucasians; people with darker skin normally have yellow sclera.*

- Unusual redness may indicate an inflammatory state as a result of trauma, allergies, or infection.
- Yellow discoloration of the sclera in clients with fair skin may be seen in conditions involving the liver, such as hepatitis.
- Bright red areas in the sclera are often subconjunctival hemorrhages and may indicate trauma or bleeding disorders. They may also occur spontaneously.

Eye and Vision Assessment (continued)

Technique/Normal Findings	Abnormal Findings
Inspect the cornea. *The cornea is normally transparent.*	■ Dullness, opacities, or irregularities of the cornea may be abnormal. ■ Corneal arcus is a thin, grayish white arc seen toward the edge of the cornea. It is normal in older clients.
Assess corneal sensitivity. *Lightly touch a wisp of cotton to the client's cornea. This action should cause a corneal reflex (blinking the eye).*	■ Failure of the corneal reflex may indicate a neurologic disorder.
Inspect the iris. *The iris is normally round, flat, and evenly colored.*	■ Lack of clarity of the iris may indicate a cloudiness of the cornea. ■ Constriction of the pupil accompanied by pain and circumcorneal redness indicates acute iritis.
Internal Eye Assessment	
Assess internal structures of the eye by using the ophthalmoscope, an instrument that allows visualization of the lens, the vitreous humor, and the retina. Box 11–1 provides guidelines for using the ophthalmoscope.	
Inspect for the red reflex. *The red reflex should be clearly visible.*	■ Absence of a red reflex often indicates improper position of the ophthalmoscope, but also may indicate total opacity of the pupil by a cataract or a hemorrhage into the vitreous humor.
Inspect the lens and vitreous body. *The lens should be clear.*	■ A cataract is an opacity of the lens, often seen as a dark shadow on ophthalmoscopic examination. It may be due to aging, trauma, diabetes, or a congenital defect.
Inspect the retina. *There should be no visible hemorrhages, exudate, or white patches.*	■ Areas of hemorrhage, exudate, and white patches may be a result of diabetes or long-standing hypertension.
Inspect the optic disc. *The optic disc should be round to oval in shape with clear, well-defined borders.*	■ Loss of definition of the optic disc, as well as an increase in the size of the physiologic cup, is seen in papilledema from increased intracranial pressure.
Inspect the blood vessels of the retina. *The retinal blood vessels should be distinct.*	■ Glaucoma often results in displacement of blood vessels from the center of the optic disc due to increased intraocular pressure. ■ Hypertension may cause a narrowing of the vein where an arteriole crosses over. ■ Engorged veins may occur with diabetes, atherosclerosis, and blood disorders.
Inspect the retinal background. *The retina should be a consistent red-orange color, becoming lighter around the optic disc.*	■ Variations in color or a pale color overall may indicate disease.
Inspect the macula. *The macula should be visible on the temporal side of the optic disc.*	■ Absence of the fovea centralis is common in older clients. It may indicate macular degeneration, a cause of loss of central vision.
Palpate over the lacrimal glands, puncta, and nasolacrimal duct. *There should be no tenderness, drainage, or excessive tearing.*	■ Tenderness over any of these areas or drainage from the puncta may indicate an infectious process. (Wear gloves if you see any drainage.) ■ Excessive tearing may indicate a blockage of the nasolacrimal duct.

To assess a health care environment that produces excessive stimuli, the nurse considers, for example, bright lights, noise, therapeutic measures, and frequency of assessments and procedures.

Social Support Network

The degree of isolation a person feels is significantly influenced by the quality and quantity of support from family members and friends. The nurse assesses (a) whether the client lives alone, (b) who visits and when, and (c) any signs indicating social deprivation. Signs of social deprivation may include withdrawal from contact with others to avoid embarrassment or dependence on others; negative self-image; reports of lack of meaningful communication with others; and absence of opportunities to discuss fears or concerns that facilitate coping mechanisms.

Physical Assessment

Physical assessment determines whether the senses are impaired. During the physical examination, the nurse assesses vision (including color vision) and hearing, and the olfactory, gustatory, tactile, and kinesthetic senses. The examination should reveal the client's specific visual and hearing abilities; perception of heat, cold, light touch, and pain in the limbs; and awareness of the position of the body parts. Specific sensory tests include the following:

- Visual acuity, using a Snellen chart or other reading material such as a newspaper, and visual fields, and picture charts for those with limited reading or language proficiency
- Hearing acuity, by observing the client's conversation with others and by performing the whisper test and the Weber and Rinne tuning fork tests
- Olfactory sense, by identifying specific aromas

- Gustatory sense, by identifying three tastes such as lemon, salt, and sugar
- Tactile sense, by testing light touch, sharp and dull sensation, two-point discrimination, hot and cold sensation, vibration sense, position sense, and stereognosis

If the client uses sensory adaptive devices such as eyeglasses or a hearing aid, the nurse should determine whether or not these function properly and if the client is compliant in using them.

Ear and Hearing Assessment

Hearing Assessment

Tuning forks are used to determine whether a hearing loss is conductive or perceptive (sensorineural). Hold the tuning fork at the base and make it ring softly by stroking the prongs or by lightly tapping them on the heel of the opposite hand. The vibrating tuning fork emits sound waves of a particular frequency, measured in hertz (Hz). Tuning forks with a frequency of 512–1024 Hz are preferred for auditory evaluation, because that range corresponds to the range of normal speech.

Technique/Normal Findings	Abnormal Findings
Perform the Weber test. Place the base of a vibrating tuning fork on the midline vertex of the client's head (Figure 11–11 ■). Ask whether the client hears the sound equally in both ears or better in one than the other. *Sound is normally heard equally in both ears.*	■ Sound heard in, or lateralized to, one ear indicates either a conductive loss in that ear or a sensorineural loss in the other ear. The sound will be louder on the impaired side with a conductive hearing loss. The sound will be softer on the impaired side with a sensorineural hearing loss. Conductive losses may be due to a buildup of cerumen, an infection such as otitis media, or perforation of the eardrum.

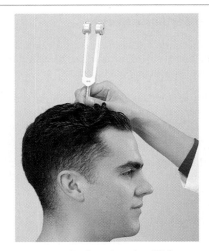

Figure 11–11 ■ Performing the Weber test with a tuning fork.

Perform the Rinne test. Place the base of a vibrating tuning fork on the client's mastoid bone. Ask the client to indicate when the sound is no longer heard. When the client does so, quickly reposition the tuning fork in front of the client's ear close to the ear canal. Ask whether the client can hear the sound. If the client says yes, ask the client to indicate when the sound is no longer heard. Repeat over the opposite mastoid bone (Figure 11–12 ■). *The client with no conductive hearing loss will hear the sound twice as long by air conduction as by bone conduction.*

■ Bone conduction is greater than air conduction in the ear with a conductive loss. The normal pattern is AC > BC (air conduction greater than bone conduction).

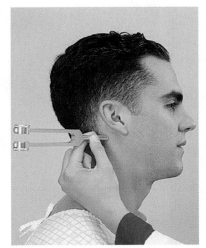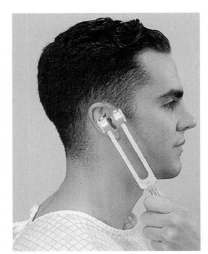

Figure 11–12 ■ Performing the Rinne test with a tuning fork.

Ear and Hearing Assessment (continued)

Technique/Normal Findings

Perform the whisper test. Ask the client to occlude one ear with a finger. Stand 1–2 feet away from the client, on the side of the unoccluded ear. Softly whisper numbers and ask the client to repeat them. Repeat the procedure, having the client occlude the other ear. Note whether you need to raise your voice or to stand closer to make the client hear you.

Use a tympanogram to measure the pressure of the middle ear and observe the tympanic membrane's response to waves of pressure. Insert the device into the ear canal. Ask the client not to speak, move, swallow, or jump when hearing a sound. Tell the client he or she will hear a loud tone as the measurements are taken. The normal pressure inside the middle ear is a 100 daPa (a very small amount). Repeat for the other ear.

Abnormal Findings

■ This test provides a rough estimate of hearing loss.

■ Abnormal findings may include fluid in the middle ear, a perforated eardrum, impacted earwax, or a tumor of the middle ear.

External Ear Assessment

Inspect the auricle. External ears are normally bilaterally equal in size, of equal color with the client's face, without redness or lesions.

■ Unusual redness or drainage may indicate an inflammatory response to infection or trauma.
■ Scales or skin lesions around the rim of the auricle may indicate skin cancer.
■ Small, raised lesions on the rim of the ear are known as tophi and indicate gout.

Inspect the external auditory canal with the otoscope. *Canal walls should be pink and smooth without lesions. Cerumen is normally present in small, odorless amounts.*

■ Unusual redness, lesions, or purulent drainage may indicate an infection.
■ Cerumen varies in color and texture, but hardened, dry, or foul-smelling cerumen may indicate an infection or an impaction of cerumen that requires removal. People with darker skin tend to have darker cerumen.

Inspect the tympanic membrane. *The tympanic membrane should be pearly gray, shiny, and translucent without bulging or retraction.*

■ White, opaque areas on the tympanic membrane are often scars from previous perforations (Figure 11–13 ■).
■ Inconsistent texture and color may be due to scarring from previous perforations caused by infection, allergies, or trauma.
■ Bulging membranes are indicated by a loss of bony landmarks and a distorted light reflex. Such bulges may be the result of otitis media or malfunctioning auditory tubes.
■ Retracted tympanic membranes are indicated by accentuated bony landmarks and a distorted light reflex. Such retraction is often due to an obstructed auditory tube.

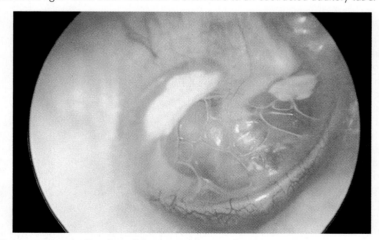

Figure 11–13 ■ Scarring of the tympanic membrane.

Source: Professor Tony Wright, Institute of Laryngology and Otology/SPL/Photo Researchers, Inc.

Palpate the auricles and over each mastoid process. *There should be no pain or swelling on palpation.*

■ Tenderness, swelling, or nodules may indicate inflammation of the external auditory canal or mastoiditis.

Cranial Nerve Assessment

Test CN I (olfactory).
Note client's ability to smell scents (e.g., soap, coffee) with each nostril. This test is usually done only if a problem with the ability to smell is reported. Sense of smell should be equal in both nostrils.

- Anosmia (an inability to smell) may be seen with lesions of the frontal lobe and may also occur with impaired blood flow to the middle cerebral artery.

Assess ability to perceive various sensations.
Touch both sides of various parts of the body (the chest, abdomen, arms, and legs) with one or more of the following:
- Cotton wisp
- Sharp object
- Dull object
- Vibrating tuning fork placed on bony prominences

Client should be able to differentiate between soft and sharp, and feel vibrations appropriately.

- Decreased sensation of pain occurs with injury to the spinothalamic tract.
- Decreased vibratory sensations are seen with injuries to the posterior column tract.
- Transient numbness of face, arm, or hand is seen with TIAs.
- Sensory loss on one side of the body is seen with lesions of higher pathways to the spinal cord.
- Bilateral sensory loss is seen in polyneuropathy (a disease in which multiple peripheral nerves are affected, such as Guillain-Barré syndrome or diabetes mellitus). Sensations are impaired with strokes, brain tumors, and spinal cord trauma or compression.

Assess sense of position (kinesthesia).
Move the client's finger or big toe up or down. Ask the client to describe the movement. Client should be able to accurately describe position of finger or toe when moved up or down.

- Lesions of the posterior column of the spinal cord may affect sense of position.

Assess ability to discriminate fine touch.
Ask the client to identify the following:
1. Object in hand, such as a coin or key (tests stereognosis)
2. Number written on hand (tests graphesthesia)
3. Two points of simultaneous pinpricks on the hand (tests two-point discrimination)
4. Where he or she is being touched (tests localization)
5. How many sensations are felt when touched simultaneously on both sides of the body (tests extinction).

Client should be able to identify and discriminate fine touch.

- Inability to discriminate fine touch (stereognosis, graphesthesia, two points, point localization, and extinction) may occur with injury to the posterior columns or sensory cortex.

Taste and Smell Assessment

One reason decreased sense of smell fails to be detected is that it is not adequately tested. Most physical examination records state "cranial nerves II–XII intact," completely omitting cranial nerve I. The nurse can examine the mucous membranes of the nares using a penlight or an otoscope and speculum, taking care not to touch the septum. The mucous membranes of the nares should be free from polyps, slightly red in color, and without ulceration or copious exudates. The nurse can then ask the patient to occlude one side of the nose, close the eyes, and identify a familiar smell such as vanilla, coffee, or an alcohol swab. This maneuver is repeated on the opposite side using a different odor. Using familiar odors enhances the validity of the test. Commercially prepared scratch-and-sniff tests are available in some smell assessment clinics. These tests contain over 40 odorants and provide more complete information regarding deficits in smell. Patients with obvious deficits in smell should be referred to their primary care provider, an otolaryngologist, and a neurologist.

DEVELOPMENTAL CONSIDERATIONS   Children

INFANT SENSORY FUNCTION

An infant's sensory function is not routinely assessed. Withdrawal responses to painful stimuli indicate normal sensory function.

SUPERFICIAL TACTILE SENSATION

Stroke the skin on the lower leg or arm with a cotton ball or a finger while the child's eyes are closed. Cooperative children over 2 years of age can normally point to the location touched.

SUPERFICIAL PAIN SENSATION

Break a tongue blade to get a sharp point. After asking the child to close the eyes, touch the child in various places on each arm and leg, alternating the sharp and dull ends of the tongue blade. A paper clip may also be used. Children over 4 years of age can normally distinguish between a sharp and dull sensation each time. To improve the child's accuracy with the test, let the child practice telling you the difference between the sharp and dull stimulation.

An inability to identify superficial touch and pain sensation may indicate sensory loss. Identify the extent of sensory loss, such as all areas below the knee. Other sensory function tests (temperature, vibratory, deep pressure pain, and position sense) are performed when sensory loss is found.

DIAGNOSTIC TESTS

Diagnostic tests of the structure and functions of the eyes are used to diagnose a specific injury, disease, or vision problem; to provide information to identify or modify the appropriate medications or assistive devices used to treat the disease or problem; and to help nurses monitor the client's responses to treatment and nursing care interventions. Diagnostic tests of the eye, especially for vision testing, are most often conducted in a health care provider's office. Diagnostic tests to assess the structure and functions of the eyes are described in the Diagnostic Tests table below and summarized in the following bulleted list.

- Refractive errors (with prescription for corrective lenses) are evaluated by retinoscopy and/or refractometry. Pupils must be dilated for accurate diagnosis.
- Tonometry is used to identify and evaluate increased intraocular pressure, characteristic of glaucoma.
- A CT scan may be used to identify foreign objects or tumors of the eye.
- Scratches or injuries from foreign matter may be assessed by staining the sclera and examining the eye with an ultraviolet light.

Hearing evaluation includes gross tests of hearing (such as the whisper test), the Rinne and Weber tests, and audiometry. Diagnostic tests of the structure and functions of the ears are used to diagnose a specific injury, disease, or hearing problem; to provide information to identify or modify the appropriate medications or assistive devices used to treat the disease or problem; and to help nurses monitor the client's responses to treatment and nursing care interventions. Diagnostic tests of the ear, especially for hearing, are most often conducted in a health care provider's office. Sometimes, however, a speech therapist or audiologist may perform diagnostic tests of the ear in a school or educational setting. Diagnostic tests to assess the structure and functions of the ears are described in the Diagnostic Tests table below and summarized in the following bulleted list.

- Rinne and Weber tests compare air and bone sound conduction. When bone conduction of sound is better than air conduction, the hearing deficit is a conductive loss. The Rinne test can identify even mild conductive hearing losses. If both air and bone conduction are impaired, a sensorineural loss is indicated.
- Audiometry identifies the type and pattern of hearing loss. Specific sound frequencies are presented to each ear by either air or bone conduction.
- Speech audiometry identifies the intensity at which speech can be recognized and interpreted. Speech discrimination evaluates the ability to discriminate among various speech sounds.
- Tympanometry is an indirect measurement of the compliance and impedance of the middle ear to sound transmission. The external auditory meatus is subjected to neutral, positive, and negative air pressure while the resultant sound energy flow is monitored.
- Acoustic reflex testing uses a tone presented at various intensities to evaluate movement of the structures of the middle ear.

Regardless of the type of diagnostic test, the nurse is responsible for explaining the procedure and any special preparation needed, for assessing for any medication use that might affect the outcome of the tests, for supporting the client during the examination as necessary, for documenting the procedures as appropriate, and for monitoring the results of the tests.

THERAPEUTIC MANAGEMENT INTERVENTIONS FOR ALTERED SENSORY PERCEPTION

Medical management of altered sensory perception is based on the cause and severity of the problem. The physician will prescribe medications or assistive devices such as eyeglasses and hearing aids. The nurse will teach the client appropriate use of any medication prescribed, and ensure that the client understands the importance of regular use of both medications and

DIAGNOSTIC TESTS   Ear Disorders

NAME OF TEST   Audiometry

PURPOSE AND DESCRIPTION   Used to evaluate and diagnose conductive and sensorineural hearing loss. Client sits in soundproof room and responds by raising a hand when sounds are heard.

RELATED NURSING CARE   No special preparation is needed.

NAME OF TEST   Auditory evoked potential (AEP)

PURPOSE AND DESCRIPTION   Used to identify electrical activity of the auditory nerve. Electrodes are placed on various areas of the ear and on the forehead and a graphic recording is made.

RELATED NURSING CARE   No special preparation is needed.

NAME OF TEST   Auditory brainstem response (ABR)

PURPOSE AND DESCRIPTION   Measures electrical activity of the auditory pathway from inner ear to brain to diagnose brainstem pathology, stroke, and acoustic neuroma.

RELATED NURSING CARE   No special preparation is needed.

NAME OF TEST   Caloric test

PURPOSE AND DESCRIPTION   Used to assess vestibular system function. Cold or warm water is used to irrigate the ear canals one at a time and the client is observed for nystagmus (repeated abnormal movements of the eyes). Normally, the nystagmus occurs opposite to the ear being irrigated. If no nystagmus occurs, the client needs further testing for brain lesions.

RELATED NURSING CARE   Assess client for use of alcohol, central nervous system depressants, and barbiturates. These chemicals may alter the test results.

---

assistive devices. The nurse will employ caring interventions to assist the patient in meeting outcomes as defined in the client's care plan.

Caring Interventions

Common outcomes for clients with sensory-perception alterations include the following:
- Preventing injury
- Maintaining the function of existing senses
- Developing an effective method of communication
- Preventing sensory overload or deprivation
- Reducing social isolation
- Performing activities of daily living independently and safely.

Nurses can assist clients with sensory alterations by promoting healthy sensory function, adjusting environmental stimuli, and helping clients to manage acute sensory deficits. This includes helping clients access the resources necessary to obtain any assistive communication devices. Nurses also teach clients and families how to find freedom within the limitations imposed by the client's sensory loss. Clients with visual impairments, for example, may find comfort and joy in attending live music performances and in downloading reading material that has been converted into spoken word via the internet. Clients with hearing impairments may experience frustration when talking on the phone, even if they have a hearing aid that works well. These clients may increase use of

DIAGNOSTIC TESTS   Eye Disorders

NAME OF TEST   Refraction, Retinoscopy, Refractometry

PURPOSE AND DESCRIPTION   Used to measure refractive error. Either a handheld retinoscope or an instrument with multiple lenses is used; with latter method, client chooses lenses that provide best vision.

RELATED NURSING CARE   No special preparation is needed; tell client that pupils will be dilated with medication and may be enlarged for several hours.

NAME OF TEST   Tonometry

PURPOSE AND DESCRIPTION   Used to diagnose increased intraocular pressure in glaucoma. A variety of methods are used, ranging from a handheld instrument (tonometer) to a computerized component of the device used to evaluate refraction. The cornea is anesthetized prior to being touched with the device. **Normal value:** 10–22 mmHg

RELATED NURSING CARE   No special preparation is needed.

NAME OF TEST   Computed tomography (CT) scan of the eye

PURPOSE AND DESCRIPTION   Radiologic examination used to identify foreign objects or tumors within the eyeball or orbit.

RELATED NURSING CARE   No special preparation is needed.

communication via e-mail and text messages in order to minimize frustration with audio communications.

PROMOTING HEALTHY SENSORY FUNCTION   Children with chronic ear infections and people who live or work in an environment where the noise level is high should receive routine auditory testing. Women who are considering pregnancy should be advised of the importance of testing for syphilis and rubella, both of which can cause hearing impairments in newborns. Periodic vision screening of all newborns and children is recommended to detect congenital blindness, strabismus, and refractive errors (Ball & Bindler, 2006, p. 251).

Healthy sensory function can be promoted with environmental stimuli that provide appropriate sensory input. This input should vary and be neither excessive nor too limited. As many senses as possible should be stimulated. Various colors, sounds, textures, smells, and body positions can provide various sensations. Nurses can teach parents to stimulate infants and children, and teach family members to stimulate an elderly person and others in the home with sensory deficits. Nurses should explain that initially there may be some trial and error as parents and caregivers learn what materials and activities stimulate the family member as well as what the family member enjoys. Exercise and social activities often help stimulate the mind and the senses.

Nurses should also teach clients at risk of sensory loss how to prevent or reduce the loss. They should teach clients general health measures, such as getting regular eye examinations and controlling chronic diseases such as diabetes. Avoidance of risk factors, such as hot temperatures for the touch-impaired individual, is also critical.

ADJUSTING ENVIRONMENTAL STIMULI   The client functions best when the environment is somewhat similar to that of the individual's ordinary daily life. Sometimes nurses need to take steps to adjust the client's environment to prevent either sensory overload or sensory deprivation.

PREVENTING SENSORY OVERLOAD   For clients who are at risk of overstimulation, nurses should assist with reducing the number and type of environmental stimuli. The nurse can counteract sensory overload by blocking stimuli and by helping the client organize the stimuli and alter responses to the stimuli.

Dark glasses with ultraviolet (UV) light protection can partially block light rays, and a window shade or drape can reduce visual stimulation. Earplugs reduce auditory stimuli, as do soft background music and earphones. The odor from a draining wound can be minimized by keeping the dressing dry and clean and applying a liquid deodorant with gauze near the wound.

Another method of blocking stimuli is to reduce novelty and surprise and provide rest intervals free of interruptions. Sometimes the number of visitors and the length of visits must be restricted. Also, if the nurse carries out several nursing measures together, the client may need to have a scheduled quiet period before the next activity.

By explaining sounds in the environment, the nurse can help the client organize them mentally: A bell signals a change of shift; a beep, an IV alarm. When clients understand the meaning of environmental sounds, these stimuli become less confusing and more easily ignored. People can also learn through practice and feedback to alter their responses to the stimuli. Clients can employ relaxation techniques to reduce anxiety and stress despite continual sensory stimulation.

PREVENTING SENSORY DEPRIVATION   For clients who are at risk for sensory deprivation, nurses can increase environmental stimuli in a number of ways. For example, newspapers, books, music, and television can stimulate the visual and auditory senses. Providing objects that are pleasant to touch, such as a pet to stroke, can provide tactile and interactive stimulation. Clocks that differentiate night from day by color can help orient a client to time. The olfactory sense can be stimulated by the presence of fresh flowers or plants.

Arrangements should also be made for people to visit and talk with the client regularly. Many church and community groups provide visitors to "shut-ins," that is, people who are confined to their homes or who reside in nursing homes.

MANAGING ACUTE SENSORY DEFICITS   When assisting clients who have a sensory deficit, the nurse needs to (a) encourage the use of sensory aids to support residual sensory function, (b) promote the use of other senses, (c) communicate effectively, and (d) ensure client safety.

SENSORY AIDS   Many sensory aids are available for clients who have visual and hearing deficits. Examples are listed in Box 11–1. A popular, but expensive example, are service dogs. Service dogs both protect sensory impaired individuals from risk as well as assisting them with activities of daily living, such as opening doors and fetching object. Raising and training service dogs can cause upwards of $40,000 before the dog is ready to go into active service. The cost along with the shortage of trainers sometimes results in long waiting lists for service dogs. Some training programs provide dogs to sensory-impaired individuals free of charge, but some do charge fees.

Sensory aids can be used in the health care setting as well as in the home. In all situations, the assistance of support people needs to be enlisted whenever possible to help the client deal with the deficit.

PROMOTING THE USE OF OTHER SENSES   When one sense is lost, the nurse can teach the client to use other senses to supplement the loss. This stimulation is similar to that provided to prevent sensory deprivation, discussed earlier. However, the type of stimulation needs to be adapted in accordance with the client's specific deficit. For example, for the visually impaired client, stimulation of hearing, taste, smell, and touch can be encouraged. A radio, audiotapes of music or books, clocks that chime, music boxes, and wind chimes can be used for auditory stimulation. Diets that include a variety of flavors, temperatures, and textures can be planned to stimulate the taste buds. Taking sips of water between foods and eating foods separately can enhance the taste sensation. Fresh flowers, scented candles (safely used), room fragrances, brewing coffee, and baking can

Box 11–1 Sensory Aids for Visual and Hearing Deficits

Visual

- Eyeglasses of the correct prescription, clean and in good repair
- Adequate room lighting, including night-lights
- Sunglasses or shades on windows to reduce glare
- Bright contrasting colors in the environment
- Magnifying glass
- Phone dialer with large numbers
- Clock and wristwatch with large numbers
- Color code or texture code on stoves, washer, medicine containers, and so on
- Colored or raised rims on dishes
- Reading material with large print
- Braille or recorded books
- Seeing-eye dog

Hearing

- Hearing aid in good order
- Lip reading
- Sign language
- Amplified telephones
- Telecommunication device for the deaf (TDD)
- Amplified telephone ringers and doorbells
- Flashing alarm clocks
- Flashing smoke detectors

stimulate the sense of smell. Clients can also be encouraged to remember pleasant or familiar odors such as the perfume of sweet peas. Measures such as providing a hug, massage, hair brushing, grooming, different textures in clothing and upholstery fabrics, and pets can be taken to stimulate touch receptors.

COMMUNICATING EFFECTIVELY Communication with clients who have sensory deficits should convey respect, enhance the person's self-esteem, and ensure the exchange of correct information. A person with a hearing impairment has to concentrate more than other people and therefore tires more readily. Fatigue compounded by an illness can further reduce the person's ability to hear. A person with impaired vision is unable to observe most nonverbal cues during communication and relies largely on the spoken word and tone of voice. Guidelines for communicating with people who are visually or hearing impaired are shown in Box 11–2.

SAFETY CONSIDERATIONS Client teaching regarding safety for the sensory impaired client is a critical intervention for the nurse. Safety prevention techniques and devices vary depending on the nature of the impairment.

Impaired Vision For clients with visual impairments, nurses should provide (in a health care setting) and teach clients and families the importance of (for use at home) the following:

- An uncluttered environment with plenty of lighting
- Clear pathways (chairs pushed under tables, things put away); furniture should not be arranged without orienting the client
- Organizing self-care articles within the client's reach
- Orienting the client to a new location when traveling or running errands
- Keeping call lights and assistive devices within easy reach
- Assisting with ambulation (as necessary) by standing at the client's side, walking about one foot ahead, and allowing the person to grasp your arm. Confirm whether the client prefers grasping your arm with the dominant or nondominant hand.

Box 11–2 Communicating with Clients Who Have a Visual or Hearing Deficit

Visual Deficit

- Always announce your presence when entering the client's room and identify yourself by name.
- Stay in the client's field of vision if the client has a partial vision loss.
- Speak in a warm and pleasant tone of voice. Some people tend to speak louder than necessary when talking to a blind person.
- Always explain what you are about to do before touching the person.
- Explain the sounds in the environment.
- Indicate when the conversation has ended and when you are leaving the room.

Hearing Deficit

- Before initiating conversation, convey your presence by moving to a position where you can be seen or by gently touching the person.
- Decrease background noises (e.g., television) before speaking.
- Talk at a moderate rate and in a normal tone of voice. Shouting does not make your voice more distinct and in some instances makes understanding more difficult.
- Address the person directly. Do not turn away in the middle of a remark or story. Make sure the person can see your face easily and that it is well lighted.

- Avoid talking when you have something in your mouth, such as chewing gum. Avoid covering your mouth with your hand.
- Keep your voice at about the same volume throughout each sentence without dropping the voice at the end of each sentence.
- Always speak as clearly and accurately as possible. Articulate consonants with particular care.
- Do not "overarticulate"; mouthing or overdoing articulation is just as troublesome as mumbling. Pantomime or write ideas, or use sign language or finger spelling as appropriate.
- Use longer phrases, which tend to be easier to understand than short ones. For example, "Would you like a drink of water?" presents much less difficulty than "Would you like a drink?" Word choice is important: "Fifteen cents" and "fifty cents" may be confused, but "half a dollar" is clear.
- Pronounce every name with care. Make a reference to the name for easier understanding, for example, "Joan, the girl from the office" or "Sears, the big downtown store."
- Change to a new subject at a slower rate, making sure that the person follows the change to the new subject. A key word or two at the beginning of a new topic is a good indicator.

Vision Impairment and Older Adults

The most common vision diseases affecting older adults are macular degeneration, glaucoma, cataract, and diabetic retinopathy.

- Age-related macular degeneration (ARMD) is the most common cause of new cases of vision impairment in people older than 65. It is the leading cause of vision impairment in adults 75 and older. The prevalence of ARMD is the same for African Americans and Caucasians up to age 75, with rates higher for Caucasians after 75.
- African Americans are three to four times more likely to have open-angle glaucoma.

- People of Asian descent and Eskimos are more likely to have closed-angle glaucoma.
- Diabetic retinopathy is more prevalent among African Americans, Hispanics, and Native Americans than Caucasians.

Source: From "The prevalence and consequences of vision impairment in later life," by A. Horowitz, 2004, *Topics in Geriatric Rehabilitation, 20*(3), pp. 185–195. Reprinted with permission.

Research has established an association between vision impairment and greater disability in activities of daily living (e.g., bathing, dressing, eating) and instrumental tasks (e.g., shopping, housekeeping) (Horowitz, 2004). Studies have also shown that visual impairment increases the risk of depression among older adults living in the community (Horowitz, 2003, 2004). Explanations for this relationship vary. One explanation is that vision loss leads to increased disability, which leads to depression. Another explanation is that loss of vision causes fear—a fear of losing one's autonomy and becoming dependent on another or others. Visual loss also affects how a person obtains information (e.g., reading the newspaper). In addition, reading is often a leisure activity and its loss can affect a person's quality of life. It is important for the nurse to be aware of and assess for signs of depression and intervene as appropriate if an older adult is experiencing depression as a result of a visual impairment.

Impaired Hearing Clients with hearing impairments who are unable to hear the alarms of IV pumps and cardiac monitors need to be assessed frequently. They can be taught to use their visual sense to identify kinks in the IV tubing or a loose electrocardiogram (ECG) lead, and so on. For home safety, clients with impaired hearing need to obtain devices that either amplify sounds or respond with flashing lights to sounds such as a doorbell or smoke detector, a baby crying, or a burglar alarm. The sounds of doorbells and alarm clocks may be amplified or changed to a lower frequency or buzzerlike sound. These devices can be obtained from hearing aid dealers, telephone companies, and appliance stores.

Impaired Olfactory Sense Clients with an impaired sense of smell should be taught about the dangers of cleaning with chemicals such as ammonia. Because a gas leak can go undetected, clients should keep gas stoves and heaters in good working order. Strong chemicals such as ammonia used in confined spaces such as a bathroom may affect the client before they are smelled. Food poisoning is a concern with clients who have difficulty detecting spoiled meat or dairy products. Clients need to carefully inspect food for freshness (check its color and texture) and check expiration dates on food packages.

Impaired Tactile Sense Clients with an impaired sense of touch may not be aware of hot temperatures, which can cause burns, or pressure on bony prominences, which can produce pressure ulcers. Clients with decreased sensation to temperature should have the temperature adjusted on their hot water heater and test water temperature with a thermometer before bathing. Clients with decreased sensation to pressure must change their position frequently.

PHARMACOLOGIC THERAPIES

The eye is vulnerable to a variety of conditions, many of which can be prevented, controlled, or reversed with proper treatment. A simple scratch can cause the client almost unbearable discomfort as well as concern about the effect the damage may have on vision. Other eye disorders may be more bearable, but extremely dangerous—including glaucoma, one of the leading causes of preventable blindness in the world. Although medications cannot cure glaucoma, many clients with open-angle glaucoma can control intraocular pressure and preserve vision indefinitely with medications. Medications are used alone or in combination with the timing and dosage individually determined by pressure measurements. The primary pharmacologic agents used to treat glaucoma are topical beta-adrenergic blocking agents, adrenergics (mydriatics), prostaglandin analogs, or carbonic anhydrase inhibitors. An oral carbonic anhydrase inhibitor also may be used.

Clients suffering from macular degeneration may benefit from medications that slow the formation of new blood vessels. Photodynamic therapy, in which a light-activated drug is injected in the body, may be used. When macular degeneration does not improve with medications, laser surgery to destroy affected blood vessels may be indicated.

Treatment of olfactory impairment generally may be resolved by treating the underlying cause of the impairment. However, olfactory impairment sometimes presents with the onset of serious illnesses, such as diabetes, hypertension, and Parkinson's disease. Treatment of the underlying disease does not always restore olfactory function.

MEDICATIONS

Drug Classifications	Mechanism of Action	Commonly Prescribed Drugs	Nursing Considerations
Antiglaucoma Drugs			
■ Prostaglandins	Drugs for glaucoma work by one of two mechanisms: increasing the outflow of aqueous humor at the canal of Schlemm or decreasing the formation of aqueous humor at the ciliary body. Many agents for glaucoma act by affecting the autonomic nervous system	■ bimatoprost (Lumigan) ■ latanoprost (Xalatan) ■ travoprost (Travatan) ■ unoprostone isopropyl (Rescula)	■ Assess and note eye color, presence of inflammation, exudates, or pain. ■ Note vital signs and most recent liver function test results because these may be altered by the drug.
■ Beta-adrenergic blockers		■ betaxolol (Betoptic) ■ carteolol (Ocupress) ■ levobunolol (Betagan) ■ metipranolol (OptiPranolol) ■ timolol (Betimol, Timoptic, and others)	■ Assess the client for allergies or contraindications to beta-blocker therapy, including asthma, chronic obstructive pulmonary disease (COPD), heart block, and heart failure. ■ Maintain pressure over the lacrimal sac after administration to prevent systemic absorption. ■ Assess for side effects such as bradycardia, hypotension, and depression. ■ Teach about the drug, its dose, administration, and desired and side effects.
■ Alpha$_2$-adrenergic agonists		■ apraclonidine (Iopidine) ■ brimonidine tartrate (Alphagan)	■ Assess the client for contraindications and adverse reactions to adrenergic agonists, including acute angle-closure glaucoma, hypertension, cardiac dysrhythmias, and coronary heart disease. ■ Assess for central nervous system side effects of anxiety, nervousness, and muscle tremors. If these side effects are severe, notify the physician. ■ Assess for a hypersensitivity reaction, including itching, lid edema, and discharge from the eyes. Notify the physician if you notice these signs.
■ Carbonic anhydrase inhibitors		■ acetazolamide (Diamox) ■ brinzolamide (Azopt) ■ methazolamide (Neptazane)	■ Assess for allergies or other contraindications to the use of carbonic anhydrase inhibitors, including known allergy to sulfa, or severe renal or hepatic disease. ■ Monitor for increased drug interactions of amphetamines, procainamide, quinidine, tricyclic antidepressants, and ephedrine and pseudoephedrine. ■ Assess daily weight, intake and output, serum electrolytes, and vital signs in clients taking oral or parenteral carbonic anhydrase inhibitors. ■ Administer PO in the morning to prevent sleep disruption because of the diuretic effect. ■ If used with another topical ophthalmic, administer 10 minutes apart. ■ Teach the client about the drug, its dose, administration, and desired and side effects.

11.1 HEARING IMPAIRMENT

BASIS FOR SELECTION OF EXEMPLAR
Healthy People 2010

LEARNING OUTCOMES

After learning about this exemplar, you will be able to do the following:

1. Describe the pathophysiology, etiology, and clinical manifestations of hearing impairment.

2. Identify risk factors associated with hearing impairment.

3. Illustrate the nursing process in providing culturally competent care across the life span for individuals with hearing impairment.

4. Formulate priority nursing diagnoses appropriate for an individual with hearing impairment.

5. Create a plan of care for an individual with hearing impairment that includes family members and caregivers.

6. Employ evidence-based caring interventions (or prevention) for an individual with hearing impairment.

7. Assess expected outcomes for an individual with hearing impairment.

8. Discuss therapies used in the collaborative care of an individual with hearing impairment.

OVERVIEW

Approximately one million children in the United States have some form of hearing impairment. Hearing loss is present in 2 out of every 1,000 births (Moore, 2006; Yaeger et al., 2006). These hearing impairments are expressed in terms of **decibels** (dB), which are units of loudness, and rated according to severity (Table 11–4). Children who have only a mild hearing loss (35–40 dB) may miss as much as 50% of everyday conversation and are considered at high risk for difficulty in school. Anyone with a hearing loss of more than 90 dB is considered legally deaf.

Hearing loss is a significant problem for adults as well, affecting an estimated 10% of adults in the United States (Kasper et al., 2005). The problem of hearing loss is particularly significant in older adults, affecting about 30–35% of people between the ages of 65 and 74, and more than 40% of those over age 75 (National Institute on Deafness and Other Communication Disorders, 2005d). As many as 70% of nursing home residents have impaired hearing.

Hearing loss impairs the ability to communicate in a world filled with sound and hearing individuals. A hearing deficit can be partial or total, congenital or acquired. It may affect one or both ears. In some types of hearing loss, the ability to perceive sound at specific frequencies is lost. In others, hearing is diminished across all frequencies.

PATHOPHYSIOLOGY AND ETIOLOGY

Lesions in the outer ear, middle ear, inner ear, or central auditory pathways can result in hearing loss. The process of aging also can affect the structures of the ear and hearing. Hearing loss is classified as conductive, sensorineural, or mixed, depending on what portion of the auditory system is affected. Profound deafness is often a congenital condition.

Conductive Hearing Loss

Anything that disrupts the transmission of sound from the external auditory meatus to the inner ear results in a conductive hearing loss. The most common cause of conductive hearing loss is obstruction of the external ear canal. Impacted cerumen, edema of the canal lining, stenosis, and neoplasms all may lead to canal obstruction. Other causes of conductive loss include a perforated tympanic membrane, disruption or fixation of the ossicles of the middle ear, fluid, scarring, and tumors of the middle ear. Conductive loss also occurs if the tympanic membrane does not fully vibrate, as in otitis media. In these cases, loss may be restored after the infection clears. Chronic and untreated ear infections may lead to ear structural changes and permanent hearing impairment. The loss of acuity may be gradual or rapid and results in diminished hearing in all ranges.

TABLE 11–4 Severity of Hearing Loss

TYPE OF LOSS	DECIBEL LEVEL (DB)	HEARING ABILITY
Slight/mild	26–40	Some speech sounds are difficult to perceive, particularly unvoiced consonant sounds
Moderate	41–60	Most normal conversational speech sounds are missed
Severe	61–80	Speech sounds cannot be heard at a normal conversational level
Profound	81–90	No speech sounds can be heard
Deaf	> 90	No sound at all can be heard

Sensorineural Hearing Loss

Disorders that affect the inner ear, the auditory nerve, or the auditory pathways of the brain may lead to a sensorineural hearing loss. In this type of hearing loss, sound waves are effectively transmitted to the inner ear. In the inner ear, however, lost or damaged receptor cells, changes in the cochlear apparatus, or auditory nerve abnormalities decrease or distort the ability to receive and interpret stimuli. Conditions leading to sensorineural hearing loss may be congenital, genetic, or acquired. In sensorineural hearing loss, high-frequency sounds are most affected.

A significant cause of sensorineural hearing deficit is damage to the hair cells of the organ of Corti. In the United States, noise exposure is the major cause. Damage may result from either loud impulse noise (e.g., an explosion) or loud continuous noise (e.g., machinery). Exposure to a high level of noise (e.g., standing close to the stage or speakers at a rock concert) on an intermittent or continuing basis damages the hair and supporting cells of the organ of Corti. Ototoxic drugs also damage the hair cells; when combined with high noise levels, the damage is greater and resultant hearing loss more profound.

PRACTICE ALERT
Ototoxic drugs include aspirin, furosemide (Lasix), aminoglycosides, streptomycin, vancomycin (Vancocin), antimalarial drugs, and chemotherapy such as cisplatin (Platinol). Other potential causes of sensory hearing loss include prenatal exposure to rubella, viral infections, meningitis, trauma, Ménière's disease, and aging.

Tumors such as acoustic neuromas, vascular disorders, demyelinating or degenerative diseases, infections (bacterial meningitis in particular), or trauma may affect the central auditory pathways and produce a neural hearing loss.

Presbycusis

With aging, the hair cells of the cochlea degenerate, producing a progressive sensorineural hearing loss. In presbycusis, hearing acuity begins to decrease in early adulthood and progresses as long as the individual lives. Higher-pitched tones and conversational speech are lost initially.

RISK FACTORS

About 50% of hearing loss in children is genetically caused, usually with a recessive inheritance pattern with GJB2 gene abnormalities (Yaeger et al., 2006). Another 25% is due to environmental causes around the time of birth; the remainder is due to unknown causes. Although many infants with hearing loss have no known risk factors, identified risks include the following:

- Family history of congenital hearing loss*
- Positive titer for TORCH infections (toxoplasmosis, rubella, cytomegalovirus, syphilis, herpes)
- Craniofacial abnormalities
- Very low birth weight (<1500 g)*
- Bilirubin greater than 16 mg/dL
- Aminoglycoside medication administration for more than 5 days
- Low Apgar score at 1 or 5 min*

- Bacterial meningitis
- Mechanical ventilation for over 5 days
- Presence of syndromes associated with hearing loss (Down syndrome, Pierre Robin syndrome, Arnold-Chiari malformation)*

*Primary risk factors (Chu et al., 2003).

CLINICAL MANIFESTATIONS AND THERAPIES

Conductive hearing loss involves an equal loss of hearing at all sound frequencies. If the level of sound is greater than the threshold for hearing, speech discrimination is good. Because of this, the client with a conductive hearing loss benefits from amplification by a hearing aid.

Sensorineural hearing losses typically affect the ability to hear high-frequency tones more than low-frequency tones. This loss makes speech discrimination difficult, especially in a noisy environment. Hearing aids are often not useful, because they amplify both speech and background noise. The increased sound intensity may actually cause discomfort for the client.

Because the hearing loss of presbycusis is gradual, the client and family may not realize the extent of the deficit. The individual with a hearing impairment may be described as unsociable or paranoid. The family may worry that the person is becoming increasingly forgetful, absentminded, or perhaps "senile." Depression, confusion, inattentiveness, tension, and negativism have been noted in older adults with hearing impairments. Functional problems such as poor general health, reduced mobility, and impaired interpersonal communication are also associated with hearing loss. Caregivers need to be alert for signs of impaired hearing such as cupping an ear, difficulty understanding verbal communication when the person cannot see the speaker's face, difficulty following conversation in a large group, and withdrawal from social activities. Hearing aids and other amplification devices are useful for most clients with presbycusis.

Tinnitus

Tinnitus is the perception of sound or noise in the ears without stimulus from the environment. The sound may be steady, intermittent, or pulsatile and is often described as a buzzing, roaring, or ringing.

Tinnitus is usually associated with hearing loss (conductive or sensorineural); however, the mechanism producing the sound is poorly understood. It is often an early symptom of noise-induced hearing damage and drug-related ototoxicity. Tinnitus is especially associated with salicylate, quinine, or quinidine toxicity. Other etiologies include obstruction of the auditory meatus, presbycusis, middle or inner ear inflammations and infections, otosclerosis, and Ménière's disease. Most tinnitus, however, is chronic and has no pathologic importance.

Early identification of hearing loss is a key element in successful treatment. Detection of hearing loss in infants is important to ensure optimal development. Clients need to know the risk for hearing damage and how to prevent it. Awareness of the effects of noise exposure, especially when combined with the ototoxic effects of aspirin or other drugs, is important in preventing sensorineural hearing loss.

CLINICAL MANIFESTATIONS AND THERAPIES

ETIOLOGY	CLINICAL MANIFESTATIONS	CLINICAL THERAPIES
Conductive hearing loss	■ Equal loss of hearing at all sound frequencies	■ Hearing aid ■ Treat underlying condition, such as infection in otitis media ■ Surgery
Sensorineural hearing loss	■ Lesser ability to hear high-frequency tones more than low-frequency tones ■ Difficulty discriminating speech	■ Cochlear implant
Presbycusis	■ Personality manifestations, such as depression, confusion, forgetfulness, not being sociable; poor health, reduced mobility, withdrawal; signs of impaired hearing, such as cupping an ear	■ Hearing aid
Tinnitus Mechanism not fully understood, etiology varies to include noise, ototoxicity; infection or inflammation, underlying conditions such as Ménière's disease	■ Buzzing, roaring, or ringing in the ears	■ Treat underlying cause ■ Tinnitus maskers such as ambient noise

Amplification

A hearing aid or other amplification device can help many clients with hearing deficits. These assistive devices do nothing to prevent, minimize, or treat the hearing loss itself. They amplify the sound presented to the hearing apparatus of the ear, which may bring the level of sound above the hearing threshold, allowing more accurate perception and interpretation of its meaning. When sound perception is distorted, a hearing aid may be less helpful, because it simply amplifies the distorted sound.

Unfortunately, less than one-fifth of older clients with a hearing deficit have or use a hearing aid. Denial of the deficit, other health problems, poor visual acuity, decreased manual dexterity, and cost all contribute to this low usage. Cost is another factor. Typically health insurance and will cover only one pair of hearing aids within a certain time frame, and in most states Medicare does not pay for hearing aids at all. Some clients choose not to pay for hearing aids. Hearing aids must be individually prescribed by an audiologist. Proper design, proper fit, and regular maintenance are necessary for their effectiveness.

All hearing aids include a microphone, amplifier, speaker, earpiece, and volume control. Many include an option to turn off the microphone when using the telephone; others can be adjusted for the client's pattern of hearing loss. Hearing aids are available in a variety of styles, each with advantages and disadvantages:

■ Canal hearing aids (in-the-canal and completely-in-canal) are the least noticeable style, fitting in the ear canal. They are appropriate for mild to moderately severe hearing loss. These small and unobtrusive devices allow use of the telephone and can be worn during exercise. Because of their small size, the client must have good manual dexterity to insert, clean, and change the batteries in canal hearing aids.

For this reason, older clients or clients with impaired dexterity may be unable to use them.

■ The in-ear style of hearing aid fits into the external ear and is used for mild to severe hearing loss (Figure 11–14 ■). Its larger size makes manipulation somewhat easier, although it still may be difficult for less dexterous individuals. A greater degree of amplification is possible with the in-ear aid. Many have a toggle switch for telephone usage.

■ The behind-ear hearing aid allows finer adjustment of the level of amplification and is easier for the client to manipulate (Figure 11–15 ■). The device can be used by clients with mild to profound hearing loss. For the client who wears glasses, this style can be modified, with all components fitting into the temple of the eyeglasses.

■ Clients with profound hearing loss may require a body hearing aid. The microphone and amplifier of this aid are contained in a pocket-sized case that the client clips on to clothing, slips into a pocket, or carries in a harness. The receiver is attached by a cord to the case and clips onto the ear mold, which delivers the sound to the ear canal.

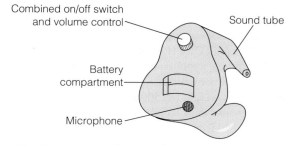

Figure 11–14 ■ An in-ear hearing aid.

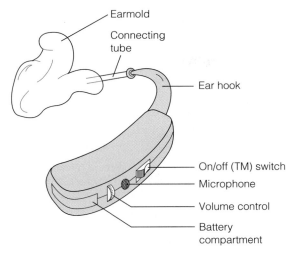

Figure 11–15 ■ A behind-ear hearing aid.

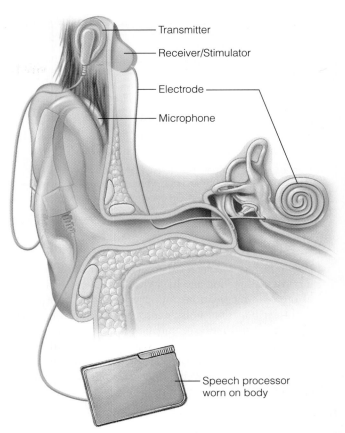

Figure 11–16 ■ A cochlear implant for sensorineural hearing loss.

With both the in-canal and in-ear style, cleaning is important. Small portals may become plugged with cerumen, interfering with sound transmission.

For the client who does not have a hearing aid, an *assistive listening device,* or "pocket talker," with a microphone and "Walkman"-type earpieces, is useful. Pocket talkers are available over-the-counter or through an audiologist and are relatively inexpensive. The earpiece requires no special fitting, and the external microphone allows the client to focus on the desired sound rather than simply amplifying all sounds. Assistive listening devices may also be used in conjunction with a hearing aid.

Clients with tinnitus may find a white noise–masking device helpful to promote concentration and rest. These devices conduct a pleasant sound to the affected ear, allowing the client to block out the abnormal sound.

TTD/TTY telephones and phones with amplifiers are available to assist deaf or hearing impaired clients in communicating with the outside world. Accessibility to the Internet can make an extraordinary difference in the quality of life to a hearing impaired individual, who can now make restaurant and airplane reservations by computer, as well as communicate by e-mail.

Surgery

Reconstructive surgeries of the middle ear, such as a stapedectomy or tympanoplasty, may help restore hearing with a conductive hearing loss. Stapedectomy is the removal and replacement of the stapes. This procedure is used to treat hearing loss related to otosclerosis.

In a tympanoplasty, the structures of the middle ear are reconstructed to improve conductive hearing deficits. Chronic otitis media with necrosis and scarring of the middle ear is a common indication for this type of surgery.

For the client with a sensorineural hearing loss, a *cochlear implant* may be the only hope for restoring sound perception. The cochlear implant consists of a microphone, speech processor, transmitter and receiver/stimulator, and electrodes (Figure 11–16 ■). Its function is more similar to the way the

ear normally receives and processes sounds than it is to that of a hearing aid. The microphone picks up sounds, sending them to the speech processor, which selects and processes those that are useful. The transmitter and receiver/stimulator receive signals from the speech processor, convert them to electrical impulses, and send these impulses to the electrodes for transmission to the brain.

Cochlear implants provide sound perception but not normal hearing. The client is able to recognize warning sounds such as automobiles, sirens, telephones, and doors opening or closing. They also receive stimuli to alert them to incoming communication so they can focus on the person speaking. Many clients learn to interpret perceived sounds as words, especially when the hearing loss is acquired as an adult.

For uncorrectable hearing loss, several approaches are used to enhance communication (Table 11–5). Clients with hearing impairment may receive speech therapy and instructions in lipreading, signing, cuing, and finger-spelling.

NURSING PROCESS

In planning and implementing nursing care for the client with a hearing deficit, the type and extent of hearing loss, the client's adaptation to the loss, and the availability of assistive hearing devices are considered, as well as the client's ability and willingness to use assistive devices.

TABLE 11–5 Communication Techniques for Clients Who Are Hearing Impaired

TECHNIQUE	DESCRIPTION
Cued speech	Supplement to lip-reading; eight hand shapes represent groups of consonant sounds and four positions about the face represent groups of vowel sounds; based on the sounds the letters make, not the letters themselves; client can "see-hear" every spoken syllable a hearing person hears.
Oral approach	Uses only spoken language for face-to-face communication; avoids use of formal signs; uses hearing aids and residual hearing.
Total communication	Uses speech and sign, finger-spelling, lip-reading, and residual hearing simultaneously; client selects communication technique depending on the situation.
Sign language	A separate or foreign language that allows the user to communicate quickly and accurately with others who understand signs. The signs or hand movements represent words or concepts. When a sign is not available, the word can be spelled out using signs. American Sign Language (ASL) is most often used; British Sign Language (BSL) is common in Europe.

Source: Ball, J. W., & Bindler, R. C., (2008). *Pediatric nursing: caring for children* (4th ed., p. 661). Upper Saddle River, NJ: Pearson Education.

Assessment

- Health history: Perceived ability to hear; effect of hearing loss on function and lifestyle; risk factors such as use of ototoxic medications; upper respiratory tract or frequent ear infection; noise exposure; presence of vertigo, tinnitus, unsteadiness, or imbalance.
- Physical examination: Apparent perception of normal speech; inspection of external ear, tympanic membrane; whisper, Rinne, and Weber tests; tests of balance and cranial nerve function.

Diagnoses

Possible nursing diagnosis for the client with hearing impairment may include the following:
- Disturbed sensory perception: Auditory
- Impaired verbal communication
- Social isolation.

Planning and Implementation

Disturbed Sensory Perception: Auditory

Whether the client's hearing deficit is partial or total, impaired sound perception is the primary problem. The client needs to understand what causes the deficit and what to expect for the future. Nursing interventions focus on maximizing available hearing and preventing further deterioration to the extent possible.

- Encourage the client to talk about the hearing loss and its effect on activities of daily living. *Hearing loss affects each individual in a different way. The client may be denying the extent of the deficit or grieving the loss. Listening and providing support encourage the client to develop coping strategies.*
- Provide information about the type of hearing loss. Refer to an audiologist for evaluation of the hearing loss and possible exploration of amplification devices. *With improved understanding of the deficit, the client can plan ways to compensate.*
- Replace batteries in hearing aids regularly and as needed. *Hearing aid batteries last approximately 1 week. If a battery is old or has been improperly stored, the life may be reduced further.*
- If the hearing aid has a toggle switch for microphone/telephone, be sure it is in the appropriate position. *This ensures proper amplification with the hearing aid.*

- Talk with the family members about techniques they can use to make communication with the client easier. The same techniques the nurse employs, as listed in Box 11–2, can be used by family members.

> **PRACTICE ALERT**
> Check hearing aids for patency, cleaning out cerumen as necessary.

Impaired Verbal Communication

A hearing deficit impairs the client's ability to receive and interpret verbal communication. A hearing loss affects the client's ability to follow conversations, use the telephone, and enjoy television or other forms of entertainment.

- Use the following techniques to improve communication:
  a. Wave the hand or tap the shoulder before beginning to speak.
  b. If the client wears corrective lenses, ensure that they are clean, and encourage the client to wear them.
  c. When speaking, face your client and keep your hands away from your face.
  d. Keep your face in full light.
  e. Reduce the noise in the environment before speaking.
  f. Use a low voice pitch with normal loudness.
  g. Use short sentences and pause at the end of each sentence.
  h. Speak at a normal rate, and do not overarticulate.
  i. Use facial expressions or gestures.
  j. Provide a magic slate for written communication.

Individuals with hearing impairments often lip-read, making good visibility of the speaker's face necessary. Excessive environmental noise interferes with the ability to perceive the message. Higher tones are typically lost with presbycusis and other types of hearing loss. Using short sentences and pausing give the client time to interpret the message. Overarticulating makes it more difficult to follow the flow and to lip-read. Nonverbal cues and written messages enhance the client's understanding.

- Be sure hearing aid is properly placed, is turned on, and has fresh batteries. *The client may not be aware that the hearing aid is not functioning well.*
- Do not place intravenous catheters in the dominant hand. *The client may need to use that hand to write.*

- Rephrase sentences when the client has difficulty understanding. Hearing losses may affect different sound tones, making some words more difficult to comprehend. Using alternative words and phrases may increase the client's ability to perceive the message.
- Repeat important information. The nurse must make sure that the client understands the information.
- Inform other staff about the client's hearing deficit and effective strategies for communication. Consistent use of effective strategies for communication decreases the client's frustration.

Social Isolation

The client with impaired hearing often becomes socially isolated. This isolation may be self-imposed because of difficulty communicating, especially in a group. Often, however, the isolation comes about gradually and without intention. The client finds social settings such as family dinners or community gatherings increasingly difficult. Friends and family become frustrated trying to communicate with someone who has a hearing impairment, and invitations to participate in social activities dwindle.

- Identify the extent and cause of the social isolation. Help to differentiate the reality of the isolation and its cause from the client's perception of isolation. Clients with impaired hearing may be unaware that they are isolated. Identifying factors that contribute to isolation may provide the needed impetus to remedy the hearing loss. Clients may also experience paranoid thinking as a result of impaired communication and believe that friends and family have purposely begun to avoid interactions.
- Encourage client to interact with friends and family on a one-to-one basis in quiet settings. Clients with impaired hearing are more successful in understanding conversations that take place in small groups and quiet settings.
- Treat client with dignity and remind friends and family that a hearing deficit does not indicate loss of mental faculties. Inappropriate responses due to a hearing deficit can cause others to perceive the client as "stupid" or demented.
- Involve client in activities that do not require acute hearing, such as checkers and chess. *The client has an opportunity to interact socially without the stress of straining to hear.*

- Obtain a pocket talker or encourage the client and family to do so.
- Refer the client to an audiologist for evaluation and possible hearing-aid fitting.
- Refer to resources such as support groups and senior citizen centers. *These groups provide new social outlets.*

Community-Based Care

Teaching for home and community-based care for the client with hearing loss focuses on managing the deficit and developing coping strategies. Referral to an audiologist for evaluation of the deficit and the usefulness of a hearing aid may be appropriate. In addition, discuss the following topics as appropriate for each client:

Evaluation

Expected outcomes of nursing care for a client with hearing impairment include the following:

- The client will demonstrate successful establishment of a communication method.
- The client will manifest growth and developmental milestones to maximum potential.
- The client and family will demonstrate positive methods of coping.

COLLABORATION

If hearing loss in a client is uncorrectable, a multidisciplinary team should be formed to assist the client and family with adaptation to the disability. Team members may include any of the following: physician, nurse, a speech/language, occupational or physical therapist, an audiologist, a teacher, a social worker, and family members and caregivers. The team may provide strategies and accommodations for a client whose loss is correctable until surgery is completed or other treatments take effect. Therapists and social workers can often assist clients in accessing assistive technology devices at relatively low cost, especially if they are not covered by insurance, as well as help the client learn how to use these tools.

REVIEW Hearing Impairment

RELATE: LINK THE CONCEPTS

Kate is deaf and had a cochlear implant at 2 years of age. She is now 5 years of age and she hears sounds, is working to integrate sounds with meaning, and attends speech therapy each week. Kate is fortunate that she has two parents who are able to attend speech therapy with her and reinforce learning at home. They are concerned about finding the best kindergarten for her to attend next year.

Linking the concept of Development with the concept of Sensory Perception:

1. Describe the normal speech patterns of a 5-year-old. How are Kate's patterns likely to differ?
2. Which immunization is especially important for Kate to receive in order to prevent a risk of meningitis with her cochlear implant? How will you counsel parents about this and help them find a resource for immunizations?

3. Provide a list of questions that Kate's parents can ask as they visit and evaluate kindergartens. What characteristics will be especially important for them to consider?

READY: GO TO COMPANION SKILLS MANUAL

1. Assessing the ears and hearing.

REFLECT: CASE STUDY

Mrs. Smith is an 87-year-old woman who recently moved into an assisted living home after hospitalization for uncontrolled diabetes. She enjoyed reading, but for a long time she has not been able to read due to poor vision acuity. During the admission assessment, the nurse also documents a hearing loss.

1. Discuss the importance of a thorough sensory assessment in older adults.
2. Describe the benefits of improving Mrs. Smith's sensory deficits.

REFERENCES

Ball, J. W., & Bindler, R. C. (2006). *Child health nursing*. Upper Saddle River, NJ: Pearson Inc.

Ball, J.W., & Bindler, R.C.(2008). *Pediatric nursing: Caring for children* (4th ed.) Upper Saddle River, NJ: Pearson, Inc.

Behrman, R. E., Kliegman, R. M., & Jenson, H. B. (2004). *Nelson textbook of pediatrics* (17th ed.). Philadelphia: Saunders.

Berman, A., Snyder, S.J., Kozier, B., & Erb, G. (2008). *Kozier & Erb's fundamentals of nursing: Concepts, process, and practice* (8th ed.). Upper Saddle River, NJ: Pearson, Inc.

Bromley, S. (2000). Smell and taste disorders: A primary care approach. *American Family Physician, 61*, 427–436, 438.

Burke, T. (2002). *A grey area: Colour specification in dementia-specific accommodation*. Retrieved December 10, 2002, from www.dementia.com.au/papers/TimBurkeFINALVERSION.htm

Centers for Disease Control and Prevention. (2002). *Trends in vision and hearing among older Americans*. Retrieved March 24, 2003, from www.cdc.gov

Centers for Disease Control and Prevention, Developmental Disabilities. (2004). *Hearing loss: Screening*. Retrieved June 28, 2006, from http://www.cdc.gov/ncbddd/dd/ddhi.htm

Centers for Disease Control and Prevention. (2006). *Frequently Asked Questions (FAQs) on General Information on Hearing Loss*. Retrieved May 7, 2009, from http://www.cdc.gov/ncbddd/ehdi/FAQ/questionsgeneralHL.htm#deaf

Chamley, C. A., Carson, P., Randall, D., & Sandwell, M. (2005). *Developmental anatomy and physiology of children*. St. Louis: Elsevier.

Chu, K., Elimian, A., Barbera, J., Ogburn, P., Spitzer, A., & Quirk, J. G. (2003) Antecedents of newborn hearing loss. *Obstetrics and Gynecology 101*, 584–588.

Committee on Sports Medicine and Fitness. (2004). Protective eyewear for young athletes. *Pediatrics, 113*, 619–622.

Curns, A. T., Holman, R. C., Shay, D. K., Cheek, J. E., Kaufman, S. F., Singleton, R. J., & Anderson, L. J. (2002). Outpatient and hospital visits associated with otitis media among American Indian and Alaska Native children younger than 5 years. *Pediatrics, 109*(3). Retrieved October 2, 2006, from http://www.pediatrics.org/cgi/content/full/109/3/e41

D'Amico, D., & Barbarito, C. (2007). *Health & physical assessment in nursing*. Upper Saddle River, NJ: Pearson, Inc.

Gordon-Salant, S. (2005). Hearing loss and aging: New research findings and clinical implications. *Journal of Rehabilitation Research & Development, 42*(4), 9–24.

Horowitz, A. (2003). Depression and vision and hearing impairment in later life. *Generations, 27*(1), 32–38.

Horowitz, A. (2004). The prevalence and consequences of vision impairment in later life. *Topics in Geriatric Rehabilitation, 20*(3), 185–195.

Joint Committee on Infant Hearing. (2000). Joint Committee on Infant Hearing 2000 position statement: Principles and guidelines for early hearing detection and intervention programs. *Pediatrics, 106*, 798–817.

Kasper, D. L., Braunwald, E., Fauci, A. S., Hauser, S. L., Longo, D. L., & Jameson, J. L. (Eds.). (2005). *Harrison's principles of internal medicine* (16th ed.). New York: McGraw-Hill.

LeMone, P., & Burke, K. (2008). *Medical-surgical nursing: Critical thinking in client care* (4th ed.). Upper Saddle River, NJ: Pearson, Inc.

Moore, J. (2006). Pediatricians need greater awareness of hearing disorders. *Infectious Diseases in Children, 19*(8), 53–54.

National Criminal Justice Reference Service. (2009). *Recognizing When a Child's Injury or Illness is Caused by Abuse: Eye Injuries*. Available from http://www.ncjrs.gov/html/ojjdp/portable_guides/abuse/eye.html

National Eye Institute, National Institutes of Health. (2003a). *Age-related macular degeneration: What you should know* (NIH Publication No. 03-2294). Bethesda, MD: Author.

National Eye Institute, National Institutes of Health. (2003b). *Cataract: What you should know* (NIH Publication No. 03-201). Bethesda, MD: Author.

National Eye Institute, National Institutes of Health. (2003c). *Diabetic retinopathy: What you should know* (NIH Publication No. 03-2171). Bethesda, MD: Author.

National Eye Institute, National Institutes of Health. (2003d). *Glaucoma: What you should know* (NIH Publication No. 03-651). Bethesda, MD: Author.

National Eye Institute, National Institutes of Health. (2004). *Statistics and data*. Retrieved from http://www.nei.nih.gov/evedata/pbd_tables.asp

National Eye Institute, National Institutes of Health. (2005a). *Facts about the cornea and corneal disease*. Retrieved from http://www.nei.nih.gov

National Eye Institute, National Institutes of Health. (2005c). *Retinal detachment*. Retrieved from http://www.nei.nih.gov

National Institute on Deafness and Other Communication Disorders, National Institutes of Health. (2005a). *Cochlear implants*. Retrieved February 23, 2005, from http://www.nidcd.nih.gov/health/hearing/coch.asp

National Institute on Deafness and Other Communication Disorders, National Institutes of Health. (2005b). *Hearing aids*. Retrieved March 1, 2005, from http://www.nidcd.nih.gov/health/hearing/hearingaid.asp

National Institute on Deafness and Other Communication Disorders, National Institutes of Health. (2005c). *Noise-induced hearing loss*. Retrieved May 4, 2005, from http://www.nidcd.nih.gov/health/hearing/noise.asp

National Institute on Deafness and Other Communication Disorders, National Institutes of Health. (2005d). *Presbycusis*. Retrieved February 23, 2005, from http://www.nidcd.nih.gov/health/hearing/presbycusis.asp

National Institute on Deafness and Other Communication Disorders, National Institutes of Health. (2009). *Taste Disorders*. Retrieved May 7, 2009, from http://www.nidcd.nih.gov/health/smelltaste/taste.asp

Nelson, D. (2001). The power of touch in facility care. *Massage & Bodywork, 16*(1), 12–18.

Prevent Blindness America, and National Eye Institute, National Institutes of Health. (2002). *Vision problems in the U.S. Prevalence of adult vision impairment and age-related eye disease in America*. Retrieved from http://www.usvisionproblems.org

Schiffman, S.S. (1997). Taste and smell losses in normal aging and disease. *Journal of the American Medical Association, 278*(16), 1357–1362.

Tierney, L. M., McPhee, S. J., & Papadakis, M. A. (Eds.). (2005). *Current medical diagnosis & treatment* (44th ed.). Stamford, CT: Appleton & Lange.

Wahl, H., Becker, S., Burmedi, D., & Schilling, O. (2004). The role of primary and secondary control in adaptation to age-related vision loss: A study of older adults with macular degeneration. *Psychology and Aging, 19*(1), 235–239.

Wahl, H., & Heyl, V. (2003). Connection between vision, hearing, and cognitive function. *Generations, 27*(1), 39–47.

Way, L. W., & Doherty, G. M. (2003). *Current surgical diagnosis & treatment* (11th ed.). New York: McGraw-Hill.

Yaeger, D., McCallum, J., Lewis, K., Soslow, L., Shah, U., Potsic, W., Stolle, C., & Krantz, I. D. (2006). Outcomes of clinical examination and genetic testing of 500 individuals with hearing loss evaluated through a genetics of hearing loss clinic. *American Journal of Medical Genetics, 140*, 827–836.

Skin and Tissue Integrity

Concept at-a-Glance

Concept Learning Outcomes

After reading about this concept, you will be able to do the following:

1. Describe the structure and physiologic processes of maintaining skin and tissue integrity.

2. Identify factors affecting skin and tissue integrity.

3. Identify commonly occurring alterations in skin and tissue integrity and their related treatments.

4. Describe common physical assessment procedures used to assess skin and tissue integrity across the life span.

5. Identify diagnostic and laboratory tests to determine the individual's skin and tissue integrity.

6. Discuss expected diagnostic test findings for alterations in skin and tissue integrity.

7. Explain management of skin and tissue integrity.

8. Apply nursing processes in providing culturally competent care across the life span for individuals with common alterations in skin and tissue integrity.

9. Identify pharmacologic interventions in caring for the individual with alterations in skin and tissue integrity.

Concept Key Terms

Alopecia, *353*

Dermis, *345*

Ecchymosis, *352*

Edema, *350*

Epidermis, *344*

Erythema, *346*

Hirsutism, *353*

Hypodermis, *345*

Integumentary system, *343*

Keratin, *344*

Lesion, *346*

Lichenification, *346*

Melanin, *344*

Pruritus, *346*

Senile purpura, *345*

Subcutaneous, *345*

Urticaria, *352*

Vitiligo, *352*

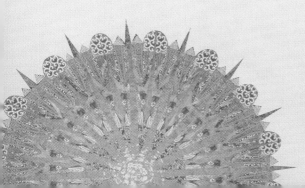

About Skin and Tissue Integrity

The largest organ in the body, the skin serves a variety of important functions in maintaining health and protecting the individual from injury. The skin is part of the body's **integumentary system**, which includes the skin, hair, and nails and the sebaceous, sweat, and mammary glands. Important nursing functions are maintaining skin integrity and promoting wound healing. Impaired skin integrity, that is, alterations to the dermis and epidermis, is not a serious problem for most healthy people but is a threat to older adults; to clients with restricted mobility, chronic illnesses, or trauma; and to those undergoing invasive health care procedures. To protect the skin and manage wounds effectively, the nurse must understand the factors that affect skin integrity, the physiology of wound healing, and specific measures that promote optimal conditions for the skin.

Tissue integrity includes integumentary, mucous membrane, corneal, or subcutaneous tissues uninterrupted by wounds. Tissue integrity is influenced by internal factors such as genetics, age, and the underlying health of the individual, as well as by external factors such as activity and injury. ●

NORMAL PRESENTATION OF THE SKIN

The skin performs several essential functions. It protects underlying tissues from invasion by microorganisms and from trauma. The nerves in the skin enable the perception of touch, pain, pressure, heat, and cold. The skin also assists the body in regulating its temperature. Dilation of blood vessels and the secretion of sweat by the eccrine sweat glands, functioning under the control of the central nervous system, enable the body to release excess heat. The sweat glands, secreting a solution of water, electrolytes, and urea, also help rid the body of toxins. The skin supplements the body's intake of vitamin D by synthesizing this vitamin from ultraviolet light.

The skin has three distinct layers: the epidermis, the dermis, and the subcutaneous fatty layer that separates the skin from the underlying tissue (Figure 12–1 ■).

Epidermis

The **epidermis**, which is the surface or outermost part of the skin, consists of epithelial cells. The epidermis has either four or five layers, depending on its location. There are five layers over the palms of the hands and the soles of the feet, and there are four layers over the rest of the body.

The stratum basale is the deepest layer of the epidermis. It contains cells known as melanocytes, which produce the pigment melanin, and keratinocytes, which produce keratin. **Melanin** forms a protective shield to protect the keratinocytes and the nerve endings in the dermis from the damaging effects of ultraviolet light. Melanocyte activity probably accounts for the difference in skin color in humans. **Keratin** is a fibrous, water-repellent protein that gives the epidermis its tough, protective quality. As keratinocytes mature, they move upward through the epidermal layers, eventually becoming dead cells at the surface of the skin. Millions of these cells are worn off by abrasion each day, but millions more are simultaneously produced in the stratum basale. The next layer of the epidermis is the stratum spinosum. Several cells thick, this layer contains abundant cells that arise from the bone marrow and migrate to the epidermis. Mitosis occurs at this layer, although not as abundantly as in the stratum basale.

The stratum granulosum is only two to three cells thick. The cells of the stratum granulosum contain a glycolipid that slows water loss across the epidermis. Keratinization, a thickening of

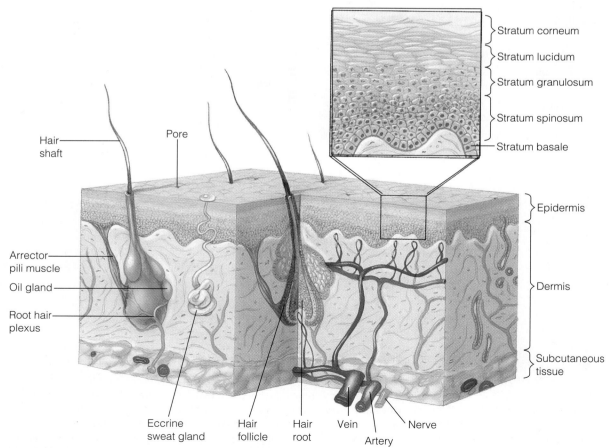

Figure 12–1 ■ Three-dimensional view of the skin, subcutaneous tissue, glands, and hairs.

the cells' plasma membranes, begins in the stratum granulosum. The stratum lucidum is present only in areas of thick skin. It is made up of flattened, dead keratinocytes.

The outermost layer of the epidermis, the stratum corneum, is also the thickest, making up about 75% of the total thickness of the epidermis. It consists of about 20–30 sheets of dead cells filled with keratin fragments arranged in "shingles" that flake off as dry skin.

Dermis

The **dermis** is the second, deeper layer of skin. Made of a flexible connective tissue, this layer is richly supplied with blood cells, nerve fibers, and lymphatic vessels. Most of the hair follicles, sebaceous glands, and sweat glands are located in the dermis. The dermis consists of a papillary and a reticular layer. The papillary layer contains ridges that indent the overlying epidermis. It also contains capillaries and receptors for pain and touch. The deeper, reticular layer contains blood vessels, sweat and sebaceous glands, deep pressure receptors, and dense bundles of collagen fibers. The regions between these bundles form lines of cleavage in the skin. Surgical incisions parallel to these lines of cleavage heal more easily and with less scarring than do incisions or traumatic wounds across cleavage lines.

Subcutaneous Tissue

The **subcutaneous** tissue (or **hypodermis**) is a loose connective tissue that stores approximately half of the body's fat cells. It cushions the body against trauma, insulates the body from heat loss, and stores fat for energy.

AGE-RELATED FACTORS

The newborn's skin is covered by vernix caseosa in utero, a greasy substance containing shed cells that cover and protect the fetal skin from amniotic fluid and urine (Chamley, 2005). It has many important properties, including anti-infective, antioxidant, moisturizing, and wound-healing agents (Stokowski, 2006).

The newborn's skin accounts for about 4% of body weight (Chamley, 2005). The infant's skin is thin, about 1 mm thick at birth, with little underlying subcutaneous fat. The skin grows to 2 mm thickness by adulthood. With thinner skin and less subcutaneous fat, the infant loses heat more rapidly, has greater difficulty regulating body temperature, and becomes chilled more quickly than an older child or an adult. The infant's thinner skin also allows increased absorption of harmful chemical substances and topical medications. The infant's skin contains more water than an adult's and has loosely attached cells. As the infant grows, the skin toughens and becomes less hydrated, making it less susceptible to bacteria.

Although changes occur in all of the body systems throughout life, skin and hair changes are the most visible and therefore greatly contribute to a person's self-perception and self-esteem. With normal aging, the thickness and elasticity of the skin decrease. These changes occur slowly, but by the seventh and eighth decades of life, they contribute to the appearance of wrinkled and sagging skin in the face, neck, and upper arms. The age-related changes in the skin's appearance correlate with changes in

function (Table 12–1). To reduce risk factors and minimize negative consequences, it is important to understand normal changes, as well as environmentally induced damage. Figure 12–2 ■ illustrates normal changes of aging in the integumentary system.

Epidermis

The epidermal cells of the older person contain less moisture. This contributes to a dry, rough skin appearance. After 50 years of age, epidermal mitosis slows by 30%, resulting in a longer healing time for the older person. This increased healing time also may contribute to infection. Rete ridges, which connect the dermis and epidermis, flatten, resulting in fewer contact areas between these two layers. This increases the risk for skin tears in response to seemingly slight friction against the skin. The number and activity of melanocytes decrease with age, contributing to a paler complexion and an increased risk of damage from ultraviolet radiation for the light-skinned older person. Remaining cells may not function normally, resulting in scattered pigmented areas such as nevi, age spots, or liver spots and an increase in the number and size of freckles.

Dermis

The dermis decreases in thickness and functionality beginning in the third decade. Elastin decreases in quality but increases in quantity, resulting in wrinkling and sagging of the skin. Collagen becomes less organized, causing a loss of turgor. Men have a thicker dermal layer than women do, which explains the more rapid age-associated changes in the female facial appearance. The vascularity of the dermis decreases with age, contributing to a paler complexion in the light-skinned older person. The capillaries become thinner and more easily damaged, leading to bruised and discolored areas known as **senile purpura**. Both touch and pressure sensations gradually decline, putting the older person at risk for injuries such as burns and pressure ulcers.

Subcutaneous Tissue

With increasing age, gradual atrophy of subcutaneous tissue occurs in some areas of the body, and a gradual increase occurs in others. Subcutaneous tissue becomes thinner in the face, neck, hands, and lower legs, resulting in more visible veins in the exposed areas and skin that is more prone to damage. A gradual hypertrophy of subcutaneous tissue in some other areas of the body leads to an overall increase in the proportion of body fat for the older person. Overall, with aging, fat distribution is more pronounced in the abdomen and thighs in women and in the abdomen in men.

ALTERATIONS IN SKIN AND TISSUE INTEGRITY

Intact skin refers to the presence of normal skin and skin layers uninterrupted by wounds. The appearance of the skin and skin integrity are influenced by internal factors such as genetics, age, and the underlying health of the individual, as well as by external factors such as activity.

Many chronic illnesses and their treatments affect skin integrity. People with impaired peripheral arterial circulation

TABLE 12–1 Age-Related Skin Changes

AGE-RELATED CHANGE	SIGNIFICANCE
Epidermis: ↓ thickness and miotic activity	■ Skin more fragile and at greater risk for tears or injury ■ Delayed wound healing ■ Hyperkeratoses and skin cancers in sun-exposed areas more evident
Epidermis: ↑ permeability, ↓ Langerhans cells	■ Increased risk of reactions to irritants ■ Decreased inflammatory response
Epidermis: ↓ number of active melanocytes	■ Increased susceptibility to sun exposure
Epidermis: hyperplasia of melanocytes, especially in sun-exposed areas	■ Small areas of hyperpigmentation (liver spots) and hypopigmentation (age spots), especially on the hands
Epidermis: ↓ vitamin D production	■ Increased risk of osteomalacia and osteoporosis
Epidermis: flattened dermal-epidermal junction	■ Increased risk of skin tears, purpura, and pressure ulcers
Dermis: ↓ perfusion	■ Greater susceptibility to dry skin ■ Decreased sensation (pain, touch, temperature, and peripheral vibration) ■ Increased risk of injury
Dermis: ↓ vasomotor response	■ Greater risk of hyperthermia and hypothermia
Dermis: elastic fiber degeneration	■ Decreased tone and elasticity, with wrinkle formation
Dermis: proliferation of capillaries	■ Cherry hemangiomas common
Subcutaneous skin layer: thinning	■ Greater risk of hypothermia ■ Increased risk of pressure ulcers
Subcutaneous skin layer: redistribution of adipose tissue	■ Cellulite formation ■ Bags over and under the eyes ■ Double chin formation ■ Increase in abdominal fat ■ Sagging of breasts ■ Skin slower to return to normal when pinched (tenting)
Glands: ↓ eccrine and apocrine activity	■ Dry skin common ■ Absent perspiration

Source: LeMone, P., & Burke, K. (2008). *Medical-surgical nursing: Critical thinking in client care* (4th ed., p. 430). Upper Saddle River, NJ: Pearson Education.

may have skin on their legs that appears shiny, has lost its hair distribution, and damages easily. Some medications, such as corticosteroids, cause thinning of the skin, making it much more easily harmed. Many medications increase sensitivity to sunlight and can predispose one to severe sunburns. Some of the most common medications that cause this kind of damage are certain antibiotics, chemotherapy drugs for cancer, and some psychotherapeutic drugs. Poor nutrition alone can interfere with the appearance and function of normal skin.

Some skin disorders have vague, generalized signs and symptoms, and others have specific and easily identifiable causes. **Pruritus**, or itching, is a general condition associated with dry, scaly skin; it may also be a symptom of mite or lice infestation. Inflammation, a characteristic of burns and other traumatic disorders, occurs when damage to the skin is extensive. Local **erythema**, or redness, accompanies inflammation and many other skin disorders. Trauma to deeper tissues may cause additional symptoms, such as bleeding, bruising, and infections.

Skin disorders are diverse and difficult to classify. These disorders are summarized in Table 12–2. One simple classification method is to group them into the following general categories:

■ *Infectious:* Bacterial, fungal, viral, and parasitic infections of the skin and mucous membranes are relatively common

and are frequently indications for anti-infective pharmacotherapy.
■ *Inflammatory:* Inflammatory disorders encompass a broad range of pathologies that includes acne, burns, eczema, dermatitis, and psoriasis.
■ *Neoplastic:* Neoplastic disease includes malignant melanoma and basal cell carcinoma.

Dermatologic signs and symptoms may reflect disease processes occurring elsewhere in the body. Skin abnormalities, including surface lesions of various colors, sizes, types, and character, and abnormal skin turgor and moisture may have systemic causes. These can include liver or renal impairment, cardiovascular insufficiency, metastatic tumors, recent injury, and poor nutritional status.

Skin **lesions** (observable changes from normal skin structure) vary in size, shape, color, and texture characteristics. Primary lesions arise from previously healthy skin and include macules, patches, papules, nodules, tumors, vesicles, pustules, bullae, and wheals. Secondary lesions result from changes in primary lesions. They include crusts, scales, **lichenification** (thickening of the skin), scars, keloids, excoriation, fissures, erosion, and ulcers. It is

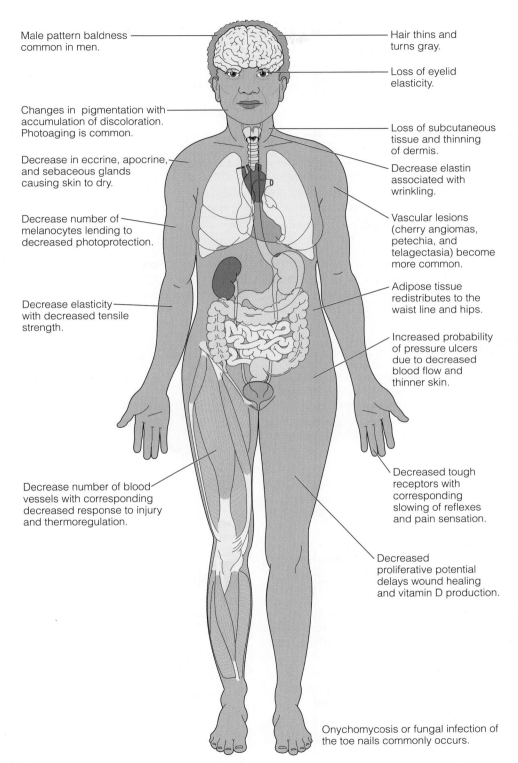

Male pattern baldness common in men.

Hair thins and turns gray.

Loss of eyelid elasticity.

Changes in pigmentation with accumulation of discoloration. Photoaging is common.

Loss of subcutaneous tissue and thinning of dermis.

Decrease in eccrine, apocrine, and sebaceous glands causing skin to dry.

Decrease elastin associated with wrinkling.

Decrease number of melanocytes lending to decreased photoprotection.

Vascular lesions (cherry angiomas, petechia, and telagectasia) become more common.

Adipose tissue redistributes to the waist line and hips.

Decrease elasticity with decreased tensile strength.

Increased probability of pressure ulcers due to decreased blood flow and thinner skin.

Decrease number of blood vessels with corresponding decreased response to injury and thermoregulation.

Decreased tough receptors with corresponding slowing of reflexes and pain sensation.

Decreased proliferative potential delays wound healing and vitamin D production.

Onychomycosis or fungal infection of the toe nails commonly occurs.

Figure 12–2 ■ Normal changes of aging in the integumentary system.

TABLE 12–2 Classification of Skin Disorders

TYPE	EXAMPLES
Infectious	Bacterial infections: boils, impetigo, infected hair follicles
	Fungal infections: ringworm, athlete's foot, jock itch, nail infection
	Parasitic infections: ticks, mites, lice
	Viral infections: cold sores, fever blisters (herpes simplex), chickenpox, warts, shingles (herpes zoster), measles (rubeola), and German measles (rubella)
Inflammatory	Injury and exposure to the sun such as sunburn and other environmental stresses
	Disorders marked by a combination of overactive glands, increased hormone production, and/or infection such as acne, blackheads, whiteheads, and rosacea
	Disorders marked by itching, cracking, and discomfort such as eczema (atopic dermatitis), other forms of dermatitis (contact dermatitis, seborrheic dermatitis, stasis dermatitis), and psoriasis
Neoplastic	Types of skin cancers: squamous cell carcinoma, basal cell carcinoma, and malignant melanoma (Malignant melanoma is the most dangerous; benign neoplasms include keratosis and keratoacanthoma.)

Source: Adams, M., & Holland, N. (2008). *Pharmacology for nurses: A pathophysiological approach* (2nd ed., p. 754). Upper Saddle River, NJ: Pearson Education.

important for the nurse to be able to identify and describe the primary and secondary skin lesions and understand their underlying cause and treatment.

Primary and secondary skin lesions are described and illustrated in Tables 12–3 and 12–4. The terms from these tables are used throughout this concept and exemplars.

TABLE 12–3 Primary Skin Lesions

Macule, Patch

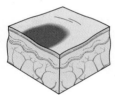

Flat, nonpalpable change in skin color. Macules are smaller than 1 cm, with a circumscribed border, and patches are larger than 1 cm and may have an irregular border.

Examples Freckles, measles, and petechiae. Patches: Mongolian spots, port-wine stains, vitiligo, and chloasma.

Papule, Plaque

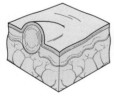

Elevated, solid, palpable mass with circumscribed border. Papules are smaller than 0.5 cm; plaques are groups of papules that form lesions larger than 0.5 cm.

Examples Elevated moles, warts, and lichen planus. Plaques: psoriasis, actinic keratosis, and also lichen planus.

Nodule, Tumor

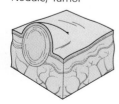

Elevated, solid, hard or soft palpable mass extending deeper into the dermis than a papule. Nodules have circumscribed borders and are 0.5–2 cm; tumors may have irregular borders and are larger than 2 cm.

Examples Small lipoma, squamous cell carcinoma, fibroma, and intradermal nevi. Tumors: large lipoma, carcinoma, and hemangioma.

Vesicle, Bulla

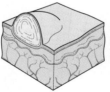

Elevated, fluid-filled, round or oval-shaped, palpable mass with thin, translucent walls and circumscribed borders. Vesicles are smaller than 0.5 cm; bullae are larger than 0.5 cm.

Examples Herpes simplex/zoster, early chickenpox, poison ivy, and small burn blisters. Bullae: contact dermatitis, friction blisters, and large burn blisters.

Wheal

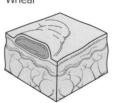

Elevated, often reddish area with irregular border caused by diffuse fluid in tissues rather than free fluid in a cavity, as in vesicles. Size varies.

Examples Insect bites and hives (extensive wheals).

Pustule

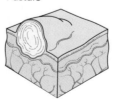

Elevated, pus-filled vesicle or bulla with circumscribed border. Size varies.

Examples Acne, impetigo, and carbuncles (large boils).

Cyst

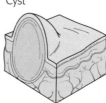

Elevated, encapsulated, fluid-filled or semi-solid mass originating in the subcutaneous tissue or dermis, usually 1 cm or larger.

Examples Varieties include sebaceous cysts and epidermoid cysts.

Source: LeMone, P., & Burke, K. (2008). *Medical-surgical nursing: Critical thinking in client care* (4th ed., p. 432). Upper Saddle River, NJ: Pearson Education.

TABLE 12–4 **Secondary Skin Lesions**

Atrophy 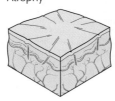	A translucent, dry, paper-like, sometimes wrinkled skin surface resulting from thinning or wasting of the skin due to loss of collagen and elastin. **Examples** Striae, aged skin.	Ulcer 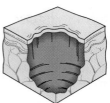	Deep, irregularly shaped area of skin loss extending into the dermis or sub cutaneous tissue. May bleed. May leave scar. **Examples** Decubitus ulcers (pressure sores), stasis ulcers, chancres.
Erosion 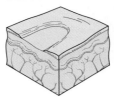	Wearing away of the superficial epidermis causing a moist, shallow depression. Because erosions do not extend into the dermis, they heal without scarring. **Examples** Scratch marks, ruptured vesicles.	Fissure 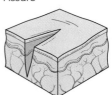	Linear crack with sharp edges, extending into the dermis. **Examples** Cracks at the corners of the mouth or in the hands, athlete's foot.
Lichenification 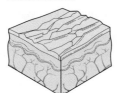	Rough, thickened, hardened area of epidermis resulting from chronic irritation such as scratching or rubbing. **Example** Chronic dermatitis.	Scar 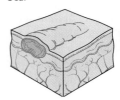	Flat, irregular area of connective tissue left after a lesion or wound has healed. New scars may be red or purple; older scars may be silvery or white. **Examples** Healed surgical wound or injury, healed acne.
Scales 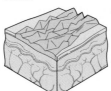	Shedding flakes of greasy, keratinized skin tissue. Color may be white, gray, or silver. Texture may vary from fine to thick. **Examples** Dry skin, dandruff, psoriasis, and eczema.	Keloid 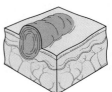	Elevated, irregular, darkened area of excess scar tissue caused by excessive collagen formation during healing. Extends beyond the site of the original injury. Higher incidence in people of African descent. **Examples** Keloid from ear piercing or surgery.
Crust 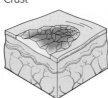	Dry blood, serum, or pus left on the skin surface when vesicles or pustules burst. Can be red-brown, orange, or yellow. Large crusts that adhere to the skin surface are called scabs. **Examples** Eczema, impetigo, herpes, or scabs following abrasion.		

Source: LeMone, P., & Burke, K. (2008). *Medical-surgical nursing: Critical thinking in client care* (4th ed., p. 433). Upper Saddle River, NJ: Pearson Education.

Wounds

Body wounds are either intentional or unintentional. *Intentional* trauma occurs during therapy; examples are operations or venipunctures. Although removing a tumor, for example, is therapeutic, the surgeon must cut into body tissues, thus traumatizing them. *Unintentional* wounds are accidental: For example, a person may fracture an arm in an automobile collision or a bicycle accident. If the tissues are traumatized without a break in the skin, the wound is closed. The wound is open when the skin or mucous membrane surface is broken.

Wounds may be described according to how they are acquired (Table 12–5). They also can be described according to the likelihood and degree of wound contamination.

- *Clean wounds* are uninfected wounds in which minimal inflammation is encountered and the respiratory, alimentary, genital, and urinary tracts are not entered. Clean wounds are primarily closed wounds.
- *Clean-contaminated wounds* are surgical wounds in which the respiratory, alimentary, genital, or urinary tract has been entered. Such wounds show no evidence of infection.
- *Contaminated wounds* include open, fresh, accidental wounds and surgical wounds that involve a major break in sterile technique or a large amount of spillage from the gastrointestinal tract. Contaminated wounds show evidence of inflammation.
- *Dirty* or *infected wounds* include wounds containing dead tissue and wounds with evidence of a clinical infection, such as purulent drainage.

TABLE 12–5 Types of Wounds

TYPE	CAUSE	DESCRIPTION AND CHARACTERISTICS
Incision	Sharp instrument (e.g., knife or scalpel)	Open wound; deep or shallow
Contusion	Blow from a blunt instrument	Closed wound; skin appearing ecchymotic (bruised) because of damaged blood vessels
Abrasion	Surface scrape, either unintentional (e.g., scraped knee from a fall) or intentional (e.g., dermal abrasion to remove pockmarks)	Open wound involving the skin
Puncture	Penetration of the skin and often the underlying tissues by a sharp instrument, either intentional or unintentional	Open wound
Laceration	Tissues torn apart, often from accidents (e.g., with machinery)	Open wound; edges often jagged
Penetrating Wound	Penetration of the skin and the underlying tissues, usually unintentional (e.g., from a bullet or metal fragments)	Open wound

Source: Berman, A., Snyder, S. J., Kozier, B., & Erb, G. (2008). *Kozier & Erb's fundamentals of nursing: Concepts, process, and practice* (8th ed., p. 904). Upper Saddle River, NJ: Pearson Education.

Wounds, excluding pressure ulcers and burns, are classified by depth, that is, the tissue layers involved in the wound (Box 12–1).

UNTREATED WOUNDS Untreated wounds usually are seen shortly after an injury (e.g., at the scene of an accident or in an emergency center). The following are guidelines for treatment:

- Control severe bleeding by (a) applying direct pressure over the wound and (b) elevating the involved extremity.
- Prevent infection by (a) cleaning or flushing abrasions or lacerations with normal saline and (b) covering the wound with a clean dressing if possible (a sterile dressing is preferred). When applying a dressing, wrap the wound tightly enough to apply pressure, and approximate the wound edges if possible. If the first layer of dressing becomes saturated with blood, apply a second layer. Do so without removing the first layer of dressing, because blood clots might be disturbed, resulting in more bleeding.
- Control swelling and pain by applying ice over the wound and surrounding tissues.

Box 12–1 Classifying Wounds by Depth

- *Partial thickness:* Confined to the skin, that is, the dermis and epidermis; heal by regeneration
- *Full thickness:* Involving the dermis, epidermis, subcutaneous tissue, and possibly muscle and bone; require connective tissue repair

Source: Berman, A., Snyder, S. J., Kozier, B., & Erb, G. (2008). *Kozier & Erb's fundamentals of nursing: Concepts, process, and practice* (8th ed., p. 904). Upper Saddle River, NJ: Pearson Education.

- If bleeding is severe or internal bleeding is suspected and if emergency equipment is available, assess the client for signs of shock (rapid, thready pulse; cold, clammy skin; pallor; lowered blood pressure).

TREATED WOUNDS Treated or sutured wounds usually need to be observed to determine the progress of healing. These wounds may be inspected when a dressing is changed. If the wound itself cannot be directly inspected, the dressing is inspected and other data regarding the wound (e.g., the presence of pain) are assessed. See exemplar 12.3, Wound Healing, for more information.

PHYSICAL ASSESSMENT

The nurse conducts an examination of the integument as part of a routine assessment and during regular care. Removing barriers to assessment is very important. Antiembolic stockings, braces, or other medical or assistive devices must be removed to assess the skin condition underneath. Examination of the skin requires good lighting to detect variations in skin color and to identify lesions.

During the review of systems as part of the nursing history, information about skin diseases, previous bruising, general skin condition, skin lesions, and usual healing of sores is obtained. Inspection and palpation of the skin focus on determining skin color distribution, skin turgor, presence of **edema** (swelling caused by excess fluid trapped in bodily tissue), and characteristics of any lesions that are present. Particular attention is paid to skin condition in areas that are most likely to break down: in skin folds such as under the breasts; in areas that are frequently moist, such as the perineum; and in areas that receive extensive pressure, such as the bony prominences.

ASSESSMENT INTERVIEW Skin and Tissue Integrity

SKIN CONDITIONS
- Have you ever had a skin problem?
- When were you diagnosed with the problem?
- What treatment was prescribed for the problem?
- Was the treatment helpful?
- What kinds of things do you do to help with the problem?
- Has the problem ever recurred (acute)?
- How are you managing the disease now (chronic)?

- Have you had an illness recently? If so, please describe it.
- Do you have or have you had a skin infection?
- When were you diagnosed with the infection?
- What treatment was prescribed for the problem?
- Was the treatment helpful? What kinds of things do you do to help with the problem?
- Has the problem ever recurred (acute)?
- How are you managing the infection now (chronic)?

ASSESSMENT INTERVIEW Skin and Tissue Integrity (continued)

SKIN CONDITION SYMPTOMS

- Do you have any sores or ulcers on your body that are slow in healing?
- Where are these?
- Do you have frequent boils or skin infections?
- Does your skin itch? If so, where?
- How severe is it?
- When does it occur?
- Have you noticed any rashes on your body? If so, please describe.
- Where on your body did the rash start? Where did it spread?
- When did you first notice it?
- Does the rash happen at the same time as any other symptoms, such as fever or chills?
- If you have a rash, do you notice it more after wearing certain clothes or jewelry? After using certain skin products?
- Did it occur soon after starting a new medication?
- Does the rash happen during or after any other activities such as gardening or washing dishes?
- Have you noticed any other lesions, lumps, bumps, tender spots, or painful areas on your body?
- If so, when did you first notice them? Where?
- Describe how they have spread and where they are located now.
- Have you noticed any drainage from any skin region?
- If so, where does the drainage come from? What does it look like? Does it have an odor?
- Is the drainage accompanied by any other symptoms? If so, please describe.
- Please describe anything you have done to treat your skin condition.
- When did you begin this treatment? How has your skin responded to the treatment?

PAIN

- Please describe any skin pain or discomfort.
- Have you experienced any pain or discomfort in any body folds, for example, between the toes, under the breasts, between the buttocks, or in the perianal area?
- Where is the pain?
- How often do you experience the pain?
- How long does the pain last?
- How long have you had the pain?
- How would you rate the pain on a scale of 1 to 10?
- Is there a trigger for the pain?
- What do you do to relieve the pain?
- Is this treatment effective?

BEHAVIORS

- Do you sunbathe?
- Have you ever sunbathed?
- Do you spend time in the sun exercising or playing sports?
- Do you work outdoors?
- How does your skin react to sun exposure?
- Do you use a lotion with sun protection factor (SPF) when spending time in the sun?
- What SPF lotion do you use? Do you reapply the lotion after several hours or after swimming?
- Do you remember having a sunburn that left blisters?
- How do you care for your skin?
- What kind of soap, cleansers, toners, or other treatments do you use?
- How do you clean your clothes?
- What kind of detergent do you use?

- How often do you bathe or shower?
- Do you now have or have you ever had a tattoo(s)?
- Have you had any problems with that area of the skin?
- Do you now have or have you ever had piercing of any part of your body?
- Where are the sites of piercing?
- How long have you had the piercing?
- Have any piercing sites closed?
- Have you ever had a problem at the piercing site?
- What was the problem?
- Did you seek treatment for the problem?
- What was the outcome of the treatment?
- What is the current condition of piercing sites?

INFANTS AND CHILDREN

- Does the child have any birthmarks? If so, where are they?
- Has the infant developed an orange hue in the skin?
- Does the child have a rash? If so, what seems to cause it?
- Have you introduced any new foods into your child's diet?
- How do you clean the child's diaper area?
- How do you wash the child's diapers?

OLDER ADULT

- What changes have you noticed in your skin in the past few years?
- Does your skin itch?
- Do you experience frequent falls?

INTERNAL ENVIRONMENT

- How would you describe your level of stress? Has it changed in the past few weeks? Few months? Describe.
- Are you now experiencing, or have you ever experienced, intermittent or prolonged anxiety or emotional upset?
- Describe the situation.
- Can you determine precipitating factors?
- Have you sought care or treatment for the problem?
- What do you do when the problem arises?
- Are you taking any prescription or over-the-counter medications?
- Have you changed your diet recently?
- Has the condition of your skin affected your social relationships in any way? Has it limited you in any way? If so, how?
- Female clients: Are you pregnant? If not, are you menstruating regularly? Describe your menstrual periods.

EXTERNAL ENVIRONMENT

- Have you been exposed recently to extremes in temperature?
- If so, when? How long was the exposure? Where did this occur?
- Describe the temperature of your home environment. Of your work environment.
- Do you work in an environment where radioisotopes or x-rays are used?
- If so, are you vigilant about following precautions and using protective gear?
- Do you wear gloves for work? If so, what types of gloves?
- How often do you travel?
- Have you traveled recently?
- If so, where?
- Have you come into contact with anyone who has a similar rash?
- Does your job or hobby require you to perform repetitive tasks? To work with any chemicals?
- Does your job or hobby require you to wear a specific type of helmet, hat, goggles, gloves, or shoes?

Source: D'Amico, D., & Barbarito, C. (2007). *Health & physical assessment in nursing.* Upper Saddle River, NJ: Pearson Education.

Integumentary Assessment

Technique/Normal Findings	Abnormal Findings
Inspect skin color and note any odors coming from the skin. *Skin color should be even, appropriate to the age and race of the client, without foul odors.*	■ A strong odor of perspiration may indicate poor hygiene and a need for client teaching. A foul odor may indicate a disorder of the sweat glands. ■ Pallor and/or cyanosis are seen with exposure to cold and with decreased perfusion and oxygenation. In cyanotic dark-skinned clients, skin loses glow and appears dull. Cyanosis may be more visible in the mucous membranes and nail beds of these clients. ■ In dark-skinned clients, jaundice may be most apparent in the sclerae of the eyes. ■ Redness, swelling, and pain are seen with various rashes, inflammations, infections, and burns. First-degree burns cause areas of painful erythema and swelling. Red, painful blisters appear in second-degree burns, whereas white or blackened areas are common in third-degree burns. ■ **Vitiligo**, an abnormal loss of melanin in patches, typically occurs over the face, hands, or groin. Vitiligo is thought to be an autoimmune disorder.
Inspect the skin for lesions and alterations, including calluses, scars, tattoos, and piercings. Include inspection of skin creases and folds. *Skin should be intact without abnormal lesions.*	■ Primary, secondary, and vascular lesions are described and shown in Tables 12–3 and 12–4. ■ Pearly edged nodules with a central ulcer are seen in basal cell carcinoma. ■ Scaly, red, fast-growing papules are seen in squamous cell carcinoma. ■ Dark, asymmetric, multicolored patches (sometimes moles) with irregular edges appear in malignant melanoma. ■ Circular lesions are usually present in ringworm and tinea versicolor. ■ Grouped vesicles may be seen in contact dermatitis. ■ Linear lesions appear in poison ivy and herpes zoster. ■ **Urticaria** (hives) appears as patches of pale, itchy wheals in an erythematous area. ■ In psoriasis, scaly red patches appear on the scalp, knees, back, and genitals. ■ In herpes zoster, vesicles appear along sensory nerve paths, turn into pustules, and then crust over. ■ Bruises (**ecchymosis**) are raised bluish or yellowish vascular lesions. Multiple bruises in various stages of healing suggest trauma or abuse.
Palpate skin temperature. *Skin should be warm.*	■ Skin is warm and red in inflammation and is generally warm with elevated body temperature. ■ Decreased blood flow decreases the skin temperature; this may be generalized, as in shock, or localized, as in arteriosclerosis.
Palpate skin texture. *Skin should be smooth.*	■ Changes in the texture of the skin may indicate irritation or trauma. ■ The skin is soft and smooth in hyperthyroidism and coarse in hypothyroidism.
Palpate skin moisture. *Skin should be dry.*	■ Excessively dry skin often is present in the older adult and in clients with hypothyroidism. ■ Oily skin is common in adolescents and young adults. Oily skin may be a normal finding, or it may accompany a skin disorder such as acne vulgaris. ■ Excessive perspiration may be associated with shock, fever, increased activity, or anxiety.
Palpate skin turgor. *Skin fold should return rapidly to normal position.*	■ Pinch the client's skin gently over the sternum or collarbone. Tenting, in which the skin remains pinched for a few moments before resuming its normal position, is common in older clients who are thin. ■ Skin turgor is decreased in dehydration. It is increased in edema and scleroderma.
Assess for edema. *No edema should be present.*	■ Assess edema (accumulation of fluid in the body's tissues) by depressing the client's skin (Figure 12–3 ■). Record findings as follows: 1+: Slight pitting, no obvious distortion 2+: Deeper pit, no obvious distortion 3+: Pit is obvious; extremities are swollen 4+: Pit remains with obvious distortion ■ Edema is common in cardiovascular disorders, renal failure, and cirrhosis of the liver. It also may be a side effect of certain drugs.

Integumentary Assessment (continued)

Technique/Normal Findings	Abnormal Findings

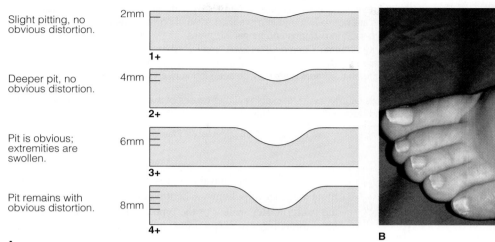

Slight pitting, no obvious distortion. — 2mm — **1+**

Deeper pit, no obvious distortion. — 4mm — **2+**

Pit is obvious; extremities are swollen. — 6mm — **3+**

Pit remains with obvious distortion. — 8mm — **4+**

A

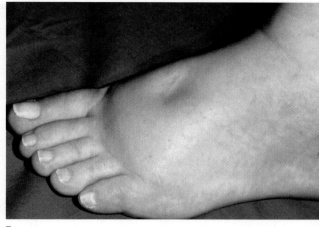

B

Figure 12–3 ■ A, Degrees of pitting in edema. B, 4+ pitting.

Source: Dr. P. Marazzi/Science Photo Library/Photo Researchers, Inc.

Inspect distribution and quality of hair. *Hair should be evenly distributed for client's gender.*

- A deviation in the normal hair distribution in the male or female genital area may indicate an endocrine disorder. **Hirsutism** (increased growth of coarse hair, usually on the face and trunk) is seen in Cushing's syndrome, acromegaly, and ovarian dysfunction. **Alopecia** (hair loss) may be related to changes in hormones, chemical or drug treatment, or radiation. In adult males whose hair loss follows the normal male pattern, the cause is usually genetic.

Palpate hair texture. *Hair should be of even texture.*

- Some systemic diseases change the texture of the hair. For instance, hypothyroidism causes the hair to coarsen, whereas hyperthyroidism causes the hair to become fine.

Inspect the scalp for lesions. *There should be no lesions on the scalp.*

- Mild dandruff is normal, but excessive, greasy flakes indicate seborrhea requiring treatment.
- Hair loss, pustules, and scales appear on the scalp in tinea capitis (scalp ringworm).
- Red, swollen pustules appear around infected hair follicles and are called folliculitis.
- Head lice may be seen as oval nits (eggs) adhering to the base of the hair shaft. Head lice are usually accompanied by itching.

Inspect nail curvature. *Nails should not be excessively curved.*

- Clubbing, in which the angle of the nail base is greater than 180 degrees, is seen in respiratory disorders, cardiovascular disorders, cirrhosis of the liver, colitis, and thyroid disease. The nail becomes thick, hard, shiny, and curved at the free end.
- The nail folds become inflamed and swollen and the nail loosens in paronychia, an infection of the nails.

Inspect the surface of the nails. *Nail surfaces should be smooth and nail folds firm, without redness.*

- Inflammation and transverse rippling of the nail are associated with chronic paronychia and/or eczema.
- The nail plate may separate from the nail bed in trauma, psoriasis, and *Pseudomonas* and *Candida* infections. This separation is called oncolysis.
- Nail grooves may be caused by inflammation, by planus, or by nail biting.
- Nail pitting may be seen with psoriasis.
- A transverse groove (Beau's line) may be seen in trachoma and/or acute diseases.
- Thin spoon-shaped nails may be seen in anemia.

Integumentary Assessment (continued)

Technique/Normal Findings	Abnormal Findings
Inspect nail color. *Nail color should be even.*	■ The sudden appearance of a pigmented band may indicate melanoma in Caucasians. Pigmented bands are normally found in more than 90% of African Americans. ■ Yellowish nails are seen in psoriasis and fungal infections. ■ Dark nails occur with trauma, *Candida* infections, and hyperbilirubinemia. ■ Blackish-green nails are apparent in injury and in *Pseudomonas* infection. ■ Red splinter longitudinal hemorrhages may be seen in injury and/or psoriasis.
Inspect nail thickness. *Nails should not be excessively thick.*	■ Trauma to the nails usually causes thickening. Other causes of thick nails include psoriasis, fungal infections, and decreased peripheral vascular blood supply.

Source: LeMone, P., & Burke, K. (2008). *Medical-surgical nursing: Critical thinking in client care* (4th ed., p. 435). Upper Saddle River, NJ: Pearson Education.

DIAGNOSTIC TESTS

The results of diagnostic tests of the structure and function of the integumentary system are used to support the diagnosis of a specific injury or disease. Diagnostic tests also provide information to identify or modify the appropriate medication or treatments used for the disease, and help nurses monitor the clients' responses to nursing care interventions. Diagnostic tests to assess the integumentary system are described in Diagnostic Tests: Integumentary System and are summarized in the following bulleted list.

■ One of the most common diagnostic tests is a skin biopsy, which is used to differentiate a benign skin lesion from a skin cancer. Skin biopsies can be obtained by using a punch technique, incision, excision, or shaving.

■ Cultures to identify infections may be conducted on tissue samples, on drainage and exudate (material, such as fluid and cells, that has escaped from blood vessels during the inflammatory process and is deposited in tissue or on tissue surfaces) from lesions, and (if an illness is generalized) on serum.

■ Tests that are used to identify infections include immunofluorescent studies, Wood's lamp, potassium hydroxide, and the Tzanck test.

■ Patch tests or scratch tests may be used to determine allergies.

Some studies are conducted to identify bacterial carriers. For example, if clients have repeated bacterial skin infections or if a health care unit or agency experiences numerous bacterial infections of clients, nasal cultures may be performed to determine whether the clients or health care workers are carriers of the bacteria. Regardless of the type of diagnostic test, the nurse is responsible for explaining the procedure to the client; explaining any special preparation needed, including fasting or avoiding allergy medications prior to testing; assessing for medication use that may affect the outcome of the tests; supporting the client during the examination as necessary; documenting the procedures as appropriate; and monitoring the results of the tests.

Laboratory data can also support the nurse's clinical assessment of a wound's progress in healing. A decreased leukocyte count can delay healing and increase the possibility of infection. A hemoglobin level below normal range indicates poor oxygen delivery to the tissues. Blood coagulation studies are also significant. Prolonged coagulation times can result in excessive blood loss and prolonged clot absorption. Hypercoagulability can lead to intravascular clotting. Intra-arterial clotting can result in a deficient blood supply to the wound area. Serum protein analysis provides an indication of the body's nutritional reserves for rebuilding cells. Albumin is an important indicator of nutritional status. A value below 3.5 g/dL indicates poor nutrition and may increase the risk of poor healing and infection. Wound cultures can either confirm or rule out the presence of infection. Sensitivity studies are helpful in the selection of appropriate antibiotic therapy. The nurse obtains a wound culture whenever an infection is suspected.

DIAGNOSTIC TESTS | Integumentary System

NAME OF TEST Punch Skin Biopsy

PURPOSE AND DESCRIPTION This biopsy is done to differentiate benign lesions from skin cancers. An instrument is used to remove a small section of dermis and subcutaneous fat. Depending on size, the incision may be sutured.

NURSING CONSIDERATIONS Explain the procedure to the client, and ensure a consent form is signed (if required). Assist with the procedure. Apply dressing and provide information about self-care and when to return for suture removal. Document the procedure and send the labeled specimen to the lab.

NAME OF TEST Incisional Skin Biopsy

PURPOSE AND DESCRIPTION This biopsy is done to differentiate benign lesions from skin cancers. An incision is made and a *part* of the lesion or tumor is removed. The incision is closed with sutures.

NURSING CONSIDERATIONS See those for punch skin biopsy.

DIAGNOSTIC TESTS Integumentary System (continued)

NAME OF TEST Excisional Skin Biopsy

PURPOSE AND DESCRIPTION This biopsy is done to differentiate benign lesions from skin cancers. An incision is made and the *entire* skin lesion or tumor is removed for analysis. The incision is closed with sutures.

NURSING CONSIDERATIONS See those for punch skin biopsy.

NAME OF TEST Shave Skin Biopsy

PURPOSE AND DESCRIPTION This skin biopsy is done to shave off superficial lesions and differentiate infectious from inflammatory lesions. A single-edged razor is used for shaving.

NURSING CONSIDERATIONS See those for punch skin biopsy.

NAME OF TEST Culture

PURPOSE AND DESCRIPTION A culture of scrapings from a lesion, from drainage, or of exudate is done to identify fungal, bacterial, or viral skin infections. Obtain the culture with a sterile Culturette swab and culture tubes.

NURSING CONSIDERATIONS Confirm physician's order. Explain the procedure to the client. Maintain strict asepsis while obtaining the culture. Document the procedure and send the labeled specimen to the lab.

NAME OF TEST Oil Slides

PURPOSE AND DESCRIPTION Oil slides are used to determine the type of skin infestation present. Scrapings of the lesion are placed on a slide with mineral oil and examined microscopically.

NURSING CONSIDERATIONS Explain the procedure to the client. Assist with or obtain the specimen and complete the slide. Document the procedure and send the labeled specimen to the lab.

NAME OF TEST Immunofluorescent Slides

PURPOSE AND DESCRIPTION Immunofluorescent studies of samples from skin and/or serum may be done to identify IgG antibodies (present in pemphigus vulgaris) and varicella in skin cells (for herpes zoster). Skin or blood samples are placed on a slide and examined microscopically.

NURSING CONSIDERATIONS See those for oil slides.

NAME OF TEST Wood's Lamp

PURPOSE AND DESCRIPTION This test uses an ultraviolet light that causes certain organisms to fluoresce (such as *Pseudomonas* organisms and fungi). The skin is examined under a special lamp.

NURSING CONSIDERATIONS Explain the procedure to the client. Document the procedure.

NAME OF TEST Potassium Hydroxide (KOH)

PURPOSE AND DESCRIPTION A specimen from hair or nails is examined for a fungal infection. The specimen is obtained by placing material from a scraping on a slide, adding a potassium hydroxide solution, and examining it microscopically.

NURSING CONSIDERATIONS Explain the procedure to the client. Assist with or obtain the specimen and complete the slide. Document the procedure and send the labeled specimen to the lab.

NAME OF TEST Tzanck Test

PURPOSE AND DESCRIPTION This test is used to diagnose herpes infections, but it does not differentiate herpes simplex from herpes zoster. Fluid and cells from the vesicles are obtained, put on a slide, stained, and examined microscopically.

NURSING CONSIDERATIONS Explain the procedure to the client. Use sterile procedure to assist with or obtain the specimen and complete the slide. Document the procedure and send the labeled specimen to the lab.

NAME OF TEST Patch Tests, Scratch Tests

PURPOSE AND DESCRIPTION These tests are used to determine a specific allergen. In a patch test, a small amount of the suspected material is placed on the skin under an occlusive bandage. In a scratch test, a needle is used to "scratch" small amounts of potentially allergic materials on the skin surface.

NURSING CONSIDERATIONS Explain the procedure to the client, including the need to return in 48 hours to have the patch testing evaluated, or to withhold allergy medications prior to the test. Document the procedure. Typically, patch or scratch tests result in very minor discomfort to the client. However, young children and severely allergic clients may experience significant discomfort during scratch testing, and may require palliative care once the test is completed.

Source: LeMone, P., & Burke, K. (2008). *Medical-surgical nursing: Critical thinking in client care* (4th ed., p. 428). Upper Saddle River, NJ: Pearson Education.

TABLE 12–6 Topical Glucocorticoids for Dermatitis and Related Symptoms

GENERIC NAME	TRADE NAMES
Highest Level of Potency	
Betamethasone	Benisone, Diprosone, Valisone
Clobetasol	Dermovate, Temovate
Diflorasone	Florone, Maxiflor, Psorcon
Middle Level of Potency	
Amcinonide	Cyclocort
Desoximetasone	Topicort, Topicort LP
Fluocinonide	Lidex, Lidex-E, others
Halcinonide	Halog
Mometasone	Elocon
Triamcinolone	Aristocort, Kenalog, others
Lower Level of Potency	
Clocortolone	Cloderm
Fluocinolone	Fluolar, Synalar, others
Flurandrenolide	Cordran, Cordran SP
Fluticasone	Flonase
Hydrocortisone	Hytone, Locoid, Westcort, others
Lowest Level of Potency	
Alclometasone	Aclovate
Desonide	DesOwen, Tridesilon
Dexamethasone	Decaderm, Decadron, others

Source: Adams, M., & Holland, N. (2008). *Pharmacology for nurses: A pathophysiological approach* (2nd ed.). Upper Saddle River, NJ: Pearson Education.

THERAPEUTIC MANAGEMENT INTERVENTIONS FOR ALTERATIONS IN TISSUE INTEGRITY

Medical management of alterations in tissue integrity is based on the cause and severity of the condition. The goals of treatment are to control the severity of the disease, prevent infection, and promote healing. Palliative care may also be necessary, depending on the severity of the problem and the level of discomfort it presents for the client. The nurse should ask questions to determine whether the client is doing anything at home to relieve discomfort that could unintentionally inhibit healing. The nurse should also provide information about what home remedies will provide comfort while promoting healing.

Pharmacologic Therapies

There are many skin disorders; some warrant only localized or short-term pharmacotherapy. Examples include lice infestation, sunburn with minor irritation, and acne. Eczema, dermatitis, and psoriasis are more serious disorders that require extensive and sometimes prolonged therapy. Table 12–6 identifies some topical agents that are used to treat skin disorders, listed according to their level of potency. Some clients may use complementary therapies to treat skin lesions, as listed in the Alternative Therapies: Skin Lesions feature.

ALTERNATIVE THERAPIES Skin Lesions

Skin Condition	Complementary Therapy
Atopic eczema	Evening primrose oil (oral)
Wound healing, superficial burns, and abrasions	Aloe vera gel (topical)
Skin inflammation	Chamomile (topical cream or ointment)

Source: Data from National Center for Complementary and Alternative Medicine. (2006). *Herbs at a glance.* Retrieved December 2, 2007, from http://nccam.nih.gov/health.

12.1 CONTACT DERMATITIS

KEY TERMS

Allergic contact dermatitis, *357*
Contact dermatitis, *357*
Irritant contact dermatitis, *357*
Patch testing, *358*

BASIS FOR SELECTION OF EXEMPLAR

Frequency of office-based visits

LEARNING OUTCOMES

After learning about this exemplar, you will be able to do the following:

1. Describe the pathophysiology, etiology, clinical manifestations, and direct and indirect causes of contact dermatitis.

2. Identify risk factors associated with contact dermatitis.

3. Apply nursing process in providing culturally competent and caring interventions across the life span for individuals with contact dermatitis.

4. Identify priority nursing diagnoses that are appropriate for an individual with contact dermatitis.

5. Develop a plan of care for individuals with contact dermatitis that includes their family members.

6. Identify and analyze expected outcomes for an individual with contact dermatitis.

7. Discuss therapies used in the collaborative care of an individual with contact dermatitis.

8. Use evidence-based care (or prevention) for an individual with contact dermatitis.

OVERVIEW

Contact dermatitis is an inflammation of the skin that occurs in response to direct contact with an allergen or irritant. The major sources known to cause contact dermatitis are dyes, perfumes, poison plants (ivy, oak, sumac), chemicals, and metals (Box 12–2). Latex (glove) dermatitis is a contact dermatitis that is common in the health care field.

PRACTICE ALERT

- The increased use of latex gloves among health care providers has resulted in increased reporting of latex allergies. It is estimated that 10–17% of health care providers are allergic to latex (Porth, 2005).
- The most common type of allergic response to latex gloves is type IV, T cell-mediated contact dermatitis.
- Type I, IgE-mediated hypersensitivity, manifested by urticaria, rhinoconjunctivitis, asthma, or anaphylaxis, is far more serious than the T cell-mediated type.
- All clients with a latex allergy should be treated in a latex-free environment.
- Health care providers with severe allergic responses to latex may have to seek a different type of employment.

Source: LeMone, P., & Burke, K. (2008). *Medical-surgical nursing: Critical thinking in client care* (4th ed., p. 456). Upper Saddle River, NJ: Pearson Education.

PATHOPHYSIOLOGY AND ETIOLOGY

Allergic contact dermatitis is a cell-mediated or delayed hypersensitivity to a wide variety of allergens. Sensitizing antigens include microorganisms, plants, chemicals, drugs, metals, and foreign proteins. On initial contact with the skin, the allergen binds to a carrier protein, forming a sensitizing antigen. The antigen is processed and carried to the T cells, which in turn become sensitized to the antigen. The first exposure is the sensitizing contact: the individual does not experience manifestations until subsequent exposures. Manifestations include erythema, swelling, and pruritic vesicles in the area of allergen contact. For example, a person who is hypersensitive to metal may have lesions under a ring or watch.

Irritant contact dermatitis is an inflammation of the skin from irritants; it is not a hypersensitivity response. Common sources of irritant contact dermatitis include chemicals (such as acids), soaps, and detergents. The skin lesions are similar to those seen in allergic contact dermatitis.

Risk Factors

Risk factors for contact dermatitis include allergies, family history of eczema, regular exposure to a moist environment, burns, exposure to plants, chemicals, and metals, occupations that require frequent hand washing. The elderly are also at greater risk for contact dermatitis.

Clinical Manifestations and Therapies

Allergic contact dermatitis is characterized by erythema, edema, pruritus, vesicles, or bullae that rupture, ooze, and crust (Figure 12–4 ■). The rash is usually limited to the area of

---

Box 12–2 **Common Causes of Contact Dermatitis**

- Acids
- Alkalis: soaps, detergents, household ammonia, lye, cleaners
- Bromide
- Chlorine
- Cosmetics: perfumes, dyes, oils
- Dusts of lime, arsenic, wood
- Hydrocarbons: crude petroleum, lubricating oil, mineral oil, paraffin, asphalt, tar
- Iodine
- Insecticides
- Fabrics: wool, polyester, dyes, sizing
- Metal salts: calcium chloride, zinc chloride, copper, mercury, nickel, silver
- Plants: ragweed, poison oak, poison sumac, poison ivy, pine
- Coloring agents
- Rubber products
- Soot

Source: LeMone, P., & Burke, K. (2008). *Medical-surgical nursing: Critical thinking in client care* (4th ed., p. 456). Upper Saddle River, NJ: Pearson Education.

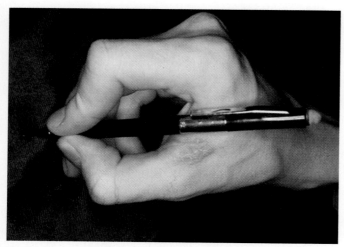

Figure 12–4 ■ Contact dermatitis.

Source: Copyright-protected material used with permission of Jane Ball and the University of Iowa's Virtual Hospital, http://www.vh.org.

contact; for example, the rash may be linear where a poison ivy leaf brushed against the skin. Symptoms of allergic contact dermatitis can develop several hours to 3 days after exposure, when the immunologic response has been activated. The rash takes 2–4 weeks to resolve naturally without treatment (Amer & Fischer, 2006).

In contrast, irritant contact dermatitis is a discrete area of redness that corresponds to the exposure location. The rash usually develops within a few hours of contact, peaks within 24 hours, and quickly resolves with removal of the irritant. Reactions to irritants include painful erythema, edema, vesiculation, dryness of the skin, scaling, fissuring, and necrosis.

The distribution of the lesions provides clues about the source and identity of the allergen or irritant (Table 12–7). The diagnosis is often based on the manifestations of the disorder and a history of exposure to a known allergen. Scratch tests and intradermal tests are used to identify a specific allergen.

TABLE 12–7 Distribution of Lesions by Type of Allergen

DISTRIBUTION OF LESION	ALLERGEN
Face, eyelids	Cosmetics, skin care products, nail cosmetics
Earlobes, neck	Nickel, fragrances
Lips, mouth	Oral hygiene products, gum, lipstick
Dorsal aspects of toes and feet	Rubber or leather chemical in shoes
Trunk	Snaps on pants, moisturizers, cleansers, sunscreens

Source: Adapted from Timm-Knudson, V. L., Johnson, J. S., Ortiz, K. J., & Yiannias, J. A. (2006). Allergic contact dermatitis to preservatives. *Dermatology Nursing, 18*(2), 130–136.

Patch testing, in which an adhesive patch with common allergens is placed on the back between the scapulae, may be used to identify the allergen.

PRACTICE ALERT

The patch for allergy testing stays on for 48–72 hours, and the client is not permitted to shower or exercise to the point of perspiring while the patch is in place. If severe pruritus develops, the health care provider should be contacted to remove the patch early to prevent skin sloughing (Mark & Slavin, 2006).

Treatment involves removing the offending agent (e.g., clothes, plant, soap). Calamine lotion can be applied to the affected skin. Cool compresses with aluminum acetate (Burow's solution) promote drying. Wet dressings or colloidal oatmeal soaks relieve itching. Antihistamines may be given to reduce itching or for a sedative effect when the itching makes the client too uncomfortable to sleep.

Acute allergic contact dermatitis is managed with medium-potency topical corticosteroids when less than 10% of the body surface area is affected; however, this topical medication should not be applied to open lesions. The topical corticosteroids limit the production of cytokines, stop lymphocyte proliferation, and limit the inflammatory response to the allergens. The topical corticosteroid is applied to the affected area twice a day for 2–3 weeks. Stopping the treatment too soon can cause rebound dermatitis. Reactions to poison ivy or other allergens covering more than 10% of the body surface area require treatment with oral corticosteroids for 7–10 days and a tapered dose over another 7–10 days. An antibiotic may be required if the area becomes infected (Table 12–8).

TABLE 12–8 Medications Used to Treat Skin Disorders

TYPE	USE	EXAMPLES
Creams	Moisturize the skin	Aquacare Curel Nutraderm
Ointments	Lubricate the skin Retard water loss	Aquaphor Vaseline
Lotions	Moisturize the skin Lubricate the skin	Alpha-Keri Dermassage Lubriderm
Anesthetics	Relieve itching	Xylocaine
Antibiotics	Treat infection	Bacitracin Polysporin Gentamicin Silvadene
Corticosteroids	Suppress inflammation Relieve itching	Dexamethasone Hydrocortisone Clocortolone Desonide

Source: LeMone, P., & Burke, K. (2008). *Medical-surgical nursing: Critical thinking in client care* (4th ed., p. 441). Upper Saddle River, NJ: Pearson Education.

NURSING PROCESS

Assessment

A health assessment interview for a condition such as contact dermatitis focuses on a chief complaint (e.g., itching or a rash). If the client has a skin problem, the nurse analyzes its onset, characteristics and course, severity, and precipitating and relieving factors; the nurse also notes the timing and circumstances of any associated symptoms. The following are specific questions to ask the client:

- What type of itching have you experienced? When did it begin?
- Have you changed any household products lately? Have you changed any personal products lately, such as soap?
- Have you been anywhere unusual, for example, hiking in a new place?
- Do you have any allergies? Have you been in contact with anything to which you are allergic?

Ask about any change in health, rashes, itching, color changes, and the presence of lesions. Possible precipitating causes, such as medications, the use of new soaps and detergents, skin care agents, cosmetics, pets, travel, stress, or dietary changes should be explored.

The examination should be conducted in a warm, private room. The client removes all clothing and puts on a gown or drape. Fully expose the area to be examined, but protect the client's modesty by keeping other areas covered. The client may be standing, sitting, or lying down at various times in the examination. Wear disposable gloves when palpating open lesions, skin surfaces that are suggestive of infections or infestations, or discharge from lesions of the skin and mucous membranes. Adhere to standard precautions when conducting a skin assessment. Use a ruler to measure the size of the lesions and a flashlight to help examine them.

Diagnosis

Possible nursing diagnoses for the client with contact dermatitis may include the following:

- Impaired Skin Integrity related to contact dermatitis as evidenced by pruritus and rash
- Deficient Knowledge

Planning

Client education for home care management focuses on care of the skin, treatment of the current manifestation, and prevention of future exposures. Teaching the client how to avoid exposure to the allergen or irritant is an important nursing role.

Implementation

Nursing care of the client with contact dermatitis focuses primarily on providing information for self-care at home. The client is responsible for managing skin problems and requires education and support. The nurse should address the following topics:

- Medications and treatments do not cure the disease; they only relieve the symptoms. Caution clients that using oatmeal soaks will make the tub slippery. Advise them to pat themselves dry to leave the oatmeal film in place. Wet dressings may be soothing and can help to loosen crusts. Applying Burow's or Domeboro solution to blistered or oozing lesions for 20 minutes daily helps dry lesions (Allen, 2004). Familiarize clients with the symptoms of infection in the affected area (e.g., increased redness, oozing, fever), and tell them when to return for follow-up care.
- Dry skin increases pruritus, which stimulates scratching. Scratching may in turn cause excoriation, which increases the risk of infection.
- It may be necessary to change the diet or environment to avoid contact with allergens. If a nickel allergy exists, make sure nickel jewelry and belt buckles are not used.
- Remove clothing worn after outside activities where suspected allergens may be present, and shower immediately after those activities.
- Wash all clothes before the first wearing, and rinse clothes an extra time to remove all soap. Mild soap should be used to clean the skin.
- Place a barrier between the allergen and the skin. For example, cover all metal snaps on clothing with cloth, and wear socks to avoid exposure to tanning chemicals left on shoe leather. If barriers do not reduce the dermatitis, then it may be necessary to try to find clothing without nickel or shoes with specific tanning chemicals.
- Apply topical corticosteroids, and keep using the ointment for 2–3 weeks, even when the skin shows signs of healing. When using steroid preparations, apply only a thin layer to

---

CLIENT TEACHING   How to Reduce Dry Skin and Relieve Pruritus

- Wash clothing in a mild detergent and rinse twice; do not use fabric softeners.
- Avoid using perfumes and lotions containing alcohol.
- Apply skin lubricants after a bath to help retain moisture.
- Because soaps and hot water are drying, clean the skin with tepid water and either a mild soap or cleansing creams. If soap is used, rinse it off carefully.
- It is not necessary to take a bath every day.
- If bath oils are used, add them to the bath water at the end of the bath (the moist skin is more likely to retain the oil). Bath oils make the tub surface slippery, so they may be contraindicated for use by clients with poor balance or who are already at risk for falls.

- Use a humidifier to humidify the air.
- Apply creams and lotions when the skin is slightly damp after bathing.
- Increase fluid intake.
- Keep nails trimmed short, wear loose clothing, and keep the environment cool.
- A brief application of pressure or cold may relieve pruritus.
- Cotton gloves may be worn at night if scratching during sleep causes skin excoriation.
- Distraction or relaxation techniques may prove helpful.

Source: LeMone, P., & Burke, K. (2008). *Medical-surgical nursing: Critical thinking in client care* (4th ed., p. 441). Upper Saddle River, NJ: Pearson Education.

slightly damp skin (e.g., after taking a bath). If using oral corticosteroids, never stop taking the medication abruptly. Follow instructions to taper the dosage gradually.

- If occlusive dressings are necessary, a plastic suit may be used.
- Antihistamines cause drowsiness. When using these medications, avoid alcohol and use caution when driving or working around machinery.

See Client Teaching: How to Relieve Reduce Dry Skin and Relieve Pruritus for suggestions on how to avoid drying of skin and how to relieve pruritus.

Evaluation

Expected outcomes of nursing care include the following:
- Control of the dermatitis is maintained, and no infection occurs.

- Triggers are identified and eliminated.
- The client's sleep is minimally disturbed by itching.

COLLABORATION

Collaborative care may be required for the client who experiences repeated episodes of contact dermatitis. For example, if a client is exposed to irritants at work, the nurse may need to encourage the client to speak with his or her employer or to contact an organization that provides training in OSHA regulations. A client who has repeated episodes due to allergy may need to be referred to an allergist for further testing and evaluation. A nurse working with a school-age child might want to speak with the school nurse or the child's classroom teacher to ensure that follow-up care is maintained at school and that the child is adequately hydrated.

REVIEW Contact Dermatitis

RELATE: LINK THE CONCEPTS

Mrs. Henderson comes to the urgent care clinic. She rolls up her sleeves. The skin on her forearms is red and inflamed, with some darker red patches. Mrs. Henderson tells the nurse that she and her husband recently moved into their new home. She was outside the day before, trimming bushes and weeding. Mrs. Henderson says that she wore gloves, a short-sleeve shirt, and jeans while working in the yard.

Linking the concepts of Immunity and Infection with the concept of Tissue Integrity:

1. What assessment questions should the nurse ask Mrs. Henderson?
2. What are some possible NANDA diagnoses that the nurse could make?
3. On the basis of your answers to questions 1 and 2, what treatments would you suggest? Under what circumstances would treatment that includes an oral antibiotic be warranted?

READY: GO TO COMPANION SKILLS MANUAL

1. Aseptic technique
2. Applying dressings
3. Administering topical medication

REFLECT: CASE STUDY

A 21-year-old female college student reported "an itchy rash" on the right side of her face. Examination revealed erythema, vesicles, and pruritus below her ear. Testing revealed a reaction to nickel. However, the client wore no nickel items. During the course of the assessment, the client took three calls on a cell phone; placement of the phone covered the rash.

1. Is it possible that the cell phone cause the reaction? Explain.
2. What kind of testing would determine a nickel allergy?
3. What can the client do to avoid further episodes?

12.2 PRESSURE ULCERS

KEY TERMS

Debridement, *370*
Eschar, *362*
Excoriation, *361*
Immobility, *361*
Maceration, *361*
Necrosis, *361*
Pressure ulcers, *361*
Shearing forces, *361*

BASIS FOR SELECTION OF EXEMPLAR

Institute of Medicine (IOM)

LEARNING OUTCOMES

After learning about this exemplar, you will be able to do the following:

1. Describe the pathophysiology, etiology, clinical manifestations, and direct and indirect causes of pressure ulcers.
2. Identify risk factors associated with pressure ulcers.
3. Illustrate the nursing process in providing culturally competent care across the life span for individuals with pressure ulcers.
4. Formulate priority nursing diagnoses appropriate for an individual with pressure ulcers.
5. Create a plan of care for individuals with pressure ulcers that includes family members.
6. Assess expected outcomes for an individual with pressure ulcers.
7. Discuss therapies used in the collaborative care of an individual with pressure ulcers.
8. Use evidence-based care (or prevention) for an individual with pressure ulcers.

OVERVIEW

Pressure ulcers are ischemic lesions of the skin and underlying tissue caused by external pressure that impairs the flow of blood and lymph (Porth, 2005). The ischemia causes tissue **necrosis** (dead tissue) and eventual ulceration. These ulcers, also called bedsores or decubitus ulcers, tend to develop over a bony prominence (such as the heels, greater trochanter, sacrum, and ischia), but they may appear on the skin of any part of the body that is subjected to external pressure, friction, or shearing forces.

The incidence of pressure ulcers in hospitals, long-term care facilities, and home settings is high enough to warrant concern among health care providers. The incidence in hospitals has been reported to be as high as 8%, whereas the incidence in long-term care facilities is reported to range from 2.4–23% (Porth, 2005). Little research has been done to determine the extent of the problem in the home setting. However, with increasing numbers of clients (and especially older adult clients) being cared for in the home, it is probable that the incidence is great enough to warrant plans of care to prevent their occurrence.

PATHOPHYSIOLOGY AND ETIOLOGY

Pressure ulcers develop from external pressure that compresses blood vessels or from friction and shearing forces that tear and injure vessels. Both types of pressure cause traumatic injury and initiate the process of pressure ulcer development.

External pressure that is greater than capillary pressure and arteriolar pressure interrupts blood flow in capillary beds. When pressure is applied to skin over a bony prominence for 2 hours, tissue ischemia and hypoxia from external pressure cause irreversible tissue damage. For example, when the body is in the supine position, the body's weight applies pressure to the sacrum. A given amount of pressure causes more damage when it is applied to a small area than when it is distributed over a large surface.

Shearing forces result when one tissue layer slides over another. The stretching and bending of blood vessels cause injury and thrombosis. Clients in hospital beds are subject to shearing forces when the head of the bed is elevated and the torso slides down toward the foot of the bed. Pulling the client up in bed also subjects the client to shearing forces. (For this reason, always lift clients up in bed instead of pulling.) In both cases, friction and moisture cause the skin and superficial fascia to remain fixed to the bedsheet, while the deep fascia and bony skeleton slides in the direction of body movement.

When a person lies or sits in one position for an extended length of time without moving, pressure on the tissue between a bony prominence and the external surface of the body distorts capillaries and interferes with normal blood flow. If the pressure is relieved, blood flow to the area increases, and a brief period of reactive hyperemia occurs without permanent damage. If the pressure continues, platelets aggregate in the endothelial cells surrounding the capillaries and form microthrombi. These microthrombi impede blood flow, resulting in ischemia and

hypoxia of tissues. Eventually, the cells and tissues of the immediate area of pressure and of the surrounding area die and become necrotic.

Alterations in the involved tissue depend on the depth of the injury. Injury to superficial layers of skin results in blister formation; injury to deeper structures causes the pressure ulcer area to appear dark reddish-blue. As the tissues die, the ulcer becomes an open wound that may be deep enough to expose the bone. The necrotic tissue elicits an inflammatory response, and the client experiences increases in temperature, pain, and white blood cell count. Secondary bacterial invasion is common. Enzymes from bacteria and macrophages dissolve necrotic tissue, resulting in a foul-smelling drainage.

Risk Factors

Although a pressure ulcer may develop in any adult who has impaired mobility, those who are most at risk are older adults with limited mobility, people with quadriplegia, and clients in the critical care setting (Porth, 2005).

Several factors contribute to the formation of pressure ulcers: immobility and inactivity, inadequate nutrition, fecal and urinary incontinence, decreased mental status, diminished sensation, excessive body heat, advanced age, and the presence of certain chronic conditions.

IMMOBILITY **Immobility** refers to a reduction in the amount and control of a person's movement. Normally, people move when they experience discomfort from pressure on an area of the body. Healthy people rarely exceed their tolerance to pressure. However, paralysis, extreme weakness, pain, or any cause of decreased activity can hinder a person's ability to change positions independently and relieve the pressure, even if the person can perceive the pressure.

INADEQUATE NUTRITION Prolonged inadequate nutrition causes weight loss, muscle atrophy, and the loss of subcutaneous tissue. These reduce the amount of padding between the skin and the bones, thus increasing the risk of pressure ulcer development. More specifically, inadequate intake of protein, carbohydrates, fluids, zinc, and vitamin C contributes to pressure ulcer formation.

Hypoproteinemia (abnormally low protein content in the blood), due to either inadequate intake or abnormal loss, predisposes the client to dependent edema. Edema (swelling caused by excess fluid trapped in bodily tissue) makes skin more prone to injury by decreasing its elasticity, resilience, and vitality. Edema increases the distance between the capillaries and the cells, thereby slowing the diffusion of oxygen to the tissue cells and of metabolites away from the cells.

FECAL AND URINARY INCONTINENCE Moisture from incontinence promotes skin **maceration** (tissues softened by prolonged wetting or soaking) and makes the epidermis more easily eroded and susceptible to injury. Digestive enzymes in feces, gastric tube drainage, and urea in urine also contribute to skin **excoriation** (area of loss of the superficial layers of the skin also known as *denuded* area). Any accumulation of secretions or excretions is irritating to the skin, harbors microorganisms, and makes the skin prone to breakdown and infection.

DECREASED MENTAL STATUS Individuals with a reduced level of awareness, including those who are unconscious, heavily sedated, or have dementia, are at risk for pressure ulcers because they are less able to recognize and respond to pain associated with prolonged pressure.

DIMINISHED SENSATION Paralysis, stroke, or other neurologic disease may cause loss of sensation in a body area. Loss of sensation reduces a person's ability to respond to trauma, to injurious heat and cold, and to the tingling ("pins and needles") that signals loss of circulation. Sensory loss also impairs the body's ability to recognize and provide healing mechanisms for a wound.

EXCESSIVE BODY HEAT Body heat is another factor in the development of pressure ulcers. An elevated body temperature increases the metabolic rate, thus increasing the cells' need for oxygen. This increased need is particularly severe in the cells of an area under pressure, which are already oxygen deficient. Severe infections with accompanying elevated body temperatures may affect the body's ability to deal with the effects of tissue compression.

ADVANCED AGE The aging process brings about several changes in the skin and its supporting structures, making the older person more prone to impaired skin integrity. These changes include the following:

- Loss of lean body mass
- Generalized thinning of the epidermis
- Decreased strength and elasticity of the skin due to changes in the collagen fibers of the dermis
- Increased dryness due to a decrease in the amount of oil produced by the sebaceous glands

- Diminished pain perception due to a reduction in the number of cutaneous end organs responsible for the sensation of pressure and light touch
- Diminished venous and arterial flow due to aging vascular walls

CHRONIC MEDICAL CONDITIONS Certain chronic conditions such as diabetes and cardiovascular disease are risk factors for skin breakdown and delayed healing. These conditions compromise oxygen delivery to tissues, resulting in poor and delayed healing and increase risk of pressure sores.

OTHER FACTORS Other factors contributing to the formation of pressure ulcers are poor lifting and transferring techniques, incorrect positioning, hard support surfaces, and incorrect application of pressure-relieving devices.

Clinical Manifestations and Therapies

Pressure ulcers are graded or staged to classify the degree of damage. The stages are listed in Box 12–3. Diagnostic tests are conducted to determine the presence of a secondary infection and to differentiate the cause of the ulcer. If the ulcer is deep or appears infected, drainage or biopsied tissue is cultured to determine the causative organism.

Topical and systemic antibiotics specific to the infectious organism eradicate any infection present. Additionally, a variety of topical products promote healing. Examples are listed in Table 12–9.

Surgical debridement may be necessary if the pressure ulcer is deep, if subcutaneous tissues are involved, or if an **eschar** (a scab or dry crust consisting of dried plasma proteins and dead cells that forms over skin damaged by burns, infections, or excoriations) has formed over the ulcer, preventing healing by granulation. Large wounds may require skin grafting for complete closure.

TABLE 12–9 Products Used to Treat Pressure Ulcers

STAGE	PRODUCT	PURPOSE
I	Skin Prep	Toughens intact skin and preserves skin integrity.
	Granulex	Prevents skin breakdown, increases blood supply, adds moisture, contains trypsin to aid in removal of necrotic tissue.
	Hydrocolloid dressing (e.g., DuoDerm)	Prevents skin breakdown and promotes healing without the formation of a crust over the ulcer; is permeable to air and water vapor; prevents the growth of anaerobic organisms.
	Transparent dressing (e.g., Tegaderm)	Prevents skin breakdown; prevents entrance of moisture and bacteria but allows oxygen and moisture vapor permeability.
II	Transparent dressing	Enhances healing (see transparent dressing in stage I).
	Hydrocolloid dressing	Enhances healing (see hydrocolloid dressing in stage I). (*Note:* If infection is present, these types of dressings are contraindicated. A sterile dressing should be applied instead.)
III	Wet-to-dry gauze dressing with sterile normal saline	Allows necrotic material to soften and adhere to the gauze, so that the wound is debrided.
	Hydrocolloid dressing	Enhances healing (see above).
	Proteolytic enzymes (such as Elase)	Serve as debriding agents in inflamed and infected lesions.
IV	Wet-to-dry gauze dressing with sterile normal saline	Enhances healing (see above). (*Note:* Transparent or hydrocolloid dressings or skin barriers are contraindicated.
	Vacuum-assisted closure (V.A.C.)	Creates a negative pressure to help reduce edema, increase blood supply and oxygenation, and decrease bacterial colonization; it also helps promote moist wound healing and the formation of granulation tissue.

Source: LeMone, P., & Burke, K. (2008). *Medical-surgical nursing: Critical thinking in client care* (4th ed., p. 474). Upper Saddle River, NJ: Pearson Education.

Box 12–3 **Pressure Ulcer Staging**

STAGE I

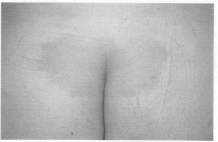

Nonblanchable erythema of intact skin; the heralding lesion of skin ulceration. Identification of stage I pressure ulcers may be difficult in clients with darkly pigmented skin.

Note: Reactive hyperemia can normally be expected to be present for one-half to three-fourths as long as the pressure occluded blood flow to the area. This should not be confused with stage I pressure ulcer.

STAGE II

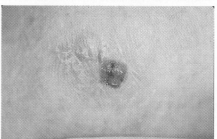

Partial-thickness skin loss involving epidermis and/or dermis. The ulcer is superficial and presents clinically as an abrasion, blister, or shallow crater.

STAGE III

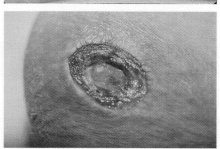

Full-thickness skin loss involving damage or necrosis of subcutaneous tissue that may extend down to, but not through, underlying fascia. The ulcer presents clinically as a deep crater with or without undermining of adjacent tissue.

STAGE IV

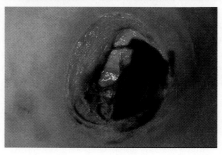

Full-thickness skin loss with extensive destruction, tissue necrosis, or damage to muscle, bone, or supporting structures (for example, tendon or joint capsule). Sinus tracts may also be associated with stage IV ulcers.

Note: When eschar is present, accurate staging of the pressure ulcer is not possible until the eschar has sloughed or the wound has been debrided.

Source: Text is from *Pressure Ulcers in Adults: Prediction and Prevention* by the Agency for Health Care Policy and Research, 1992 Rockville, MD: U.S. Department of Health and Human Services. Photos courtesy of Karen Lou Kennedy, RN, FPN, www.kennedyterminalulcer.com.

NURSING PROCESS

Prevention is the goal for the client at risk for pressure ulcers. The client with one or more pressure ulcers not only has impaired skin integrity, but also is at increased risk for infection, pain, and decreased mobility. Pressure ulcers prolong treatment for other health problems, increase health care costs, and diminish the client's quality of life.

Assessment

Ensure that the lighting is good; natural or fluorescent lighting is preferable, because incandescent lights can create a transilluminating effect. Regulate the environment before beginning the assessment so that the room is neither too hot nor too cold. Heat can cause the skin to flush; cold can cause the skin to blanch or become cyanotic.

Inspect pressure areas for discoloration, which can result from impaired blood circulation to the area. The pressure areas should have brisk capillary refill or blanch response when gently palpated with the end of a finger or thumb.

Inspect pressure areas for abrasions and excoriations (Figure 12–5 ■). An abrasion can occur when skin rubs against a sheet (e.g., when the client is pulled). Excoriations can occur when the skin has prolonged contact with body secretions or excretions or with dampness in skin folds.

Palpate the surface temperature of the skin over the pressure areas (warm hands first). Normally, the temperature is the same as that of the surrounding skin. Increased temperature is abnormal and may be due to inflammation or blood trapped in the area. Palpate over bony prominences and dependent body areas for the presence of edema, which feels spongy or boggy. If a pressure ulcer is open or visibly infected, wear gloves during the examination.

If a pressure ulcer is present, the nurse notes the following:

- Location of the ulcer, related to a bony prominence
- Size of ulcer in centimeters (Measure length, width, and depth, beginning with length [head to toe] and then width [side to side]. To measure depth, insert a sterile applicator swab at the deepest part of the wound, and then measure it against a measuring guide.)
- Presence of undermining or sinus tracts, assessed as face on a clock, where 12 o'clock is the client's head
- Stage of the ulcer (see Box 12–3)
- Color of the wound bed and location of necrosis or eschar
- Condition of the wound margins
- Integrity of surrounding skin

- Clinical signs of infection, such as redness, warmth, swelling, pain, odor, and exudate (note color of exudate)
- Client complaints of pain or discomfort at the wound site
- Signs of infection such as fever, chills, or elevated white blood cell count (WBC)

Document the status of the client's skin and wounds on the standard agency form. It is important to be able to determine how these change over time.

Several risk assessment tools are available that provide the nurse with systematic means of identifying clients at high risk for pressure ulcer development. The Panel for the Prediction and Prevention of Pressure Ulcers in Adults (PPPPUA, 1992a) has recommended that the tools include data collection in the areas of immobility, incontinence, nutrition, and level of consciousness.

In 1987, Bergstrom, Braden, Laguzza, and Holman published the Braden Scale for Predicting Pressure Sore Risk. Their scale consists of six subscales: sensory perception, moisture, activity, mobility, nutrition, and friction and shear (Figure 12–6 ■). A total of 23 points is possible. An adult who scores below 18 points is considered at risk (Folkedahl & Frantz, 2002b). For best results, nurses should be trained in proper use of the scale.

CARE SETTINGS **Assessing Common Pressure Sites**

- Ensure the lighting is good, preferably natural or fluorescent, because incandescent lights can create a transilluminating effect.
- Regulate the environment before beginning the assessment so that the room is neither too hot nor too cold. Heat can cause the skin to flush; cold can cause the skin to blanch or become cyanotic.
- Inspect pressure areas (see Figure 12–5) for discoloration. This can be caused by impaired blood circulation to the area. The pressure areas should have brisk capillary refill or blanch response when gently palpated with the end of a finger or thumb.

- Inspect pressure areas for abrasions and excoriations. An abrasion can occur when skin rubs against a sheet (e.g., when the client is pulled). Excoriations can occur when the skin has prolonged contact with body secretions or excretions or with dampness in skin folds.
- Palpate the surface temperature of the skin over the pressure areas (warm your hands first). Normally, the temperature is the same as that of the surrounding skin. Increased temperature is abnormal and may be due to inflammation or blood trapped in the area.
- Palpate over bony prominences and dependent body areas for the presence of edema, which feels spongy or boggy.

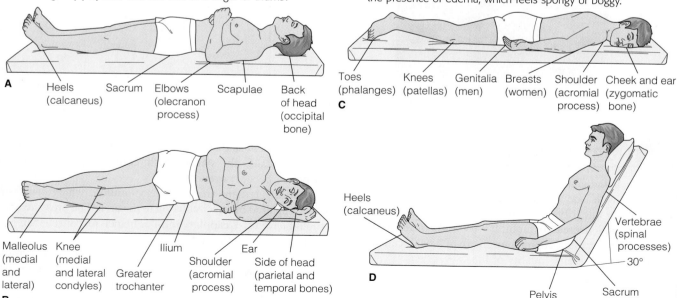

Figure 12–5 ■ Body pressure areas in *A,* supine position; *B,* lateral position; *C,* prone position; *D,* Fowler's position.

BRADEN SCALE FOR PREDICTING PRESSURE SORE RISK

Patient's Name _____ Evaluator's Name _____ Date of Assessment

	1	2	3	4
SENSORY PERCEPTION Ability to respond meaningfully to pressure-related discomfort	**1. Completely Limited:** Unresponsive (does not moan, flinch, or grasp) to painful stimuli, due to diminished level of consciousness or sedation. OR limited ability to feel pain over most of body surface.	**2. Very Limited:** Responds only to painful stimuli. Cannot communicate discomfort except by moaning or restlessness, OR has a sensory impairment which limits the ability to feel pain or discomfort over 1/2 of body.	**3. Slightly Limited:** Responds to verbal commands but cannot always communicate discomfort or need to be turned, OR has some sensory impairment which limits ability to feel pain or discomfort in 1 or 2 extremities.	**4. No Impairment:** Responds to verbal commands. Has no sensory deficit which would limit ability to feel or voice pain or discomfort.
MOISTURE Degree to which skin is exposed to moisture	**1. Constantly Moist:** Skin is kept moist almost constantly by perspiration, urine, etc. Dampness is detected every time patient is moved or turned.	**2. Moist:** Skin is often but not always moist. Linen must be changed at least once a shift.	**3. Occasionally Moist:** Skin is occasionally moist, requiring an extra linen change approximately once a day.	**4. Rarely Moist:** Skin is usually dry; linen requires changing only at routine intervals.
ACTIVITY Degree of physical activity	**1. Bedfast:** Confined to bed.	**2. Chairfast:** Ability to walk severely limited or nonexistent. Cannot bear own weight and/or must be assisted into chair or wheelchair.	**3. Walks Occasionally:** Walks occasionally during day but for very short distances, with or without assistance. Spends majority of each shift in bed or chair.	**4. Walks Frequently:** Walks outside the room at least twice a day and inside room at least once every 2 hours during waking hours.
MOBILITY Ability to change and control body position	**1. Completely Immobile:** Does not make even slight changes in body or extremity position without assistance.	**2. Very Limited:** Makes occasional slight changes in body or extremity position but unable to make frequent or significant changes independently.	**3. Slightly Limited:** Makes frequent though slight changes in body or extremity position independently.	**4. No Limitations:** Makes major and frequent changes in position without assistance.
NUTRITION Usual food intake pattern	**1. Very Poor:** Never eats a complete meal. Rarely eats more than 1/3 of any food offered. Eats 2 servings or less of protein (meat or dairy products) per day. Takes fluids poorly. Does not take a liquid dietary supplement, OR is NPO and/or maintained on clear liquids or IV's for more than 5 days.	**2. Probably Inadequate:** Rarely eats a complete meal and generally eats only about 1/2 of any food offered. Protein intake includes only 3 servings of meat or dairy products per day. Occasionally will take a dietary supplement, OR receives less than optimum amount of liquid diet or tube feeding.	**3. Adequate:** Eats over half of most meals. Eats a total of 4 servings of protein (meat, dairy products) each day. Occasionally will refuse a meal, but will usually take a supplement if offered, OR is on a tube feeding or TPN regimen, which probably meets most of nutritional needs.	**4. Excellent:** Eats most of every meal. Never refuses a meal. Usually eats a total of 4 or more servings of meat and dairy products. Occasionally eats between meals. Does not require supplementation.
FRICTION AND SHEAR	**1. Problem:** Requires moderate to maximum assistance in moving. Complete lifting without sliding against sheets is impossible. Frequently slides down in bed or chair, requiring frequent repositioning with maximum assistance. Spasticity, contractures, or agitation leads to almost constant friction.	**2. Potential Problem:** Moves feebly or requires minimum assistance. During a move skin probably slides to some extent against sheets, chair, restraints, or other devices. Maintains relatively good position in chair or bed most of the time but occasionally slides down.	**3. No Apparent Problem:** Moves in bed and in chair independently and has sufficient muscle strength to lift up completely during move. Maintains good position in bed or chair at all times.	

Total Score

Figure 12–6 ■ Braden Scale for Predicting Pressure Sore Risk.

Source: Clinical Practice Guideline, Pressure Ulcers in Adults: Prediction and Prevention, by U.S. Department of Health and Human Services, PPPPUA Pub No. 92-0047, pp. 16–17, 1992, Rockville, MD: Public Health Service. Copyright © Barbara Braden and Nancy Bergstrom, 1988. Reprinted with permission.

Norton's Pressure Area Risk Assessment Form Scale includes the categories of general physical condition, mental state, activity, mobility, and incontinence. A category of medications was added in 1987, resulting in a possible score of 24. Scores of 15 or 16 should be viewed as indicators, not predictors, of risk. The Braden and Norton tools should be used when the client first enters the health care agency and whenever the client's condition changes. In some long-term care facilities, a risk assessment scale such as the Braden or Norton scale is used on admission and then on a regular basis, usually weekly. This increases awareness of specific risk factors and provides assessment data to use in planning goals and interventions to either maintain or improve skin integrity.

Diagnoses

The following NANDA diagnoses may be appropriate for the client with a pressure ulcer:

- Risk for Impaired Skin Integrity
- Impaired Skin Integrity
- Risk for Infection
- Imbalanced Nutrition: Less than Body Requirements
- Risk for Compromised Human Dignity
- Situational Low Self-Esteem

Planning

Outcomes to be developed in collaboration with the client and caregivers include the following:

- Client who is immobile or on bed rest will be repositioned every two hours. Appropriate positioning devices may be used.
- Client who is mobile will maintain or improve activity levels.
- Client will report any alterations such as changes in pain level, redness, numbness, tingling, or increased drainage.
- Client will articulate the importance of maintaining adequate nutrition and hydration.
- Client will describe measures to protect and heal tissue.

Implementation

Risk for Impaired Skin Integrity / Impaired Skin Integrity

In order to assist the client at risk for or with Impaired Skin Integrity, the nurse should consider the following:

- *Conduct a systematic skin inspection at least once a day, paying particular attention to the bony prominences. Systematic, comprehensive, and routine skin care may decrease pressure ulcer incidence (although the exact role is unknown).* Skin inspection provides data the nurse uses in designing interventions to reduce risk and in evaluating outcomes of those interventions.
- *Clean the skin at the time of soiling and at routine intervals, as frequently as the client's need or preference dictates. Avoid hot water, use a mild cleansing agent, and clean the skin gently, applying as little force and friction as possible.* Metabolic wastes and environmental contaminants accumulate on the skin; these potentially irritating substances should be removed frequently. Feces and urine cause chemical irritation and should be removed as soon as possible. Hot water may cause skin injury. Mild cleansing agents are less likely to remove the skin's natural barrier.
- *Minimize environmental factors leading to skin drying, such as low humidity and exposure to cold. Treat dry skin with moisturizers.* Well-hydrated skin resists mechanical trauma. Hydration decreases as the ambient air temperature decreases, especially when the air humidity is low. Poorly hydrated skin is less pliable, and severe dryness is associated with fissuring and cracking of the stratum corneum. Moisturizers reduce dry skin.
- *Avoid massage over bony prominences.* Although massage has been practiced for years, evidence now suggests that massage over bony prominences may lead to deep tissue trauma in clients at risk for, or with beginning, skin manifestations of a pressure ulcer.
- *Minimize skin exposure to moisture due to incontinence, perspiration, or wound drainage. When these sources of moisture cannot be controlled, use underpads or briefs made of materials that absorb moisture and present a quick-drying surface to the skin. Change underpads and briefs frequently. Do not place plastic directly against the skin.* Moisture from incontinence, perspiration, or wound drainage may contain factors that irritate the skin; moisture alone can increase the susceptibility of the skin to injury.
- *To minimize skin injury due to friction and shearing forces, use proper positioning, transferring, and turning techniques. Lubricants (such as cornstarch or creams), protective films (such as transparent dressings and skin sealants), protective dressings (such as hydrocolloids), and protective padding may also reduce friction injuries.* Shear injury occurs when skin remains stationary and the underlying tissue shifts. This shift diminishes the blood supply to the skin, resulting in ischemia and tissue damage. Proper positioning, however, can eliminate most shear injuries. Friction injuries occur when the skin moves across a coarse surface, such as bed linens. Most friction injuries can be avoided by using appropriate techniques to move clients so that their skin is never dragged across the linens. Any agent that eliminates contact or decreases the friction between the skin and the linens reduces the potential for injury.
- For the client who is immobile or on bedrest, provide interventions against the adverse effects of external mechanical forces of pressure, friction, and shear:
  a. Reposition all at-risk clients at least every 2 hours, using a written schedule for systematic turning and repositioning.
  b. For clients on bedrest, use positioning devices, such as pillows or foam wedges, to protect bony prominences.
- For completely immobile clients, use devices to totally relieve pressure on the heels (the most common method is to raise the heels off the bed). Do not use doughnut-type devices.
- Avoid placing clients in the side-lying position directly on the trochanter.
- Maintain the head of the bed at the lowest degree of elevation consistent with the client's medical condition and

other restrictions. Limit the amount of time the head of the bed is elevated.

- Use assistive devices, such as a trapeze or bed linen, to move clients in bed who cannot assist during transfers and position changes.
- *Place any at-risk client on a pressure-reducing device, such as foam, static air, alternating air, gel, or water mattress.* Data indicate that the more spontaneous movements that bedridden, older adult clients make, the lower the incidence of pressure ulcers. Studies reveal that fewer pressure ulcers develop in at-risk clients who are turned every 2–3 hours. Proper positioning can reduce pressure on bony prominences. It is difficult to redistribute pressure under heels; suspending the heels is the best method. Do not use doughnut cushions, which are more likely to cause than to prevent pressure ulcers. Shearing forces are exerted on the body when the head of the bed is elevated. Lifting (rather than dragging) is less likely to cause injury from friction. Pressure-reducing devices and beds can reduce the incidence of pressure ulcers.
- *For chair-bound clients, use pressure-reducing devices. Consider postural alignment, distribution of weight, balance and stability, and pressure relief when positioning these clients. Avoid uninterrupted sitting in a chair or wheelchair. Reposition the client every hour. Teach clients who can do so to shift their weight every 15 minutes. Use a written plan for positioning, movement, and the use of positioning devices. Do not use doughnut devices.* Prolonged, uninterrupted mechanical pressure results in tissue breakdown. The client's weight should be shifted at least every hour.

Risk for Infection

Untreated pressure ulcers can become infected quickly. The nurse working with a client who is at risk for pressure ulcers should teach the client to guard against infection by doing the following:

- Maintaining skin hygiene
- Maintaining appropriate nutrition and hydration
- Recognizing the early stages of a pressure ulcer
- Contacting the officer at the earliest appearance of a pressure ulcer or change in skin integrity
- Maintaining or improving current activity levels.

Imbalanced Nutrition: Less than Body Requirements

Although the role nutrition plays in the development of (and to a lesser degree, the healing of) pressure ulcers is not understood, poor dietary intake of kilocalories, protein, and iron has been associated with the development of pressure ulcers. The nurse should do the following:

- Assess factors involved in inadequate dietary intake of protein or kilocalories.
- Offer nutritional supplements, and support the client during mealtimes as necessary to insure adequate dietary intake.
- If dietary intake remains inadequate, consult with a dietitian about other dietary interventions.

Risk for Compromised Human Dignity / Situational Low Self-Esteem

The immobile or nearly immobile client is at the mercy of those caring for him or her. If family members or caregivers do not effect interventions necessary to inhibit the growth of pressure

---

EVIDENCE-BASED PRACTICE | Treating Pressure Ulcers

Despite advances in health care to extend life and improve functional status, older adults with chronic illnesses are at increased risk of developing pressure ulcers. The older adult, with age-related compromised cellular activity, is especially vulnerable to impaired healing of injured tissue, including pressure ulcers. Frantz (2004) describes an evidence-based protocol designed to enhance the healing of pressure ulcers in older clients by using evidence-based interventions. The following interventions are recommended:

- Assess all individuals admitted to a health care facility with a pressure ulcer for the risk of developing additional pressure ulcers by using a standardized risk assessment scale.
- Perform a complete history and physical examination, combined with a detailed assessment of the ulcer characteristics (location, stage, type of tissue, presence of tunneling or tracts, exudate, odor, and condition of skin around the ulcer).
- Remove necrotic tissue and debris from the ulcer to decrease the growth of bacteria. Remove foreign materials, such as exudates and metabolic wastes.
- Provide a moist wound environment to promote reepithelialization and healing.
- Control bacterial levels in the wound by using cleansing and debridement, as well as systemic and topical antibiotics.
- Supply essential substrates for tissue repair, including protein, calories, vitamins, and minerals. Maintain a positive nitrogen balance.

- Manage tissue loads by positioning to avoid external force on the ulcer.

Implications for Nursing

The design and implementation of a pressure ulcer prevention and treatment plan is essential for any person at risk, including older adults, those with debilitating or multiple illnesses, and those with health problems limiting mobility. To implement a plan effectively, it is important to prepare providers to use a standard protocol, and to monitor indicators of improvement or deterioration in the ulcer and presence or absence of new ulcers. These outcomes should be assessed and recorded on a weekly basis.

Critical Thinking in Client Care

1. Consider the activities to treat pressure ulcers. What would you do about the following:
   a. What level of health care provider would you delegate to care for the client?
   b. How much time in an 8-hour period would be needed for nursing care?
   c. What would you teach family caregivers about providing care at home?

Source: Franz, R. (2004). Treatment of pressure ulcers. *Journal of Gerontological Nursing, 30*(5), 4–10. Used with permission.

ulcers and maintain client hygiene, the client is at risk for compromised human dignity. This can effect a client's moods and perception of self, in turn putting the client at risk for situational low self-esteem. Depression can follow quickly. The nurse can assist the client in these areas by doing the following:

- Conducting a physical examination at each health care interaction that includes examining the client for indicators of abuse or neglect.
- Develop a caring, trusting relationship with the client so that you will be able to get him or her to discuss issues related to human dignity and self-esteem. Refer for counseling as appropriate.
- Teaching family members and caregivers the importance of repositioning the client every two hours and teaching them about skin hygiene and how to position the client properly.
- Assisting family members and caregivers with obtaining supportive devices to assist in maintaining appropriate positioning of the client.

Evaluation

For clients who are immobile or on bed rest, the treatment plan may need to be evaluated and modified as often as daily, depending on the assessment of the client's skin integrity, client comfort and pain level, and whether or not the written repositioning plan has been followed. Clients who are in bed for long periods of time can experienced diminished appetites. If a client is not maintaining adequate dietary intake even if changes to the nutrition plan have been made, the nurse may need to arrange to consult with a nutritionist or dietician. For clients who are mobile, the nurse should provide instructions when to call the office if there is another appearance of a potential pressure ulcer or change in skin integrity.

Preventing Pressure Ulcers

To reduce the likelihood of pressure ulcers developing in all clients, the nurse employs a variety of preventive measures (i.e., skin hygiene and pressure relief devices) to maintain the skin integrity and instructs the client, support people, and caregivers in how to prevent pressure ulcers.

PROVIDING NUTRITION Because an inadequate intake of calories, protein, vitamins, and iron is believed to be a risk factor for pressure ulcer development, nutritional supplements should be considered for nutritionally compromised clients. The diet should be similar to that which supports wound healing, as discussed earlier. The nurse should monitor weight regularly to help assess nutritional status. Pertinent lab work should also be monitored, including lymphocyte count, protein (especially albumin), and hemoglobin.

MAINTAINING SKIN HYGIENE The nurse should obtain baseline data using the established tool and then reassess the skin at least daily in the hospital and weekly at home. When bathing the client, the nurse should minimize the force and friction applied to the skin, using mild cleansing agents that minimize irritation and dryness and that do not disrupt the skin's "natural barriers." Also, the nurse should avoid using hot water, which increases skin dryness and irritation. Nurses can minimize dryness by avoiding exposure to cold and low humidity. Dry skin is best treated with moisturizing lotions applied while the skin is moist after bathing. The client's skin should be kept clean and dry and free of irritation and maceration by urine, feces, sweat, or incomplete drying after a bath. The nurse applies skin protection if indicated. Dimethicone-based creams or alcohol-free barrier films, which are available in liquid, spray, and moist wipe format, are very effective in preventing moisture or drainage from collecting on the skin. In most cases, the nurse can apply these without a primary care provider's order. Petroleum-based creams and ointments are no longer advised because of poor overall skin protection and interference with diaper/incontinence product absorption.

AVOIDING SKIN TRAUMA Providing the client with a smooth, firm, and wrinkle-free foundation on which to sit or lie helps prevent skin trauma. To prevent injury due to friction and shearing forces, clients must be positioned, transferred, and turned correctly. For bedridden clients, shearing force can be reduced by elevating the head of the bed to no more than 30 degrees, if this position is not contraindicated by the client's condition. (For example, clients with respiratory disorders may find it easier to breathe in Fowler's position.) When the head of the bed is raised, the skin and superficial fascia stick to the bed linen while the deep fascia and skeleton slide down toward the bottom of the bed. As a result, blood vessels in the sacral area become twisted, and the tissues in the area can become ischemic and necrotic. Baby powder and cornstarch are never used as friction or moisture prevention. These powders create harmful abrasive grit that is damaging to tissues and are considered a respiratory hazard when airborne. Instead, use moisturizing creams and protective films, such as transparent dressings and alcohol-free barrier films.

Frequent shifts in position, even if only slight, effectively change pressure points. The client who is able should shift weight 10–15 degrees every 15–30 minutes and, whenever possible, exercise or ambulate to stimulate blood circulation.

When lifting a client to change position, nurses should use a lifting device such as a trapeze rather than dragging the client across or up in bed. The friction that results from dragging the skin against a sheet can cause blisters and abrasions, which may contribute to more extensive tissue damage. Therefore, using devices that lift the client's weight off the bed surface is the method of choice. To deter shearing forces, the nurse should place a draw sheet that covers the bed from an individual's chest to buttocks and is folded to be wide enough to tuck under the mattress on either side when not in use.

Any at-risk client who is confined to bed—even when a special support mattress is used—should be repositioned at least every 2 hours, depending on the client's need, to allow another body surface to bear the weight. Six body positions can usually be used: prone, supine, right and left lateral (side-lying), and right and left Sims' positions. When a lateral position is used, the nurse should avoid positioning the client directly on the trochanter and should instead position the client on a 30-degree angle. A written schedule should be established for turning and repositioning.

PROVIDING SUPPORTIVE DEVICES For circulation to remain uncompromised, pressure on the bony prominences should remain below capillary pressure for as much time as possible through a combination of turning, positioning, and use of

NURSING CARE PLAN   The Client With a Pressure Ulcer

A registered nurse who works for a home health agency has been assigned to Mrs. Krebs, a 75-year-old client with a chronic stage III ulcer on her heel that has shown no progress in the last 3 months. The nurse notes that Mrs. Krebs has a smoking history of 40 pack years and has not followed her diet instruction. The supervisor of the home health agency has warned the nurse that if Mrs. Krebs does not improve, the insurance company will not continue to pay for the visits and treatment. Mrs. Krebs has refused to be admitted to the hospital for ulcer care and feels that the nurses and physician do not understand her situation.

ASSESSMENT

On the first visit, the nurse did a complete assessment and discussed the client's history, which includes peripheral vascular disease and hypertension. Mrs. Krebs's physical examination showed blood pressure 140/82 mmHg, pulse 76 beats/min, respirations 20 breaths/min, and temperature 98°F. On examination of the heel ulcer, the nurse noted a 4-cm by 6-cm stage III ulcer with a minimal amount of serous drainage and no local signs of inflammation.

Mrs. Krebs is eating poorly, mostly freezer and canned foods with little protein and high sodium. She admits that she is smoking and not following her diet. She states, "I lost my husband 6 months ago and have not been able to take care of things. I tried to quit smoking but it only lasted 5 days. I have been smoking for 40 years, and it is just too hard to stop. I'm doing the best I can."

DIAGNOSIS

The current nursing diagnoses for Mrs. Krebs include the following:
- *Impaired skin integrity:* stage III ulcer, related to prolonged pressure, inadequate nutrition, decreased vascular perfusion
- *Ineffective management of therapeutic regimen related to complex regimen:* limited resources and impaired adjustment as manifested by client self-assessment of poor dietary intake, inability to rest and elevate foot, and smoking behavior
- *Risk for altered nutrition—less than body requirements:* related to lack of physical and economic resources, and increased nutritional requirements related to ulcer

EXPECTED OUTCOMES

The expected outcomes for the plan specify that Mrs. Krebs will do the following:
- Describe measures to protect and heal the tissue, including wound care.
- Report any additional symptoms, such as pain, redness, numbness, tingling, or increased drainage.
- Demonstrate an understanding of nutritional needs, including the need for supplemental protein drink and vitamins.
- Collaborate with the nurse to develop a therapeutic plan that is congruent with her goals and present lifestyle.

PLANNING AND IMPLEMENTATION

The following nursing interventions may be appropriate for Mrs. Krebs:
- Establish a trusting relationship with Mrs. Krebs.
- Begin to explore what the client's goals are in relation to her health care.
- Determine her daily habits and schedule, and find some small measures that can be started for health improvement.
- Begin to determine ways to work with Mrs. Krebs's family to motivate her toward a healthier lifestyle (i.e., nutrition, smoking cessation, foot care).
- Set priorities of care that Mrs. Krebs will agree to, such as (1) ulcer improvement, (2) diet adjustments, and (3) smoking reductions.

EVALUATION

The nurse hopes to develop a long-term relationship with Mrs. Krebs and make an impact on her health and well-being. The nurse will consider the plan a success on the basis of the following criteria:
- Mrs. Krebs will develop a trusting relationship and develop a plan with the nurse to improve her health.
- A family member will agree to assist Mrs. Krebs with her wound care and shopping issues.
- Mrs. Krebs will begin a smoking reduction effort.
- Mrs. Krebs will agree that if the ulcer is not healing in 4 weeks, she will seek inpatient treatment.

CRITICAL THINKING AND THE NURSING PROCESS

1. What are the intrinsic and extrinsic factors that can cause skin problems in older adults? Make a list with two columns, and see how many factors you can identify.
2. How important is nutrition to the dermatologic health of your skin?
3. What type of dressings do you see used in your clinical rotations with older people? Are they consistent with current guidelines and recommendations?
4. What positioning techniques have you seen used in your clinical rotations?

pressure-relieving surfaces. Mean capillary pressure can be estimated at 20 mmHg, although this varies. Some research has evaluated the effectiveness of pressure-reducing support surfaces in preventing pressure ulcers in clients at low, intermediate, or high risk; however, the results have been inconclusive (Cullum, McInnes, Bell-Syer, & Legood, 2005). The nurse should review the manufacturer's product descriptions that report the amount of time that the pressure between the surface and the bony prominence is above or below specified levels and determine whether this is adequate to protect a particular client.

For clients who are confined to bed, three types of support surfaces can be used to relieve pressure:

1. The overlay mattress is applied on top of the standard bed mattress. Use a replacement mattress instead of the standard mattress; most are made of foam and gel combinations.
2. Specialty beds replace hospital beds. They provide pressure relief, eliminate shearing and friction, and reduce moisture. Examples are high-air-loss beds, low-air-loss beds, and beds that provide kinetic therapy.
3. Kinetic beds provide continuous passive motion or oscillation therapy, both of which are intended to counteract the effects of a client's immobility.

When a client is confined to bed or to a chair, pressure-reducing devices, such as pillows made of foam, gel, air, or a combination of these, can be used. When the client is sitting, weight should be distributed over the entire seating surface so that pressure does not center on just one area. To protect a client's heels in bed, supports such as wedges or pillows can be used to raise the heels completely off the bed. Doughnut-type devices should not be used, since they limit blood flow and can cause tissue damage to the areas in direct contact with the device. Table 12–10 lists mechanical devices for reducing pressure on body parts.

Treating Pressure Ulcers

Pressure ulcers are a challenge for nurses because of the number of variables involved (e.g., risk factors, types of ulcers, and degrees of impairment) and the numerous treatment measures advocated. Existing and potential infections are the most serious complications of pressure ulcers. In treating pressure ulcers, nurses should follow the agency protocols and the primary care provider's orders, if any. Prompt treatment can prevent further tissue damage and pain and facilitate wound healing. See Box 12–4 regarding treating pressure ulcers.

Some wounds are covered with thick necrotic tissue, or eschar. These wounds require **debridement** (removal of the necrotic material). Nonviable tissue must be removed from a wound before the wound can be staged or heal. There are four types of debridement: sharp, mechanical, chemical, and autolytic. In *sharp debridement*, a scalpel or scissors are used to separate and remove dead tissue. In many settings, specially trained nurses (wound ostomy continence nurses, or WOCNs), physical therapists, and physician's assistants are permitted to perform sharp debridement. *Mechanical debridement* is accomplished through scrubbing force or moist-to-moist dressings. *Chemical debridement* is more selective than sharp or mechanical techniques. Collagenase enzyme agents such as papain-urea are currently most often recommended for this use. In *autolytic debridement*, dressings that contain wound moisture, such as hydrocolloid and clear absorbent acrylic dressings, trap the wound drainage against the eschar. The body's own enzymes in the drainage break down the necrotic tissue. Although this method takes longer than the other three, it is the most selective and therefore causes the least damage to healthy surrounding and healing tissues. Recently, the use of fly larvae (maggots, *Phaenicia sericata*) has received increased attention. Larval therapy can be extremely effective in cleansing chronic wounds because the maggots secrete enzymes that break down

TABLE 12–10 Mechanical Devices for Reducing Pressure on Body Parts

DEVICE	DESCRIPTION/COMMENTS
Gel flotation pads	Polyvinyl, silicone, or Silastic™ pads filled with a gelatinous substance similar to fat
Pillows and wedges (foam, gel, air, fluid)	Support positioning and offloads bone on bone contact
Heel protectors (sheepskin boots, padded splints, off-loading inflatable boots, foam blocks)	Can raise or "float" a body part (e.g., heels) off the or surface; prevent shearing and limit pressure on heel area
Memory foam mattress/chair pad	Distributes weight over bony areas evenly; molds to the body
Alternating pressure mattress	Composed of a number of cells in which the pressure alternately increases and decreases; uses a pump
Water bed	Support surface filled with water; water temperature controllable
Static low-air-loss (LAL) bed	Consists of many air-filled cushions divided into four or five sections (Separate controls permit each section to be inflated to a different level of firmness; thus pressure can be reduced on bony prominences but increased under other body areas for support.)
Active or second-generation LAL bed	Like the static LAL but in addition gently pulsates or rotates from side to side, thus stimulating capillary blood flow and facilitating movement of pulmonary secretions
Air-fluidized (AF) bed (static high-air-loss bed)	Forced temperature-controlled air circulated around millions of tiny silicone-coated beads, producing a fluidlike movement; provides uniform support to body contours; decreases skin maceration by its drying effect (Moisture from the client penetrates the linens and soaks the beads. Air flow forces the beads away from the client and rapidly dries the sheet. A major disadvantage is that the head of the bed cannot be elevated. Some beds are a unique combination of air fluidized therapy and low-air-loss therapy on an articulating frame. These are used with clients who require head elevation.)

Source: Berman, A., Snyder, S. J., Kozier, B., & Erb, G. (2008). *Kozier & Erb's fundamentals of nursing: Concepts, process, and practice* (8th ed., p. 921). Upper Saddle River, NJ: Pearson Education.

Box 12–4 **Treating Pressure Ulcers**

- Minimize direct pressure on the ulcer. Reposition the client at least every 2 hours. Make a schedule, and record position changes on the client's chart. Provide devices to minimize or float pressure areas.
- Clean the pressure ulcer with every dressing change. The method of cleaning depends on the stage of the ulcer, products available, and agency protocol.
- Clean and dress the ulcer using surgical asepsis. Never use alcohol or hydrogen peroxide, as they are cytotoxic to tissue beds.
- If the pressure ulcer is infected, obtain a sample of the drainage to culture and test for sensitivity to antibiotic agents.
- Teach the client to move, even if only slightly, to relieve pressure.
- Provide range-of-motion (ROM) exercises and mobility out of bed as the client's condition permits.

Source: Berman, A., Snyder, S. J., Kozier, B., & Erb, G. (2008). *Kozier & Erb's fundamentals of nursing: Concepts, process, and practice* (8th ed., p. 920). Upper Saddle River, NJ: Pearson Education.

necrotic tissue (while leaving healthy tissue untouched), eat bacteria, and reduce bacterial growth by increasing surface pH that results from their presence (Sosin, 2005).

Evaluation

For clients who are immobile or on bed rest, the treatment plan may need to be evaluated and modified as often as daily, depending on the assessment of the client's skin integrity, client comfort and pain level, and whether or not the written repositioning plan has been followed. Clients who are in bed

for long periods of time can experienced diminished appetites. If a client is not maintaining adequate dietary intake even if changes to the nutrition plan have been made, the nurse may need to arrange to consult with a nutritionist or dietician. For clients who are mobile, the nurse should provide instructions when to call the office if there is another appearance of a potential pressure ulcer or change in skin integrity.

COLLABORATION

Nurses may find themselves collaborating with a number of individuals when providing care for a client who has or is at risk for pressure ulcers. Nurses frequently collaborate with physical therapists, especially in hospitals, rehabilitation centers, and nursing homes. When caring for a client who is living at home, the nurse will often collaborate with the individual's primary caregiver, be that a family member or a hired professional. Because many clients with pressure ulcers are older or have other serious illnesses, a caregiver may require teaching on such topics as the following:

- Definition and description of pressure ulcers
- Common locations of pressure ulcers
- Risk factors for the development of pressure ulcers
- Skin care
- Ways to avoid injury
- Diet

Depending on the stage of the pressure ulcer, the nurse teaches the client or caregiver how to care for ulcers that are already present: how to change dressings, apply skin barriers, and avoid injury and infection. Referrals to a home health agency or community health department can help the family through the lengthy healing process.

REVIEW **Pressure Ulcers**

RELATE: **LINK THE CONCEPTS**

Linking the concepts of Infection and Mobility with the concept of Tissue Integrity:

1. What are the manifestations of infection in a pressure ulcer?
2. What measures will you take to minimize the risk of infection in a client with a pressure ulcer?
3. For an 80-year-old client with limited mobility? For a 30-year-old client in a coma? For a 10-year-old child who is chair-bound?

READY: **GO TO COMPANION SKILLS MANUAL**

1. Moving and positioning clients in bed
2. Performing safe and effective lifting and transfer techniques
3. Maintaining body alignment
4. Applying body mechanics
5. Moving a client up in bed
6. Using a turn or lift sheet

REFLECT: **CASE STUDY**

Lydia Ocampo is a 69-year-old widow who has recently been moved from a rehabilitation center to the skilled

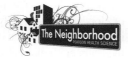

nursing wing of a nursing facility. She is still receiving care related to surgery on a broken hip a couple of months before. Before that,

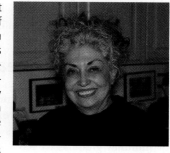

she had lived in the home that she shared with her husband of 50 years. Her husband died a few weeks ago. Lydia has Alzheimer's disease. At the nursing home, she exhibits intermittent confusion and is alternately passive and uncooperative with the staff. Over the course of the next month, her condition deteriorates. She eats very little and is fairly unresponsive to caregivers. She sleeps often.

1. What data suggest that Lydia is particularly vulnerable to pressure ulcer development?
2. What additional information do you need in order to use the Braden scale to determine Lydia's potential for pressure ulcer development?
3. What independent measures can you take to protect Lydia's skin from further breakdown?
4. Considering that Lydia does not have any areas of skin breakdown, why is it important to institute treatment for pressure ulcers at this time?

12.3 WOUND HEALING

LEARNING OUTCOMES

After learning about this exemplar, you will be able to do the following:

1. Describe the pathophysiology, etiology, clinical manifestations, and direct and indirect causes of wound healing.

2. Identify risk factors associated with wound healing.

3. Illustrate the nursing process in providing culturally competent care across the life span for individuals with wound healing.

4. Formulate priority nursing diagnoses appropriate for an individual with wound healing.

5. Create a plan of care for individuals with wound healing that includes their family members.

6. Assess expected outcomes for an individual with wound healing.

7. Discuss therapies used in the collaborative care of an individual with wound healing.

8. Employ evidence-based care (or prevention) for an individual with wound healing.

BASIS FOR SELECTION OF EXEMPLAR

Institute of Medicine (IOM)

OVERVIEW

Healing is a quality of living tissue; it is also referred to as **regeneration** (renewal) of tissues. Healing can be considered in terms of *types of healing*, having to do with the caregiver's decision on whether to allow the wound to seal itself or to purposefully close the wound, and *phases of healing*, which refer to the steps in the body's natural processes of tissue repair. The phases are the same for all wounds, but the rate of healing depends on factors such as the type of healing, the location and size of the wound, and the client's health.

Types of Wound Healing

There are two types of healing, each influenced by the amount of tissue loss. **Primary intention healing** occurs where the tissue surfaces have been **approximated** (closed) and there is minimal or no tissue loss; it is characterized by the formation of minimal granulation tissue and scarring. It is also called *primary union* or *first intention healing*. An example of wound healing by primary intention is a closed surgical incision. Another example would be the use of tissue adhesive, a liquid "glue," to seal clean lacerations or incisions, which may result in better appearing scars (Coulthard, Worthington, Esposito, van der Elst, & van Waes, 2005).

A wound that is extensive and involves considerable tissue loss and in which the edges cannot or should not be approximated, heals by **secondary intention healing**. An example of wound healing by secondary intention is a pressure ulcer. Secondary intention healing differs from primary intention healing in three

ways: (a) The repair time is longer, (b) the scarring is greater, and (c) the susceptibility to infection is greater.

Those wounds that are left open for 3–5 days to allow edema or infection to resolve or to permit exudate to drain and then are closed with sutures, staples, or adhesive skin closures, **tertiary intention healing**. This is also called delayed primary intention.

PATHOPHYSIOLOGY AND ETIOLOGY

Wound healing can be broken down into three phases: inflammatory, proliferative, and maturation or remodeling (Figure 12–7 ■).

Phases of Wound Healing

INFLAMMATORY PHASE The *inflammatory phase* is initiated immediately after injury and lasts 3–6 days. Two major processes occur during this phase: hemostasis and phagocytosis.

Hemostasis (the cessation of bleeding) results from vasoconstriction of the larger blood vessels in the affected area, retraction (drawing back) of injured blood vessels, the deposition of **fibrin** (connective tissue), and the formation of blood clots in the area. The blood clots, formed from blood platelets, provide a matrix of fibrin that becomes the framework for cell repair. A scab also forms on the surface of the wound. Consisting of clots and dead and dying tissue, the scab aids hemostasis and inhibits contamination of the wound by microorganisms. Below the scab, epithelial cells migrate into the wound from the edges. The epithelial cells serve as a barrier between the body and the environment, preventing the entry of microorganisms.

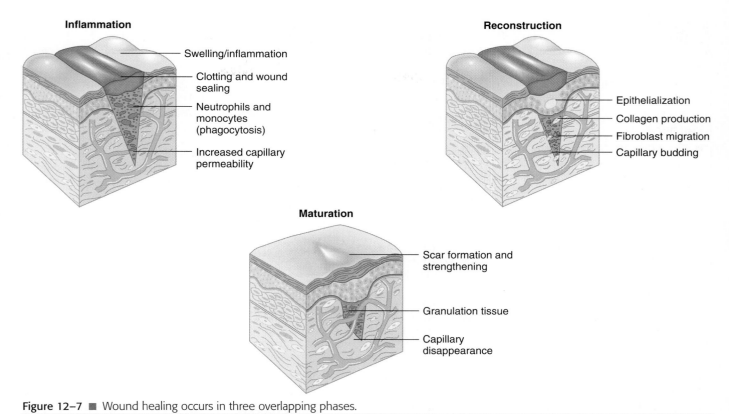

Inflammation
- Swelling/inflammation
- Clotting and wound sealing
- Neutrophils and monocytes (phagocytosis)
- Increased capillary permeability

Reconstruction
- Epithelialization
- Collagen production
- Fibroblast migration
- Capillary budding

Maturation
- Scar formation and strengthening
- Granulation tissue
- Capillary disappearance

Figure 12–7 ■ Wound healing occurs in three overlapping phases.

Source: Data from Nicol, N. H., Heuther, S. E., & Weber, R. (2006). Structure, function, and disorders of the integument. In K. L. McCance & S. E. Huether, *Pathophysiology: The biologic basis for disease in adults and children* (5th ed., pp. 1573–1607). St. Louis: Elsevier Mosby.

The inflammatory phase also involves vascular and cellular responses intended to remove any foreign substances as well as dead and dying tissues. The blood supply to the wound increases, bringing with it oxygen and nutrients needed in the healing process. As a result, the area appears reddened and edematous. Exudate of fluid and cell debris is a normal accumulation and helps cleanse the wound. Overproduction of this exudate and other factors can impair wound healing, especially in chronic wounds (Hanson, Langemo, Thompson, Anderson, & Hunter, 2005).

During cell migration, leukocytes (specifically, neutrophils) move into the interstitial space. These are replaced about 24 hours after injury by **macrophages** (large cells of the immune system that remove waste and harmful microorganisms), which arise from the blood monocytes. These macrophages engulf microorganisms and cellular debris by a process known as **phagocytosis**. The macrophages also secrete an angiogenesis factor, which stimulates the formation of epithelial buds at the end of injured blood vessels. The microcirculatory network that results sustains the healing process and the wound during its life. This inflammatory response is essential to healing. Measures that impair inflammation, such as steroid medications, can place the healing process at risk.

PROLIFERATIVE PHASE The *proliferative phase,* the second phase in healing, extends from day 3 or 4 to about day 21 postinjury. Fibroblasts (connective tissue cells), which migrate into the wound starting about 24 hours after injury, begin to synthesize collagen. **Collagen** is a whitish protein substance that adds tensile strength to the wound. As the amount of collagen increases, so does the strength of the wound; thus the chance that the wound will remain closed increases progressively. If the wound is sutured, a raised "healing ridge" appears under the intact suture line. In a wound that is not sutured, the new collagen is often visible.

Capillaries grow across the wound, increasing the blood supply. Fibroblasts move from the bloodstream into the wound, depositing fibrin. As the capillary network develops, the tissue becomes a translucent red. This tissue, called **granulation tissue**, is fragile and bleeds easily.

When the skin edges of a wound are not sutured, the area must be filled in with granulation tissue. When the granulation tissue matures, marginal epithelial cells migrate to it, proliferating over this connective tissue base to fill the wound. If the wound does not close by epithelialization, the area becomes covered by a scab or dry crust formed by dried plasma proteins and dead cells. This is called *eschar.* Initially, wounds healing by secondary intention seep blood-tinged (serosanguineous) drainage. Later, if they are not covered by epithelial cells, they become covered with thick, gray, fibrinous tissue that is eventually converted into dense scar tissue.

MATURATION PHASE The *maturation phase* begins about day 21 and can extend 1 or 2 years after the injury. Fibroblasts continue to synthesize collagen. The collagen fibers themselves, which were initially laid in a haphazard fashion, reorganize into a more orderly structure. During maturation, the wound is remodeled and contracted. The scar becomes stronger, but the repaired

DEVELOPMENTAL CONSIDERATIONS **Wound Care**

INFANTS

- The skin of infants is more fragile than that of older children and adults and is more susceptible to infection, shearing from friction, and burns.

CHILDREN

- *Staphylococcus* and fungus are two major infectious agents affecting the skin of children. Abrasions or small lacerations, commonly experienced by children, provide an entry in the skin for these organisms. Clean minor wounds with warm, soapy water, and covered with a sterile bandage. Instruct children not to touch the wound.
- With more serious skin lesions, remind the child not to touch the wound, drains, or dressing. Cover with an appropriate bandage that will remain intact during the child's usual activities. Cover a transparent dressing with opaque material if viewing the site is distressing to the child. Restrain the child only when all alternatives have been tried and when absolutely necessary.
- For younger children, demonstrate wound care on a doll. Reassure the child that the wound will not be permanent and that nothing will fall out of the body.

OLDER ADULTS

- Hold wrinkled skin taut during application of a transparent dressing. Obtain assistance if needed.
- Skin is more fragile and can easily tear with removal of tape (especially adhesive tape). Use paper tape and tape remover as indicated, keeping tape use to the minimum required. Use extreme caution during tape removal.
- Older adults in long-term care facilities often have the following factors: immobility, malnutrition, and incontinence—all of which increase the risk for development of skin breakdown.
- Skin breakdown can occur as quickly as within 2 hours, so assessments should be done with each repositioning of the client.
- A thorough assessment of a client's heels should be done every shift. The skin can break down quickly from friction of movement in bed.

Source: Berman, A., Snyder, S. J., Kozier, B., & Erb, G. (2008). *Kozier & Erb's fundamentals of nursing: Concepts, process, and practice* (8th ed., p. 927). Upper Saddle River, NJ: Pearson Education.

---

area is never as strong as the original tissue. In some individuals, particularly dark-skinned persons, an abnormal amount of collagen appears. This can result in a hypertrophic scar, or **keloid**.

Complications of Wound Healing

Several untoward events can interfere with the healing of a wound. These include hemorrhage, infection, and dehiscence and evisceration.

HEMORRHAGE   Some escape of blood from a wound is normal. **Hemorrhage** (massive bleeding), however, is abnormal. A dislodged clot, a slipped stitch, or erosion of a blood vessel may cause severe bleeding.

Internal hemorrhage may be detected by swelling or distention in the area of the wound and, possibly, by sanguineous drainage from a surgical drain. Some clients will have a **hematoma**, a localized collection of blood underneath the skin that may appear as a reddish blue swelling (bruise). A large hematoma may be dangerous because it can place pressure on blood vessels, thereby obstructing blood flow.

The risk of hemorrhage is greatest during the first 48 hours after surgery. Hemorrhage is an emergency; the nurse applies pressure dressings to the area and monitors the client's vital signs. In many instances, the client must be taken to the operating room for surgical intervention.

INFECTION   Contamination of a wound surface with microorganisms (colonization) is an inevitable result. Because the colonizing organisms compete with new cells for oxygen and nutrition and because their byproducts can interfere with a healthy surface condition, the presence of contamination can impair wound healing and lead to infection. When the microorganisms colonizing the wound multiply excessively or invade tissues, infection occurs. Infection suggested by the presence of a change in wound color, pain, or drainage is confirmed by performing a culture of the wound. Severe infection

causes fever and elevated white blood cell count. Clients who are immunosuppressed, such as those with HIV or those receiving myelosuppressive treatment for cancer, are especially susceptible to wound infections.

A wound can be infected with microorganisms at the time of injury, during surgery, or postoperatively. Wounds that occur as a result of injury (e.g., bullet and knife wounds) are most likely to be contaminated at the time of injury. Surgery involving the intestines can also result in infection from the microorganisms inside the intestine. Surgical infection is most likely to become apparent 2–11 days postoperatively.

DEHISCENCE WITH POSSIBLE EVISCERATION   **Dehiscence** is the partial or total rupturing of a sutured wound. Dehiscence usually involves an abdominal wound in which the layers below the skin also separate. **Evisceration** is the protrusion of the internal viscera through an incision. A number of factors, including obesity, poor nutrition, multiple trauma, failure of suturing, excessive coughing, vomiting, and dehydration heighten a client's risk of wound dehiscence. Wound dehiscence is more likely to occur 4–5 days postoperatively, before extensive collagen is deposited in the wound.

Sudden straining, such as coughing or sneezing, may precede dehiscence. It is not unusual for a client to feel that "something has given way." When dehiscence or evisceration occurs, the wound should be supported quickly by large sterile dressings soaked in sterile normal saline. The nurse should place the client in bed with knees bent to decrease pull on the incision. The surgeon must be notified because immediate surgical repair of the area may be necessary.

Factors Affecting Wound Healing

Characteristics of the individual such as age, nutritional status, lifestyle, and medications influence the speed of wound healing.

DEVELOPMENTAL CONSIDERATIONS   Factors Inhibiting Wound Healing

OLDER ADULTS

- Vascular changes associated with aging, such as atherosclerosis and atrophy of capillaries in the skin, can impair blood flow to the wound.
- Collagen tissue is less flexible, which increases the risk of damage from pressure, friction, and shearing.
- Scar tissue is less elastic.
- Changes in the immune system may reduce the formation of the antibodies and monocytes necessary for wound healing.
- Nutritional deficiencies may reduce the numbers of red blood cells and leukocytes, thus impeding the delivery of oxygen and

the inflammatory response essential for wound healing. Oxygen is needed for the synthesis of collagen and the formation of new epithelial cells.

- Having diabetes, chronic lung disease, or cardiovascular disease increases the risk of delayed healing due to impaired oxygen delivery to these tissues.
- Cell renewal is slower, resulting in delayed healing.

Source: Berman, A., Snyder, S. J., Kozier, B., & Erb, G. (2008). *Kozier & Erb's fundamentals of nursing: Concepts, process, and practice* (8th ed., p. 912). Upper Saddle River, NJ: Pearson Education.

DEVELOPMENTAL CONSIDERATIONS Healthy children and adults often heal more quickly than do older adults, who are more likely to have chronic diseases that hinder healing. For example, reduced liver function can impair the synthesis of blood clotting factors. See Developmental Considerations: Wound Care for factors specific to children and to older adults and Developmental Considerations: Factors Inhibiting Wound Healing for factors inhibiting wound healing in older adults.

NUTRITION Wound healing places additional demands on the body. Clients require a diet rich in protein, carbohydrates, lipids, vitamins A and C, and minerals such as iron, zinc, and copper. Malnourished clients may require time to improve their nutritional status before surgery, if possible. Obese clients are at increased risk of wound infection and slower healing because adipose tissue usually has a minimal blood supply.

LIFESTYLE People who exercise regularly tend to have good circulation. Because blood brings oxygen and nourishment to the wound, clients who exercise regularly are more likely to heal quickly. Smoking reduces the amount of functional hemoglobin in the blood, thus limiting the oxygen-carrying capacity of the blood, and constricts arterioles. As a result, smokers are at risk for delayed healing.

MEDICATIONS Anti-inflammatory drugs (e.g., steroids and aspirin) and antineoplastic agents interfere with healing. Prolonged use of antibiotics may make a person susceptible to wound infection by resistant organisms.

Clinical Manifestations and Therapies

Exudate is material, such as fluid and dead phagocytic cells, that has escaped from blood vessels during the inflammatory process and is deposited in tissue or on tissue surfaces. The nature and amount of exudate vary according to the tissue involved, the intensity and duration of the inflammation, and the presence of microorganisms.

There are three major types of exudate: serous, purulent, and sanguineous (hemorrhagic). A **serous exudate** typically accompanies mild inflammation and presents as clear or straw colored. It is thin and watery and has few cells. An example is the fluid in a blister from a burn.

A **purulent exudate** is thicker than serous exudate and consists of a large quantity of cells and necrotic debris; it is

usually opaque or milky in appearance. The formation of purulent exudate, commonly referred to as **pus**, is referred to as **suppuration**, and the bacteria that produce pus are called **pyogenic bacteria**. Not all microorganisms are pyogenic. Purulent exudates can vary in color, some acquiring tinges of blue, green, or yellow. The color may depend on the causative organism.

A **sanguineous (hemorrhagic) exudate** consists of large amounts of red blood cells, indicating damage to capillaries that is severe enough to allow the escape of red blood cells from plasma. This type of exudate is frequently seen in open wounds. Mixed types of exudates are often observed. A **serosanguineous exudate** (consisting of clear and blood-tinged drainage) is commonly seen in surgical incisions. A *purosanguineous* discharge (consisting of pus and blood) is often seen in a new wound that is infected.

> **PRACTICE ALERT**
> A bright sanguineous exudate indicates fresh bleeding, whereas dark sanguineous exudate denotes older bleeding.

NURSING PROCESS

Assessment

Nurses commonly assess both untreated and treated wounds. Untreated wounds usually are seen shortly after an injury (e.g., at the scene of an accident or in an emergency center). Assessment for these wounds is as follows:

- Assess the location and extent of tissue damage (e.g., partial thickness or full thickness). Measure the length, width, and depth of the wound.
- Inspect the wound for bleeding. The amount of bleeding varies according to the type of wound and location. Penetrating wounds may cause internal bleeding.
- Inspect the wound for foreign bodies (soil, broken glass, shreds of cloth, or other foreign substances).
- Assess associated injuries such as fractures, internal bleeding, spinal cord injuries, or head trauma.
- If the wound is contaminated with foreign material, determine when the client last had a tetanus toxoid injection. A tetanus immunization or booster may be necessary.

NURSING CARE PLAN   A Client Undergoing Surgery

Martha Overbeck is a 74-year-old widow of German descent who lives alone in a senior citizens' housing complex. She is active there, as well as in the Lutheran church. She has been in good health and is independent, but she has become progressively less active as a result of arthritic pain and stiffness. Mrs. Overbeck has degenerative joint changes that have particularly affected her right hip. On the recommendation of her physician and following a discussion with her friends, Mrs. Overbeck has been admitted to the hospital for an elective right total hip replacement. Her surgery has been scheduled for 8:00 a.m. the following day.

Mrs. Eva Jackson, a close friend and neighbor, accompanies Mrs. Overbeck to the hospital. Mrs. Overbeck explains that her friend will help in her home and assist her with the wound care and prescribed exercises.

ASSESSMENT

Gloria Nobis, RN, is assigned to Mrs. Overbeck's care on return to her room. Ms. Nobis performs a complete head-to-toe assessment and determines that Mrs. Overbeck is drowsy but oriented. Her skin is pale and slightly cool. Mrs. Overbeck states that she is cold and requests additional covers. Ms. Nobis places a warmed cotton blanket next to Mrs. Overbeck's body, adds another blanket to her covers, and adjusts the room's thermostat to increase the room temperature. Mrs. Overbeck states that she is in no pain and would like to sleep. She has even, unlabored respirations and stable vital signs in comparison to preoperative readings.

Mrs. Overbeck is NPO. An intravenous solution of dextrose and water is infusing at 100 mL/h per infusion pump. No redness or edema is noted at the infusion site. Ms. Nobis notes that the antibiotic ciprofloxacin hydrochloride (Cipro) is to be administered by mouth when the client is able to tolerate fluids. Mrs. Overbeck has a large gauze dressing over her right upper lateral thigh and hip with no indications of drainage from the wound. Tubing protrudes from the distal end of the dressing and is attached to a passive suctioning device (Hemovac). Ms. Nobis empties 50 mL of dark red drainage from the suctioning device and records the amount and characteristics on a flow record. Mrs. Overbeck has a Foley catheter in place with 250 mL of clear, light amber urine in the dependent gravity drainage bag.

When assessing Mrs. Overbeck's lower extremities, Ms. Nobis finds her feet slightly cool and pale with rapid capillary refill time bilaterally. Dorsalis pedis and posterior tibial pulses are strong and equal bilaterally. Ms. Nobis notes slight pitting edema in the right foot and ankle compared with the left extremity. She also notes sensation and ability to move both feet and toes, without numbness or tingling (paresthesia).

Ms. Nobis records the preceding findings on a postoperative flowsheet. After ensuring that Mrs. Overbeck is safely positioned and can reach her call light, Ms. Nobis gives a progress report to Mrs. Overbeck's friend, Mrs. Jackson, who is in a waiting room nearby. They then go into Mrs. Overbeck's room.

DIAGNOSES

Ms. Nobis makes the following postoperative nursing diagnoses for Mrs. Overbeck:
- Risk for infection of right hip wound related to disruption of normal skin integrity by the surgical incision
- Risk for injury related to potential dislocation of right hip prosthesis secondary to total hip replacement
- Pain related to right hip incision and positioning of arthritic joints during surgery

EXPECTED OUTCOMES

The expected outcomes established in the plan of care specify that Mrs. Overbeck will do the following:
- Regain skin integrity of the right hip incision without experiencing signs or symptoms of infection.
- Demonstrate (along with Mrs. Jackson) proper aseptic technique while performing the dressing change.
- Verbalize signs and symptoms of infection to be reported to her physician.
- Describe measures to be taken to prevent dislocation of right hip prosthesis.
- Report control of pain at incision and in arthritic joints.
- Remain afebrile.

PLANNING AND IMPLEMENTATION

Ms. Nobis develops a care plan that includes the following interventions to assist Mrs. Overbeck during her postoperative recovery:
- Use aseptic technique while changing dressing.
- Monitor temperature and pulse every 4 hours to assess for elevation.
- Assess wound every 8 hours for purulent drainage and odor. Assess edges of wound for approximation, edema, redness, or inflammation in excess of expected inflammatory response.
- Teach Mrs. Overbeck and Mrs. Jackson how to use aseptic technique while assessing the wound and performing the dressing change.
- Teach Mrs. Overbeck and Mrs. Jackson the signs and symptoms of infection and when to report findings to the physician.
- Review and discuss with Mrs. Overbeck the written materials on total hip replacement.
- Convey empathetic understanding of Mrs. Overbeck's incisional and arthritic joint pain.
- Medicate Mrs. Overbeck every 4 hours (or as ordered) to maintain a therapeutic analgesic blood level.

NURSING CARE PLAN A Client Undergoing Surgery (continued)

EVALUATION

Throughout Mrs. Overbeck's hospitalization, Ms. Nobis works with Mrs. Overbeck and Mrs. Jackson to ensure that Mrs. Overbeck can care for herself after discharge from the hospital. Five days after her surgery, Mrs. Overbeck is discharged with a well-approximated incision with no indications of an infection. Before discharge, Ms. Nobis is confident that, with Mrs. Jackson's help, Mrs. Overbeck can properly assess the incision. With minimal help, Mrs. Overbeck is able to replace the dressing using aseptic technique. She can cite the signs and symptoms of an infection, take her own oral temperature, and describe preventive measures to decrease the chances of dislocating her prosthetic hip. Because of her reduced mobility over the past 5 days, Mrs. Overbeck says she can tell that the arthritis in her "old bones" is "acting up." She reports less pain in her right hip than before the surgery. Mrs. Overbeck tells Ms. Nobis that she will be back the following winter to have her left hip replaced.

PLANNING FOR HOME CARE

Increasingly, wound care is provided in the home rather than in health care facilities. The client and family assume much of the responsibility for assessing and treating existing wounds and for helping to prevent pressure ulcers. The accompanying Home Care Assessment feature outlines appropriate assessment for clients who have wounds or pressure ulcers or are at risk for developing pressure ulcers. In planning for client discharge, nurses are accountable for teaching the client and family wound preventive and care measures, including maintaining intact skin and promoting wound healing.

MAINTAINING INTACT SKIN

- Discuss the relationship between adequate nutrition (especially fluids, protein, vitamins B and C, iron, and calories) and healthy skin.
- Demonstrate appropriate positions for pressure relief.
- Establish a turning or repositioning schedule.
- Demonstrate application of appropriate skin protection agents and devices.
- Instruct to report persistent reddened areas.
- Identify potential sources of skin trauma and means of avoidance.

PROMOTING WOUND HEALING

- Discuss the importance of adequate nutrition (especially fluids, protein, vitamins B and C, iron, and calories).
- Instruct in wound assessment and provide mechanism for documenting.
- Emphasize principles of asepsis, especially hand hygiene and proper methods of handling used dressings.
- Provide information about signs of wound infection and other complications to report.
- Reinforce appropriate aspects of pressure ulcer prevention.
- Demonstrate wound care techniques such as wound cleansing and dressing changing.
- Discuss pain control measures, if needed.

Source: LeMone, P., & Burke, K. (2008). *Medical-surgical nursing: Critical thinking in client care* (4th ed., pp. 80–81). Upper Saddle River, NJ: Pearson Education.

Assessment of a treated (sutured) wound involves observation of its appearance, size, drainage, and the presence of swelling, pain, and status of drains or tubes. In some long-term facilities, home care situations, and outpatient clinics, photographs are taken weekly for a visual record of the progress of pressure ulcers and wounds. Other assessments are documented and dated along with the photograph.

Estimating the amount of wound drainage can be difficult. One recommendation is to describe the degree to which the dressing is saturated. Minimal drainage only stains the dressing; moderate drainage saturates the dressing without leakage prior to scheduled dressing changes; and heavy drainage overflows the dressing prior to scheduled changes (Brown, 2006). These terms, plus the description of the drainage and the amount and type of dressing material used, should be well understood by all care providers.

Sometimes the wound reaches under the skin surface (called *undermining*). The edges of the wound around an open center may be raw or appear healed, but the undermining can result in a sinus tract or tunnel that extends the wound many centimeters beyond the main wound surface. To assess the size of the wound, gently explore the undermined area with a thin, flexible probe. Do not use a cotton-tipped swab, since it can leave fibers in the wound. Once the end of the tract is reached, gently raise the probe so that the bulge created by the end can be seen and its length can be measured on the skin surface. Sinus tracts are often caused by infection and have significant drainage. They may be treated by using antibiotics, irrigation, surgical incision to open and drain the tract, or vacuum therapy for large tracts.

Diagnosis

The following nursing diagnoses relate to clients who have skin wounds or who are at risk for skin breakdown:

- Risk for Impaired Skin Integrity
- Impaired Skin Integrity
- Impaired Tissue Integrity

Impaired Skin Integrity commonly applies to pressure ulcers and wounds that extend through the epidermis but not through the dermis. *Impaired Tissue Integrity* applies to pressure ulcers and wounds that extend into subcutaneous tissue, muscle, or bone. Additional nursing diagnoses may be appropriate for clients with existing impaired skin or tissue integrity, including the following examples:

- *Risk for Infection* if the skin impairment is severe, the client is immunosuppressed, or the wound is caused by trauma
- *Pain* related to nerve involvement within the tissue impairment or as a consequence of procedures used to treat the wound

Planning

The major goals for clients at *Risk for Impaired Skin Integrity* are to maintain skin integrity and avoid potential associated risks. Clients with *Impaired Skin Integrity* need goals to demonstrate progressive wound healing and regain intact skin within a specified time. Client education for home care management focuses on maintaining skin integrity.

Implementation

The four major areas in which nurses can help clients develop optimal conditions for wound healing are maintaining moist wound healing, providing sufficient nutrition and hydration, preventing wound infections, and proper positioning.

Moist Wound Healing

The dressing and frequency of change should support moist wound bed conditions. Wound beds that are too dry or disturbed too often fail to heal.

Nutrition and Fluids

Clients should be assisted to take in at least 2,500 mL of fluids a day unless other health conditions contraindicate this amount. Although there is no evidence that excessive doses of vitamins or minerals enhance wound healing, adequate amounts are extremely important. The nurse should ensure that clients receive sufficient protein, vitamins C, A, B, and B5, and zinc. Obtaining a consultation with a registered dietitian helps to ensure that correct supplementation needs are met. Nurses and those planning the client's meals should take into account both the client's personal and religious food preferences.

Preventing Infection

There are two main aspects to controlling wound infection: preventing microorganisms from entering the wound and preventing the transmission of bloodborne pathogens to or from the client to others.

Positioning

To promote wound healing, clients must be positioned to keep pressure off the wound (sometimes referred to as *off-loading*). Changes of position and transfers can be accomplished without shear or friction damage. In addition to proper positioning, the client should be assisted to be as mobile as possible because activity enhances circulation. If the client cannot move independently, range-of-motion exercises and a turning schedule are implemented. See the accompanying Nursing Care Plan and Care Settings: Home Care Assessment.

Evaluation

The major goals for clients at Risk for Impaired Skin Integrity are to maintain skin integrity and to avoid potential associated risks. Clients with Impaired Skin Integrity need goals to demonstrate progressive wound healing and regain intact skin within a specified time.

Expected outcomes of nursing care include the following:
- Skin and tissue integrity is maintained.
- Wound decreases in size.
- Client demonstrates understanding of preventive care measures.

CARE SETTINGS Home Care Assessment

WOUND CARE AND PREVENTION OF PRESSURE ULCERS

Client and Environment
- Current level of knowledge: Understanding of the cause of the wound or risk for developing a pressure ulcer; prevention or treatment strategies
- Self-care abilities for mobility: Physical ability to change position, ambulate, and transfer including the use of assistive devices
- Self-care abilities for wound care: Manual dexterity and visual acuity necessary to perform skin assessments and wound treatments
- Facilities: Presence of running water, garbage container, bathroom needed to perform wound care and contain potentially infectious materials
- Current level of nutrition: Eating habits and preferences, laboratory values indicating need for teaching or other intervention

Family
- Caregiver availability, skills, and responses: Understanding of the cause of the wound or risk for developing a pressure ulcer,

prevention or treatment strategies, willingness to assist with wound care, and actions to prevent pressure ulcers
- Family role changes and coping: Effect on financial status, parenting and spousal roles, sexuality, and social roles
- Alternative potential primary or respite caregivers: For example, other family members, volunteers, church members, paid caregivers, or housekeeping services; available community respite care (adult day care, senior centers, etc.)

Community
- Resources: Availability and familiarity with possible sources of assistance such as equipment and supply companies, organizations that offer medical supplies or financial assistance, home health agencies, and transportation to and from medical appointments, if needed

Source: Berman, A., Snyder, S. J., Kozier, B., & Erb, G. (2008). *Kozier & Erb's fundamentals of nursing: Concepts, process, and practice* (8th ed., p. 917). Upper Saddle River, NJ: Pearson Education.

COLLABORATION

The client with a wound receives care from a number of health care providers. Surgeons, nurses, scrub persons, anesthetists, phlebotomists, x-ray technicians, registration clerks, and emergency transporters are often involved in securing the safety and health of clients. Case managers and social workers are available based on client needs postdischarge. This interdisciplinary approach focuses on placing the client in the best possible health status to achieve successful wound healing.

REVIEW Wound Healing

RELATE: **LINK THE CONCEPTS**

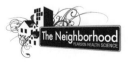

Mrs. James, a 65-year-old widow who lives alone, presents at the geriatric nursing clinic at the local senior center with a wound on her ankle about the size of a quarter. The wound is sore, with yellowish drainage. The skin around the wound is red and inflamed. Mrs. James says that she's had the sore about three weeks and that she treated it with butter for a while but that that seemed to make it worse. Mrs. James says that her foot hurts when she walks on it. The nurse at the clinic smells the cigarette smoke on Mrs. James clothing. When asked, Mrs. James reports that she smokes about a pack a day. In response to a question from the nurse, Mrs. James says that she has diabetes and high blood pressure. Mrs. James is not able to say what medicines she takes but estimates that she takes "about four different ones."

Linking the concept of Infection with the concept of Tissue Integrity:

1. What NANDA diagnoses might be appropriate for Mrs. James?
2. What treatment does Mrs. James need for the wound on her ankle?
3. What caring interventions should the nurse working with Mrs. James put in place?

READY: **GO TO COMPANION SKILLS MANUAL**

1. Obtaining a specimen of wound drainage
2. Irrigating a wound
3. Dressing wounds

REFLECT: **CASE STUDY**

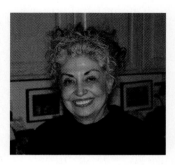

Lydia Ocampo, 69, wakes during the night to urinate but falls on the way to the bathroom. An ambulance takes her to the emergency department, where she is diagnosed with a left hip fracture. She is sent to the operating room for an open reduction internal fixation of the left hip. She is admitted to the medical-surgical floor following surgery.

Mrs. Ocampo remains at the hospital because she has developed an infection in her incision and needs intravenous antibiotics and dressing changes. Her oral intake has been inadequate, but she has been well hydrated by the intravenous fluids. She has been incontinent ever since the Foley catheter was removed. Attempts at physical therapy have been unproductive. The physical therapists are successful at transferring her from the bed to a chair, but this requires nearly full assistance.

1. Identify priority nursing diagnosis for Mrs. Ocampo.
2. List factors that put Mrs. Ocampo at risk for impaired tissue integrity.

REFERENCES

Agency for Health Care Policy and Research. (1992). *Pressure ulcers in adults: Prediction and prevention.* Rockville, MD: U.S. Department of Health and Human Services.

Agency for Health Care Policy and Research. (1994). *Treatment of pressure ulcers.* Rockville, MD: U.S. Department of Health and Human Services.

Allen, P. L. J. (2004). Leaves of three, let them be: If it were only that easy! *Pediatric Nursing, 30*(2), 129–135.

Amer, A., & Fischer, H. (2006). Linear rash leaves your patient itching. *Contemporary Pediatrics, 23*(10), 20, 23.

The Braden Scale for Predicting Pressure Sore Risk. *Nursing Research, 36*(4):205–210.

Brown, G. (2006). Wound documentation: Managing risk. *Advances in Skin and Wound Care, 19*, 155–165.

Chamley, C. A. (2005). Development of the integumentary system. In C. A. Chamley, P. Carson, D. Randall, & M. Sandwell, *Developmental anatomy and physiology of children: A practical approach* (pp. 37–58). Edinburgh, UK: Elsevier Churchill Livingstone.

Coulthard, P., Worthington, H., Esposito, M., van der Elst, M., & van Waes, O. J. F. (2005). Tissue adhesives for closure of surgical incisions. *The Cochrane Library* (ID #CD004287).

Cullum, N., McInnes, E., Bell-Syer, S. E. M., & Legood, R. (2005). Support surfaces for pressure ulcer prevention. *The Cochrane Library* (ID #CD001735).

Folkedahl, B. A., & Frantz, R. (2002b). *Treatment of pressure ulcers.* Iowa City: University of Iowa Gerontological Nursing Interventions Research Center, Research Dissemination Core. Retrieved June 9, 2006, from http://www.guideline.gov/summary/summary.aspx?view_id=1&doc_id=3457&nbr=2683

Frantz, R. (2004). Treatment of pressure ulcers. *Journal of Gerontological Nursing, 30* (5), 4–10.

Frantz, R. A., Tang, J. H., & Titler, M. G. (2004). Evidence-based protocol: Prevention of pressure ulcers. *Journal of Gerontological Nursing, 30* (5), 4–11.

Hanson, D., Langemo, D., Thompson, P., Anderson, J., & Hunter, S. (2005). Understanding wound fluid and the phases of healing. *Advances in Skin & Wound Care 18*, 360–362.

Mark, B. J., & Slavin, R. G. (2006). Allergic contact dermatitis. *Medical Clinics of North America, 90*, 169–185.

National Center for Complementary and Alternative Medicine. (2006). *Herbs at a glance.* Retrieved December 2, 2007, from http://nccam.nih.gov/health

Panel for the Prediction and Prevention of Pressure Ulcers in Adults. (1992a). *Clinical practice guideline, pressure ulcers in adults: Prediction and prevention* (Publication No. 92–0047). Rockville, MD: Agency for Health Care Policy and Research, Public Health Service, U.S. Department of Health and Human Services.

Porth, C. (2005). *Pathophysiology: Concepts of altered health states* (7th ed.). Philadelphia: Lippincott Williams & Wilkins.

Sosin, J. (2005). Ancient remedy heals today's wounds. *Nursing Spectrum, 14* (6), 32–33.

Stokowski, L. A. (2006). Neonatal skin: Back to nature? *Medscape Pediatrics.* Retrieved January 3, 2006, from http://www.medscape.com/viewarticle/519767?src=mp

Timm-Knudson, V. L., Johnson, J. S., Ortiz, K. J., & Yiannias, J. A. (2006). Allergic contact dermatitis to preservatives. *Dermatology Nursing, 18*(2), 130–136.

U.S. Department of Health and Human Services. (2000). *Healthy people 2010: Understanding and improving health* (2nd ed.). Washington, DC: U.S. Government Printing Office.

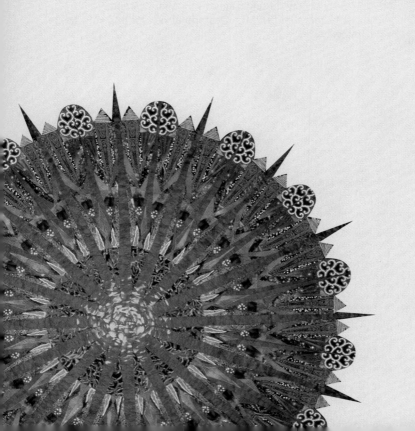

Thermoregulation 13

Concept at-a-Glance

Concept Learning Outcomes

After reading about this concept, you will be able to do the following:

1. Contrast the body regulatory processes that increase heat production with those that increase heat loss.
2. Predict the impact of alterations to any of the three parts of the body temperature regulation process.
3. Apply the factors that affect body temperature to client care needs.
4. Select the best site to choose for measuring core temperature based on client needs and conditions.
5. Contrast the different types of thermometers that may be used for measuring core temperature.
6. Convert temperature measurements between the Celsius and Fahrenheit scales.

Concept Key Terms

Afebrile, *384*
Basal metabolic rate, *382*
Body temperature, *381*
Chemical thermogenesis, *382*
Conduction, *382*
Convection, *383*
Febrile, *384*
Fever, *382*
Heat balance, *382*
Hyperpyrexia, *384*
Hyperthermia, *382*

Hypothermia, *382*
Insensible heat loss, *383*
Insensible water loss, *383*
Neutral thermal environment, *384*
Pyrexia, *384*
Radiation, *382*
Surface temperature, *381*
Thermoregulation, *382*
Vaporization, *383*

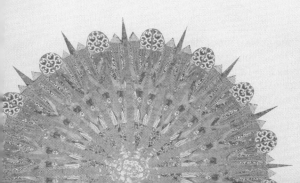

About Thermoregulation

Body temperature reflects the balance between the heat produced and the heat lost from the body, and is measured in heat units called degrees. The body's **surface temperature**—the temperature of the skin, subcutaneous tissues, and fat—fluctuates in response to environmental factors and is therefore unreliable for monitoring a client's health status. The nurse should monitor core body temperatures (or the deep tissues of the body) for a more reliable assessment. This temperature remains relatively constant at about 37°C, or 98.6°F.

Sensors in the hypothalamus regulate the body's core temperature. When these hypothalamic sensors detect heat, they signal the body to decrease heat production and increase heat loss by vasodilation and sweating. When sensors in the hypothalamus detect cold, they signal the body to increase heat production and decrease heat loss by shivering, vasoconstriction, and inhibition of sweating.

Much of the care nurses deliver is mysterious and new to clients who do not fully understand what is being done or why unless the nurse explains it. Thermoregulation is different in that most, if not all, adult clients understand what a temperature is; many can tell you exactly how they felt when their temperature began to change. Almost everyone has experienced shivering when cold or perspiring when hot. Most people want to know what the results are when their temperature is measured, especially if they are not feeling well or suspect they have a **fever** (temperature elevation). Have you ever heard someone say, "My temperature is normally low, so if I measure my temperature and it's 98.6 it means I have a fever"? Do you think this is true? If the person saying this was your client, would you feel like you needed to treat this temperature of 98.6°? ●

NORMAL PRESENTATION

Thermoregulation is the body process that balances heat production and heat loss to maintain the body's temperature. There are two kinds of body temperature: core temperature and surface temperature. Core temperature remains relatively constant. The normal core body temperature is a range (Figure 13–1 ■). The surface temperature rises and falls in response to the environment. The body continually produces heat as a byproduct of metabolism. When the amount of heat produced by the body equals the amount of heat lost, the person is in **heat balance** (Figure 13–2 ■). If the body produces more heat than is lost, the client displays **hyperthermia**. If more heat is lost than produced, the client displays **hypothermia**.

A number of factors affect the body's heat production. The most important are these five:

1. *Basal metabolic rate (BMR).* The **basal metabolic rate (BMR)** is the rate of energy utilization the body requires to maintain essential activities such as breathing. Metabolic rates decrease with age. In general, the younger the person, the higher the BMR.
2. *Muscle activity.* Muscle activity, including shivering, increases the metabolic rate. All muscle activity produces heat.
3. *Thyroxine output.* Increased thyroxine output increases the rate of cellular metabolism throughout the body. This effect is called **chemical thermogenesis**, the stimulation of heat production in the body through increased cellular metabolism.
4. *Epinephrine, norepinephrine, and sympathetic stimulation/stress response.* These hormones are neurotransmitters that mount a sympathetic nervous system response that can immediately increase the rate of cellular metabolism in many body tissues. Epinephrine and norepinephrine directly affect liver and muscle cells, thereby increasing cellular metabolism.
5. *Fever.* Fever is a protective immune response to foreign antigens within the body that increases the cellular metabolic rate thus increasing the body's temperature.

Heat is lost from the body through radiation, conduction, convection, and vaporization. **Radiation** is the transfer of heat from the surface of one object to the surface of another without contact between the two objects, usually in the form of infrared rays. **Conduction** is the transfer of heat from one molecule to a molecule of lower temperature. Because conductive

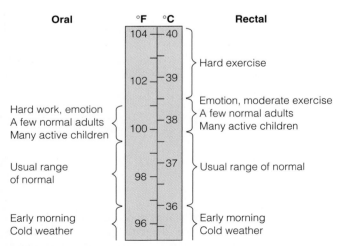

Figure 13–1 ■ Estimated ranges of body temperature in normal persons.

Source: From *Fever and the Regulation of Body Temperature*, by E.F. DuBois, 1948, Springfield, IL: Charles C. Thomas. Reprinted with permission.

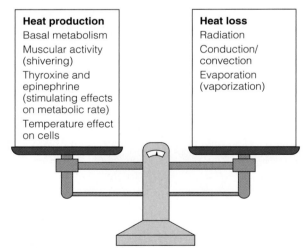

Figure 13–2 ■ As long as heat production and heat loss are properly balanced, body temperature remains constant. Factors contributing to heat production (and temperature rise) are shown on the left side of the scale; those contributing to heat loss (and temperature fall) are shown on the right side of the scale.

Source: From *Human Anatomy and Physiology*, 7th ed. (p. 985), by E. N. Marieb and K. Hoehn, 2007, San Francisco: Pearson Benjamin Cummings. Adapted with permission.

transfer cannot take place without contact between the molecules, it normally accounts for minimal heat loss except, for example, when a body is immersed in cold water. The amount of heat transferred depends on the temperature difference and the amount and duration of the contact.

Convection is the dispersion of heat by air currents. The body usually has a small amount of warm air adjacent to it. Because this warm air rises and is replaced by cooler air, people always lose a small amount of heat through convection. **Vaporization** is continuous evaporation of moisture from the respiratory tract, the mucosa of the mouth, and the skin. This continuous and unnoticed water loss is called **insensible water loss**; the accompanying heat loss is called **insensible heat loss**. Insensible heat loss accounts for about 10% of basal heat loss. When the body temperature increases, vaporization accounts for greater heat loss. Perspiration also results in vaporation of water and a cooling of body temperature.

Regulation of Body Temperature

The system that regulates body temperature has three main parts: sensors in the shell and in the core, an integrator in the hypothalamus, and an effector system that adjusts the production and loss of heat. Most sensors or sensory receptors are in the skin. The skin has more receptors for cold than warmth; therefore, skin sensors detect cold more efficiently than warmth.

When the skin becomes chilled over the entire body, three physiologic processes occur as the body attempts to regulate its temperature:

1. Shivering increases heat production.
2. Sweating is inhibited to decrease heat loss.
3. Vasoconstriction decreases heat loss.

The hypothalamic integrator, the center that controls the core temperature, is located in the preoptic area of the hypothalamus. When the sensors in the hypothalamus detect heat, they send out signals intended to reduce the temperature, that is, to decrease heat production and increase heat loss. In contrast, when the cold sensors are stimulated, they send out signals to increase heat production and decrease heat loss.

The signals from the cold-sensitive receptors of the hypothalamus initiate effectors such as vasoconstriction, shivering, and the release of epinephrine. Epinephrine increases cellular metabolism and, therefore, heat production. When the warmth-sensitive receptors in the hypothalamus are stimulated, the effector system sends out signals that initiate sweating and peripheral vasodilation. In addition to the body's thermoregulation responses, individuals consciously make appropriate adjustments, such as putting on additional clothing in response to cold or turning on a fan in response to heat.

Factors Affecting Body Temperature

Nurses should be aware of the factors that can affect a client's body temperature. They should also be able to recognize normal temperature variations as well as understand the significance of body temperature measurements that deviate from normal. The following are some factors that affect body temperature:

1. *Age.* Infants are greatly influenced by the temperature of the environment and must be protected from extreme changes. Until they reach puberty, children's temperatures continue to be more variable than those of adults. Many older people, particularly those over 75 years, are at risk of hypothermia (temperatures below 36°C, or 96.8°F) for a variety of reasons, including inadequate diet, loss of subcutaneous fat, lack of activity, and reduced thermoregulatory efficiency. Older adults are particularly sensitive to extremes in the environmental temperature due to decreased thermoregulatory controls.

2. *Diurnal variations (circadian rhythms).* Body temperatures normally change throughout the day, varying as much as 1.0°C (1.8°F) between the early morning and the late afternoon. The point of highest body temperature is usually reached between 4:00 and 6:00 p.m.) (Mackowiak, Wasserman, & Levine, 1992), and the lowest point is reached during sleep between 4:00 and 6:00 a.m.). (See Figure 13–3 ■).

3. *Exercise.* Hard work or strenuous exercise can increase body temperature to as high as 38.3–40°C (101–104°F), measured rectally, secondary to the heat produced by muscle action and increased metabolic rate.

4. *Hormones.* Women usually experience more fluctuations in hormone levels than men. In women, progesterone secretion at the time of ovulation raises body temperature by approximately 0.3–0.6°C (0.5–1.0°F) above basal temperature.

5. *Stress.* Stimulation of the sympathetic nervous system can increase the production of epinephrine and norepinephrine, thereby increasing metabolic activity and heat production. Nurses may anticipate that a highly stressed or anxious client could have a mildly elevated body temperature due to stress.

6. *Environment.* Extremes in environmental temperatures can affect a person's thermoregulation. In a very warm room, if a person's body temperature cannot be modified by convection, conduction, or radiation, his or her temperature will be elevated. Similarly, if a client has been outside in cold weather without suitable clothing, or if there is a medical condition preventing the client from controlling

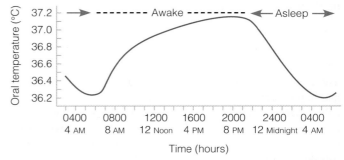

Figure 13–3 ■ Range of oral temperatures during 24 hours for a healthy young adult.

the temperature in the environment (e.g. the client has altered mental status or cannot dress self), her body temperature may be low.

Newborns are *homeothermic*; they attempt to stabilize their internal (core) body temperatures within a narrow range in spite of significant temperature variations in their environment. Thermoregulation in the newborn is closely related to the rate of metabolism and oxygen consumption. Within a specific environmental temperature range, called the **neutral thermal environment (NTE)** zone, the rates of oxygen consumption and metabolism are minimal, and internal body temperature is maintained because of thermal balance. For an unclothed, full-term newborn, the NTE is an ambient environmental temperature range of 32–34°C (89.6–93.2°F) within 50% relative humidity. The limits for an adult are 26–28°C (78.8–82.4°F) (Polin, Fox, & Abman, 2004). Thus, the normal newborn requires higher environmental temperatures to maintain a thermoneutral environment. Several newborn characteristics affect the establishment of thermal stability:

- The newborn has less subcutaneous fat than an adult and a thin epidermis.
- Blood vessels in the newborn are closer to the skin than those of an adult. Therefore, the newborn's circulating blood is more influenced by changes in environmental temperature and in turn influences the hypothalamic temperature-regulating center.
- The flexed posture of the term newborn decreases the surface area exposed to the environment, reducing heat loss. Size and age may also affect the establishment of an NTE. For example, the preterm or small-for-gestational-age (SGA) newborn has less adipose tissue and is hypoflexed, therefore requiring higher environmental temperatures to achieve an NTE. Larger, well-insulated newborns may be able to cope with lower environmental temperatures. If the environmental temperature falls below the lower limits of the NTE, the newborn responds with increased oxygen consumption and metabolism, which results in greater heat production. Prolonged exposure to the cold may result in depleted glycogen stores and acidosis. Oxygen consumption also increases if the environmental temperature is above the NTE.

Because neonates are adversely affected by heat loss through convection, be sure to place padding on any surface used for diapering or examination of the newborn.

ALTERATIONS

There are two primary alterations in body temperature: pyrexia and hypothermia. A body temperature above the usual range is called **pyrexia**, hyperthermia, or (in lay terms) fever. A very high fever, such as 41°C (105.8°F), is called **hyperpyrexia** (Figure 13–4 ■). The client who has a fever is referred to as **febrile**; one who does not is **afebrile**. Hypothermia is a core body temperature below the lower limit of normal. The three

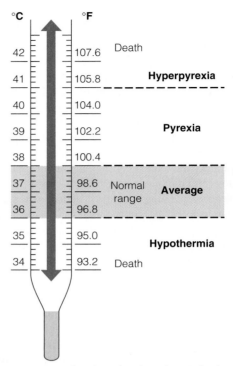

Figure 13–4 ■ Terms used to describe alterations in body temperature (oral measurements) and ranges in Celsius (centigrade) and Fahrenheit scales.

physiologic mechanisms of hypothermia are (a) excessive heat loss, (b) inadequate heat production to counteract heat loss, and (c) impaired hypothalamic thermoregulation (Figure 13–5 ■).

PHYSICAL ASSESSMENT

Thermoregulation is assessed primarily by measuring body temperature. The body temperature is measured in degrees on two scales: Celsius (centigrade) and Fahrenheit. Sometimes a nurse needs to convert a Celsius reading to Fahrenheit, or vice

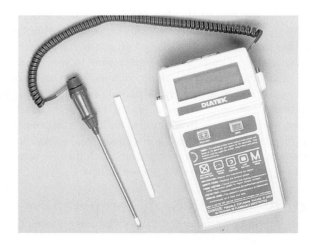

Figure 13–5 ■ An electronic thermometer. Note the probe and probe cover.

ALTERATIONS AND TREATMENTS

Alteration	Description	Treatment
Hypothermia	Decrease in body temperature as a result of more heat lost than produced	▪ Monitor vital signs. ▪ Assess skin color and temperature. ▪ Apply warm blankets or warm clothing. ▪ Provide warm environment. ▪ Provide dry clothing if heat loss is due to conduction. ▪ Keep limbs close to body. ▪ Cover scalp with cap or turban. ▪ Use hyperthermia blanket. ▪ Administer warmed oral or IV fluids. ▪ Use heat lamps, hot water bottles, or heating pad.
Hyperthermia	Increase in temperature as a result of more heat produced than lost	▪ Monitor vital signs. ▪ Assess skin color and temperature. ▪ Monitor white blood cell count, hematocrit value, and other pertinent laboratory reports for indication of infection or dehydration. ▪ Reduce covering (clothing, blankets, etc) to allow heat loss. ▪ Lower room temperature. ▪ Administer antipyretic medications. ▪ Increase fluid intake and provide adequate nutrition. ▪ Measure intake and output. ▪ Reduce physical activity to limit heat production. ▪ Provide oral hygiene to keep mucous membranes moist. ▪ Administer tepid sponge bath to increase heat loss through conduction. ▪ Provide dry clothing and bed linens if client is perspiring. ▪ Use hypothermia blanket.

versa. Although the conversion can be accomplished using several formulas, the most common is described here. To convert from Fahrenheit to Celsius, deduct 32 from the Fahrenheit reading and then multiply by the fraction 5/9:

$$C = (\text{Fahrenheit temperature} - 32) \times 5/9$$

For example, when the Fahrenheit reading is 100,

$$C = (100 - 32) \times 5/9 = (68) \times 5/9 = 37.8$$

To convert from Celsius to Fahrenheit, multiply the Celsius reading by the fraction 9/5 and then add 32:

$$F = (\text{Celsius temperature} \times 9/5) + 32$$

For example, when the Celsius reading is 40,

$$F = (40 \times 9/5) + 32 = (72 + 32) = 104$$

If using a calculator, the simplest way to convert Fahrenheit to Celsius will be to subtract 32 from the Fahrenheit temperature, divide the result by 9, and then multiply by 5. To convert Celsius to Fahrenheit, do exactly the opposite: Multiply by 9, divide by 5, and then add 32.

The most common sites for measuring body temperature are oral, rectal, axillary, tympanic membrane, and skin/temporal artery. Each of the sites has advantages and disadvantages (see Table 13–1).

The body temperature may be measured *orally*. If a client has been smoking or taking cold or hot food or fluids, the nurse should wait 30 minutes before taking the temperature orally. This ensures that the temperature of the mouth is not affected by the temperature of the warm smoke, food, or fluid.

Rectal temperature readings are considered to be very accurate. In some agencies, taking temperatures rectally is contraindicated for clients with myocardial infarction. It is believed that inserting a rectal thermometer can produce vagal stimulation, which can cause abnormal heart rhythms. However, not all authorities share this belief. Rectal temperatures are contraindicated for clients who are undergoing rectal surgery, have diarrhea or diseases of the rectum, are immunosuppressed, have a clotting disorder, or have significant hemorrhoids.

The *axilla* is the preferred site for measuring temperature in newborns because it is accessible and safe. However, some research indicates that the axillary method is inaccurate when assessing a fever (Bindler & Ball, 2003). Nurses should check agency protocol before they take the temperature of newborns, infants, toddlers, and children. Adult clients for whom the axillary method of temperature assessment is appropriate include those for whom other temperature sites are contraindicated.

The *tympanic membrane*, or nearby tissue in the ear canal, is a frequent site for estimating core body temperature. Like

TABLE 13–1 Advantages and Disadvantages of Sites for Body Temperature Measurement

SITE	ADVANTAGES	DISADVANTAGES
Oral	Accessible and convenient	Thermometers can break if bitten. Inaccurate if client has just ingested hot or cold food or fluid or smoked. Could injure the mouth following oral surgery.
Rectal	Reliable measurement	Inconvenient and more unpleasant for clients; difficult for client who cannot turn to the side. Could injure the rectum following rectal surgery. Presence of stool may interfere with thermometer placement. If the stool is soft, the thermometer may be embedded in stool rather than against the wall of the rectum.
Axillary	Safe and noninvasive	The thermometer must be left in place a long time to obtain an accurate measurement.
Tympanic membrane	Readily accessible; reflects the core temperature Very fast	Can be uncomfortable and involves risk of injuring the membrane if the probe is inserted too far. Repeated measurements may vary. Right and left measurements can differ. Presence of cerumen can affect the reading.
Temporal artery	Safe and noninvasive; very fast	Requires electronic equipment that may be expensive or unavailable; variation in technique needed if the client has perspiration on the forehead.

the sublingual oral site, the tympanic membrane has an abundant arterial blood supply, primarily from branches of the external carotid artery. Because temperature sensors applied directly to the tympanic membrane can be uncomfortable and involve risk of membrane injury or perforation, noninvasive infrared thermometers are used. Electronic tympanic thermometers are found extensively in both inpatient and ambulatory care settings.

The temperature may also be measured on the forehead using a chemical thermometer or a temporal artery thermometer. Forehead temperature measurements are most useful for infants and children for whom a more invasive measurement is not necessary.

Types of Thermometers

Traditionally, body temperatures were measured using mercury-in-glass thermometers. Glass thermometers can be hazardous if they crack or break because of the risk for exposure to mercury, which is toxic to humans, and the broken glass. In 1998, the U.S. Environmental Protection Agency and the American Hospital Association agreed on the goal of eliminating mercury from health care environments. Hospitals no longer use mercury-in-glass thermometers, and several cities have banned their sale and manufacture. Some modern versions of the thermometer have replaced glass with plastics and mercury with safer chemicals. However, the nurse may still encounter this type of thermometer.

The amount of mercury in a thermometer is minimal, but cleanup, should it break, involves several "dos and don'ts." Unsealed mercury slowly vaporizes into the air. The nurse should keep children and pets away from the area. Wearing rubber gloves, the nurse can wipe mercury beads off clothing, skin, or disposable items with a paper towel, and immediately place it into a plastic bag and discard. If the spill is on a porous material that cannot be discarded (e.g., carpet), a contractor trained in mercury disposal may be needed. If the mercury is on a hard surface, the nurse should use folded stiff cardboard to slowly gather the beads and pour them into a wide-mouthed container. The nurse should use a flashlight to search for the beads, since the light reflects off mercury, and then dispose of all items used in the cleanup in a plastic bag, which should then be sealed with tape. The nurse should shower or wash well after cleaning up, and keep the area well ventilated for several days. Vacuum cleaners or brooms should not be used since these will disperse the mercury and become contaminated. The mercury should not be poured down a toilet or drain; any contaminated materials should not be washed or reused.

PRACTICE ALERT
Whenever mercury-in-glass thermometers are encountered, the nurse should recommend their immediate replacement with less hazardous thermometers and their safe disposal.

Depending on the model, an electronic thermometer can provide a reading in only 2–60 seconds. The equipment consists of a battery-operated portable electronic unit, a probe that the nurse attaches to the unit, and a probe cover, which is usually disposable (Figure 13–5 ■). Some models have a different circuits and probes for oral and rectal measurement.

Basal and hypothermia thermometers are two specific types of oral thermometers that can be glass or electronic. A basal thermometer is calibrated with 0.1°F intervals and is used for fertility purposes, as it indicates the temperature rise associated with ovulation. Hypothermia thermometers have a greater low range than everyday thermometers, usually measuring temperatures from 81 to 108°F.

Chemical disposable thermometers are also used to measure body temperatures. Chemical thermometers using liquid crystal dots or bars or heat-sensitive tape or patches applied to the forehead change color to indicate temperature. Some of these are for single use; others may be reused several times. One type that has small chemical dots at one end is shown in Figure 13–6 ■. To read the temperature, the nurse notes the highest reading among the dots that have changed color.

Temperature-sensitive tape may also be used to obtain a general indication of body surface temperature. It does not indicate the core temperature. When the tape is applied to the skin, usually on the forehead or abdomen, the temperature digits respond by changing color (Figure 13–7 ■). The skin area should be dry. After the length of time specified by the manufacturer (e.g., 15 seconds), a color appears on the tape. This method is particularly useful at home and for use with infants.

Infrared thermometers sense body heat in the form of infrared energy produced by a heat source. In the ear canal, this source is the tympanic membrane (Figure 13–8 ■). The infrared thermometer makes no contact with the tympanic membrane.

Temporal artery thermometers determine temperature using a scanning infrared thermometer that compares temperature in the temporal artery of the forehead to the temperature in the room and then calculates the heat balance to approximate the core temperature of the blood in the pulmonary artery (Roy, Powell, & Gerson, 2003). The probe is placed in the middle of the forehead and then drawn laterally to the hairline. If the client has perspiration on the forehead, the probe is also touched behind the earlobe so the thermometer can compensate for evaporative cooling (Figure 13–9 ■).

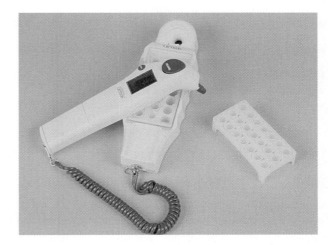

Figure 13–8 ■ An infrared (tympanic) thermometer used to measure the tympanic membrane temperature.

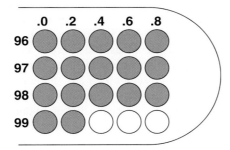

Figure 13–6 ■ A chemical thermometer showing a reading of 99.2°F.

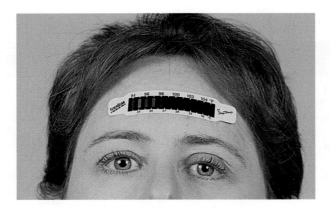

Figure 13–7 ■ A temperature-sensitive skin tape.

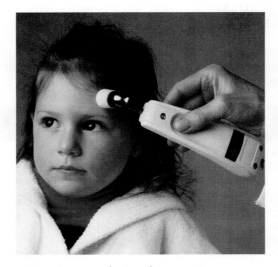

Figure 13–9 ■ A temporal artery thermometer.

DEVELOPMENTAL CONSIDERATIONS **Temperature**

INFANTS

- The body temperature of newborns is extremely labile; newborns must be kept warm and dry to prevent hypothermia.
- Using the axillary site, you need to hold the infant's arm against the chest.
- The axillary route may not be as accurate as other routes for detecting fevers in children (Bindler & Ball, 2003).
- The tympanic route is fast and convenient. Place the infant supine and stabilize the head. Pull the pinna straight back and slightly downward. Direct the probe tip anteriorly and insert it far enough to seal the canal. The tip will not touch the tympanic membrane.
- Avoid the tympanic route in a child with active ear infections or tympanic membrane drainage tubes.
- The tympanic membrane route may be more accurate in determining temperature in febrile infants (Liu, Chang, & Chang, 2004; Nimah, Bshesh, Callahan, & Jacobs, 2006).
- When using a temporal artery thermometer, it is necessary only to touch the forehead or behind the ear.
- The rectal route is least desirable in infants.

CHILDREN

- Tympanic or temporal artery sites are preferred.
- For the tympanic route, have the child held on an adult's lap with the child's head held gently against the adult for support. Pull the pinna straight back and upward for children over age 3.

- Avoid the tympanic route in a child with active ear infections or tympanic membrane drainage tubes.
- The oral route may be used for children over age 3, but nonbreakable, electronic thermometers are recommended.
- For a rectal temperature, place the child prone across your lap or in a side-lying position with the knees flexed. Insert the thermometer 1 inch into the rectum.

OLDER ADULTS

- Older adults' temperatures tend to be lower than those of middle-aged adults.
- Older adults' temperatures are strongly influenced by both environmental and internal temperature changes. Their thermoregulation control processes are not as efficient as those of younger adults, and they are at higher risk for both hypothermia and hyperthermia.
- Older adults can develop significant buildup of ear cerumen that may interfere with tympanic thermometer readings.
- Older adults are more likely to have hemorrhoids. Inspect the anus before taking a rectal temperature.
- Older adults' temperatures may not be a valid indication of the seriousness of the pathology of a disease. They may have pneumonia or a urinary tract infection and exhibit only a slight temperature elevation. Other symptoms, such as confusion and restlessness, may be presented and need follow-up to determine if there is an underlying process.

DIAGNOSTIC TESTS

Diagnostic tests may be indicated if the cause of fever is not obvious on physical examination. For example, a client suspected of having an infection might require a complete blood count with differential to diagnose the type of infection, or a client whose fever is believed to be related to head trauma may require imaging studies to determine degree and location of trauma.

THERAPEUTIC MANAGEMENT INTERVENTIONS

Support the client's environment to maintain thermoregulatory mechanisms. Elderly clients and young infants may require a warmer environmental temperature than other clients. Infants and children should wear a hat when exposed to temperature extremes; they can gain and lose more heat through their disproportionately larger heads. Adequate hydration should be maintained, especially when ambient temperatures are very hot. Dehydration can present with a low-grade fever that will resolve when hydration status is corrected. Teach the client the importance of maintaining adequate hydration during times of strenuous exercise. Nurses should monitor the temperature of the highly stressed or anxious client for potential temperature elevation.

 CARE SETTINGS **Temperature**

- Teach the client accurate use and reading of the type of thermometer to be used. Examine the thermometer the client uses in the home for safety and proper functioning. Facilitate the replacement of mercury-in-glass thermometers with other types. See page 386 for instructions regarding management of a broken mercury-in-glass thermometer.
- Observe the client or caregiver taking and reading a temperature. Reinforce the importance of reporting the site and type of thermometer used and the value of using these consistently.
- Discuss means of keeping the thermometer clean, such as warm water and soap, and avoiding cross-contamination.

- Ensure that the client has water-soluble lubricant when using a rectal thermometer.
- Instruct the client or family member to notify the health care provider if the temperature is 37.7°C (100°F) or higher.
- When making a home visit, take a thermometer with you in case the clients do not have a functional thermometer of their own.
- Check that the client knows how to record the temperature. Provide a recording chart/table if indicated.
- Discuss environmental control modifications that should be taken during illness or extreme climate conditions (e.g., heating, air conditioning, appropriate clothing and bedding).

13.1 HYPOTHERMIA

Basis for Selection of Exemplar

Nursing Skills B & I

LEARNING OUTCOMES

After learning about this exemplar, you will be able to do the following:

1. Describe the pathophysiology, etiology, and risk factors for hypothermia.
2. Apply an understanding of the danger and indications of hypothermia to the needs of clients throughout the life span.
3. Create a nursing plan of care using the nursing process for clients experiencing hypothermia with or without frostbite.

OVERVIEW

Hypothermia is a condition in which the core body temperature falls below 35°C (95°F). This occurs when the heat the body produces is less than the heat lost. Hypothermia can be a life-threatening emergency, and can occur in any season and any geographic location.

PATHOPHYSIOLOGY AND ETIOLOGY

Hypothermia may be induced or accidental. Induced hypothermia is the deliberate lowering of the body temperature to decrease metabolic rate, reducing the body's need for oxygen. Accidental hypothermia may occur as the result of immersion in cold water, exposure to cold environments, or damage to the body's thermoregulatory processes.

As the body's core temperature falls, the body tries to conserve the core temperature at the expense of the extremities. Two major routes of heat loss are from the internal core of the body to the body surface and from the external surface to the environment. The core temperature is usually higher than the skin temperature, resulting in continuous transfer or conduction of heat to the surface. The greater the difference in temperature between core and skin, the more rapidly heat transfers. The transfer is accomplished through an increase in oxygen consumption, depletion of glycogen stores, and, in the newborn, metabolization of brown fat.

Induced Hypothermia

Hypothermia may be induced for a variety of reasons, but the most frequent reason for this treatment is to reduce metabolic rates and lower the cellular demand for oxygen in the tissues, particularly in the brain. Historically, induced hypothermia has been used to reduce neurological damage following head trauma, strokes, or during cardiac surgery. Kozik (2007) reports that elevated body temperatures following cardiac arrest increase the risk and amount of neurological damage from anoxia during the event. This study found that the lower the body temperature, the greater the neurological recovery will be. Based on this and other study results, the American Heart Association now recommends induced hypothermia in clients post–cardiac arrest. Research is being conducted to determine if there are benefits to emergency responders initiating hypothermia in the field (Clumpner & Mobley, 2008).

Cooling is initiated with iced saline gastric lavage and ice packs in the axilla and groin until the cooling blanket is started at 5°C. The goal is a client temperature of 33°C. After 24 hours, the temperature is gradually increased by one degree every 2–4 hours. It is important to stop all potassium administration during the rewarming phase: Potassium released by damaged cells will be circulated and serum potassium levels will rise. Clients are sedated and paralytic medications are administered to prevent the body's natural response to cold (shivering), which produces heat and reduces the effectiveness of the induced hypothermia (Kozik, 2007).

Etiology

Accidental hypothermia can result from (a) exposure to a cold environment, (b) immersion in cold water, or (c) lack of adequate clothing, shelter, or heat. Hypothermia is associated with near-drowning episodes because body heat is lost more quickly in water than in air. Other causes of hypothermia include ingestion of alcohol or barbiturates, trauma or a brain disorder that interferes with temperature regulation, and overwhelming sepsis. If skin and underlying tissues are damaged by freezing cold, frostbite results.

A newborn is at a distinct disadvantage in maintaining a normal temperature. With a large body surface in relation to mass and a limited amount of insulating subcutaneous fat, the full-term newborn loses about four times more heat than an adult. The newborn's poor thermal stability is primarily due to excessive heat loss rather than impaired heat production. Because of the risk of hypothermia and possible cold stress, minimizing heat loss in the newborn after birth is essential. Once the infant has been dried after birth, the highest losses of heat generally result from radiation and convection because of the newborn's large body surface compared with weight. Thermal conduction is also a risk because of the marked difference between the newborn's core temperature and skin temperature. The newborn can respond to the cooler environmental temperature with adequate peripheral vasoconstriction, but this mechanism is not entirely effective because of the minimal amount of fat insulation present, the large body surface, and ongoing thermal conduction. Minimizing the baby's heat loss and preventing hypothermia are imperative.

The newborn has several physiologic mechanisms that increase heat production, or thermogenesis. These mechanisms include increased basal metabolic rate, muscular activity, and

chemical thermogenesis (also called **nonshivering thermogenesis** or NST) (Rosenberg, 2007). NST is an important mechanism of heat production unique to the newborn. It occurs when skin receptors perceive a drop in the environmental temperature and, in response, transmit sensations to stimulate the sympathetic nervous system. NST uses the newborn's stores of **brown adipose tissue (BAT)** (also called brown fat) to provide heat. Brown fat receives its name from its dark color, which is caused by its enriched blood supply, dense cellular content, and abundant nerve endings. These characteristics of brown fat cells promote rapid metabolism, heat generation, and heat transfer to the peripheral circulation. The large numbers of brown fat cells increase the speed with which triglycerides are metabolized to produce heat.

NST from BAT is the primary source of heat in the hypothermic newborn. It first appears in the fetus at about 26–30 weeks' gestation and continues to increase until 2–5 weeks after the birth of a term infant, unless the fat is depleted by cold stress. Brown fat is deposited in the midscapular area, around the neck, and in the axillas, with deeper placement around the trachea, esophagus, abdominal aorta, kidneys, and adrenal glands (Figure 13–10 ■). BAT constitutes 2–6% of the newborn's total body weight.

Shivering, a form of muscular activity common in the cold adult, is rarely seen in the newborn, although it has been observed at ambient temperatures of 15°C (59°F) or less (Polin et al., 2004). If the newborn shivers, it means the newborn's metabolic rate has already doubled. The extra muscular activity does little to produce needed heat. Thermographic studies of newborns exposed to cold show an increase in the skin heat produced over the newborn's brown fat deposits between 1 and 14 days of age (Polin et al., 2004). However, if the brown fat

supply has been depleted, the metabolic response to cold is limited or lacking. An increase in basal metabolism as a result of hypothermia results in an increase in oxygen consumption. A decrease in the environmental temperature of 2°C, from 33 to 31°C, is sufficient to double the oxygen consumption of a term newborn. Keeping the normal newborn warm promotes normal oxygen requirements, whereas chilling can cause signs of respiratory distress in the newborn.

When exposed to cold, the normal term newborn is usually able to cope with the increase in oxygen requirements. The preterm newborn, however, may be unable to increase ventilation to the necessary level of oxygen consumption. Because oxidation of fatty acids depends on the availability of oxygen, glucose, and adenosine triphosphate (ATP), the newborn's ability to generate heat can be altered by pathologic events. Such events include hypoxia, acidosis, and hypoglycemia or by medications that block the release of norepinephrine.

Meperidine (Demerol) given to a laboring woman or as a newborn analgesic can slow or prevent metabolism of newborn brown fat and lead to a greater decrease in the newborn's body temperature during the neonatal period. This effect of meperidine on brown fat is lessened if the mother and the newborn are well hydrated and in a neutral thermal environment. Newborn hypothermia prolongs as well as potentiates the effects of many analgesic and anesthetic drugs in the newborn.

The core temperature of infants is highly responsive to changes in the external environment; therefore, infants need extra protection from even mild variations in temperature. The core body temperature of children is more stable than that of infants but less so than that of adolescents or adults. However, older adults are more sensitive than middle adults to variations in environmental temperature. This increased sensitivity may be due to the decreased thermoregulatory control and loss of subcutaneous fat common in older adults, or it may be due to environmental factors such as lack of activity, inadequate diet, or lack of central heating. Illness or a central nervous system disorder may impair the thermostatic function of the hypothalamus.

FROSTBITE **Frostbite** is an injury of the skin resulting from freezing. If the exposure to freezing temperatures is limited, only the skin and subcutaneous tissues become involved. However, as exposure increases, deeper structures freeze. The skin freezes when the temperature drops to 14–24.8°F (21°–24°C). Frostbite is most common on exposed or peripheral areas of the body, such as the nose, ears, feet, and hands.

As human tissues freeze, ice crystals form, increasing intracellular sodium content. Small blood vessels initially vasoconstrict but then vasodilate and become more permeable, causing cells and tissues to swell. With continued exposure, vasoconstriction and increased viscosity of the blood cause infarction and necrosis of the affected tissue.

Superficial frostbite causes numbness, itching, and prickling. The skin appears cyanotic, reddened, or white. Deeper frostbite causes stiffness and paresthesias. As the skin and tissues thaw, the skin becomes white or yellow and loses its elasticity. The client experiences burning pain. Edema, blisters, necrosis, and gangrene may appear.

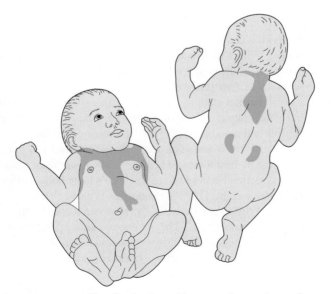

Figure 13–10 ■ The distribution of brown adipose tissue (brown fat) in the newborn.

Source: Adapted from Davis, V. (1980, November–December). Structure and function of brown adipose tissue in the neonate. *Journal of Obstetric, Gynecologic, and Neonatal Nursing, 9,* p.364.

Rapid thawing may significantly decrease tissue necrosis. The following are general guidelines for rewarming areas of frostbite:

- Outdoors, treat superficial frostbite by applying firm pressure with a warm hand or by placing frostbitten hands in the axillae. If the feet are frostbitten, remove wet footwear, dry the feet, and put on dry footwear. Do not rub the areas with snow.

- In the hospital, rapidly rewarm affected areas in circulating warm water, 104–105°F (40–40.5°C) for 20–30 minutes. Do not rub or massage the areas.

Following rewarming, the client should kept on bedrest, with the affected parts elevated. Administer pain medications and anti-inflammatory agents and debride any blisters. Whirlpool therapy may be used to clean the skin and debride necrotic tissue. Recovery from frostbite is usually complete if the involved area has not become necrotic. Necrotic tissue may require amputation.

PRACTICE ALERT
Frostbite can also occur if a chemical ice pack (found in many first aid kits) is left in contact with the skin for too long. Avoid using these chemical packs in children if possible. When using a chemical ice pack, cover it with a few layers of clothing or towel and monitor the skin under the pack frequently. Remove the chemical ice pack if the skin starts to looks white or has decreased sensation. Remove the ice pack periodically to allow the skin to rewarm.

Risk Factors

Certain clients are at greater risk for accidental hypothermia. As people age, metabolic rate slows, placing the older adult at risk of hypothermia. This can be complicated further by reduced sensory perception, use of medications such as sedatives, and financial issues resulting in the inability to adequately heat their homes. Many suffer and die each year from hypothermia. A lowered metabolism and loss of normal insulation from thinning subcutaneous tissue decrease the older client's ability to retain heat. Older clients frequently prefer a warmer environment than younger adults. The older adult who spends time outdoors in cold weather or does not turn on the heat in the home is at significant risk for hypothermia.

Infants and young children are at risk because of immature temperature regulatory mechanisms, thinner skin, limited subcutaneous fat, and high ratios of skin surface area to body mass. Adolescents are at risk due to risk-taking behaviors including drug and alcohol use and engaging in remote outdoor activities without proper equipment or clothing. Alcohol causes peripheral vasodilation, which exposes the circulating bloodstream to more rapid cooling, resulting in a faster decrease in temperature. Drug and alcohol use may reduce the ability to sense cold, further exacerbating risk.

Other risk factors include damage to the hypothalamus, decreased ability to shiver, decreased metabolic rate, evaporation from skin in cool environments, exposure to a cool environment, illness, inactivity, inadequate clothing, malnutrition,

CLINICAL MANIFESTATIONS AND THERAPIES

ETIOLOGY	CLINICAL MANIFESTATION	CLINICAL THERAPIES
Reduction in temperature results in decreased metabolic rate and reduced oxygen demands, slowing respirations and pulse rate.	Decreased body temperature, pulse, and respirations	■ Provide a warm environment. ■ Provide dry clothing. ■ Apply warm blankets. ■ Keep limbs close to body.
The body's compensatory mechanism initiates shivering to produce heat from muscle activity.	Severe shivering (initially)	■ Cover the client's scalp with a cap or turban. ■ Supply warm oral or intravenous fluids.
	Feelings of cold and chills	■ Apply warming pads.
Hypothermia causes vasoconstriction to reduce exposure of the circulating bloodstream to the cold environment.	Pale, cool, waxy skin	
Vasoconstriction caused by hypothermia reduces peripheral circulation.	Frostbite (nose, fingers, toes)	■ Rapidly rewarm affected areas in circulating warm water, 104–105°F (40–40.5°C) for 20–30 minutes. ■ Do not rub or massage the areas.
Reduced heart rate reduces cardiac output.	Hypotension	■ Following rewarming, keep on bedrest with the affected parts elevated.
Blood flow to the kidneys is reduced.	Decreased urinary output	■ Administer analgesics and anti-inflammatory agents.
Blood flow to the brain is reduced secondary to slowed metabolic rate and reduced cardiac output.	Lack of muscle coordination	■ Debride blisters. ■ Administer whirlpool therapy to clean skin and debride necrotic tissue. ■ Necrotic tissue may require amputation.
	Disorientation	■ Support respiratory and cardiac function. ■ Place on cardiorespiratory monitor.
	Drowsiness progressing to coma	■ Reduce handling as this increases the risk of cardiac fibrillation.

medications, and trauma (NANDA, 2009). Hypothyroidism, immaturity of a newborn's temperature regulatory system, and ineffective thermoregulation can all contribute to hypothermia.

Clinical Manifestations and Therapies

Symptoms of mild hypothermia (32–35°C [90–95°F]) include fatigue, slurred speech, poor coordination and clumsiness, confusion and poor judgment, inappropriate behavior, shivering, tachycardia, and tachypnea. Symptoms of moderate hypothermia (28–32°C [82–90°F]) include depressed mental status, no shivering, depressed respirations, slow pulse or irregular heartbeat, low blood pressure, pale or cyanotic color, hallucinations, and coma. Profound hypothermia (body temperature below 28°C [82°F]) results in absence of respirations and pulse, ventricular fibrillation, dilated and unresponsive pupils, and coma.

PRACTICE ALERT

It is important to note that a client who is hypothermic should not be declared dead. Hypothermia reduces oxygen demands, and clients with hypothermia can survive cardiac arrest for far longer than those at normal temperature. As a result, clients in cardiac arrest who are hypothermic should be warmed and resuscitated. Only if resuscitation fails after warming should the client be declared dead.

NURSING PROCESS

Assessment

The nurse assesses the client for defining characteristics of hypothermia, including the following:

- Lowered body temperature below normal range
- Cool skin
- Cyanotic nail beds due to vasoconstriction, resulting from the body's attempt to raise temperature and prevent further heat loss
- Hypertension
- Pallor
- **Piloerection** (goosebumps)
- Shivering
- Slowed capillary refill
- Tachycardia

Diagnosis

Potential NANDA nursing diagnoses (NANDA, 2009) for the client with hypothermia include the following:

- Imbalanced Body Temperature
- Hypothermia

Planning

Prevention is a primary nursing goal. Suggested Nursing Outcome Classifications recommends the following outcomes:

- Thermoregulation: balance among heat production, heat gain, and heat loss

- Thermoregulation in Neonate: balance among heat production, heat gain, and heat loss during the first 28 days of life
- Vital signs: extent to which temperature is within normal range

Implementation

Managing hypothermia involves removing the client from the cold and rewarming the client's body. For mild hypothermia, warm the client by applying blankets; for severe hypothermia, apply a **hyperthermia blanket** (an electronically controlled blanket that provides a specified temperature) and give warm intravenous fluids. Wet clothing, which increases heat loss because of the high conductivity of water, should be replaced with dry clothing. See the Clinical Manifestations and Therapies box for nursing interventions used to treat clients with hypothermia. Monitor vital signs and urine output during active rewarming and assess the client for cold-related injuries.

Newborns

The amount of heat an infant loses depends to a large extent on the actions of the nurse or caregiver. During the transfer of a newborn in the neonatal intensive care unit (NICU) from one bed to another, a transient (although not significant) decrease in temperature may be noted for up to 1 hour. Prevention of heat loss is especially critical in the very-low-birth-weight (VLBW) infant. Placing the VLBW newborn in a polyethylene wrapping immediately following birth can decrease the postnatal drop in temperature that normally occurs. Using head coverings made of insulated fabrics, wool, polyolefin, or lined with Gamgee can significantly decrease heat loss after childbirth (Blackburn, 2007). Convective, radiant, and evaporative heat losses can all be reduced (Blackburn, 2007). Swaddling and nesting maintain flexion, which reduces exposed surface area and thus convective and radiant losses. The nurse observes all newborns for signs of cold stress, including increased movement and respirations, decreased skin temperature and peripheral perfusion, development of hypoglycemia, and possible development of metabolic acidosis. Vasoconstriction is the initial response to cold stress; because it initially decreases skin temperature, the nurse should monitor and assess skin temperature instead of rectal temperature. A decrease in rectal temperature means that the infant has longstanding cold stress. By monitoring skin temperature, a possible decrease will become apparent before the infant's core temperature is affected. If a decrease in skin temperature is noted, the nurse determines whether hypoglycemia is present. Hypoglycemia is a result of the metabolic effects of cold stress and is suggested by glucometer values below 40 mg/dL, tremors, irritability or lethargy, apnea, or seizure activity.

If hypothermia occurs with a newborn, the following nursing interventions should be initiated (Blackburn, 2007; Cloherty, Eichenwald, & Stark, 2008):

- Maintain a neutral thermal environment (NTE); adjust based on the gestational age and postnatal age.
- Warm the newborn slowly because rapid temperature elevation may cause hypotension and apnea.
- Increase the air temperature in hourly increments of 1°C (33.8°F) until the infant's temperature is stable.

NURSING CARE PLAN Hypothermia

ASSESSMENT DATA

Jerry Karpinski, an 87-year-old Caucasian male, is brought to the emergency room after his son found him unresponsive. The son reports the client has lived alone in a single family home in Minnesota since his wife died 3 years ago. Mr. Karpinski depends on his Social Security income as his sole means of financial support and has been trying to keep his utility bills low by setting his thermostat to 15.6°C (60°F). His son checks on him every day and found him lying on the kitchen floor near the stove. He has a history of hypothyroidism and hypertension. He recently began taking sedatives to help him sleep at night.

NURSING DIAGNOSIS

Hypothermia as evidenced by rectal temperature of 29°C

DESIRED OUTCOMES

Mr. Karpinski will demonstrate thermoregulation as evidenced by the following indicators:
- Increased skin temperature
- Skin color becoming pink and less pale
- Presence of piloerection when cold
- Shivering when cold
- Reported thermal comfort

PHYSICAL EXAMINATION

Vital signs: 29°C rectal – 52-6 BP: 82/36
Height: 183 cm (6′)
Weight: 72.7 kg (160 lb)
Skin pale, cool to touch, nail beds cyanotic, breath sounds diminished throughout, pulse weak and thready
Nonresponsive to voice or stimulation (deep pain response not evaluated secondary to hypothermia)

DIAGNOSTIC DATA

TSH—6.7 (0.35–5.5 mIu/mL)
T_4—2.9 (5–12 mcg/dl)
T_3—78 (80–200 ng/dl)
Arterial blood gas: pH—7.28,
  PaO_2—50, $PaCO_2$—44,
  HCO_3—7720

NURSING INTERVENTIONS/SELECTED ACTIVITIES

NURSING INTERVENTIONS/SELECTED ACTIVITIES	RATIONALE
Gradual rewarming using a heating blanket until temperature reaches 36°C	*Client should be rewarmed gradually to prevent shock and acidosis.*
Warm IV solutions to maintain hydration	*Warmed IV solutions will help to raise core temperature.*
Assessing for symptoms of hypothermia	*Bradycardia, bradypnea, and hypotension are the result of vasoconstriction, reduced cardiac output, and lower metabolic rate. Pallor, lack of shivering and piloerection, and unresponsiveness are the result of poor perfusion.*
Instituting use of a continuous core temperature monitoring device	*Continuous monitoring of the client's core temperature is important to evaluating the effectiveness of the treatment regimen.*
Continuous monitoring and recording of vital signs and cardiac rhythm on cardiorespiratory monitor	*This client is at risk for ventricular fibrillation and cardiac arrest, so continuous monitoring of cardiac rhythm and vital signs is essential.*
Social service referral	*The client requires financial assistance to maintain adequate living conditions, including help with paying utility bills to prevent recurrence of hypothermia.*
Teaching client and family actions to prevent hypothermia	*Explain the vulnerability of older adults to hypothermia, the importance of maintaining an ambient temperature of at least 21.1°C (70°F), dressing warmly, and maintaining adequate hydration to prevent reoccurrence of hypothermia.*
Teaching indications of hypothermia and appropriate emergency treatment	*If the client recognizes the early symptoms of hypothermia, it can be treated before it becomes severe.*
Assessment data	*Avoiding intramuscular or subcutaneous injections.*
Reducing manual stimulation	*Rough handling or excessive stimulation of clients in a state of severe hypothermia increases the risk of ventricular fibrillation because the cardiac muscle is in a hyperexcitable state.*

(continued)

NURSING CARE PLAN Hypothermia (continued)

EVALUATION

As Mr. Karpinski's core temperature approaches normal range, he becomes increasingly more alert and vital signs return to normal ranges. Mr. Karpinski was at increased risk for hypothermia due to his age and poorly controlled hypothyroidism. Prior to discharge, Mr. Karpinski and his son were able to explain signs of early hypothermia, strategies for preventing hypothermia, and the importance of taking his thyroid hormone supplement every day. Social services contacted a local agency that can help the client pay for his prescription medications, freeing him to pay his utility bills while maintaining an acceptable environmental temperature.

APPLYING CRITICAL THINKING

1. What factors contributed to Mr. Karpinski's development of hypothermia?
2. The care plan focuses on the acute care of Mr. Karpinski's hypothermia. Once the client's temperature returns to normal range, what nursing care will this client require? Why will that care be required?
3. What client teaching (other than that mentioned in the plan of care) would the nurse initiate and why?
4. Does this event indicate the client is no longer to care for himself? Explain the assessments you would perform to reach a decision about the client's competence for self-care.

- Monitor skin temperature every 15–30 minutes to determine if the newborn's temperature is increasing.
- Remove plastic wrap, caps, and heat shields while rewarming the infant so that cool air as well as warm air is not trapped.
- Warm intravenous fluids before infusion.
- Initiate efforts to block heat loss by evaporation, radiation, convection, and conduction; maintain the newborn in NTE such as a heated incubator for transport and radiant heater for procedures.

The nurse assesses for the presence of anaerobic metabolism and initiates interventions for the resulting metabolic acidosis. Attempts to burn brown fat increase oxygen consumption, lactic acid levels, and metabolic acidosis. Hypoglycemia may be reversed by adequate glucose intake.

Children

Parents should be educated to layer children's clothing and use hats in cold climates, recognize signs of hypothermia, decrease time of exposure to cold, and know how to treat mild hypothermia. The nurse teaches school-age children and adolescents who go on camping and hunting trips how to recognize and manage hypothermia in themselves and others. Teach preventive techniques, such as avoiding riding snow mobiles or walking on ice that may not be deep enough to support the child's weight. First aid for hypothermia includes moving the child to a dry area, removing any wet clothing, and protecting the child from further environmental exposure. The nurse should wrap the child in dry blankets or dress the child in warm, dry clothing, and encourage the child to drink a warm, high-calorie liquid, if able.

Older Adults

Older adults are at increased risk for hypothermia because their bodies are less able to maintain a constant internal temperature. Chronic conditions (problems with the circulatory or neurological systems, hypothyroidism, etc), medication use, reduced sensory perception, and cognitive disorders can all increase risk still further. Initial treatment is similar to treatment for hypothermia at any age, including removing wet clothing, increasing environmental temperatures, applying more clothing

or blankets, and providing warm liquids. However, once the initial hypothermia is resolved, the nurse should assess for other issues that may place the geriatric client at increased risk for recurrent hypothermia. These may include nutritional status, financial concerns limiting their ability to heat their homes, and self-care deficits.

Evaluation

Evaluation criteria include determining that the client will:

- not exhibit piloerection or shivering,
- maintain core temperature within normal ranges,
- report thermal comfort,
- describe adaptive measures to minimize fluctuations in body temperature, and
- report early signs and symptoms of hypothermia (Wilkinson & Ahern, 2009).

COLLABORATION

Clients with severe hypothermia may require hemodialysis, peritoneal dialysis, or colonic irrigation in order to increase core body temperature. These interventions are typically used when hypothermia is the result of damage to the hypothalamus, usually due to trauma or cerebrovascular accidents (CVA). Such damage to the hypothalamus may make return of thermoregulation physiologically impossible.

Social service referrals may be indicated to assess the parents' ability to meet newborn or infant home care needs as well as for the client who experiences hypothermia because he or she is unable to provide a comfortable environmental temperature due to financial constraints or homelessness.

Free clinics and manufacturer prescription programs may be able to assist patients with limited incomes in getting some of their medications free or at reduced cost.

Health Care

Further information regarding disparity in availability of health care may be found in Concept Health Policy. Health promotion issues for the newborn and older adult can be found in Concept Safety.

REVIEW Hypothermia

RELATE: LINK THE CONCEPTS
Linking the concept of Safety with the concept of Thermoregulation:
1. The nurse is teaching a class on safety at a long-term care facility. When covering the topic of safety for the elderly, what information should the nurse include regarding prevention of hypothermia in the geriatric client?

READY: GO TO COMPANION SKILLS MANUAL
1. Assess body temperature

REFLECT: CASE STUDY
Baby girl Cho is born at 34 weeks' gestation to Mr. and Mrs. Cho. This is their first child. They attended Lamaze classes because they wanted to deliver the baby using natural childbirth methods and avoided all medications during labor. The baby has made a successful transition to extrauterine life and is breathing independently and maintaining oxygenation without assistance. After spending 30 minutes bonding with her parents, the baby is brought to the newborn nursery. The baby's axillary temperature is 34.2°C and she begins to demonstrate mild substernal and intercostal retractions and nasal flaring. Respiratory rate is 52 and apical pulse is 148.
1. What factors may contribute to the baby's development of respiratory distress?
2. What are the priority nursing interventions for this newborn?
3. What nursing interventions would be appropriate to warm the newborn?

13.2 HYPERTHERMIA

KEY TERMS
CHCT, *397*
Constant fever, *395*
Endogenous pyrogens, *396*
Febrile seizure, *398*
Fever spike, *395*
Heat exhaustion, *395*
Heat stroke, *395*
Intermittent fever, *395*
Malignant hyperthermia, *396*
Relapsing fever, *395*
Remittent fever, *395*

LEARNING OUTCOMES
After learning about this exemplar, you will be able to do the following:
1. Contrast the four common types of fevers.
2. Relate the pathophysiology of fevers to the nursing care indicated at each phase.
3. Contrast malignant hyperthermia to other forms of hyperthermia, and relate the nursing care required.
4. Plan nursing care for clients throughout the life span with hyperthermia resulting from various etiologies.
5. Predict the collaborative care required for a client with hyperthermia.

Basis for Selection of Exemplar
Nursing Skills B & I

OVERVIEW

To review, a body temperature above the usual range is called pyrexia, hyperthermia, or (in lay terms) fever. A very high fever, such as 41°C (105.8°F), is called hyperpyrexia (Figure 13–11 ■). The client who has a fever is referred to as febrile; the one who does not is afebrile.

Four common types of fevers are intermittent, remittent, relapsing, and constant. During an **intermittent fever**, the body temperature alternates at regular intervals between periods of fever and periods of normal or subnormal temperatures. Intermittent fever is common with some illnesses, such as malaria. During a **remittent fever**, such as with a cold or influenza, a wide range of temperature fluctuations (more than 2°C [3.6°F]) occurs over the 24-hour period, all of which are above normal. In a **relapsing fever**, short febrile periods of a few days are interspersed with periods of 1 or 2 days of normal temperature. During a **constant fever**, the body temperature fluctuates minimally but always remains above normal. This can occur with typhoid fever. A temperature that rises to fever level rapidly following a normal temperature and then returns to normal within a few hours is called a **fever spike**. Bacterial blood infections often cause fever spikes.

In some conditions, an elevated temperature is not a true fever. Two examples are heat exhaustion and heat stroke. **Heat exhaustion** is a result of excessive heat exposure and dehydration. Signs of heat exhaustion include paleness, dizziness, nausea, vomiting, fainting, and a moderately increased temperature (101–102°F). Persons experiencing **heat stroke**, a more serious form of heat exhaustion which can be life-threatening, generally have been exercising in hot weather, have warm, flushed skin, and often do not sweat. They usually have a temperature of 106°F or higher, and may be delirious, unconscious, or having seizures.

PATHOPHYSIOLOGY AND ETIOLOGY

The clinical signs of fever vary with the onset, course, and abatement stages. These signs occur as a result of changes in the set-point of the temperature control mechanism regulated by the hypothalamus. Under normal conditions, whenever the core temperature rises, the rate of heat loss increases, resulting in a decrease in temperature toward the set-point level. Conversely, when the core temperature falls, the rate of heat production is increased, resulting in a rise in temperature toward the set-point.

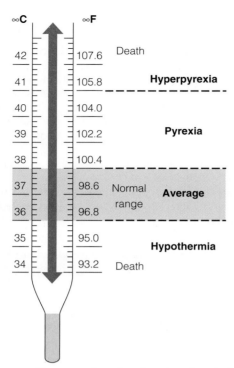

Figure 13–11 ■ Terms used to describe alterations in body temperature (oral measurements) and ranges in Celsius (centigrade) and Fahrenheit scales.

In a fever, however, the set-point of the hypothalamic thermostat changes suddenly from the normal level to a higher than normal value (e.g., 39.5°C [103.1°F]). This results from the effects on the hypothalamus of tissue destruction, pyrogenic substances, or dehydration. Although the set-point changes rapidly, the core body temperature (i.e., the blood temperature) reaches this new set-point only after several hours. During this interval, the usual heat production responses that elevate the body temperature occur: chills, feeling of coldness, cold skin due to vasoconstriction, and shivering. This is referred to as the chill phase.

When the core temperature reaches the new set-point, the client feels neither cold nor hot and no longer experiences chills (the plateau phase). Depending on the degree of temperature elevation, other signs may occur during the course of the fever. Very high temperatures, such as 41–42°C (106–108°F), damage the parenchyma of cells throughout the body, particularly in the brain where destruction of neuronal cells is irreversible. Damage to the liver, kidneys, and other body organs can also be great enough to disrupt functioning and eventually cause death.

When the cause of the high temperature is suddenly removed, the set-point of the hypothalamic thermostat is suddenly reduced to a lower value, perhaps even back to the original normal level. In this instance, the hypothalamus now attempts to lower the temperature, and the usual heat loss responses causing a reduction of the body temperature occur: excessive sweating and a hot, flushed skin due to sudden vasodilaation. This is referred to as the flush phase.

In response to an infection, macrophages release **endogenous pyrogens** (interleukins, interferons, and tumor necrosis factor). These pyrogens travel through the circulatory system to the hypothalamus, the control center for body temperature regulation. In the hypothalamus, the pyrogens trigger the production of prostaglandins, which are believed to raise the body's thermoregulatory set-point, thus causing the fever to occur (Crocetti & Serwint, 2005). See Figure 13–12 ■.

Heat loss from the body is reduced and the body temperature rises to the new temperature set-point. When the temperature is elevated, the heart rate increases. One degree of temperature elevation causes an increase in respiratory rate by four breaths per minute and increases the metabolic need for oxygen by 7%. Vasodilation occurs and the skin flushes, becoming warm to the touch.

Malignant hyperthermia (MH) is frequently inherited, and is a rare but serious reaction to volatile inhalational anesthetic gases and succinylcholine, a depolarizing neuromuscular

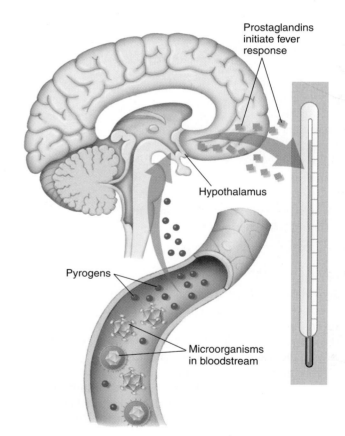

Figure 13–12 ■ The hypothalamus functions as the body's thermostat, directing the body to conserve or dissapate heat. When microorganisms invade the body, endogenous pyrogens are released into the bloodstream. These substances travel to the hypothalamus where they trigger the production and release of prostaglandins, which initiate the fever response. Blood is diverted from the extremities to more central vessels. This helps increase the core body temperature by decreasing heat loss. Shivering increases the metabolic action and heat production. The hypothalamus then maintains the temperature at the new set-point.

blocker. The client manifests the following signs and symptoms: unexplained rise in end-tidal carbon dioxide that does not respond to ventilation, hyperthermia, tachypnea, tachycardia, and sustained skeletal muscle contraction (Carter-Templeton, 2005). If unchecked, the condition will progress to hyperkalemia, myoglobinuria, disseminated intravascular coagulation, congestive heart failure, bowel ischemia, and compartment syndrome in the limbs. Dantrolene sodium is the drug that inhibits the muscular pathology and prevents death.

Because the condition is inherited, susceptibility testing is available, but the testing is expensive and the most accurate test is invasive. The "gold standard" involves biopsy of thigh skeletal muscle tissue to determine sensitivity to caffeine and halothane (**CHCT**) (Litman & Rosenberg, 2005). Genetic testing is not as sensitive and reliable as CHCT, but will improve with the discovery of more causative mutations. Clients with muscle myopathies, such as muscular dystrophy, sometimes experience early signs of MH and respond well to dantrolene. Because the symptoms of MH may manifest with other pathologies, it is important for clients to know if they have a genetic susceptibility to MH, which could affect all members of the family (Brandom, 2005).

MH can develop during an operation or when the client returns to the postanesthetic care unit (PACU). If the early symptoms of MH (e.g., escalating temperature, increased carbon dioxide production) are suspected, the nurse should immediately administer 100% oxygen with a nonrebreather mask, stay with the patient, ensure good intravenous (IV) access, and summon the anesthesia provider. The anesthesia provider will order 2.5 mg/kg of dantrolene, which can be given via IV push. The dantrolene can be repeated up to 10 mg/kg until the signs and symptoms of MH diminish. Measures to decrease core body temperature should be started at once and continued until core temperature is 36.0°C. A urinary catheter should be placed to monitor urine output, and blood drawn for testing. Blood gases should be drawn to measure pH; sodium bicarbonate is given to correct metabolic acidosis. Insulin may be ordered to decrease serum potassium. Expect this client to be transferred to the ICU for continued monitoring and doses of dantrolene every 4–6 hours.

Etiology

Hyperthermia may occur in response to viral or bacterial infections, or from tissue breakdown following myocardial infarction, malignancy, surgery, or trauma.

Risk Factors

Clients at risk for fever are those at risk for conditions resulting in fever. Diminished immune response increases the risk of infection, which increase the risk for fever. The very young and very old have diminished immunity, placing them at risk for fever. Adolescents who practice risky behavior resulting in infections or neurological trauma are also at risk for resulting fevers.

Fevers are most frequently seen in children, especially those in day care or exposed to many other children, because they have not developed immunity to common contagious diseases of childhood. Infections such as otitis media, upper respiratory infections, chickenpox, and other common diseases of childhood frequently result in fevers.

Clinical Manifestations

The clinical manifestations of fever are frequently due, at least in part, to the cause of the fever. Signs and symptoms common to all fevers include flushing, skin that is warm or hot to the touch, increased metabolic rate resulting in an increased need for fluids, tachycardia, and tachypnea. Fatigue, malaise, weakness, decreased responsiveness, difficulty concentrating, skin rash, poor appetite, malaise, vomiting and/or diarrhea, and body aches are some common signs and symptoms that may accompany a fever.

Treatment for fever is not always indicated. A fever can be a beneficial physiologic response, helping to slow the growth of organisms that thrive at lower body temperatures. A fever helps mobilize the immune response by increasing neutrophil production and T-cell proliferation (Crocetti & Serwint, 2005). Fever is not inherently harmful until it reaches 41°C (105.9°F). For this reason, medical management may include postponing treatment of low-grade fevers under 38.9°C (102°F) in otherwise healthy children (101°F in adults) to promote the body's natural defenses against an infection. Fevers are more likely to be treated if associated with discomfort.

Acetaminophen and ibuprofen are the preferred antipyretics for children. Aspirin is no longer recommended for children because of its association with Reye's syndrome. Antipyretics reduce fever by inhibiting prostaglandin synthesis, which results in lowering of the body's temperature set-point.

Antibiotics may also be administered for infectious diseases. Antibiotics have been responsible for decreases in morbidity and mortality from infections among children. However, some strains of bacteria have developed resistance to many antibiotics. Children with chronic illnesses such as cystic fibrosis, sickle-cell disease, and AIDS are particularly susceptible to infection by drug-resistant pathogens.

PRACTICE ALERT

The practice of alternating acetaminophen with ibuprofen in the care of children with fever is not based on scientific evidence. Both medications are effective in managing fever. However, because they have different durations of action (4 hours for acetaminophen and 6 hours for ibuprofen) and many preparations, there is risk for overdosing the child if the administration schedule is not strictly adhered to. In addition, combining the two medications in an alternating schedule has a potentially synergistic effect on the kidneys that can cause renal tubular toxicity. An important patient safety initiative is to use only one antipyretic to manage fever, especially in children (Carson, 2003).

 ALTERNATIVE THERAPIES Hot and Cold Theory

Many cultures subscribe to the hot and cold theory of disease causation. "Hot" and "cold" do not refer to temperature, but to categories. Fever, a hot condition, is treated by giving the patient cold substances (foods or medicines). Cold foods include vegetables, fruits, and fish. Cold medicines include orange flower water, linden, and sage.

CLINICAL MANIFESTATIONS AND THERAPIES

CLINICAL MANIFESTATION	THERAPY	RATIONALE
Flushing	Correction of temperature elevation	As body temperature rises the blood vessels vasodilate to bring more blood flow to the surface of the body. This allows cooler environmental temperatures to reduce the temperature of the blood flow as heat dissipates through convection.
Warm skin	Correction of temperature elevation	As body temperature raises, the blood vessels vasodilate to bring more blood flow to the surface of the body. This causes the skin to feel warm secondary to the warmth of the blood flow.
Tachycardia	Correction of temperature elevation	With the increase in temperature, there is an increased metabolic rate resulting in increased pulse rate and respiratory rate.
Tachypnea	Correction of temperature elevation	With the increase in temperature, there is an increased metabolic rate resulting in increased pulse rate and respiratory rate.
Increased fluid requirement	Increasing oral fluid intake or provide intravenous fluids; monitoring hydration status	Insensible water loss increases as the result of perspiration, tachypnea, and increased metabolic rate. Dehydration can occur quickly, especially in young children and older adults, if extra fluid intake is not provided.
Elevated body temperature	Ranges from no treatment for a low-grade fever (>102°F in children, >101°F in adults) to the following for higher temperatures: ■ Antipyretic ■ Tepid bath ■ Reducing clothing and skin covering ■ Increasing fluid intake (at least 2000 mL per day with additional fluids in hot weather or during strenuous exercise) ■ Applying cool washcloths or ice bags to axilla, groin, forehead, and nape of neck ■ Cooling blanket ■ For malignant hyperthermia, keeping emergency equipment nearby ■ Using a circulating fan in client's room	

Source: Wilkinson, J. M., & Ahern, N. R. (2009). *Nursing diagnosis handbook* (9th ed.). Upper Saddle River, NJ: Prentice Hall.

Febrile seizures are generalized seizures that usually occur in children as the result of rapid temperature rise above 39°C (102°F) in association with an acute illness. No evidence of intracranial infection or other defined cause is found. These seizures are usually seen in children between the ages of 3 months and 5 years, with a peak incidence between 17 and 24 months of age. There is often a family history of febrile seizures. In addition, children who have one febrile seizure have a 30–50% greater chance of having future seizures (Gill & Gieron-Korthals, 2002). The lower convulsive threshold of infants may explain this type of seizure.

NURSING PROCESS

Assessment

The nurse assesses the client's hydration status and fluid intake, vital signs, comfort level, and appetite, and observes for seizures and a toxic appearance (lethargy, poor perfusion, hypoventilation or hyperventilation, and cyanosis), especially in the pediatric client. The client with a fever may be irritable and restless, sleep fitfully, and have nonspecific muscular pain.

The nurse should identify those clients who may be at higher risk for a serious illness in association with a fever, the following in particular:

- Infants and children with a toxic appearance
- Neonates under 28 days of age with a temperature over 38°C (100.4°F)
- Children under 4 years of age with a temperature over 41°C (105.8°F)
- Children with conditions such as a ventriculoperitoneal shunt, congenital heart disease, asplenia, and sickle-cell disease
- Clients with immunosuppression, such as those receiving chemotherapy, undergoing organ transplantation, or diagnosed with HIV/AIDS
- Clients with chronic conditions such as diabetes mellitus, congestive heart failure, or pulmonary diseases

The client should be observed for other signs of infection, such as a rash, nausea and vomiting, and/or diarrhea, as well as generalized symptoms of a poor appetite and malaise.

Diagnosis

Examples of nursing diagnoses that may be appropriate for clients with febrile illnesses include the following:

- Hyperthermia related to infectious disease process
- Risk for Deficient Fluid Volume related to hypermetabolic state
- Impaired Skin Integrity related to hyperthermia and self-mutilation of skin lesions
- Impaired Oral Mucous Membrane related to infectious disease process
- Deficient Fluid Volume related to repeated episodes of vomiting and diarrhea

Planning

Care is planned for the client with hyperthermia based on the specific needs of the client and the cause of the temperature elevation. Goals specific to fever may include the following:

- Temperature will approach normal limits within 60 minutes of administration of antipyretic.
- Temperature will remain within normal limits within 48–72 hours of beginning antibiotic therapy.
- Temperature will be maintained within acceptable limits within 4 hours of application of hypothermia blanket.
- Client or parent will describe temperature elevations to be reported to the provider immediately.

Client or parent will recognize symptoms requiring consultation with health care provider.

Implementation

Nursing interventions for a client who has a fever are designed to support the body's normal physiologic processes, provide comfort, and prevent complications. During the course of fever, the nurse needs to monitor the client's vital signs closely.

Nursing measures during the chill phase are designed to help the client decrease heat loss. At this time, the body's physiologic processes are attempting to raise the core temperature to the new set-point temperature. During the flush or crisis phase, the body processes are attempting to lower the core temperature to the reduced or normal set-point temperature. At this time, the nurse takes measures to increase heat loss and decrease heat production. Nursing interventions for a client with fever are shown in Boxes 13–1 and 13–2.

Box 13–1 Identifying Nursing Diagnoses, Outcomes, and Interventions

IMBALANCED BODY TEMPERATURE

Nursing diagnosis: Definition	Sample desired outcomes: Definition	Indicators*	Selected interventions: Definition†	Sample activities (also see Box 13–2)
Risk for Imbalanced Body Temperature/At risk for failure to maintain body temperature within normal range	Hydration [0602]/ Adequate water in the intracellular and extracellular compartments of the body	■ Moist mucous membranes ■ Urine output	Temperature Regulation [3900]/Attaining and/or maintaining body temperature within a normal range	Monitor temperature every 2 hours, as appropriate. Promote adequate fluid and nutritional intake.
Hyperthermia/Body temperature elevated above normal range	Thermoregulation [0800]/*Balance among heat production, heat gain, and heat loss*	■ Skin temperature in expected range ■ Body temperature in expected range ■ Sweating when hot	Fever Treatment [3740]/ *Management of a patient with hyperpyrexia caused by nonenvironmental factors*	Monitor intake and output. Apply ice bag covered with a towel to groin. Cover the patient with only a sheet.

*The NOC # for desired outcomes and the NIC # for nursing interventions are listed in brackets following the appropriate outcome or intervention. Outcomes, indicators, interventions, and activities selected are only a sample of those suggested by NOC and NIC and should be further individualized for each client.
†The measurement scale for these indicators ranges from *extremely compromised* to *not compromised*.

Nursing care for treatment of fever includes administering antipyretics, removing unnecessary clothing, and careful continued monitoring of temperature progression. Identify clear fluids the client prefers to drink, and encourage the intake of extra fluids.

Care in the Community

The nurse teaches parents to care for their child at home, including how and when to give antipyretics. Parents often fear a fever, believing it is a disease rather than a symptom of an illness. Their greatest fears about the harmful effects of fever include seizure, brain damage, and death (Nativio, 2005). The nurse should provide information and reassurance, helping parents to recognize signs of the child's worsening condition in association with the child's specific disease (see Families Want to Know: Evaluating and Treating Fever in Children).

Evaluation

Expected outcomes of nursing care include the following:
- The client's fever is effectively managed with antipyretics.
- The client maintains adequate hydration as evidenced by skin turgor, moist mucous membranes, and hematocrit within normal range.

COLLABORATION

Collaboration related to hyperthermia or fever will generally revolve around the underlying cause of the fever. For a child with a history of febrile seizures, the nurse from the child's pediatrician's office should collaborate with the child's preschool or classroom teacher, to ensure that any staff working with the child know what to do in the event the child has a seizure, and how to prevent the onset of a febrile seizure. Adequate hydration, shortened periods outside during hot weather, and shade are just some of the measures school staff can use to help prevent febrile seizures in children.

Box 13–2 Evaluating and Treating Fever in Children

ABOUT FEVERS
- A fever is not a disease; it is the body's response to an infection. It means the child's body is using natural defenses to fight an infection.
- If the child has a fever and does not look sick, it may be better to let the child use the body's natural defenses to fight off the virus or bacteria causing the fever. Follow guidelines about when to contact the child's health care provider.

TREATING THE FEVER
- Use a thermometer to check the child's temperature every 4–6 hours.
- Administer either acetaminophen or ibuprofen to lower a fever. Check the label to make sure the correct dosage is given—drops and syrups do not have the same concentration. Do not alternate medications.
- Remove all but a light layer of the child's clothing.
- Monitor the child's behavior and response to fever medication. The fever medication will reduce the child's temperature, but the temperature may not return to normal until the child is recovering from the illness.
- If sponging the child, give fever medication first, and then use tepid water to sponge the child. Cool water may increase shivering and discomfort. Alcohol should not be used.
- The temperature may rise again 4 hours after acetaminophen or 6 hours after ibuprofen is given. Check the temperature and give another dose of fever medicine. Follow the recommendations on the bottle for the maximum number of doses allowed per day.

CALL YOUR HEALTH CARE PROVIDER IMMEDIATELY IF ANY OF THE FOLLOWING OCCUR
- The infant is under 2 months old and has a fever over 38.0°C (100.4°F).
- The child has a fever over 40.1°C (104.2°F) and any of the symptoms below are present:
- The child is crying inconsolably or whimpering. The child cries when moved or otherwise touched by the parent or other family members.
  - The child is difficult to awaken.
  - The child's neck is stiff.
  - There are purple spots present on the skin.
  - Breathing is difficult and no better after the nose is cleared.
  - The child is drooling saliva and is unable to swallow anything.
  - The child has a convulsion or seizure.
  - The child acts or looks very sick.

CALL YOUR HEALTH CARE PROVIDER WITHIN 24 HOURS IF ANY OF THE FOLLOWING OCCUR
- The child is 2–4 months old (unless fever occurs within 48 hours of a DTaP shot and the infant has no other serious symptoms).
- The fever is higher than 40.1°C (104.2°F) (especially if the child is under 3 years old).
- The child complains of burning or pain with urination.
- The fever has been present for more than 24 hours without an obvious cause or location of infection.
- The fever went away for more than 24 hours and then returned.

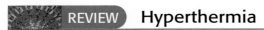 **REVIEW** Hyperthermia

RELATE: LINK THE CONCEPTS

Linking the concept of Infection with the concept of Thermoregulation:

1. Clients with infection frequently present with an elevated temperature. When caring for a client with an elevated temperature and suspected unknown infection, what nursing interventions would be important to reduce exposure of other clients to the infection?
2. What nursing interventions would be indicated if the infection was suspected of being contagious?
3. Do all infections cause fevers?
4. What infections can you think of that would be unlikely to result in hyperthermia?
5. Clients with what infections would you expect to have an elevated temperature?

READY: GO TO COMPANION SKILLS MANUAL

1. Use of a hypothermia blanket
2. Assessing body temperature

REFLECT: CASE STUDY

Matt Larkinson is a 32-year-old man diagnosed with AIDS who presents to the community clinic with a temperature of 38.8°C (101.8°F). The client reports he felt lethargic all day yesterday but had no other symptoms; this morning he awoke with a fever. He is currently taking several antiviral medications, which have helped him maintain a normal T-cell count since his initial diagnosis 2 years ago. He is accompanied to the clinic by his life partner who reports the client woke him this morning with severe shivering and chills. They took the client's temperature at that time and it was only 37.6°C (99.6°F), but 30 minutes later, when they rechecked the temperature, it was 40°C (104°F). The client took 650 mg of acetaminophen and came to the clinic to find the cause of the temperature elevation.

1. When examining the client what will the nurse assess for?
2. What laboratory and diagnostic tests will the nurse anticipate receiving orders for from the physician?
3. What client teaching will the nurse provide the client and his partner regarding care of the client if chills recur?

REFERENCES

Ball, J.W., & Bindler, R.C.(2008). *Pediatric nursing: Caring for children* (4th ed.). Upper Saddle River, NJ: Pearson, Inc.

Berman, A., Snyder, S.J., Kozier, B., & Erb, G. (2008). *Kozier & Erb's fundamentals of nursing: Concepts, process, and practice* (8th ed.). Upper Saddle River, NJ: Pearson, Inc.

Bindler, R. C., & Ball, J. W. (2003). *Clinical skills manual for pediatric nursing: Caring for children* (3rd ed.). Upper Saddle River, NJ: Prentice Hall Health.

Blackburn, S. T. (2007). *Maternal, fetal, & neonatal physiology: A clinical perspective* (3rd ed.). St. Louis: W.B. Saunders.

Brandom, B. W. (2005). The genetics of malignant hyperthermia. *Anesthesiology Clinics of North America, 23*, 615–619.

Carson, S. M. (2003). Alternating acetaminophen and ibuprofen in the febrile child: Examining the evidence regarding efficacy and safety. *Pediatric Nursing, 29*(5), 379–382.

Carter-Templeton, H. (2005). Malignant hyperthermia. *Nursing, 35*(6), 88.

Cloherty, J. P., Eichenwald, E. C., & Stark, A. R.(2008). *Manual of neonatal care* (6th ed.). Philadelphia: Lippincott Williams & Wilkins.

Clumpner, M., & Mobley, J. (2008). Raising the dead: Prehospital hypothermia for cardiac arrest victims may improve neurological outcome and survival to discharge. *EMS Magazine, 37*(9), 52–60.

Crocetti, M. T., & Serwint, J. R. (2005). Fever: Separating fact from fiction. *Contemporary Pediatrics, 22*(1), 34–41.

DuBois, E. F. (1948). *Fever and the regulation of body temperature.* Springfield, IL: Charles C. Thomas.

Gieron-Korthals, M., & Gill, J. K. (2002). Febrile convulsions: An ever changing story. What every pediatrician should know about it. *Contemporary Pediatrics, 19*(5):139-144.

Kozik, T. M. (2007). Induced hypothermia for patients with cardiac arrest: Role of a clinical nurse specialist. *Critical Care Nurse, 27*(5), 41–42.

Ladewig, P. W., London, M. L., & Davidson, M. R. (2010). *Contemporary maternal-newborn nursing care* (7th ed.). Upper Saddle River, NJ: Pearson, Inc.

LeMone, P., & Burke, K. (2008). *Medical-surgical nursing: Critical thinking in client care* (4th ed.). Upper Saddle River, NJ: Pearson, Inc.

Litman, R. S., & Rosenberg, H. (2005). Malignant hyperthermia: Update on susceptibility testing. *Journal of the American Medical Association, 293*(23), 2918–2924.

Liu, C. C., Chang, R. E., & Chang, W. C. (2004). Limitations of forehead infrared body temperature detection for fever screening for severe acute respiratory syndrome. *Infection Control Hospital Epidemiology, 25*, 1109–1111.

Mackowiak, P. A., Wasserman, S. S., & Levine, M. M. (1992). A critical appraisal of 98.6 degrees F, the upper limit of the normal body temperature, and other legacies of Carl Reinhold August Wunderlich. *Journal of the American Medical Association, 268*, 1578–1580.

Marieb, E. N. & Hoehn, K. (2007). *Human anatomy and physiology* (7th ed.). San Francisco: Benjamin Cummings.

NANDA International. (2009). *Nursing diagnoses: Definitions and classification 2009-2011.* Chichester, West Sussex, UK: Wiley-Blackwell.

Nativio, D. G. (2005). Understanding fever in children. *American Journal for Nurse Practitioners, 9*(11/12), 47–52.

Nimah, M. M., Bshesh, K., Callahan, J., & Jacobs, B. R. (2006). Infrared tympanic thermometry in comparison with other temperature measurement techniques in febrile children. *Pediatric Critical Care Medicine, 7*, 48–55.

Polin, R. A., Fox, W.W., & Abman, S. H. (2004). *Fetal and neonatal physiology* (3rd ed.). Philadelphia: W.B. Saunders.

Rosenberg, A. A. (2007). The neonate. In S. G. Gabbe, J. R. Niebyl, & J. L. Simpson (Eds.). *Obstetrics: Normal and problem pregnancies* (5th ed., pp. 523–565). Philadelphia: Churchill Livingstone/Elsevier.

Roy, S., Powell, K., & Gerson, L. W. (2003). Temporal artery temperature measurements in healthy infants, children, and adolescents. *Clinical Pediatrics, 42*, 433–437.

Smith, L. S. (2004). Temperature measurement in critical care adults: A comparison of thermometry and measurement routes. *Biological Research for Nursing, 6*(2), 117–125.

Smith, L. S. (2004). Temperature monitoring in newborns, a comparison of thermometry and measurement sites. *Journal of Neonatal Nursing, 10*, 157–165.

Sund Levander, M., Grodzinsky, E., Loyd, D., & Wahren, L. K. (2004). Errors in body temperature assessment related to individual variation, measuring technique and equipment. *International Journal of Nursing Practice, 10*, 216–223.

Wilkinson, J. M., & Ahern, N. R. (2009). *Nursing diagnosis handbook* (9th ed.). Upper Saddle River, NJ: Prentice Hall.

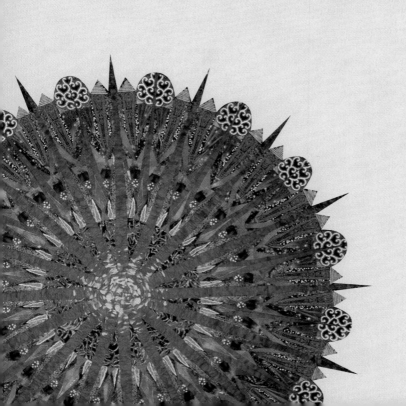

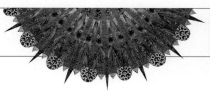